Handbook of Parkinson's Disease

Handbook of Parkinson's Disease

Edited by Aubrey Walsh

hayle
medical

New York

Hayle Medical,
750 Third Avenue, 9th Floor,
New York, NY 10017, USA

Visit us on the World Wide Web at:
www.haylemedical.com

ISBN: 978-1-63241-675-9

Cataloging-in-Publication Data

Handbook of Parkinson's disease / edited by Aubrey Walsh.
    p. cm.
Includes bibliographical references and index.
ISBN 978-1-63241-675-9
1. Parkinson's disease. 2. Brain--Diseases. I. Walsh, Aubrey.
RC382 .H35 2019
616.833--dc23

Table of Contents

Preface

Over the recent decade, advancements and applications have progressed exponentially. This has led to the increased interest in this field and projects are being conducted to enhance knowledge. The main objective of this book is to present some of the critical challenges and provide insights into possible solutions. This book will answer the varied questions that arise in the field and also provide an increased scope for furthering studies.

A degenerative condition of the central nervous system, which affects the motor system, is called Parkinson's disease (PD). The symptoms of this disease are mostly with respect to motor abilities and expressed in terms of rigidity, shaking, difficulty in walking and slowness of movement. These motor difficulties are collectively termed as 'parkinsonism'. When parkinsonism occurs with no identifiable cause, it is termed as 'idiopathic parkinsonism'. When neurodegenerative disorders occur with parkinsonism, it may termed as 'atypical parkinsonism'. These include dementia with Lewy bodies, multiple system atrophy, corticobasal degeneration, etc. Some of the identifiable causes of Parkinson's disease include infections, exposure to toxins, side effects of drugs, brain lesions and metabolic derangement. This book provides comprehensive insights into Parkinson's disease. While understanding the long-term perspectives of the topics, the book makes an effort in highlighting their impact in advancing the understanding of this disease. It is appropriate for students seeking detailed information in this area as well as for experts.

I hope that this book, with its visionary approach, will be a valuable addition and will promote interest among readers. Each of the authors has provided their extraordinary competence in their specific fields by providing different perspectives as they come from diverse nations and regions. I thank them for their contributions.

Editor

1

The Association between E326K of *GBA* and the Risk of Parkinson's Disease

Yongpan Huang,[1,2] Langmei Deng,[3] Yanjun Zhong,[4] and Minhan Yi ⓘ[1,5]

[1]*Information Security and Big Data Research Institute, Central South University, Changsha, Hunan, China*
[2]*Department of Pharmacology, Institute of Chinese Medicine, Hunan Academy of Chinese Medicine, Changsha, Hunan, China*
[3]*Department of Emergency, The Third Xiangya Hospital and School of Life Sciences, Central South University, Changsha, Hunan, China*
[4]*ICU Centre, The Second Xiangya Hospital, Central South University, Changsha, Hunan, China*
[5]*Department of Ecology and Evolutionary Biology, University of Michigan, Ann Arbor, MI, USA*

Correspondence should be addressed to Minhan Yi; minhan@csu.edu.cn

Academic Editor: Fabrizio Stocchi

It is reported that both the homozygous and heterozygous states of GBA mutations which are the causes of Gaucher disease (GD) are linked to the risk of PD. However, the GBA variant p.E326K (c.1093G > A, rs2230288), which does not result in GD in homozygous carriers, has triggered debate among experts studying Parkinson's disease (PD). In order to determine if the E326K variant of GBA is associated with the risk of PD, a standard meta-analysis was conducted by searching and screening publications, data extraction, and statistical analysis. Finally, a total of 15 publications, containing 5,908 PD patients and 5,605 controls, were included in this analysis. The pooled OR of the E326K genotype analysis was 1.99 (95% CI: 1.57–2.51). The minor allele frequencies of E326K for PD patients and controls were 1.67% and 1.03%, respectively. The pooled OR for the minor allele A was 1.99 (95% CI: 1.58–2.50). According to the subgroup analysis, we found that the significant differences between PD patients and controls for both genotype and allele of E326K also exist in Asians and Caucasians, respectively. In this study, we found that E326K of GBA is associated with the risk of PD in total populations, Asians, and Caucasians, respectively. Further studies are needed to clarify the role of GBA in the pathogenesis of PD.

1. Introduction

Parkinson's disease (PD) is a common neurodegenerative disorder, with a prevalence of 1% in a population greater than 60 years old [1]. Though the etiology of PD remains unclear, it is understood that genetic, environmental, and aging factors play a role in the occurrence of PD [2].

Pathogenetic mutations in the glucocerebrosidase gene (*GBA*), encoding lysosomal enzyme glucocerebrosidase (GCase), are the cause of Gaucher disease (GD) [3]. It is reported that both the homozygous and heterozygous states of these mutations are linked to the risk of PD [4]. Moreover, PD patients with *GBA* mutations are more likely to have an early age onset, initial bradykinesia, and a family history of dementia [5]. Furthermore, screening of *GBA* in PD patients has found other potentially related variants, including p.E326K (c.1093G > A, rs2230288). E326K was

named in accordance with the tradition nomenclature, which was excluded the first 39-residue signal peptide of *GBA* protein and is widely used in this field. In fact, it is the same as p.E365K, which was the recommendation of HGVS nomenclature. In the studies conducted by Ziegler's team of researchers [6] and Duran and his colleagues [7], the E326K variant increased the risk of PD. This association, however, was not observed in other studies [4, 8]. In order to evaluate the association of E326K with risk of PD, we performed a meta-analysis to clarify the general findings of large-scale results.

2. Methods

2.1. Literature Search. Databases that included PubMed, Embase, and Web of Knowledge were utilized up to July 30, 2017, with the following key words: ("parkinson*" or "PD")

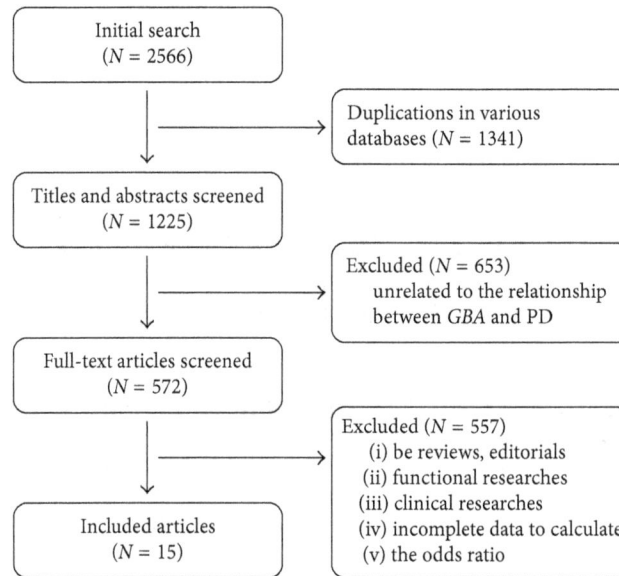

FIGURE 1: Flowchart of included publications.

TABLE 1: The characteristics of all included publications.

First author, year	NOS	Genetic method	Country	Total number (N^{a})		Genotype (GG/GA/AA)	
				Cases	Controls	Cases	Controls
Bras, 2009 [10]	9	PCR and Sanger sequencing	Portugal	230	430	228/2/0	427/3/0
Clark, 2007 [11]	9	PCR and Sanger sequencing	America	278	179	277/1/0	178/1/0
Spitz, 2008 [12]	8	RFLP	Brazil	65	267	64/1/0	267/0/0
Ziegler, 2007 [6]	8	PCR and Sanger sequencing	China	92	92	74/18/0	92/0/0
Nichols, 2009 [13]	8	PCR and TaqMan allelic-discrimination assays	North America	450	359	422/28/0	348/11/0
Kalinderi, 2009 [14]	7	NA	Greece	172	132	171/1/0	131/1/0
Lesage, 2011 [4]	7	PCR and Sanger sequencing	France	1391	391	1390/1/0	391/0/0
Lesage, 2011 [15]	7	NA	North Africa	194 (193)	177	192/1/0	176/1/0
Duran, 2013 [7]	7	PCR and Sanger sequencing	UK	185	283	171/12/2	283/0/0
Yu, 2015 [16]	8	PCR and Sanger sequencing	China	184	130	183/1/0	130/0/0
Han, 2016 [17]	8	PCR and Sanger sequencing	Canada	225	110	221/4/0	106/4/0
Ran, 2016 [8]	8	Pyrosequencing	Sweden	1625 (1540)	2025 (1937)	1450/90/0	1872/65/0
Crosiers, 2016 [18]	8	PCR and Sanger sequencing	Flanders-Belgian	266	536	254/12/0	521/15/0
Jesús, 2016 [19]	8	HRM and direct resequening	Spain	532	542	516/16/0	529/13/0
Barkhuizen, 2017 [20]	8	PCR and Sanger sequencing	South Africa	105	40	100/5/0	39/1/0

NOS: Newcastle–Ottawa Scale; NA: not available; PD: Parkinson's disease; [a]number of patients whose sequencing results for E326K were available.

and ("*GBA*" or "glucocerebrosidase"). EndNote was used to manage and organize all searched publications.

2.2. Inclusion and Exclusion Criteria. All eligible studies had to fulfill the following inclusion criteria: (1) case-control design; (2) all PD cases diagnosed accurately according to reported criteria; (3) none of the controls had PD or a neurological disease; and (4) the genotype results of E326K

were named by traditional nomenclatures, and HGVS nomenclatures were converted to traditional for both case and control groups. The exclusion criteria were as follows: (1) duplicate articles found in different databases; (2) different manuscripts using an overlapping study population; (3) genetic screening results lacking sufficient data to calculate the odds ratio (OR) and 95% confidence interval (CI); and (4) reviews. Overlapping articles from different databases were excluded with the help of electronic and manual

| Study or subgroup | Experimental | | Control | | Weight | Odds Ratio | Odds Ratio |
	Events	Total	Events	Total		M-H, Fixed, 95% CI	M-H, Fixed, 95% CI
5.3.1 Asian							
2007 Shira G. Ziegler	18	92	0	92	0.4%	45.94 (2.72, 775.00)	
2014 Zhe Yu	1	184	0	130	0.6%	2.13 (0.09, 52.79)	
Subtotal (95% CI)		**276**		**222**	**1.0%**	**20.02 (2.83, 141.56)**	
Total events	19		0				

Heterogeneity: $\chi^2 = 2.20$, df $= 1$ $(P = 0.14)$; $I^2 = 55\%$
Test for overall effect: $Z = 3.00$ $(P = 0.003)$

5.3.2 Caucasian							
2007 Jose Bras	2	230	3	430	2.0%	1.25 (0.21, 7.53)	
2007 L. N. Clark	1	278	1	179	1.2%	0.64 (0.04, 10.34)	
2007 Mariana Spitz	1	65	0	267	0.2%	12.44 (0.50, 308.96)	
2008 W. C. Nichols	28	450	11	359	11.2%	2.10 (1.03, 4.28)	
2009 Kallirhoe Kalinderi	1	172	1	132	1.1%	0.77 (0.05, 12.36)	
2011 S. Lesage(2)	1	193	1	177	1.0%	0.92 (0.06, 14.77)	
2013 Raquel Duran	14	185	0	283	0.4%	47.94 (2.84, 808.75)	
2015 Fabin Han	4	225	4	110	5.2%	0.48 (0.12, 1.96)	
2016 Caroline Ran	90	1540	65	1937	53.1%	1.79 (1.29, 2.48)	
2016 David Crosiers	12	266	15	536	9.3%	1.64 (0.76, 3.56)	
2016 Silvia Jesús	16	532	13	542	12.2%	1.26 (0.60, 2.65)	
Subtotal (95% CI)		**4136**		**4952**	**96.9%**	**1.82 (1.43, 2.32)**	
Total events	170		114				

Heterogeneity: $\chi^2 = 12.46$, df $= 10$ $(P = 0.26)$; $I^2 = 20\%$
Test for overall effect: $Z = 4.85$ $(P < 0.00001)$

5.3.3 African							
2011 Suzanne Lesage(1)	1	1391	0	391	0.8%	0.84 (0.03, 20.78)	
2017 Melinda Barkhuizen	5	105	1	40	1.4%	1.95 (0.22, 17.23)	
Subtotal (95% CI)		**1496**		**431**	**2.1%**	**1.55 (0.26, 9.29)**	
Total events	6		1				

Heterogeneity: $\chi^2 = 0.18$, df $= 1$ $(P = 0.67)$; $I^2 = 0\%$
Test for overall effect: $Z = 0.48$ $(P = 0.63)$

Total (95% CI)		**5908**		**5605**	**100.0%**	**1.99 (1.57, 2.51)**	
Total events	195		115				

Heterogeneity: $\chi^2 = 18.83$, df $= 14$ $(P = 0.17)$; $I^2 = 26\%$
Test for overall effect: $Z = 5.75$ $(P < 0.00001)$
Test for subgroup differences: $\chi^2 = 5.73$, df $= 2$ $(P = 0.06)$; $I^2 = 65.1\%$

0.001 0.1 1 10 1000
Favours (experimental)   Favours (control)

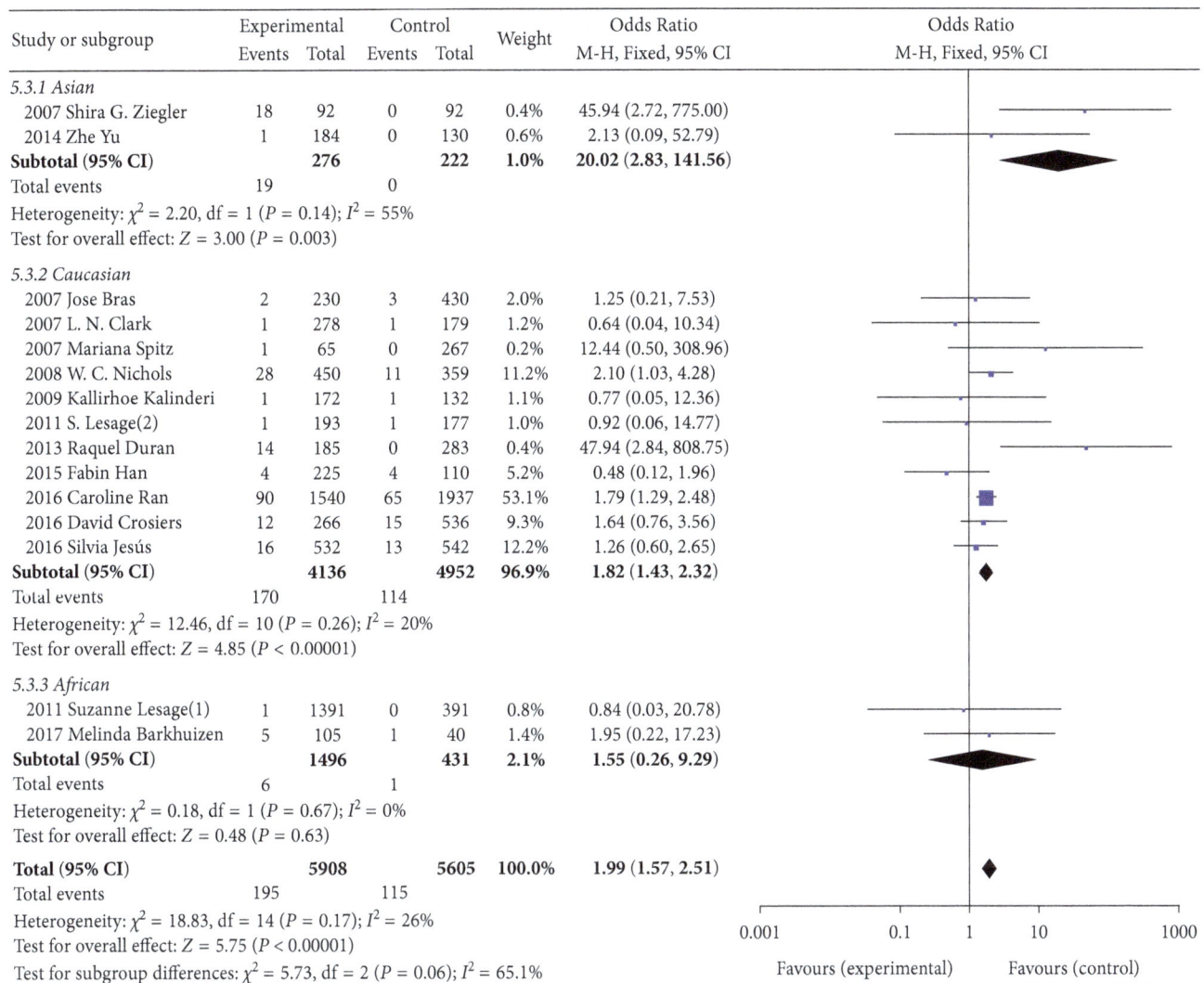

FIGURE 2: Forest plot of genotype analysis for E326K in PD.

checking. Two researchers performed the search independently. In the case of opposing opinions or decisions, a third researcher was asked to arbitrate.

2.3. Data Extraction. Two authors independently performed extraction of the following information from studies meeting inclusion criteria: publication date (year), first author, country of origin, sequencing method, total numbers, and responsive number of E326K genotypes (GG/GA/AA) and alleles (G/A) in PD patients and controls. If there were conflicts, a third party was asked to make a final decision. In terms of the assessment of a publication's quality, the Newcastle–Ottawa Scale (NOS) [9] was used.

2.4. Statistical Analysis. All statistical analyses were conducted in RevMan 5.3 software. Pooled odds ratio (OR) and 95% confidence interval (CI) were applied to measure the strength of associations between E326K and PD. Heterogeneity among all studies was calculated with a standard Q test. A fixed model (FM) was applied when

the heterogeneity was not significant ($P > 0.1$; $I^2 \leq 50\%$), or a random model (RM) was used. Publication bias was measured through funnel plot analysis. Sensitivity analysis was conducted by removing each individual publication from the pool of all the included studies and then reanalyzed the remaining pool to measure the stability of the results.

3. Results

According to the standard steps of meta-analysis, a total of 15 publications containing 5,908 PD patients and 5,605 controls were included. The flowchart of screening publications and characteristics of all studies included in the final stages of screening are shown in Figure 1 and Table 1. The NOS scores of each study ranged from 7 to 9, indicating that all of the studies were of good quality.

In total, there were 195 E326K carriers in the group of PD cases, 2 of which were homozygous, while the other 193 cases were heterozygous. The dominant model (GA +AA/GG) was used to compare the association of E326K

| Study or subgroup | Experimental | | Control | | Weight | Odds Ratio | Odds Ratio |
	Events	Total	Events	Total		M-H, Fixed, 95% CI	M-H, Fixed, 95% CI
5.4.1 Asian							
2007 Shira G. Ziegler	18	184	0	184	0.4%	41.00 (2.45, 685.66)	
2014 Zhe Yu	1	368	0	260	0.6%	2.13 (0.09, 52.41)	
Subtotal (95% CI)		**552**		**444**	**1.0%**	**19.06 (2.67, 136.03)**	
Total events	19		0				
Heterogeneity: $\chi^2 = 2.08$, df = 1 ($P = 0.15$); $I^2 = 52\%$							
Test for overall effect: $Z = 2.94$ ($P = 0.003$)							
5.4.2 Caucasian							
2007 Jose Bras	2	460	3	860	2.0%	1.25 (0.21, 7.49)	
2007 L. N. Clark	1	556	1	358	1.2%	0.64 (0.04, 10.32)	
2007 Mariana Spitz	1	130	0	534	0.2%	12.38 (0.50, 305.71)	
2008 W. C. Nichols	28	900	11	718	11.3%	2.06 (1.02, 4.17)	
2009 Kallirhoe Kalinderi	1	344	1	264	1.1%	0.77 (0.05, 12.32)	
2011 S. Lesage(2)	1	386	1	354	1.0%	0.92 (0.06, 14.71)	
2013 Raquel Duran	16	370	0	566	0.4%	52.73 (3.15, 881.74)	
2015 Fabin Han	4	450	4	220	5.1%	0.48 (0.12, 1.95)	
2016 Caroline Ran	90	3080	65	3874	53.4%	1.76 (1.28, 2.44)	
2016 David Crosiers	12	532	15	1072	9.3%	1.63 (0.76, 3.50)	
2016 Silvia Jesús	16	1064	13	1084	12.1%	1.26 (0.60, 2.63)	
Subtotal (95% CI)		**8272**		**9904**	**96.9%**	**1.82 (1.43, 2.31)**	
Total events	172		114				
Heterogeneity: $\chi^2 = 12.85$, df = 10 ($P = 0.23$); $I^2 = 22\%$							
Test for overall effect: $Z = 4.92$ ($P < 0.00001$)							
5.4.3 African							
2011 Suzanne Lesage(1)	1	2782	0	782	0.7%	0.84 (0.03, 20.74)	
2017 Melinda Barkhuizen	5	210	1	80	1.3%	1.93 (0.22, 16.75)	
Subtotal (95% CI)		**2992**		**862**	**2.1%**	**1.54 (0.26, 9.14)**	
Total events	6		1				
Heterogeneity: $\chi^2 = 0.18$, df = 1 ($P = 0.67$); $I^2 = 0\%$							
Test for overall effect: $Z = 0.48$ ($P = 0.63$)							
Total (95% CI)		**11816**		**11210**	**100.0%**	**1.99 (1.58, 2.50)**	
Total events	197		115				
Heterogeneity: $\chi^2 = 19.01$, df = 14 ($P = 0.16$); $I^2 = 26\%$							
Test for overall effect: $Z = 5.81$ ($P < 0.00001$)							
Test for subgroup differences: $\chi^2 = 5.45$, df = 2 ($P = 0.07$); $I^2 = 63.3\%$							

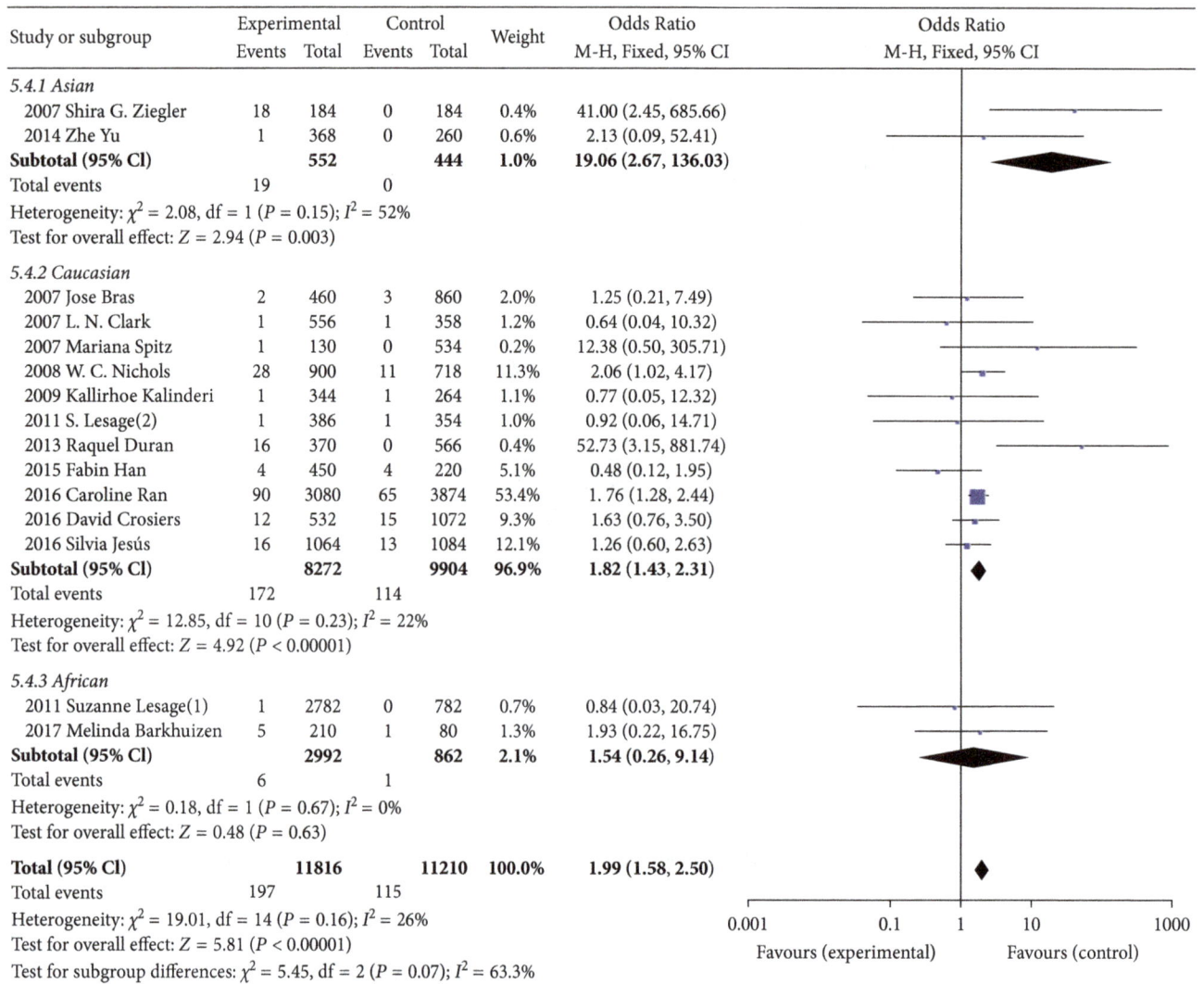

0.001   0.1   1   10   1000
Favours (experimental)   Favours (control)

FIGURE 3: Forest plot of allele analysis for E326K in PD.

and PD. The heterogeneity was acceptable, with a result of $I^2 = 26\%$. Then, the FM was adopted to calculate the genotype association of E326K. The pooled OR of E326K genotype analysis was 1.99, with a 95% CI range from 1.57 to 2.51, as shown in Figure 2, which indicated that E326K is a modest risk factor for PD. In terms of allele frequency comparison between cases and controls, there was no significant difference in heterogeneity ($P = 0.16$ and $I^2 = 26\%$). Additionally, the minor allele frequencies of E326K were 1.67% and 1.03%, for PD patients and controls, respectively. The pooled OR for the minor allele A was 1.99, and the 95% CI was 1.58 to 2.50 (Figure 3), which reflects an increased risk of PD. We conducted the subgroup analysis according to Asians, Caucasians, and Africans. We found a significant difference between PD patients and controls for both genotype and allele of E326K in Asians and Caucasians.

The funnel plots of genotype and allele analyses had a small tendency toward negative results (Figures 4 and 5). When all high quality studies were combined, the pooled ORs were significantly different. By deleting each individual article one at a time, the pooled ORs and 95% CI of each analysis remained stable.

4. Discussion

Our meta-analysis demonstrated that a higher proportion of E326K carriers developed PD and the minor allele A was a risk factor for PD. Previously, over 300 variants of *GBA* were reported in PD. However, the replications of those risk variants mostly were not conducted well. For example, after sequencing the a cohort of 519 PD patients and 544 controls, Mitsui et al. [21] found that R120W could increase the risk of PD, which reportedly had no relationship with PD in either Caucasian or Asian [4, 17, 22, 23]. Such cases include H255Q, T369M, D409H, and so on. All these studies were done independently with small sample size, which limited the power to detect the positive relationships between the target variants and PD. Through the method of meta-analysis, we conducted a multicenter, large sample size study. Our study's results were convincing for the following reasons: First, it was conducted with a large, multicenter PD

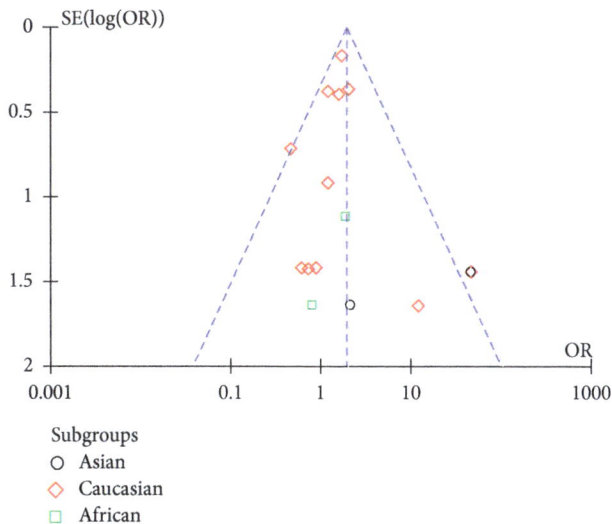

FIGURE 4: Funnel plot of genotype analysis for E326K in PD.

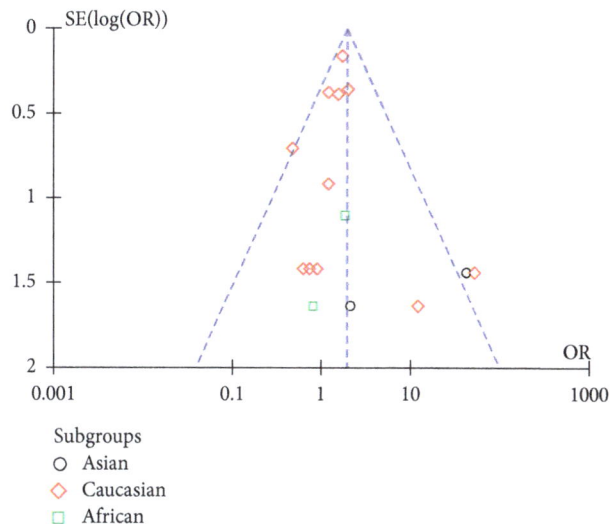

FIGURE 5: Funnel plot of allele analysis for E326K in PD.

cohort worldwide including 5,908 PD patients and 5,605 controls. Second, all the included publications were of high quality without obvious heterogeneity. Third, even though there was a slight negative reporting bias, the final pooled ORs had positive results. Fourth, the minor allele frequency of E326K among controls in this meta-analysis was 1.03%, which is similar to the allele frequency in the Exome Aggregation Consortium (0.98%).

The *GBA* gene has 11 exons, and the common risk variants N370S and L444P were located near E326K. The OR for E326K was 1.99, which indicates a mild risk for PD when compared with mutations manifesting strong effects, such as N370S and L444P. In a multicenter genetic analysis of *GBA* within the PD population, conducted in 2009 by Sidransky et al. [24], the ORs for N370S and L444P in non-Ashkenazi PD were 3.30 and 9.68, respectively. In Ashkenazi PD patients, the ORs for N370S and L444P were 5.62 and 4.95, respectively. In addition, E326K commonly coexists with other mutations such as N370S and L444P [25]. Moreover, in vitro experiments showed that the GCase activity of both E326K and the L444P variant were lower than that of a single L444P mutation [26]. All of these relationships indicate that E326K has a mild modifying effect on enzyme activity that can participate in the development of PD in a manner similar to other common variants found in genome-wide association studies. Furthermore, in a genetic and phenotypic analysis for a 733 PD patient cohort [27], E326K predicted a more rapid progression of cognitive decline and motor symptom dysfunction, which supports the effect of E326K on the onset of PD.

However, there are some inevitable limitations in this study. First, we did not conduct subgroup analysis according to ethnicity, age at onset, and other related factors due to limited information regarding subgroups. Also, subgroup analysis with an insufficient number of publications may produce a false-positive result. Second, some publications of higher quality were not included due

to insufficient data to calculate the ORs and 95% CI. Third, the study did not adjust for age, gender, environment, or other factors.

5. Conclusion

In this study, we found that E326K of *GBA* is associated with the risk of PD in total populations, Asians, and Caucasians, respectively. Further studies are needed to clarify the role of *GBA* in the pathogenesis of PD.

Authors' Contributions

Yongpan Huang, Langmei Deng and Yanjun Zhong contributed equally to this work.

Acknowledgments

This work was supported by the National Natural Science Foundation of China (nos. 31500999 and 81701962) and Hunan Provincial Natural Science Foundation of China (nos. 2017JJ3404 and 2017JJ2343) and the International Postdoctoral Exchange Fellowship Program (no. 20160029).

References

[1] O. B. Tysnes and A. Storstein, "Epidemiology of Parkinson's disease," *Journal of Neural Transmission*, vol. 124, no. 8, pp. 901–905, 2017.

[2] L. V. Kalia and A. E. Lang, "Parkinson's disease," *The Lancet*, vol. 386, no. 9996, pp. 896–912, 2015.

[3] K. S. Hruska, M. E. LaMarca, C. Ronald Scott, and E. Sidransky, "Gaucher disease: mutation and polymorphism spectrum in the glucocerebrosidase gene (GBA)," *Human Mutation*, vol. 29, no. 5, pp. 567–583, 2008.

[4] S. Lesage, M. Anheim, C. Condroyer et al., "Large-scale screening of the Gaucher's disease-related glucocerebrosidase gene in Europeans with Parkinson's disease," *Human Molecular Genetics*, vol. 20, no. 1, pp. 202–210, 2011.

[5] Y. Zhang, Q.-y. Sun, Y.-w. Zhao et al., "Effect of GBA mutations on phenotype of parkinson's disease: a study on Chinese population and a meta-analysis," *Parkinson's Disease*, vol. 2015, Article ID 916971, 10 pages, 2015.

[6] S. G. Ziegler, M. J. Eblan, U. Gutti et al., "Glucocerebrosidase mutations in Chinese subjects from Taiwan with sporadic Parkinson disease," *Molecular Genetics and Metabolism*, vol. 91, no. 2, pp. 195–200, 2007.

[7] R. Duran, N. E. Mencacci, A. V. Angeli et al., "The glucocerobrosidase E326K variant predisposes to Parkinson's disease, but does not cause Gaucher's disease," *Movement Disorders*, vol. 28, no. 2, pp. 232–236, 2013.

[8] C. Ran, L. Brodin, L. Forsgren et al., "Strong association between glucocerebrosidase mutations and Parkinson's disease in Sweden," *Neurobiology of Aging*, vol. 45, pp. 212 e5–212 e11, 2016.

[9] A. Stang, "Critical evaluation of the Newcastle-Ottawa scale for the assessment of the quality of nonrandomized studies in meta-analyses," *European Journal of Epidemiology*, vol. 25, no. 9, pp. 603–605, 2010.

[10] J. Bras, C. Paisan-Ruiz, R. Guerreiro et al., "Complete screening for glucocerebrosidase mutations in Parkinson disease patients from Portugal," *Neurobiology of Aging*, vol. 30, no. 9, pp. 1515–1517, 2009.

[11] L. N. Clark, B. M. Ross, Y. Wang et al., "Mutations in the glucocerebrosidase gene are associated with early-onset Parkinson disease," *Neurology*, vol. 69, no. 12, pp. 1270–1277, 2007.

[12] M. Spitz, R. Rozenberg, L. da Veiga Pereira, and E. R. Barbosa, "Association between Parkinson's disease and glucocerebrosidase mutations in Brazil," *Parkinsonism & Related Disorders*, vol. 14, no. 1, pp. 58–62, 2008.

[13] W. C. Nichols, N. Pankratz, D. K. Marek et al., "Mutations in GBA are associated with familial Parkinson disease susceptibility and age at onset," *Neurology*, vol. 72, no. 4, pp. 310–316, 2009.

[14] K. Kalinderi, S. Bostantjopoulou, C. Paisan-Ruiz, Z. Katsarou, J. Hardy, and L. Fidani, "Complete screening for glucocerebrosidase mutations in Parkinson disease patients from Greece," *Neuroscience Letters*, vol. 452, no. 2, pp. 87–89, 2009.

[15] S. Lesage, C. Condroyer, N. Hecham et al., "Mutations in the glucocerebrosidase gene confer a risk for Parkinson disease in North Africa," *Neurology*, vol. 76, no. 3, pp. 301–303, 2011.

[16] Z. Yu, T. Wang, J. Xu et al., "Mutations in the glucocerebrosidase gene are responsible for Chinese patients with Parkinson's disease," *Journal of Human Genetics*, vol. 60, no. 2, pp. 85–90, 2015.

[17] F. Han, D. A. Grimes, F. Li et al., "Mutations in the glucocerebrosidase gene are common in patients with Parkinson's disease from Eastern Canada," *International Journal of Neuroscience*, vol. 126, no. 5, pp. 415–421, 2016.

[18] D. Crosiers, A. Verstraeten, E. Wauters et al., "Mutations in glucocerebrosidase are a major genetic risk factor for Parkinson's disease and increase susceptibility to dementia in a Flanders-Belgian cohort," *Neuroscience Letters*, vol. 629, pp. 160–164, 2016.

[19] S. Jesus, I. Huertas, I. Bernal-Bernal et al., "GBA variants influence motor and non-motor features of Parkinson's disease," *PLoS One*, vol. 11, no. 12, Article ID e0167749, 2016.

[20] M. Barkhuizen, D. G. Anderson, F. H. van der Westhuizen, and A. F. Grobler, "A molecular analysis of the GBA gene in Caucasian South Africans with Parkinson's disease," *Molecular Genetics & Genomic Medicine*, vol. 5, no. 2, pp. 147–156, 2017.

[21] J. Mitsui, I. Mizuta, A. Toyoda et al., "Mutations for Gaucher disease confer high susceptibility to Parkinson disease," *Archives of Neurology*, vol. 66, no. 5, pp. 571–576, 2009.

[22] Y. Li, T. Sekine, M. Funayama et al., "Clinicogenetic study of GBA mutations in patients with familial Parkinson's disease," *Neurobiology of Aging*, vol. 35, no. 4, pp. 935 e3–935 e8, 2014.

[23] Y. R. Wu, C.-M. Chen, C.-Y. Chao et al., "Glucocerebrosidase gene mutation is a risk factor for early onset of Parkinson disease among Taiwanese," *Journal of Neurology, Neurosurgery & Psychiatry*, vol. 78, no. 9, pp. 977–979, 2007.

[24] E. Sidransky, M. A. Nalls, J. O. Aasly et al., "Multicenter analysis of glucocerebrosidase mutations in Parkinson's disease," *New England Journal of Medicine*, vol. 361, no. 17, pp. 1651–1661, 2009.

[25] M. Horowitz, M. Pasmanik-Chor, I. Ron, and E. H. Kolodny, "The enigma of the E326K mutation in acid beta-glucocerebrosidase," *Molecular Genetics and Metabolism*, vol. 104, no. 1-2, pp. 35–38, 2011.

[26] M. Montfort, A. Chabás, L. Vilageliu, and D. Grinberg, "Functional analysis of 13 GBA mutant alleles identified in Gaucher disease patients: pathogenic changes and "modifier" polymorphisms," *Human Mutation*, vol. 23, no. 6, pp. 567–575, 2004.

[27] M. Y. Davis, C. O. Johnson, J. B. Leverenz et al., "Association of GBA mutations and the E326K polymorphism with motor and cognitive progression in Parkinson disease," *JAMA Neurology*, vol. 73, no. 10, pp. 1217–1224, 2016.

Assessment of Atrial Conduction Times in Patients with Newly Diagnosed Parkinson's Disease

Yiğit Çanga ⓘ,[1] Ayşe Emre,[1] Gülbün Asuman Yüksel,[2] Mehmet Baran Karataş,[1] Nizamettin Selçuk Yelgeç,[1] Ufuk Gürkan,[1] Ali Nazmi Çalık ⓘ,[1] Hülya Tireli,[2] and Sait Terzi[1]

[1]Department of Cardiology, Dr. Siyami Ersek Cardiovascular and Thoracic Surgery Center, Istanbul, Turkey
[2]Department of Neurology, Haydarpasa Numune Training and Research Hospital, Istanbul, Turkey

Correspondence should be addressed to Yiğit Çanga; canga81@hotmail.com

Academic Editor: Jan Aasly

Background. An increased risk of ischemic stroke has been reported in patients with Parkinson's disease (PD). Atrial fibrillation (AF) is strongly associated with ischemic stroke. Prolonged atrial electromechanical delay (EMD) is an independent predictor for the development of AF. *Aims.* The aim of the present study was to evaluate the atrial conduction parameters in patients with PD and to assess their relation with the severity of PD. *Study design.* We prospectively enrolled 51 consecutive patients with newly diagnosed PD and 31 age- and sex-matched non-PD subjects. *Methods.* To assess atrial electromechanical coupling (PA), the time intervals from the onset of p wave on ECG to the late diastolic wave at the septal (PAs) and lateral (PAl) mitral annulus and lateral tricuspid annulus (PAt) were measured on Tissue Doppler Echocardiography (TDE). The difference between PAs-PAl, PAs-PAt, and PAl-PAt were defined as left intra-atrial, right intra-atrial, and interatrial EMD, respectively. P-wave dispersion (PWD) was calculated from the 12-lead ECG. *Results.* PWD, PAs, PAl, and PAt durations were significantly prolonged in the PD group (all $p < 0.001$). Interatrial, right, and left intra-atrial EMD were also significantly longer in PD patients ($p < 0.001$, $p < 0.001$ and $p = 0.002$, resp.). There were significant positive correlations between disease severity (UPDRS score) and PWD ($r = 0.34$, $p = 0.041$), left intra-atrial ($r = 0.39$, $p = 0.005$), and interatrial EMD ($r = 0.35$, $p = 0.012$). By multivariate analysis, PWD (OR: 1.13, 95% CI: 1.02–1.25; $p = 0.017$), LA volume index (OR: 1.19, 95% CI: 1.02–1.37; $p = 0.021$), left intra-atrial (OR: 1.12, 95% CI: 1.01–1.24; $p = 0.041$), and interatrial EMD (OR: 1.08, 95% CI: 1.01–1.16; $p = 0.026$) were found as independent predictors of PD. *Conclusion.* Atrial conduction times were longer and correlated with the severity of disease in PD patients. Prolonged inter- and intra-atrial-EMD intervals were also found as independent correlates of PD. These findings may suggest an increased predisposition to atrial fibrillation in PD.

1. Introduction

Parkinson's disease (PD) has been associated with an increased risk of ischemic stroke and stroke-related mortality [1–3]. A recent population-based, propensity score-matched longitudinal follow-up study demonstrated that newly diagnosed PD was related with an increased risk of developing ischemic stroke [4]. Patients with atrial fibrillation have about 3- to 5-fold higher risk of stroke even after adjustment for risk factors [5]. Atrial fibrillation has been associated with stroke in different patient populations [6]. Prediction of atrial fibrillation may be crucial for risk stratification of PD patients with regard to ischemic stroke.

Prolonged atrial conduction times have been related to both onset and recurrence of atrial fibrillation [7, 8]. Tissue Doppler Echocardiography (TDE) has been used to determine atrial electromechanical coupling and electromechanical delay (EMD) intervals between different regions as indicators of electrical and/or structural remodeling of atria and as predictors of atrial fibrillation [9]. Regional changes in atrial conduction times might have a different influence on surface p waves leading to an interlead variation in p-wave duration called p-wave dispersion (PWD) [10]. In the present study, we investigated atrial conduction parameters in patients with newly diagnosed PD and also evaluated their relationship with the severity of PD.

2. Methods

2.1. Study Population. Fifty-one consecutive patients with newly diagnosed PD and 31 age- and sex-matched non-PD subjects were prospectively enrolled between January 1st, 2015 and December 31, 2015. Patients with PD were diagnosed according to the UK Parkinson's Disease Society Brain Bank Criteria [11]. The severity of PD was assessed by Unified Parkinson's Disease Rating Scale (UPDRS) [12]. Patients with a previous diagnosis of PD, stroke, other extrapyramidal disease, abnormal movement disorder, cerebral degeneration, cardiac arrhythmia, valvular heart disease, heart failure, coronary artery disease, chronic obstructive pulmonary disease, chronic renal failure, thyroid disease, active infectious disease, poor echocardiographic image quality, and a history of cardiac surgery or implanted device were excluded from the study. Baseline history, medication, and electrocardiography were recorded at the beginning of enrollment. PWD was defined as the difference between the maximum and minimum p-wave duration from multiple surface ECG leads [10]. The study was approved by the local ethics committee. Written informed consents were obtained from all participants.

2.2. Echocardiography. All patients were evaluated by transthoracic M mode, two dimensional, pulsed wave, continuous wave, colour flow, and TDE using the GE Vivid 3 system (GE Vingmed, Horten, Norway) with a 2.5–3.5 MHz transducer. Continuous single lead ECG was obtained from each participant during echocardiography.

LV diameter and wall thickness were measured by M-mode echocardiography. LV ejection fraction was calculated by Simpson's method according to the American Society of Echocardiography guidelines [13]. The mitral valve inflow pattern (E wave, A wave, E-wave deceleration time, E/A ratio, and isovolumic relaxation time) was measured by pulsed wave Doppler. LA volume was obtained from apical four and two chamber views by a disc method and indexed to body surface area [13].

TDE was performed by adjusting the pulsed Doppler signal filters to acquire the Nyquist limit of 15–20 cm/s and using the minimal optimal gain. Motions were recorded simultaneously with electrocardiogram in lead II to assess the relation between atrial electrical phases and myocardial motion. To assess atrial electromechanical coupling (PA), the time intervals from the onset of p wave on ECG to the late diastolic wave at the septal (PAs), and lateral (PAl) mitral annulus and lateral tricuspid annulus (PAt) were measured on TDE. The difference between PAs-PAl, PAs-PAt, and PAl-PAt were defined as left intra-atrial, right intra-atrial and interatrial EMD, respectively [7, 9]. Echocardiographic measurements were performed by two cardiologists. Patients with $a > 5\%$ difference between the measurements of two cardiologists were not included.

2.3. Statistical Analysis. Statistical analysis was performed using SPSS 16.0 (SPSS, Inc. Chicago, Illinois). A two-tailed p value < 0.05 was considered statistically significant.

Categorical variables were expressed as frequencies (percentages). Continuous variables were presented as mean ± standard deviation (tested for normality with Shapiro–Wilk test). Categorical variables were compared using the chi-square or Fischer's exact tests. Group means for continuous variables were compared using independent sample t-test. Pearson's correlation test was performed to assess the correlation between atrial conduction times and the severity of PD. Multivariate regression analysis was used to identify independent predictors of PD. Age, gender, hypertension, diabetes, LA volume index, PWD, and EMD intervals were included in the multivariate models.

3. Results

Fifty-one consecutive PD patients (mean age: 66.3 ± 12.4 years and 71% men) and 31 non-PD subjects (mean age: 69.8 ± 12.7 years and 52% men) entered the study. Mean UPDRS score of the PD group was 35.3 ± 17.9 (range, 10 to 75). Baseline demographic and clinical characteristics of the PD and non-PD groups are provided in Table 1. There was no statistically significant difference in all the baseline characteristics between the PD and non-PD groups.

Echocardiographic parameters are provided in Table 2. LA volume index was significantly higher in the PD group ($p = 0.006$). Mitral E/A was lower and mitral E-wave deceleration time was higher in the PD group, but both failed to reach statistical significance ($p = 0.057$ and $p = 0.058$, resp.). The remaining standard echocardiographic parameters were comparable between the two groups.

Atrial conduction time intervals are shown in Table 2. PWD, PAs, PAl, and PAt durations were significantly prolonged in the PD group (all $p < 0.001$). Left intra-atrial, right intra-atrial, and interatrial EMD were significantly longer in PD patients ($p < 0.001$, $p < 0.001$, and $p = 0.002$, resp.). PWD showed significant correlations with left intra-atrial ($r = 0.57$, $p < 0.001$) and interatrial EMD ($r = 0.54$, $p < 0.001$).

There were significant positive correlations between disease severity (UPDRS score) and PWD ($r = 0.36$, $p = 0.008$), left intra-atrial ($r = 0.34$, $p = 0.015$), and interatrial EMD ($r = 0.43$, $p = 0.002$) (Figure 1). By multivariate analysis, PWD (OR: 1.13, 95% CI: 1.02–1.25; $p = 0.017$), LA volume index (OR: 1.19, 95% CI: 1.02–1.37; $p = 0.021$), left intra-atrial (OR: 1.12, 95% CI: 1.01–1.24; $p = 0.041$), and interatrial EMD (OR: 1.08, 95% CI: 1.01–1.16; $p = 0.026$) were found to be independent predictors of PD (Table 3).

4. Discussion

The major findings of the present study are (1) patients with newly diagnosed PD are more likely to have abnormal atrial conduction times as assessed by prolonged PWD, PAs, PAl, PAt, intra-atrial, and interatrial EMD; (2) prolonged atrial conduction times were significantly correlated with the severity of PD as assessed by the UPDRS score, and (3) PWD, left intra-atrial, and interatrial EMD were found to be independent predictors of PD.

TABLE 1: Baseline demographic and clinical data of the study patients.

Characteristics	PD ($n = 51$)	Control ($n = 31$)	p value
Age, years	68.1 ± 10.4	67.2 ± 13.5	0.819
Male, n (%)	36 (71)	16 (52)	0.135
Hyperlipidemia, n (%)	12 (24)	8 (26)	0.816
DM, n (%)	8 (16)	5 (16)	0.958
Hypertension, n (%)	14 (27)	11 (35)	0.604
Smoking, n (%)	9 (18)	4 (13)	0.796
BMI (kg/m^2)	23.5 ± 2.7	23.0 ± 2.5	0.356
BSA (m^2)	1.94 ± 0.1	1.93 ± 0.12	0.659
Medications			
ASA, n (%)	6 (12)	5 (16)	0.820
ACEI, n (%)	5 (10)	5 (16)	0.617
ARB, n (%)	5 (10)	7 (23)	0.206
Calcium channel blocker, n (%)	7 (14)	5 (16)	0.765
Diuretic, n (%)	7 (14)	8 (25)	0.281
Statin, n (%)	8 (16)	6 (19)	0.900
OAD, n (%)	5 (10)	5 (16)	0.617
Insulin, n (%)	4 (8)	3 (10)	0.773
SBP (mmHg)	132.7 ± 19.8	135.5 ± 14.1	0.498
DBP (mmHg)	78.9 ± 8.4	83.1 ± 12.1	0.065
HR (bpm)	80 ± 11	79 ± 14	0.750
PWD (ms)	44.9 ± 6.1	40.0 ± 5.5	<0.001

PD, Parkinson's disease; DM, diabetes mellitus; BMI, body mass index; BSA, body surface area; ASA, acetylsalicylic acid; ACEI, angiotensin converting enzyme inhibitor; ARB, angiotensin receptor blocker; OAD, oral antidiabetic; SBP, systolic blood pressure; DBP, diastolic blood pressure; HR, heart rate; PWD, p-wave dispersion.

TABLE 2: Echocardiographic data and atrial conduction time intervals of the study patients.

Characteristics	PD ($n = 51$)	Control ($n = 31$)	p value
LVDD (mm)	44.6 ± 4.2	45.6 ± 2.9	0.232
LVSD (mm)	26.5 ± 4.9	27.2 ± 3.3	0.481
IVS (mm)	9.9 ± 1.9	9.3 ± 1.6	0.137
PW (mm)	9.1 ± 1.3	8.8 ± 0.8	0.179
LV EF (%)	60 (6)	60 (5)	0.782
LA volume index (cm^3/m^2)	17.1 ± 6.4	13.6 ± 2.5	0.006
DT (ms)	277 (91)	239 (67)	0.058
IRT (ms)	98.5 ± 15.9	102.6 ± 17.7	0.279
E/A ratio	0.9 ± 0.4	1.1 ± 0.4	0.057
Atrial conduction times			
ML-PA (ms)	63.1 ± 15.0	49.5 ± 9.0	<0.001
MS-PA (ms)	47.3 ± 9.9	35.0 ± 7.3	<0.001
TL-PA (ms)	55 (25)	37 (10)	<0.001
Intra-LA EMD (ms)	19 (10)	14 (8)	<0.001
Intra RA EMD (ms)	15 (15)	5 (7)	<0.001
Interatrial EMD (ms)	18 (19)	13 (12)	0.002

LVDD, left ventricular diastolic diameter; LVSD, left ventricular systolic diameter; IVS, interventricular septum thickness; PW, posterior wall thickness; LV, left ventricle; EF, ejection fraction; LA, left atrium; A, mitral inflow late diastolic velocity; E, mitral inflow early diastolic velocity; DT, left ventricular deceleration time; IRT, isovolumic relaxation time; ML-PA, mitral lateral annulus PA duration; MS-PA; mitral septal annulus PA duration; TL-PA, tricuspid lateral annulus PA duration; EMD, electromechanical delay; RA, right atrium.

Atrial fibrillation is the most common sustained arrhythmia in clinical practice [14]. Electrophysiological studies have revealed prolonged atrial conduction times as predictors of atrial fibrillation [15, 16]. In a previous study examining atrial conduction times with TDE, Deniz et al. have found significant correlations regarding left intra-atrial and interatrial conduction times detected by TDE and by electrophysiological study [9]. PWD and left intra-atrial conduction time detected by TDE were found to be independent predictors of inducibility of sustained atrial fibrillation in their study. Sequential analysis of atrial electromechanical coupling to evaluate the mechanisms of paroxysmal atrial fibrillation showed that atrial electromechanical coupling at the interventricular septum, left lateral mitral annulus, and right lateral tricuspid annulus was significantly longer in patients with paroxysmal atrial fibrillation (with or without underlying heart disease) compared to control subjects [7]. Left intra-atrial EMD was significantly prolonged even after correction for age in patients with atrial fibrillation [7]. The juxtaposition of atrial fibrotic lesions with normal atrial fibers has been suggested as a mechanism for nonhomogeneity of atrial conduction in atrial fibrillation [17]. Prolongation of atrial electromechanical coupling might be due to the time delay from atrial electric activation to myocardial contraction and/or left atrial enlargement [8]. In our study, PAs, PAl, and PAt durations were significantly prolonged and interatrial, right intra-atrial, and left intra-atrial EMD were significantly longer in patients with newly diagnosed PD. LA volume index was also increased in patients with PD.

Previous clinical studies have shown electrocardiographic PWD to be a predictor of paroxysmal atrial fibrillation [10]. PWD reflects inhomogeneous atrial conduction via variation in p-wave duration between different surface ECG leads [18, 19]. PWD was significantly prolonged in PD patients in our study. Furthermore, we demonstrated that PWD had significant correlations with left intra-atrial and interatrial EMD durations in PD patients.

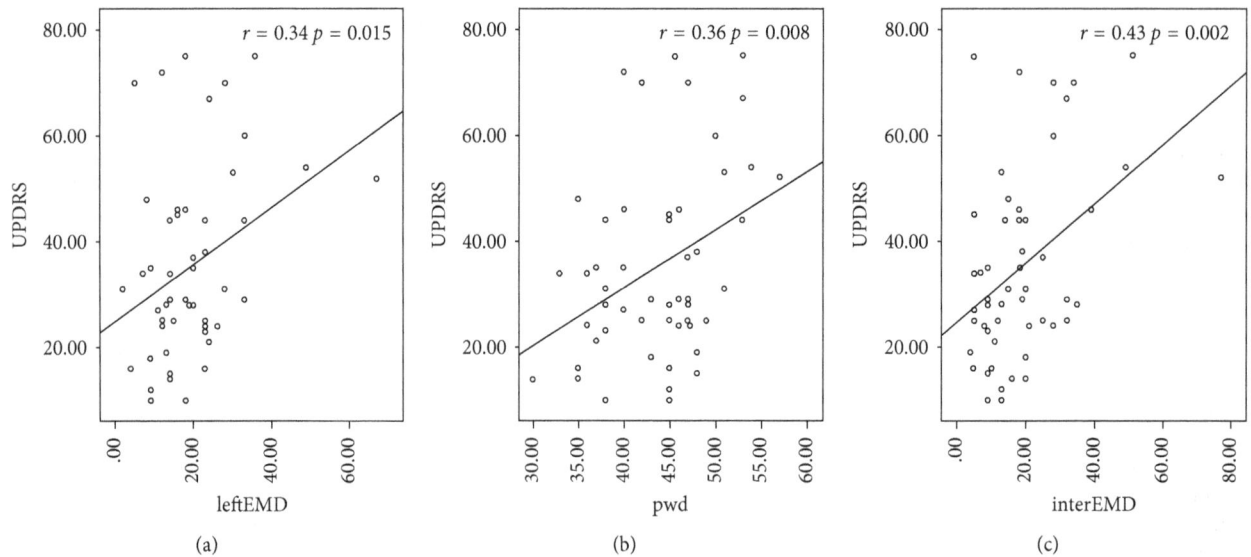

FIGURE 1: (a) Correlation between left intra-atrial EMD and the severity of Parkinson's disease (UPDRS score). (b) Correlation between p-wave dispersion and the severity of Parkinson's disease. (c) Correlation between interatrial EMD and the severity of Parkinson's disease UPDRS, Unified Parkinson's Disease Rating Scale; EMD, electromechanical delay.

TABLE 3: Multivariate analyses of variables associated with Parkinson's disease.

Variables	OR	95% CI	p value
PWD	1.13	1.02–1.25	0.017
LA volume index	1.19	1.02–1.37	0.021
Intra-LA EMD	1.12	1.01–1.24	0.041
Interatrial EMD	1.08	1.01–1.16	0.026
Intra-RA EMD	1.15	1.05–1.25	0.001

OR, odds ratio; CI, confidence interval; PWD, p-wave dispersion; LA, left atrium; EMD, electromechanical delay; RA, right atrium.

Patients with atrial fibrillation have an increased risk of stroke even after adjustment for risk factors [5]. PD has also been related with an increased risk of stroke [1–3]. Therefore, prediction of development of atrial fibrillation might be vital for risk stratification of PD patients with regard to ischemic stroke. Indeed, prolonged atrial conduction times were found to be significantly correlated with the severity of PD in our study.

Several potential explanations may be postulated for the pathophysiologic mechanisms by which atrial fibrillation and PD may be related. First, both atrial fibrillation and PD are associated with an increased inflammatory state [20–23]. Neuroinflammation plays an important role in the pathogenesis of PD and contributes to the progressive loss of nigral dopaminergic neurons [20]. Inflammatory responses mediated by activated glial cells, T cell infiltration, and increased expression of inflammatory cytokines are described as features of PD [20]. Likewise, the prevalence and prognosis of atrial fibrillation have been associated with increased levels of inflammatory markers [21, 22]. Moreover, high-sensitivity C-reactive protein levels have shown significant positive correlations with stroke risk factors in atrial fibrillation patients and have been associated with a composite endpoint of ischemic stroke, myocardial infarction, and death

[23]. Second, oxidative stress plays an important role in the pathogenesis of atrial fibrillation and PD [24, 25]. Oxidative stress has been shown to increase dopamine cell degeneration in PD [24]. Increased oxidative stress measured by the redox potentials of glutathione has been found to be an independent predictor of atrial fibrillation after adjustment for risk factors, heart failure, coronary artery disease, and high-sensitivity C-reactive protein levels [25]. Third, dysfunction of the autonomic nervous system is a common occurrence in atrial fibrillation and PD [26–29]. Symptoms of cardiovascular dysautonomia such as orthostatic hypotension have been frequently reported in PD [26]. Likewise, increased vagal tone has been related to the onset of paroxysmal atrial fibrillation both through cholinergic and noncholinergic pathways [27, 28]. An interaction between sympathetic and parasympathetic nervous system demonstrated via recording activities from stellate ganglia and vagal nerve has been shown to play a role in the development of atrial fibrillation [29].

A limitation of our study might be that the study population was not followed up in terms of development of atrial fibrillation. Another limitation might be that data regarding inflammatory and oxidative markers were not studied. Also because of the limited number of patients included in the study, our findings require validation and further studies with larger patient groups with follow-up for arrhythmias are needed.

In conclusion, the present study showed that atrial conduction times were prolonged in patients with newly diagnosed PD. Furthermore, atrial conduction parameters were significantly correlated with the severity of PD. Our findings might contribute to risk stratification of PD patients with regard to atrial fibrillation.

Disclosure

The manuscript was presented as an oral presentation at "14th International Congress of Update in Cardiology and Cardiovascular Surgery" and published as abstract at the supplement of *The American Journal of Cardiology* (Volume 121, Issue 8, Supplement, 15 April 2018, Page e54).

References

[1] C. Becker, S. S. Jick, and C. R. Meier, "Risk of stroke in patients with idiopathic Parkinson's disease," *Parkinsonism & Related Disorders*, vol. 16, no. 1, pp. 31–35, 2010.

[2] Y. Ben-Shlomo and M. G. Marmot, "Survival and cause of death in a cohort of patients with parkinsonism: possible clue to etiology?," *Journal of Neurology, Neurosurgery & Psychiatry*, vol. 58, no. 3, pp. 293–299, 1995.

[3] J. M. Gorel, C. C. Johnson, and B. A. Rybicki, "Parkinson's disease and its comorbid disorders: an analysis of Michigan mortality data, 1970 to 1990," *Neurology*, vol. 44, no. 10, pp. 1865–1868, 1994.

[4] Y.-P. Huang, L.-S. Chen, M.-F. Yen et al., "Parkinson's disease is related to an increased risk of ischemic stroke-a population-based propensity score-matched follow-up study," *PLoS One*, vol. 8, no. 9, Article ID e68314, 2013.

[5] P. A. Wolf, T. R. DAwber, H. E. Thomas Jr., and W. B. Kannel, "Epidemiologic assessment of chronic atrial fibrillation and risk of stroke: The Framingham Study," *Neurology*, vol. 28, no. 10, pp. 973–977, 1978.

[6] T. A. Manolio, R. A. Kronmal, G. L. Burke, D. H. O'leary, and T. R. Price, "Short-term predictors of incident stroke in older adults: the Cardiovascular Health Study," *Stroke*, vol. 27, no. 9, pp. 1479–1486, 1996.

[7] Q. Q. Cui, W. Zhang, H. Wang et al., "Assessment of atrial electromechanical coupling and influential factors in non-rheumatic paroxysmal atrial fibrillation," *Clinical Cardiology*, vol. 31, no. 2, pp. 74–78, 2008.

[8] W. Omi, H. Nagai, M. Takamura et al., "Doppler tissue analysis of atrial electromechanical coupling in paroxysmal atrial fibrillation," *Journal of the American Society of Echocardiography*, vol. 18, no. 1, pp. 39–44, 2005.

[9] A. Deniz, D. Y. Sahin, and M. Kanadasi, "Conduction characteristics in atrial fibrillation," *Herz*, vol. 39, no. 1, pp. 137–141, 2014.

[10] S. Okutucu, K. Aytemir, and A. Oto, "P-wave dispersion: what we know till now?," *JRSM Cardiovascular Disease*, vol. 5, article 2048004016639443, 2016.

[11] A. J. Hughes, S. E. Daniel, L. Kilford, and A. J. Lees, "Accuracy of clinical diagnosis of idiopathic Parkinson's disease: a clinico-pathological study of 100 cases," *Journal of Neurology, Neurosurgery and Psychiatry*, vol. 55, no. 3, pp. 181–184, 1992.

[12] Movement Disorder Society Task Force on Rating Scales for Parkinson's Disease, "The Unified Parkinson's Disease Rating Scale (UPDRS): status and recommendations," *Movement Disorders*, vol. 18, no. 7, article 738750, 2003.

[13] R. M. Lang, M. Bierig, F. A. Flachskampf et al., "Recommendations for chamber quantification: a report from the American society of Echocardiography's guidelines and standards committee and the chamber quantification writing group, developed in conjunction with the European association of Echocardiography, a branch of the European Society of Cardiology," *Journal of the American Society of Echocardiography*, vol. 18, no. 12, pp. 1440–1463, 2005.

[14] C. R. C. Wyndham, "Atrial fibrillation: the most common arrhythmia," *Texas Heart Institute Journal*, vol. 27, no. 3, pp. 257–267, 2000.

[15] JC. Daubert, D. Pavin, G. Jauvert, and P. Mabo, "Intra- and interatrial conduction delay: implications for cardiac pacing," *Pacing and Clinical Electrophysiology*, vol. 27, no. 4, pp. 507–525, 2004.

[16] P. Papageorgiou, K. Monahan, N. G. Boyle et al., "Site-dependent intra-atrial conduction delay: relationship to initiation of atrial fibrillation," *Circulation*, vol. 94, no. 3, pp. 384–389, 1996.

[17] M. Allessie, J. Ausma, and U. Schotten, "Electrical, contractile and structural remodeling during atrial fibrillation," *Cardiovascular Research*, vol. 54, no. 2, pp. 230–246, 2002.

[18] P. E. Dilaveris and J. E. Gialafos, "P-wave dispersion: a novel predictor of paroxysmal atrial fibrillation," *Annals of Noninvasive Electrocardiology*, vol. 6, no. 2, pp. 159–165, 2001.

[19] P. E. Dilaveris, E. J. Gialafos, S. K. Sideris et al., "Simple electrocardiographic markers for the prediction of paroxysmal idiopathic atrial fibrillation," *American Heart Journal*, vol. 135, no. 5, pp. 733–738, 1998.

[20] K. U. Tufekci, R. Meuwissen, S. Genc, and K. Genc, "Inflammation in Parkinson's disease," *Advances in Protein Chemistry and Structural Biology*, vol. 88, pp. 69–132, 2012.

[21] Y. Guo, G. Y. Lip, and S. Apostolakis, "Inflammation in atrial fibrillation," *Journal of the American College of Cardiology*, vol. 60, no. 22, pp. 2263–2270, 2012.

[22] J. A. Vilchez, V. Roldan, M. Hernandez-Romero, M. Valdes, G. Y. Lip, and F. Marin, "Biomarkers in atrial fibrillation: an overview," *International Journal of Clinical Practice*, vol. 68, no. 4, pp. 434–443, 2014.

[23] J. Hermida, F. L. Lopez, R. Montes, K. Matsushita, B. C. Astor, and A. Alonso, "Usefulness of high-sensitivity C-reactive protein to predict mortality in patients with atrial fibrillation," *American Journal of Cardiology*, vol. 109, no. 1, pp. 95–99, 2012.

[24] P. Jenner, "Oxidative stress in Parkinson's disease," *Annals of Neurology*, vol. 53, no. S3, pp. S26–S38, 2003.

[25] A. Samman Tahhan, P. B. Sandesara, S. S. Hayek et al., "Association between oxidative stress and atrial fibrillation," *Heart Rhythm*, vol. 14, no. 12, pp. 1849–1855, 2017.

[26] T. Ziemssen and H. Reichmann, "Cardiovascular dysautonomia in de novo Parkinson's disease," *Journal of the Neurological Sciences*, vol. 289, no. 1-2, pp. 74–80, 2010.

[27] H. E. Hoff and L. A. Geddes, "Cholinergic factor in auricular fibrillation," *Journal of Applied Physiology*, vol. 8, no. 2, pp. 177–192, 1955.

[28] D. Yang, Y. Xi, T. Ai et al., "Vagal stimulation promotes atrial electrical remodeling induced by rapid atrial pacing in dogs: evidence of a noncholinergic effect," *Pacing and Clinical Electrophysiology*, vol. 34, no. 9, pp. 1092–1099, 2011.

[29] P. S. Chen, L. S. Chen, M. C. Fishbein et al., "Role of the autonomic nervous system in atrial fibrillation: pathophysiology and therapy," *Circulation Research*, vol. 114, no. 9, pp. 1500–1515, 2014.

3

A Randomized Controlled Trial of Chinese Medicine on Nonmotor Symptoms in Parkinson's Disease

Ka-Kit Chua,[1,2] Adrian Wong,[3] Kam-Wa Chan,[1] Yin-Kei Lau,[3] Zhao-Xiang Bian,[1,2] Jia-Hong Lu,[4] Liang-Feng Liu,[1,2] Lei-Lei Chen,[1,2] Ka-Ho Chan,[1] Kim-Pong Tse,[1] Anne Chan,[3] Ju-Xian Song,[1,2] Justin Wu,[3] Li-Xing Zhu,[5] Vincent Mok,[3] and Min Li[1,2]

[1]School of Chinese Medicine, Hong Kong Baptist University, Kowloon, Hong Kong
[2]Mr. & Mrs. Ko Chi Ming Centre for Parkinson's Disease Research, Hong Kong Baptist University, Kowloon, Hong Kong
[3]Institutes of Integrative Medicine, Department of Medicine and Therapeutics, The Chinese University of Hong Kong,
  Sha Tin, Hong Kong
[4]State Key Laboratory of Quality Research in Chinese Medicine, Institute of Chinese Medical Sciences, University of Macau, Macau
[5]Department of Mathematics, Statistics Research & Consultancy Centre, Faculty of Science, Hong Kong Baptist University,
  Kowloon, Hong Kong

Correspondence should be addressed to Vincent Mok; vctmok@cuhk.edu.hk and Min Li; limin@hkbu.edu.hk

Academic Editor: Hélio Teive

Nonmotor symptoms (NMS) of Parkinson's disease (PD) have devastating impacts on both patients and their caregivers. Jiawei-Liujunzi Tang (JLT) has been used to treat some NMS of PD based on the Chinese medicine theory since Qing dynasty. Here we report a double-blind, randomized, placebo-controlled, add-on clinical trial aiming at evaluating the efficacy and safety of the JLT in treating NMS in PD patients. We randomly assigned 111 patients with idiopathic PD to receive either JLT or placebo for 32 weeks. Outcome measures were baseline to week 32 changes in Movement Disorder Society-Sponsored Revision of Unified PD Rating Scale (MDS-UPDRS) Parts I–IV and in NMS assessment scale for PD (NMSS). We observed improvements in the NMSS total score ($p = 0.019$), mood/cognition ($p = 0.005$), and reduction in hallucinations ($p = 0.024$). In addition, post hoc analysis showed a significant reduction in constipation ($p < 0.001$). However, there was no evidence of improvement in MDS-UPDRS Part I total score ($p = 0.216$) at week 32. Adverse events (AEs) were mild and comparable between the two groups. In conclusion, long-term administration of JLT is well tolerated and shows significant benefits in improving NMS including mood, cognition, and constipation.

1. Introduction

Parkinson's disease (PD) is the second most common neurodegenerative disease in the world, with a prevalence rate of 1% in the population over age of 60 [1]. Increasing attention has been paid to nonmotor aspects which might precede motor symptoms [2]. Common nonmotor symptoms (NMS) of PD include fatigue, mood disorders, hallucinations, constipation, and sleep disorders [3]. Though not fatal, they reduce quality of life for both patients and their caregivers [4]. The most common treatment for PD is levodopa. However, levodopa primarily treats motor symptoms and it typically generates adverse events after long-term use [5]. As a result of both the failure of levodopa improving NMS and its side effects, patients often seek alternative treatments [6].

Traditional Chinese medicine (TCM) is one of the most investigated streams of alternative medicine [7, 8]. It has been used to treat PD throughout China [9]. In TCM theory, patients are divided into categories according to the signs and symptoms presented [10]. The concept is similar to using factor analysis and cluster analysis in modern statistics to classify patients with different clinical patterns [11]. According to Chinese medicine theory, PD patients who present with fatigue, constipation, and/or mood disorder are classified in the subgroup of "Spleen Qi Deficiency." Treatment typically involves different herbal formulas to "Replenish Spleen Qi." Randomized controlled trials (RCT) have been conducted to examine the efficacy and safety of using various TCM formulas to treat PD. However, the quality of most of these RCT is compromised by methodological defects including poor randomization, insufficient masking, lack of proper sample size calculation, and/or improper data analysis [12].

Our group previously reported that a Chinese herbal medicine formula, Jiawei-Liujunzi Tang (JLT), relieved some nonmotor complications after 24 weeks of treatment [13]. It has been used to treat some PD-like NMS since Qing dynasty [13]. Recently, our team demonstrated that corynoxine B (Cory B), an active compound isolated from the Chinese medicine *Uncaria rhynchophylla* (Miq.) Jacks. (Gouteng in Chinese), which is one of the principal herbs in the JLT, efficiently promotes the clearance of α-synuclein (α-syn) aggresomes in vitro and in vivo via inducing autophagy which protects neurons in PD [14]. Cory B rescues α-syn-induced impairment of autophagy, possibly through blocking α-syn-HMGB1 (high mobility group box 1, HMGB 1) interaction [15]. Moreover, our group investigated corynoxine (Cory), another active compound isolated from Gouteng, and found that it can promote the clearance of α-syn via Akt/mTOR (Akt murine thymoma viral oncogene homolog 1, Akt; mammalian target of rapamycin, mTOR) pathway [16]. We also found that more than 90% of PD patients are having DSQ [17]. JLT may be suitable for most PD patients if it is workable.

Given the number of people using Chinese medicine, it is critical to test the efficacy of JLT in clinical trials. In this trial, we aimed to study the efficacy and safety of using JLT to treat NMS in idiopathic PD patients.

2. Methods

2.1. Participants

Inclusion Criteria. Adults between 18 and 80 years of age who (1) had been diagnosed with idiopathic PD based on UK Brain Bank criteria with Hoehn and Yahr (H&Y) stages 1–4 by conventional medicine physicians [18] and (2) presented symptoms classified as Deficiency of Spleen Qi (diagnosis of DSQ, Supplementary Material 1, available online at https://doi.org/10.1155/2017/1902708) based on Guidance for Clinical Research of New Chinese Herbal Medicine published by China [19] during a screening visit were eligible. The diagnostic criteria of DSQ included presentation of dyspepsia, fatigue, and abdominal distention. Other inclusion criteria included stable daily administration of levodopa and permitted antiparkinsonian drugs (dopamine agonists, selegiline, rasagiline, entacapone, amantadine, and anticholinergic drugs) for at least 4 weeks before the start of treatment and normal liver and renal function.

Exclusion Criteria. Patients who had atypical or drug-induced parkinsonism, a score of <24 on the Mini-Mental State Examination (MMSE), history of psychosis, history of Chinese herbal medicine allergy, concurrent intake of antidepressants, a history of suicide attempts, or unstable medical disorders were excluded. Those who had participated in other trials within 30 days of the start of this trial as well as women who were pregnant or were breastfeeding were also excluded.

This clinical study was carried out at the Hong Kong Baptist University (HKBU) Chinese Medicine Specialty Centre. It was approved by the Ethics Committee of the HKBU's Institutional Review Board (code: HASC/09-10/09) and registered on the Chinese Clinical Trial Registry (ChiCTR-TRC-13003085). Written informed consent was obtained from every patient before they participated in any study-related activity. This study report followed the guidelines of Consolidated Standards of Reporting Trials (CONSORT).

2.2. Sample Size Calculation. According to our previous pilot study [13], the management team estimated an effect size of 0.626 and a standard deviation of 1.99 with G-Power version 3.1. At least 105 patients (1 : 1) were required to provide an 80% power of detecting a difference with a 2-sided α-level of 0.05 with a maximum of 20% attrition rate. No covariates or center effects were used in power calculation.

2.3. Randomization and Masking. This study was a double-blind, randomized, placebo-controlled, add-on trial. Patients were randomly assigned to receive 32 weeks of either active herbal treatment or placebo and followed up for a further 6-week observation period without treatment. The randomization sequence was generated by "Random Allocation Software." The sequence was password-protected and kept in a computer by Lei-Lei Chen. Group allocation was stratified block randomization according to their H&Y stages at the screening. The sequential number was contained in a sealed opaque envelop and distributed to assessors. Patients, investigators, and all sponsoring parties were masked to treatment allocation until the end of the study.

2.4. Study Medication. The active herbal medicine under study was JLT (Supplementary Table 1, composition of JLT). The granules were produced in a single batch (JLT batch number: A120065; Placebo batch number: A120153), mixed, and packed to ensure the stability and homogeneity of the composition by PuraPharm Pharmaceuticals Company Limited, a GMP plant, as previously reported [13]. The placebo was made of caramel, gardenia yellow pigment, sunset yellow, permicol egg yellow, cocoa brown, citric acid, sodium cyclamate, dextrin, and broadleaf holly leaf [20]. The herbal granules and the placebo granules had identical appearance and smell, and both were sealed in plastic bags. All herbal and placebo granules were distributed by Kim-Pong Tse with both written and verbal instructions for each participant. They were instructed to take the granules orally, twice per day, 11 g each time (a dosage equivalent to 55 g herbs), at least two hours apart from taking any routine Western medication.

2.5. Outcome Measurements and Its Assessment. The primary outcome of this study was the Movement Disorder Society-Sponsored Revision of Unified PD Rating Scale (MDS-UPDRS) [21] Part I total score. MDS-UPDRS Part I subscores, nonmotor symptom assessment scale (NMSS) for Parkinson's disease [22] total score, and total scores of each domain as well as the total score of other parts of MDS-UPDRS (Parts II–IV) were used as secondary outcomes.

Outcome measurements were carried out during the study visits at weeks 0, 16, 32 (end of treatment), and 38 (end of observation period). Assessments were carried out in the "on" state. Safety assessment, which included reporting of adverse events (AEs) and measurement of vital signs and physical examination, was carried out throughout the study. In addition, laboratory safety screening of liver and renal function was performed at week 32. Both bilingual assessors, that is, Ka-Kit Chua and Yin-Kei Lau, were blind to the allocation and were trained by the same neurology specialist Vincent Mok and qualified by the online training program of the Movement Disorder Society.

A home diary was given to the patients or their caregivers to monitor their medical condition. Formal instruction for the home diary was given during the first visit. Compliance to treatment was defined by the record of the diary with reference to the amount of the returned medicine/placebo packages.

2.6. Statistical Analysis. Demographic and clinical data were compared between the JLT and placebo groups using independent sample t-test or Chi-squared test as appropriate. Changes in primary and secondary outcomes, between baseline and week 32, were compared between the JLT and placebo groups using independent sample t-tests.

Missing data were input in the last-observation-carried-forward (LOCF) manner. All patients randomized with at least one postrandomization measurement were included in the primary analysis to follow the intention-to-treat principle. Analyses were done with SPSS 19.0 package (SPSS, Chicago, IL).

To avoid inflation of type-1 errors due to multiple-endpoint testing, analyses of the primary outcomes were performed with a hierarchical approach. To begin, the scores of MDS-UPDRS Part I at week 32 for the JLT and placebo groups were compared. If the difference was deemed statistically significant at a 2-sided α-level of 0.05, the scores of MDS-UPDRS Part I at week 16 and week 38 were compared between groups. The hierarchical order was as follows: (1) MDS-UPDRS Part I total score at week 32; (2) MDS-UPDRS Part I total score at weeks 16 and 38. Secondary outcomes were analyzed in the same manner as the primary outcome.

A post hoc analysis was performed to test any possible effect of JLT by analyzing all the subscores of each domain of NMSS in the same manner as the primary outcome.

3. Results

Figure 1 is a flow chart depicting the participant screening and recruitment in this study. Demographic data and baseline scores are summarized in Table 1. A total of 234 patients were screened for eligibility, and 116 participants were enrolled. Five patients withdrew from the study due to personal reasons after randomization and before the start of treatment. Among the remaining 111 patients (73 males; 38 females;

mean ages: 62.69 ± 9.11 years; mean duration of PD: 5.95 ± 3.97 years), 56 were assigned to the JLT group and 55 were assigned to the placebo group. Twenty participants dropped out during the study due to reasons listed in Figure 1. Forty-five participants in the JLT group and 46 in the placebo group completed the study.

In the primary analysis, we observed a trend of improvement; a decreased score was obtained at week 32 in JLT group which suggested an improvement in NMS in the MDS-UPDRS Part I total score in the JLT group relative to the placebo group, though the difference was not statistically significant (mean diff. = −1.30; 95% CI: −3.37 to 0.77; p = 0.215). In comparison, an increased score was obtained at week 32 in the placebo group, which suggested worsening. Further analyses performed on the subscores of MDS-UPDRS Part I between the two groups revealed that the JLT group showed nonsignificant trends of reduction in constipation (mean diff. = −1.09; 95% CI: −2.30 to 0.13; p = 0.079) and in hallucination (mean diff. = −0.18; 95% CI: −0.38 to 0.19; p = 0.075) compared to the placebo group (Table 2).

In the secondary analysis, the data indicate a significant difference in NMSS for Parkinson's disease total score between JLT group and placebo group (mean diff. = −14.05; 95% CI: −25.71 to −2.39; p = 0.019) after 32 weeks of treatment. A trend of improvement in the JLT group was also noted by the hierarchical approach in week 16 (mean diff. = −8.87; 95% CI: −18.78 to 1.04; p = 0.079) and the improvement persisted at 38 weeks (mean diff. = −11.70; 95% CI: −23.12 to −0.28; p = 0.045). Further analyses of the NMSS subscores showed that the PD patients in the JLT group experienced improvement in mood/cognition (mean diff. = −6.66; 95% CI: −11.24 to −2.09; p = 0.005) and reduction in hallucinations (mean diff. = −1.58; 95% CI: −2.96 to −0.21; p = 0.024) compared to those in the placebo group at week 32. Relative to the control group, the JLT group showed a trend of improvement in the gastrointestinal tract (mean diff. = −1.84; 95% CI: −3.87 to −0.20; p = 0.076) as well as a significant reduction in constipation which persisted from week 16 (mean diff. = −2.49; 95% CI: −3.75 to −1.23; p < 0.001) to week 38 (mean diff. = −2.17; 95% CI: −3.53 to −0.82; p = 0.002) (Table 3). There were no significant differences in other subscores between the two groups at week 16 and the end of treatment in other domains. No statistically significant differences were found in other parts (II–IV) of MDS-UPDRS in week 32.

For the withdrawal and adverse events, twenty patients (11 (19.6%) [JLT] versus 9 (16.4%) [placebo], p = 0.65) discontinued treatment after randomization. Among these 20 patients, 4 in each group withdrew because of AEs. During the treatment phase, two patients (3.57%) in the JLT group and four patients (7.27%) in the placebo group had serious AEs: one patient had hypoglycemia (placebo), one had sepsis (placebo), one had finger sarcoma (placebo), two had coronary heart disease (one in placebo and one in JLT), and one had breast cancer (JLT). No deaths were recorded during the trial. AEs were reported by at least 5% of patients in each group; these are presented in Table 4.

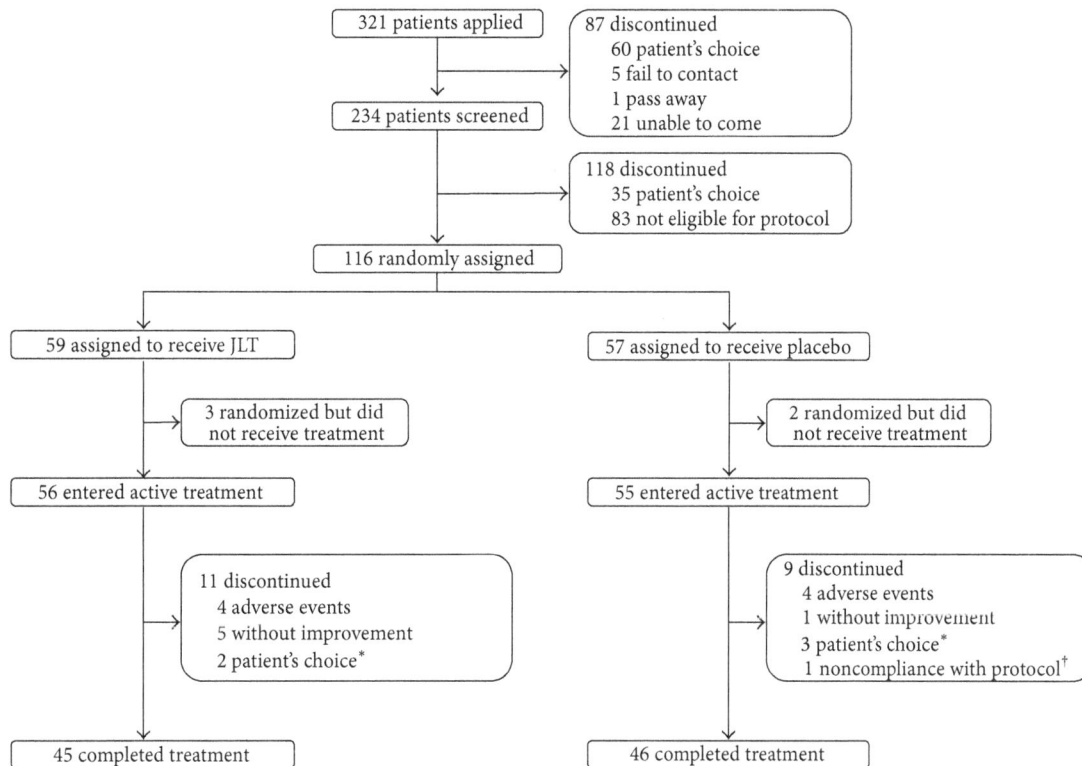

* Participation in the study could be discontinued because of noncompliance with dosing or visits.

† Patient's choice to discontinue was for reasons unrelated to the study drug.

FIGURE 1

4. Discussion

In this RCT, there was no evidence supporting the hypothesis that JLT can reduce NMS as represented by improvement in the overall MDS-UPDRS Part I score (the NMS of PD). However, a reduction in NMS was noted by the secondary outcome of the NMSS total score, even after the patients had stopped medication. Also, improvement in the form of reduction in hallucinations and constipation was suggested by secondary analysis of MDS-UPDRS Part I subscore. Improvement in the mood, hallucinations, and constipation, without effect on the motor features of PD, was found by secondary analysis and post hoc analysis of the NMSS subscore. JLT was well tolerated. Discontinuation due to AEs occurred with the same frequency in the JLT group (4 patients) as in the placebo group (4 patients). Further targeted studies on the effect of JLT on mood and gastrointestinal condition could confirm these observations.

TCM has long been used to treat symptoms similar to PD in China [23]. According to TCM theory, JLT replenishes and facilitates circulation of "spleen and stomach Qi," which is related to PD NMS. Depletion and stagnation of "spleen and stomach Qi" would lead to NMS such as constipation, nausea, sleep disruption, and mood disorder. In this trial,

the improvement of NMS assessed by the NMSS showed continual effect even after the patients had stopped the medication for 6 weeks. It suggested that the effect of JLT may not be just symptomatic; instead, it may alter some pathophysiological processes underlying NMS.

JLT is an herbal formula composed mainly of *Codonopsis pilosula* (Franch.) Nannf. (Dangshen in Chinese), *Rehmannia glutinosa* Libosch. (Dihuang in Chinese), *Poria cocos* (Schw.) Wolf. (Fuling in Chinese), and *Uncaria rhynchophylla* (Miq.) Jacks. (Gouteng in Chinese) [13]. Jung et al. found that Gouteng extract is an effective anxiolytic agent and acts via the serotonergic nervous system [24]. Lee et al. showed that triterpenoids in Fuling may regulate the expressed 5-hydroxytryptamine 3A (5-HT$_{3A}$) receptors which have close relationship to the gastric system and nervous system [25]. These suggest that the effect of JLT, which includes improvement in mood and reduction of constipation, may be due to the increased levels or stimulation of serotonin receptors.

Serotonin or 5-hydroxytryptamine (5-HT) is a monoamine neurotransmitter with a significant role in mood and appetite regulation [26]. It is synthesized in both serotonergic neurons of the central nervous system (CNS) to regulate mood and appetite and in the alimentary canal to regulate intestinal movements [27]. Neurotransmitters in general,

TABLE 1: Baseline characteristics.

Parameter	JLT group (n = 56)	Control group (n = 55)	p value[a]
Age (years)	63.48 ± 9.72	63.31 ± 8.20	0.919[b]
Gender (M/F)	35/21	38/17	0.464[c]
Disease duration (years)	6.42 ± 4.15	5.42 ± 3.77	0.096[b]
Duration of Levodopa treatment (years)	5.17 ± 4.42	3.94 ± 3.13	0.187[b]
Total Levodopa dosage (mg/day)	459.82 ± 350.90	374.55 ± 257.46	0.148[b]
Medication use			
Levodopa, n (%)	53 (94.6)	50 (90.9)	0.447[c]
Dopaminergic agonist, n (%)	23 (41.1)	17 (30.9)	0.265[c]
Anticholinergic, n (%)	18 (32.1)	21 (38.2)	0.505[c]
COMT inhibitor, n (%)	14 (25.0)	4 (7.3)	0.011[c]
MAO-B inhibitor, n (%)	17 (30.4)	12 (21.8)	0.306[c]
Amantadine, n (%)	5 (8.9)	4 (7.3)	0.749[c]
Senna, n (%)	5 (8.9)	6 (10.9)	0.727[c]
Lactulose, n (%)	4 (7.1)	3 (5.5)	0.714[c]
Baseline scores			
H&Y score	2.07 ± 0.60	2.02 ± 0.59	0.639[b]
NMSS total	65.52 ± 49.77	47.42 ± 35.70	0.030[b]
MDS-UPDRS part I	10.21 ± 7.06	8.76 ± 6.63	0.267[b]
MDS-UPDRS part II	14.71 ± 7.95	11.58 ± 7.51	0.035[b]
MDS-UPDRS part III	33.21 ± 15.39	33.27 ± 14.27	0.983[b]
MDS-UPDRS part IV	4.00 ± 4.45	2.78 ± 3.70	0.120[b]

Data are expressed as mean ± S.D; [a]p value was comparing the difference between two groups in baseline; [b]treatment group compared with placebo group by independent t-test; [c]treatment group compared with placebo group by Chi-square test with continuity correction.

5-HT in particular, may be involved in the NMS of PD, including mood disorder, psychosis, and constipation [28].

For the limitations, the improvement of NMS was just supported by the NMSS total score (p = 0.019), the secondary outcome, but not the MDS-UPDRS Part I total score (p = 0.216), the primary outcome. Also, constipation was improved by JLT as suggested by the post hoc analyses of NMSS. We are aware that the evidence suggesting improvements in constipation (p = 0.079) by the MDS-UPDRS Part I, the secondary outcome, among patients taking JLT was noted to be weak. The inconsistency within the test may be due to the inadequate power of the study to measure small differences. It should be noted though that while the differences are small, to an individual patient, this small difference may still have an important impact on their quality of life. The current data suggests that a scaled-up study would be able to confirm the difference [29]. On the other hand, the scale of NMSS is more in depth in testing NMS than the MDS-UPDRS (score: 0–4). NMSS measures the severity as well as the frequency of each NMS independently and multiplies these factors to achieve an overall result (score: 0–12). This may result in a difference between the two measurements.

An attrition rate of 20% was high for PD patients at a relatively early stage of the disease. This was due to the long treatment period (32 weeks) when compared to other clinical trials [30]. As the main motivation of some PD patients to participate in a clinical trial was to obtain benefit [31], 6 patients withdrew when they believed the medication was ineffective.

Another limitation is that there was a significant difference at baseline in the number of patients using catechol O-methyltransferase (COMT) inhibitor and the total score of NMSS and MDS-UPDRS Part II even after randomization. This might be due to the use of stratified block randomization based on the H&Y stages of PD patients. PD patients were divided into difference H&Y stages based on their clinical motor symptoms, which was best shown by the total score of MDS-UPDRS Part 3. As H&Y stages do not consider the use of medication, this may result in differences in the medical history of patients. In general, the more medicines patients are taking, the more serious their condition becomes. It could induce a great variation in the assessment score even if the patients were in the same PD stage. Hence, a difference could result in the motor part and nonmotor part but not in the clinical presentation of PD symptoms, the total score of MDS-UPDRS Part 3. Larger sample size may be a possible way to minimize such problem in future.

In conclusion, although the result of MDS-UPDRS does not show significant improvement, the NMSS data does show some positive outcomes on the NMS of PD. Our data suggest that JLT could alleviate gastrointestinal problems and mood

Table 2: Efficacy result of JLT on Parkinson's disease patient at week 32.

	JLT	Placebo	Mean difference	95% confidence interval (CI)	p value[a]
Movement Disorder Society-Sponsored Revision of Unified PD Rating Scale (MDS-UPDRS)					
Part I total score (nonmotor symptom)	−0.46 ± 6.61	0.84 ± 4.09	−1.30	−3.37 to 0.77	0.215
Q.1 Cognitive	−0.07 ± 0.97	0.00 ± 0.69	−0.07	−0.39 to 0.25	0.657
Q.2 Hallucinations	−0.04 ± 0.54	0.15 ± 0.52	−0.18	−0.38 to 0.02	0.075
Q.3 Depression	−0.07 ± 1.03	0.07 ± 0.72	−0.14	−0.48 to 0.19	0.393
Q.4 Anxious	−0.14 ± 0.82	−0.02 ± 0.71	−0.13	−0.41 to 0.16	0.393
Q.5 Apathy	−0.23 ± 1.36	−0.02 ± 0.87	−0.21	−0.64 to 0.22	0.327
Q.6 Dopamine dysregulation	−0.13 ± 0.63	−0.15 ± 0.52	0.02	−0.20 to 0.24	0.854
Q.7 Sleep	0.23 ± 1.03	0.13 ± 1.06	0.11	−0.29 to 0.50	0.597
Q.8 Daytime sleep	0.16 ± 0.91	0.11 ± 0.85	0.05	−0.28 to 0.38	0.759
Q.9 Pain	−0.02 ± 1.30	0.24 ± 1.05	−0.25	−0.70 to 0.19	0.261
Q.10 Urinary	−0.02 ± 0.73	0.02 ± 0.87	−0.04	−0.34 to 0.27	0.813
Q.11 Constipation	−0.13 ± 1.45	0.96 ± 4.35	−1.19	−2.30 to 0.13	0.079
Q.12 Light headedness	0.04 ± 1.08	−0.04 ± 0.38	0.72	−0.23 to 0.38	0.641
Q.13 Fatigue	−0.04 ± 1.21	−0.02 ± 0.97	−0.05	−0.47 to 0.36	0.796
Part II total score (motor symptom)	0.45 ± 4.13	1.05 ± 4.58	−0.61	−2.25 to 1.03	0.464
Part III total score (motor examination)	−0.52 ± 10.13	1.38 ± 8.27	−1.90	−5.38 to 1.58	0.282
Part IV total score (motor complications)	0.21 ± 3.56	0.65 ± 3.42	−0.44	−1.75 to 0.87	0.508
Nonmotor Symptom Assessment Scale for Parkinson's Disease (NMSS)					
Total score	−2.27 ± 32.90	11.78 ± 28.93	−14.05	−25.71 to −2.39	0.019
D1 total cardiovascular	−0.89 ± 3.38	−0.15 ± 2.31	−0.75	−1.84 to 0.35	0.178
D2 total sleep/fatigue	3.63 ± 7.98	4.62 ± 7.08	−0.99	−3.83 to 1.84	0.490
D3 total mood/cognition	−3.54 ± 14.38	3.13 ± 9.36	−6.66	−11.23 to −2.10	0.005
D4 total perceptual/hallucinations	−0.88 ± 4.17	0.71 ± 3.04	−1.58	−2.96 to −0.21	0.024
D5 total attention/memory	−1.86 ± 6.07	−0.15 ± 7.08	−1.71	−4.20 to 0.77	0.174
D6 total gastrointestinal tract	−0.86 ± 5.15	0.98 ± 5.66	−1.84	−3.87 to 0.20	0.076
D7 total urinary	1.71 ± 7.57	1.47 ± 7.12	0.24	−2.52 to 3.01	0.863
D8 total sexual function	−0.71 ± 4.20	0.16 ± 3.81	−0.88	−2.39 to 0.63	0.251
D9 total miscellaneous	1.13 ± 6.41	1.00 ± 5.46	0.13	−2.11 to 2.36	0.912

[a] p value was comparing the score changes at week 32 between JLT group and placebo group by independent sample t-tests; values are given as mean ± S.D. Values in JLT group and placebo group are the score changed in the same group between week 32 and baseline (score at week 32 minus score at the baseline).

TABLE 3: Result of hierarchical approach.

Parameter	Week 16		Week 32		Week 38	
	JLT	Placebo	JLT	Placebo	JLT	Placebo
Total score of NMSS	−3.13 ± 29.49	5.75 ± 22.67	−2.27 ± 32.90	11.78 ± 28.93	0.48 ± 34.01	12.18 ± 26.08
	Mean difference: −8.87		Mean difference: −14.05		Mean difference: −11.70	
	95% CI: −18.78 to 1.04		95% CI: −25.71 to −2.39		95% CI: −23.12 to −0.28	
	p value = 0.079		p value = 0.019		p value = 0.045	
NMSS D3 total mood/cognition	−1.68 ± 12.12	0.93 ± 7.76	−3.54 ± 14.38	3.13 ± 9.36	−0.66 ± 15.02	3.18 ± 10.38
	Mean difference: −2.61		Mean difference: −6.66		Mean difference: −3.84	
	95% CI: −6.43 to 1.22		95% CI: −11.23 to −2.10		95% CI: −8.71 to 1.02	
	p value = 0.181		p value = 0.005		p value = 0.120	
NMSS D4 total perceptual/hallucinations	−0.64 ± 3.28	0.09 ± 0.59	−0.88 ± 4.17	0.71 ± 3.04	−0.86 ± 4.52	0.22 ± 1.76
	Mean difference: −0.73		Mean difference: −1.58		Mean difference: −1.08	
	95% CI: −1.62 to 0.16		95% CI: −2.96 to −0.21		95% CI: −2.37 to 0.22	
	p value = 0.105		p value = 0.024		p value = 0.103	
NMSS D6 Q21 constipation	−1.02 ± 3.89	1.47 ± 2.71	−1.25 ± 3.46	1.55 ± 3.40	−0.43 ± 3.68	1.75 ± 3.54
	Mean difference: −2.49		Mean difference: −2.80		Mean difference: −2.17	
	95% CI: −3.75 to −1.23		95% CI: −4.09 to −1.50		95% CI: −3.53 to −0.82	
	p value < 0.001		p value < 0.001		p value = 0.002	

p value was comparing the score changes at different time points between JLT group and placebo group by independent sample t-tests; values are given as mean ± S.D. Values in JLT group and placebo group are the score changed in the same group between different time points and baseline (score at different time points minus score at the baseline).

TABLE 4: Adverse events reported by >5% of patients in each group.

Adverse events	Number of patients (%)	
	JLT ($N = 56$)	Placebo ($N = 55$)
Abdominal pain	3 (5.36)	3 (5.45)
Dyspepsia	5 (8.93)	1 (1.82)
Diarrhea	1 (1.79)	3 (5.45)
Dizziness	3 (5.36)	7 (12.73)
Back pain	1 (1.79)	5 (9.09)
Joint pain	2 (3.57)	4 (7.27)

disorders in some PD patients over 32 weeks with minimal side effects. Also, the effect of JLT on NMS and constipation could persist 6 weeks after treatment. It appears to be both safe and effective for long-term use to treat NMS of PD. While not conclusive, this initial trial warrants future work into JLT, especially on the mood and gastrointestinal improvement of PD patients.

Authors' Contributions

Min Li conceived the project and coordinated all efforts in the clinical trial; Vincent Mok monitored the trial; Min Li, Anne Chan, Zhao-Xiang Bian, and Justin Wu contributed to the design of the trial; Ka-Kit Chua and Yin-Kei Lau helped carry out and monitor the clinical trial; Lei-Lei Chen generated the randomization sequence; Kim-Pong Tse distributed the medicine; Li-Xing Zhu, Kam-Wa Chan, Ka-Ho Chan, Liang-Feng Liu, and Adrian Wong helped with data analysis and discussion; Ka-Kit Chua, Adrian Wong, Jia-Hong Lu, Ju-Xian Song, and Min Li wrote the paper.

Acknowledgments

This work was supported by PuraPharm International (H.K.) Ltd., HMRF 08091111 and HMRF 12132091 from the Food and Health Bureau, Hong Kong Government, research grants (IRMS/12-13/1A, MPCF04-12/13, and MPCF 008-2014/2015) from HKBU, and S.H. Ho Foundation. This study was also supported by Mr. & Mrs. Ko Chi Ming Center for Parkinson's Disease Research. The authors would like to thank Dr. Feng Sun and Ms. Vicky Keng from Clinical Division, School of Chinese Medicine, HKBU, for their great support on this clinical study. The authors would also like to thank Professor David Moher for his valuable comments and Dr. Martha Dahlen for her English editing of this manuscript.

References

[1] L. M. de Lau and M. M. Breteler, "Epidemiology of Parkinson's disease," *The Lancet Neurology*, vol. 5, no. 6, pp. 525–535, 2006.

[2] T. Simuni and K. Sethi, "Nonmotor manifestations of Parkinson's disease," *Annals of Neurology*, vol. 64, supplement 2, pp. S65–S80, 2008.

[3] J. Massano and K. P. Bhatia, "Clinical approach to Parkinson's disease: features, diagnosis, and principles of management," *Cold Spring Harbor Perspectives in Medicine*, vol. 2, no. 6, Article ID a008870, 2012.

[4] K. R. Chaudhuri, P. Odin, A. Antonini, and P. Martinez-Martin, "Parkinsons disease: the non-motor issues," *Parkinsonism & Related Disorders*, vol. 17, no. 10, pp. 717–723, 2011.

Cold Spring Harbor Perspectives in Medicine, vol. 2, no. 6, Article ID a008870, 2012.

[4] K. R. Chaudhuri, P. Odin, A. Antonini, and P. Martinez-Martin, "Parkinsons disease: the non-motor issues," *Parkinsonism & Related Disorders*, vol. 17, no. 10, pp. 717–723, 2011.

[5] W. J. Weiner, "Levodopa—toxic or neuroprotective?" *Nature Clinical Practice Neurology*, vol. 2, no. 10, pp. 518–519, 2006.

[6] P. R. Rajendran, R. E. Thompson, and S. G. Reich, "The use of alternative therapies by patients with Parkinson's disease," *Neurology*, vol. 57, no. 5, pp. 790–794, 2001.

[7] P. Leung, "Development of traditional Chinese medicine in Hong Kong and its implications for orthopaedic surgery," *Hong Kong Journal of Orthopaedic Surgery*, vol. 6, no. 1, pp. 1–5, 2002.

[8] A.-P. Lu, H.-W. Jia, C. Xiao, and Q.-P. Lu, "Theory of traditional chinese medicine and therapeutic method of diseases," *World Journal of Gastroenterology*, vol. 10, no. 13, pp. 1854–1856, 2004.

[9] Y. Wang, X.-M. Lin, and G.-Q. Zheng, "Traditional Chinese medicine for Parkinson's disease in china and beyond," *Journal of Alternative and Complementary Medicine*, vol. 17, no. 5, pp. 385–388, 2011.

[10] W.-Y. Jiang, "Therapeutic wisdom in traditional Chinese medicine: a perspective from modern science," *Trends in Pharmacological Sciences*, vol. 26, no. 11, pp. 558–563, 2005.

[11] W. C. Moore, D. A. Meyers, and S. E. Wenzel, "Identification of asthma phenotypes using cluster analysis in the severe asthma research program," *American Journal of Respiratory and Critical Care Medicine*, vol. 181, no. 4, pp. 315–323, 2010.

[12] V. Chung, L. Liu, Z. Bian et al., "Efficacy and safety of herbal medicines for idiopathic Parkinson's disease: a systematic review," *Movement Disorders*, vol. 21, no. 10, pp. 1709–1715, 2006.

[13] M. Li, W. F. Kum, S. S. K. Durairajan et al., "Treatment of idiopathic Parkinson's disease with traditional chinese herbal medicine: A Randomized Placebo-Controlled Pilot Clinical Study," *Evidence-Based Complementary and Alternative Medicine*, vol. 2011, Article ID 724353, 8 pages, 2011.

[14] J.-H. Lu, J.-Q. Tan, S. S. K. Durairajan et al., "Erratum to: Lu J-H, Tan J-Q, Durairajan SSK, Liu L-F, Zhang Z-H, Ma L, et al. Isorhynchophylline, a natural alkaloid, promotes the degradation of a-synuclein in neuronal cells via inducing autophagy. Autophagy 2012; 8:98-108 (Autophagy (2012) 8, 5 (864-866))," *Autophagy*, vol. 8, no. 5, pp. 864–866, 2012.

[15] J. X. Song, J. H. Lu, L. F. Liu et al., "HMGB1 is involved in autophagy inhibition caused by SNCA/α-synuclein overexpression: a process modulated by the natural autophagy inducer corynoxine B," *Autophagy*, vol. 10, no. 1, pp. 144–154, 2014.

[16] L.-L. Chen, J.-X. Song, J.-H. Lu et al., "Corynoxine, a natural autophagy enhancer, promotes the clearance of alpha-synuclein via Akt/mTOR pathway," *Journal of Neuroimmune Pharmacology*, vol. 9, no. 3, pp. 380–387, 2014.

[17] K.-K. Chua and M. Li, "Occurrence of spleen qi deficiency as defined by chinese medicine in parkinson disease," *Journal of Traditional Chinese Medical Sciences*, 2017.

[18] A. J. Hughes, S. E. Daniel, L. Kilford, and A. J. Lees, "Accuracy of clinical diagnosis of idiopathic Parkinson's disease: a clinicopathological study of 100 cases," *Journal of Neurology Neurosurgery and Psychiatry*, vol. 55, no. 3, pp. 181–184, 1992.

[19] *The Guidance for Clinical Research of New Chinese Herbal Medicine. Chinese Medical Scientific Publishers*, Medical Scientific Publishers, Beijing, China, 2002.

[20] Xu. Tang, B. L. Q. Dong, R. Gao, and S. J. Guan, "Exploration into the Preparation of Placebos Used in Chinese Medicinal Clinical Trial," *Chinese Journal of Integrated Traditional and Western Medicine*, vol. 29, no. 7, pp. 656–658, 2009.

[21] C. G. Goetz, B. C. Tilley, S. R. Shaftman et al., "Movement disorder society-sponsored revision of the unified Parkinson's disease rating scale (MDS-UPDRS): scale presentation and clinimetric testing results," *Movement Disorders*, vol. 23, no. 15, pp. 2129–2170, 2008.

[22] K. R. Chaudhuri, P. Martinez-Martin, A. H. V. Schapira et al., "International multicenter pilot study of the first comprehensive self-completed nonmotor symptoms questionnaire for Parkinson's disease: the NMSQuest study," *Movement Disorders*, vol. 21, no. 7, pp. 916–923, 2006.

[23] G. Zheng, "Therapeutic History of Parkinson's Disease in Chinese Medical Treatises," *The Journal of Alternative and Complementary Medicine*, vol. 15, no. 11, pp. 1223–1230, 2009.

[24] J. W. Jung, N. Y. Ahn, H. R. Oh et al., "Anxiolytic effects of the aqueous extract of *Uncaria rhynchophylla*," *Journal of Ethnopharmacology*, vol. 108, no. 2, pp. 193–197, 2006.

[25] J.-H. Lee, Y. J. Lee, J.-K. Shin et al., "Effects of triterpenoids from *Poria cocos* Wolf on the serotonin type 3A receptor-mediated ion current in *Xenopus oocytes*," *European Journal of Pharmacology*, vol. 615, no. 1–3, pp. 27–32, 2009.

[26] S. N. Young, "How to increase serotonin in the human brain without drugs," *Journal of Psychiatry and Neuroscience*, vol. 32, no. 6, pp. 394–399, 2007.

[27] M. Berger, J. A. Gray, and B. L. Roth, "The expanded biology of serotonin," *Annual Review of Medicine*, vol. 60, pp. 355–366, 2009.

[28] S. H. Fox, R. Chuang, and J. M. Brotchie, "Serotonin and Parkinson's disease: on movement, mood, and madness," *Movement Disorders*, vol. 24, no. 9, pp. 1255–1266, 2009.

[29] R. Nuzzo, "Scientific method: statistical errors," *Nature*, vol. 506, no. 7487, pp. 150–152, 2014.

[30] P. Skapinakis, E. Bakola, G. Salanti, G. Lewis, A. P. Kyritsis, and V. Mavreas, "Efficacy and acceptability of selective serotonin reuptake inhibitors for the treatment of depression in Parkinson's disease: a systematic review and meta-analysis of randomized controlled trials," *BMC Neurology*, vol. 10, article 49, 2010.

[31] A. Valadas, M. Coelho, T. Mestre et al., "What motivates Parkinson's disease patients to enter clinical trials?" *Parkinsonism and Related Disorders*, vol. 17, no. 9, pp. 667–671, 2011.

4

Sirtuin-2 Protects Neural Cells from Oxidative Stress and Is Elevated in Neurodegeneration

Preeti Singh,[1,2] **Peter S. Hanson,**[1] **and Christopher M. Morris**[1,2,3]

[1]*Medical Toxicology Centre and NIHR Health Protection Research Unit in Chemical and Radiation Threats and Hazards, Newcastle University, Wolfson Building, Claremont Place, Newcastle NE2 4AA, UK*
[2]*NIHR Biomedical Research Unit in Lewy Body Disorders, Newcastle University, Edwardson Building, Institute of Neuroscience, Newcastle upon Tyne NE4 5PJ, UK*
[3]*NIHR Biomedical Research Centre in Ageing and Chronic Disease, Newcastle University, Biomedical Research Building, Campus for Ageing and Vitality, Newcastle upon Tyne NE4 5PJ, UK*

Correspondence should be addressed to Christopher M. Morris; c.m.morris@ncl.ac.uk

Academic Editor: Hélio Teive

Sirtuins are highly conserved lysine deacetylases involved in ageing, energy production, and lifespan extension. The mammalian SIRT2 has been implicated in Parkinson's disease (PD) where studies suggest SIRT2 promotes neurodegeneration. We therefore evaluated the effects of SIRT2 manipulation in toxin treated SH-SY5Y cells and determined the expression and activity of SIRT2 in postmortem brain tissue from patients with PD. SH-SY5Y viability in response to oxidative stress induced by diquat or rotenone was measured following SIRT2 overexpression or inhibition of deacetylase activity, along with α-synuclein aggregation. SIRT2 in human tissues was evaluated using Western blotting, immunohistochemistry, and fluorometric activity assays. In SH-SY5Y cells, elevated SIRT2 protected cells from rotenone or diquat induced cell death and enzymatic inhibition of SIRT2 enhanced cell death. SIRT2 protection was mediated, in part, through elevated SOD2 expression. SIRT2 reduced the formation of α-synuclein aggregates but showed minimal colocalisation with α-synuclein. In postmortem PD brain tissue, SIRT2 activity was elevated compared to controls but also elevated in other neurodegenerative disorders. Results from both in vitro work and brain tissue suggest that SIRT2 is necessary for protection against oxidative stress and higher SIRT2 activity in PD brain may be a compensatory mechanism to combat neuronal stress.

1. Introduction

The mammalian Sirtuin, SIRT2, is a nicotinamide adenine diphosphate (NAD$^+$) dependent cytoplasmic protein and an orthologue to yeast Hst2p [1]. SIRT2, though predominantly a cytoplasmic protein, shuttles between the cytoplasm and nucleus depending upon the cell cycle stage [2]. Human SIRT2 deacetylates a number of cytoplasmic and nuclear proteins and thus is a key modulator of many cellular processes including cell cycle, cell motility, autophagy, metabolic homeostasis, myelination, apoptosis, antioxidant defence mechanisms, and tumorigenesis. Although all SIRTs are expressed in the brain, SIRT2 is the most abundant [3] and is expressed in nearly all brain regions with particularly high

levels in myelin- producing oligodendrocytes (OL) [4, 5]. In the mouse, isoform 2 of SIRT2, SIRT2.2 is highly expressed in the adult brain and age related accumulation of SIRT2.2 is observed in both the mouse and human cortex [3]. SIRT2 regulates myelin formation by deacetylating alpha-tubulin (Lysine 40) in OL [4] and deacetylating Par-3 (protease activated receptor) in Schwann's cells [6]. While being a modulator of OL differentiation, SIRT2 is also suggested to have a role in regulation of neurite growth and neuronal motility in hippocampal neurones [7]. These findings indicate that SIRT2 influences axonal plasticity and plays an important role in maintenance of neuronal networks in the brain and hence may be involved in age related neurodegenerative disorders such as Parkinson's disease (PD).

Parkinson's disease is the most common neurodegenerative movement disorder [8, 9] and typically involves progressive loss of dopaminergic (DA) neurones in the substantia nigra (SN) and accumulation of cytoplasmic inclusions, Lewy bodies (LB) and Lewy neurites composed of alpha-synuclein (α-synuclein) [10]. PD is clinically characterised by tremor, rigidity, bradykinesia, postural instability, and other accompanying symptoms [11]. Given the role of SIRTs in fundamental cell processes and protection from age related changes, the role of SIRT2 has begun to be studied in neurodegeneration. Inhibition of SIRT2 in cellular and drosophila models of PD reduces α-synuclein mediated toxicity [12]. Rotenone treatment of rats which causes SN cell death appears in part to rely on SIRT2 with treatment leading to an elevation of SIRT2 in the SN leading to worsening motor impairment while inhibition of SIRT2 diminished striatal DA depletion and improved behaviour abnormality [13]. Conversely, reduction of SIRT2 causes cell death in neural PC12 cells [14] and also in BV2 microglia [15, 16], with increased SIRT2 activity rescuing microtubule dynamics in SH-SY5Y cells [17]. Ablation of SIRT2 in the brain however causes minimal effects and therefore modulation of SIRT2 activity may be important in the context of cellular and in particular neuronal stress [18].

Given the possible role of SIRT2 in PD, the present study evaluated the role of SIRT2 in oxidative stress mediated cell death and characterised its role in PD. The effects of overexpression of SIRT2 and inhibition of deacetylase activity of SIRT2 were determined in oxidative stress in SH-SY5Y cells using diquat or rotenone, which induce cellular and mitochondrial stress, respectively [19, 20]. The effect of SIRT2 on α-synuclein aggregate formation in toxin treated SH-SY5Y cells was also evaluated. We also determined the expression, activity, and localisation of SIRT2 in postmortem human brain tissue obtained from the patients with PD, PD with dementia (PDD), dementia with Lewy bodies (DLB), and Alzheimer's disease (AD).

2. Materials and Method

2.1. SH-SY5Y Cells. SH-SY5Y neuroblastoma cells were obtained from the European Collection of Cell Cultures (ECACC, Salisbury, UK) and cultured as described previously [20]. Cells were grown at 37°C in a humidified atmosphere of 95% air/5% CO_2.

2.2. SIRT2 Overexpression and Toxin Treatment in SH-SY5Y Cells. Wild type SIRT2 (SIRT2pcDNA3.1; Plasmid number 13813) was obtained from Addgene and pcDNA 3.1 was purchased from ThermoFisher Scientific. SH-SY5Y cells were seeded in 12-well plates and the cells were transfected with SIRT2pcDNA3.1 and the control group was transfected with empty pcDNA3.1 plasmid using PEI (polyethyleneimine; Invitrogen). Plasmids were incubated with cells at 37°C for 48 hours. To study the effect of SIRT2 inhibition, one set of cells transfected with SIRT2 and pcDNA3.1 were treated with either diquat (Sigma-Aldrich, UK) dissolved in PBS (Phosphate buffered saline; Sigma-Aldrich) or rotenone (Sigma-Aldrich) dissolved in DMSO (dimethyl sulphoxide, Sigma-Aldrich) at a final concentration of 0.2% PBS/DMSO

alone and a second set of cells with toxin and AGK2 as a specific SIRT2 inhibitor (25 μM; Tocris, UK; see Supplementary Figure 4 in Supplementary Material available online at https://doi.org/10.1155/2017/2643587). AGK2 was added to cells 2 hours prior to diquat or rotenone treatment and the cells were incubated overnight for 20 hours. Cell viability was determined by Alamar Blue reduction assay [20] (refer to Figures 1, 2, and 4 in supplementary files for efficiency of SIRT2 transfection and inhibition).

2.3. Western Blotting. Following toxicity determination, cell lysates were prepared by scraping the viable cells in native lysis buffer (1% 10x Tris buffered saline (TBS), 0.27 M Sucrose, 1% Triton X-100, 1x protease inhibitor cocktail). The cell lysates were sonicated for 20 seconds using a sonic probe and the total protein was determined using Bradford assay (modified from [21]). Twenty micrograms of protein in cell lysates were subjected to electrophoresis and were probed for selected antibodies as described previously [20] (see Table 1 in supplementary files for dilution and suppliers of antibodies).

2.4. Fluorescence Immunocytochemistry. SH-SY5Y cells were grown in chamber slides (BD Falcon, UK), transfected with SIRT2 plasmids, and treated with diquat or rotenone with or without AGK2. The cells were washed with PBS and slides incubated with 4% formaldehyde (Sigma-Aldrich) in warm 1x PBS for 15 minutes and then washed with PBS and stored until use in 10% glycerol (Sigma-Aldrich, UK) at 4°C. Cells were washed and blocked in 1x PBS/5% normal serum/0.3% Triton™ X-100 for an hour then incubated overnight at 4°C with SIRT2 and phospho-α-synuclein (Wako) for α-synuclein aggregates. Cells were washed with PBS and incubated with secondary antibodies for 60 minutes protected from light. Cells were washed with PBS and counterstained and mounted with ProLong Gold Antifade Mountant with DAPI (Thermo Fisher). Images were acquired using a Zeiss Axioplan 2 microscope (Zeiss, Oberkochen, Germany) with a 40x objective and images captured at 1024 × 1024 pixel resolution for analysis. Images were quantified using ImageJ (NIH, Bethesda, USA). The exposure time of the fluorescence was standardised to empty vector transfected cells with the same exposure time applied to all other sections with the SIRT2 overexpressing cells showing reduced α-synuclein staining intensity. All stained sections were quantified using ImageJ (NIH, Bethesda, USA) analysis of confocal images. The total immunostaining was analysed by importing the image to ImageJ and binarisation of the image (converted to 8-bit grey scale) and the highlighted cell area was quantified by using the "analyse particles" function. α-Synuclein aggregate immunoreactivity was also determined by using a standardised custom histogram based coloured thresholding technique and then subjected to "analyse particles." The parameters recorded were total area and percentage area of staining. α-Synuclein aggregate percentage was calculated as the total area of α-synuclein divided by the total area of immunostaining multiplied by 100.

TABLE 1: Details of brain samples used for Western blot and immunohistochemistry.

Groups	FCX	TCX	Cb	Pu	Hp	Age at death (years)	Tissue pH	PMD (hours)	Gender	
---	---	---	---	---	---	---	---	---	M	F
Control (N)	11	12	12	12	8	77.5 ± 6.98	6.17 ± 0.34	19.9 ± 6.42	7	5
PD (N)	12	12	12	12	—	77.44 ± 7.03	5.85 ± 0.06	23.44 ± 9.72	8	4
PDD (N)	8	9	12	8	—	75.93 ± 5.38	6.19 ± 0.32	24.69 ± 11.38	9	3
DLB (N)	12	12	12	12	6	77.00 ± 5.35	6.32 ± 0.29	18.0 ± 8.58	9	3
AD (N)	12	12	12	—	9	80.37 ± 5.25	6.19 ± 0.33	19.84 ± 9.30	5	7

The table summarises the case details of brain samples used in Western blot analysis and immunohistochemistry. FCX: frontal cortex; TCX: temporal cortex; Cb: cerebellum; Pu: putamen; Hp: hippocampus; PMD: postmortem delay.

2.5. Postmortem Tissue Analysis. Brain samples were obtained from Newcastle Brain Tissue Resource, a Human Tissue Authority licensed tissue bank. All aspects of the study were approved by the National Research Ethics Service. Tissue was obtained at postmortem as soon as possible after death and samples were snap frozen and stored at $-80°C$. Frozen tissue of the relevant region was identified and protein homogenates from PD, DLB, PDD, AD, and controls (Table 1) were prepared by homogenising approximately 250 mg of freshly thawed grey matter in 2.5 ml of 0.2 M triethylammonium bicarbonate (TEAB) containing 1x protease inhibitor. After addition of 10 μl of 10% SDS to 500 μl of homogenate, samples were vortexed and then sonicated using a sonic probe for 15 secs, followed by sonication on ice in a sonic bath for 40 mins. The concentration of protein was determined by Bradford assay. Western blotting was performed as previously [20].

2.6. Sirtuin Activity. Brain protein homogenates were thawed and vortexed and sonicated as previous section. Samples were spun down at 100 g at $4°C$ for 5 minutes and the protein concentration of supernatant was determined by Bradford assay. Fluorescent SIRT substrate p53 (379–382), Ac-RHKK (Ac)-AMC was synthesised by Cambridge Research Biolabs, UK. Stock peptide was prepared as a 5 mM solution in diluted SIRT Assay buffer (50 mM Tris-HCl, pH 8.0, containing 137 mM sodium chloride, 2.7 mM KCl, and 1 mM $MgCl_2$) and was stored at $-70°C$ until use. Total SIRT activity was determined by using 30 μg protein in substrate buffer containing 41.6 μM peptide, 1 mM NAD^+, and 100 nM TSA (as an HDAC inhibitor) and incubated at room temperature for 2 hours on a shaker. After 2 hours 2.5 μg/ml trypsin in 50 mM NAM was added to stop further deacetylation and to cleave the deacetylated product. The fluorescence was recorded for each well after one hour of incubation of the trypsin-NAM solution in the plate reader on excitation wavelength of 350–360 nm and emission wavelength of 450–460 nm. SIRT2 activity was determined as AGK2 (20 μM) inhibitable activity. Use of recombinant SIRT1, SIRT2, and SIRT3 showed equivalent activity with the Ac-RHKK (Ac)-AMC substrate (see supplementary files for sample and buffer preparation, and protein activity).

2.7. Determination of Cellular Localisation of SIRT2. Formalin fixed paraffin embedded brain tissue sections were used to determine distribution of SIRT2 in the CNS in disease. For immunohistochemistry, 10 μM coronal sections were sampled from the temporal cortex, hippocampus, and cerebellum. The sections were heated at $60°C$ for 10 minutes followed by 2 × 10-minute washes in xylene (Fisher Scientific) followed by rehydration in decreasing ethanol solutions (2 × 100%, 95%, 70%, 50%, and 0% ethanol in ddH_2O). Antigen retrieval was performed by boiling the sections in heated citrate buffer (pH 6) in a microwave at high power heat for 10 mins before allowing them to cool for 20 minutes and then washing them in running tap water. The sections were then quenched in 30% H_2O_2 in tap water for 20 minutes followed by 3 × 3-minute washes in TBS-T. Rabbit monoclonal antibody to SIRT2 (SantaCruz Biotechnology) dissolved in TBS-T was applied to the sections for an hour at room temperature followed by 3 × 3-minute washes in TBS-T. Sections were visualised using Menarini X-Cell Plus detection system according to the manufacturer's instructions with DAB reagent. Sections were counterstained with haematoxylin dehydrated through graded alcohols to xylene before coverslips were mounted with DPX (Fisher Scientific). Images of the sections were acquired using a Zeiss Axioplan 2 microscope (Zeiss, Oberkochen, Germany) with 10x and 63x magnifying objective and 3-chip CCD true colour camera (JVC, Yokohama, Japan) coupled to a PC.

2.8. Statistical Analyses. Statistical analysis was performed using one-way ANOVA within groups and two-way ANOVA within two groups using SPSS21 (IBM) followed by appropriate post hoc (Bonferroni) nonparametric testing. Error bars represent standard deviation ($\pm$SD). $^*p < 0.05$ was considered statistically significant. Statistical analysis of Western blotting data was performed in GraphPad prism using a two-sample t-test assuming unequal variances. Statistical significance was considered as $p < 0.05$. The results are presented as mean $\pm$SD.

3. Results

3.1. SH-SY5Y Cells

3.1.1. Overexpression of SIRT2 Protects Cells from Toxin Mediated Cell Death. Diquat and rotenone have been reported to induce oxidative stress and rotenone has been shown to induce parkinsonian symptoms in a rat model [22]. Diquat is

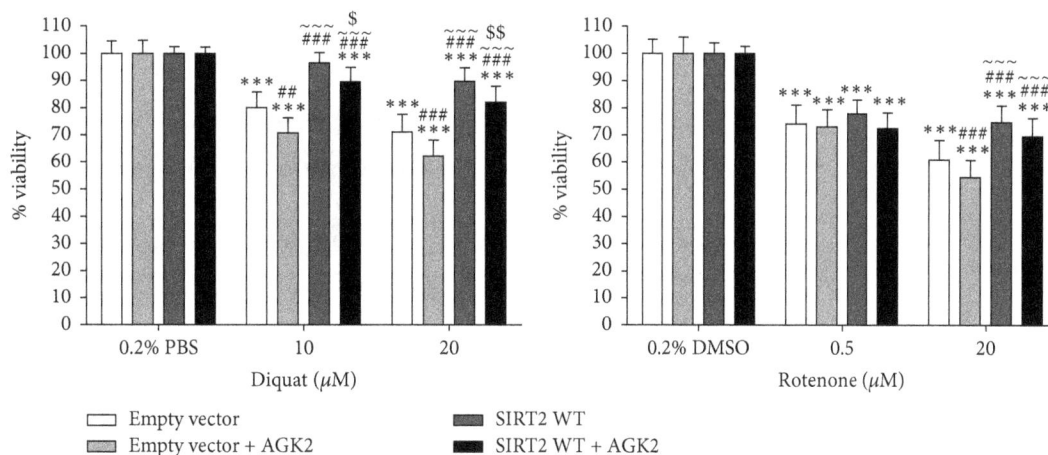

FIGURE 1: The effect of SIRT2 overexpression and inhibition was determined in toxin treated SH-SY5Y cells. SIRT2 was overexpressed in SH-SY5Y cells and control cells were transfected with empty vector following which one set of cells was treated with toxin alone and another with SIRT2 inhibitor AGK2 and toxin for 20 hours and viability measured by reduction of Alamar Blue. Toxins used: diquat (20 μM or 10 μM) or rotenone (20 μM or 0.5 μM) treated cells. Data are presented as fold- untreated ($\pm$SD) from three independent assays ($n = 3$). $^{***}p < 0.001$ when compared to 0.2% vehicle (PBS or DMSO), one-way ANOVA (Bonferroni corrected), $^{###}p < 0.001$ and $^{##}p < 0.01$ when compared to control cells, $^{\sim\sim\sim}p < 0.001$ when compared to control + AGK2 treatment, and $^{\$\$}p < 0.01$ and $^{\$}p < 0.05$ when compared to SIRT2 cells, two-way ANOVA (Bonferroni corrected).

a potent redox cycler [23] that upon entry into cells utilises molecular oxygen to generate O_2^- which can lead to lipid peroxidation in cell membranes resulting in cell death [24]. In diquat treated cells, overexpression of SIRT2 significantly increased viability compared to control cells ($p < 0.001$). A significant elevation in cytotoxicity was observed in control cells coincubated with diquat and AGK2 compared to diquat alone (20 μM diquat: $p < 0.001$ and 10 μM diquat $p < 0.001$). In cells treated with 0.5 μM rotenone, no significant effect was seen by overexpression or inhibition of SIRT2 ($p > 0.05$) but in cells treated with 20 μM rotenone, a reduction in toxicity was observed in SIRT2 overexpressing cells compared to control cells and to control cells treated with AGK2 ($p < 0.001$) (Figure 1).

3.1.2. Under Oxidative Stress, SIRT2 Induces the Expression of SOD2.
SIRT2 has been shown to increase antioxidant defence mechanisms by deacetylating FOXO3a and elevating FOXO3a DNA binding, resulting in an increased expression of SOD2 [25]. To test this possibility, the levels of SOD2 were measured in diquat or rotenone treated SH-SY5Y cells. In 20 μM diquat treated cells, SOD2 levels were elevated in control (~1.5-fold, $p < 0.001$), SIRT2 (~2-fold, $p < 0.001$), and SIRT2 + AGK2 cells (~1.6-fold; $p < 0.001$) compared to 0.2% PBS treated control cells (Figure 2). The levels of SOD2 were reduced by 28% in control + AGK2 cells ($p < 0.001$) compared to 0.2% PBS treated control cells. In 10 μM diquat treated cells, SOD2 levels were elevated in control (~1.5-fold, $p < 0.001$), SIRT2 (~1.7-fold, $p < 0.001$), and SIRT2 + AGK2 cells (~1.4-fold; $p < 0.01$) compared to 0.2% PBS treated control cells (Figure 2). The levels of SOD2 were reduced by 12% in control + AGK2 cells ($p < 0.05$) compared

to 0.2% PBS treated control cells. The expression of SOD2 was tested only in 20 μM rotenone treated cells, as 0.5 μM rotenone cells did not show significant difference in cell viability between the groups (see Figure 1). In addition, at low levels of rotenone (0.5 μM) oxidative damage may be limited to only the mitochondria leading to mitochondria-mediated cell death independent of cytoplasmic SIRT2. Higher levels of rotenone (20 μm) with increased oxidative stress and mitochondrial inhibition leading to marked depletion of cellular ATP could reduce cytoplasmic SIRT2 phosphorylation causing increased SIRT2 activation [7] leading to induction of SOD2 and other mediators. The levels of SOD2 were elevated in control (~1.3-fold, $p < 0.01$), SIRT2 (~1.6-fold, $p < 0.001$), and SIRT2 + AGK2 cells (~1.4-fold; $p < 0.001$) compared to 0.2% DMSO treated control cells. The levels of SOD2 were reduced by 17% in control + AGK2 cells ($p < 0.05$) compared to 0.2% DMSO treated control cells (Figure 2).

3.1.3. SIRT2 Shows Minimal Colocalisation with α-Synuclein.
Cells respond to stress by synthesising stress proteins and/or by relocalising the proteins to different cellular compartments. SIRT2 is a cytoplasmic protein which can translocate to the nucleus depending upon the cell cycle stage and cellular stress [2, 26]. To study the effect of cellular stress on localisation of SIRT2, SH-SY5Y cells were treated with diquat or rotenone to induce the stress and the localisation of SIRT2 was determined using immunocytochemistry and microscopy. On treatment with diquat or rotenone, SIRT2 was localised both in the nucleus and in the cytoplasm but was present prominently in the nucleus (see supplementary Figure 3). The localisation of SIRT2 in the nucleus under toxin induced oxidative stress could be attributed to the role played

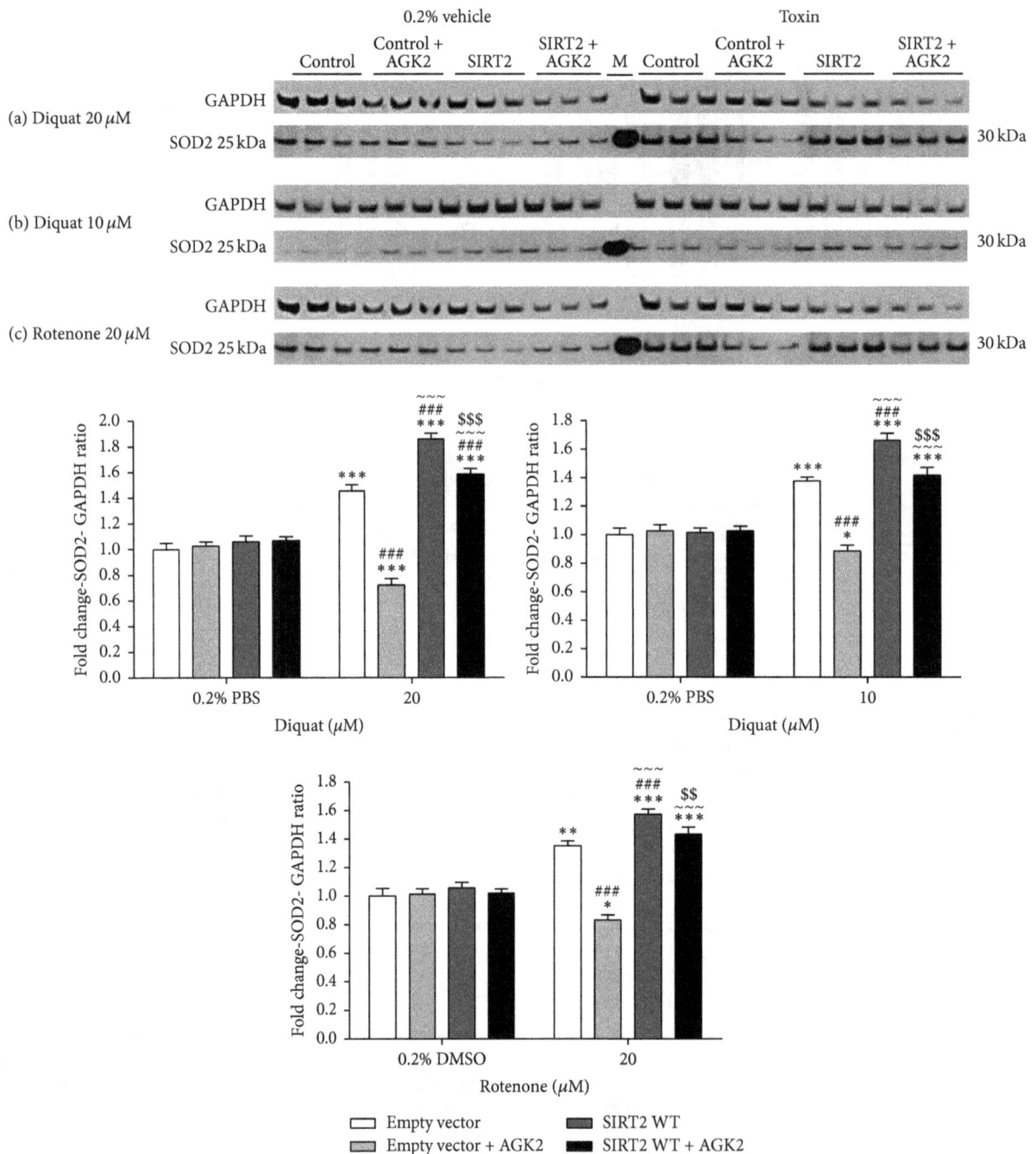

FIGURE 2: Expression of SOD2 was measured in toxin treated SH-SY5Y cells. SIRT2 was overexpressed in SH-SY5Y cells and control cells were transfected with empty vector following which one set of cells was treated with toxin alone and another with SIRT2 inhibitor AGK2 and toxin. Cells were harvested and the samples were probed for SOD2 expression. Data presented as fold-untreated (0.2% vehicle) (±SD) from three independent assays ($n = 3$). ***$p < 0.001$, **$p < 0.01$, and *$p < 0.05$ when compared to 0.2% vehicle, one-way ANOVA (Bonferroni corrected), ###$p < 0.001$ when compared to control cells, ~~~$p < 0.001$ when compared to control + AGK2 treatment, and $$$$p < 0.001$ and $$$p < 0.01$ when compared to SIRT2, two-way ANOVA (Bonferroni corrected). M indicates molecular weight marker lane.

by SIRT2 in DNA damage repair and cell cycle regulation under normal circumstances and as well as under genotoxic stress [27, 28] (Figures 3 and 4).

3.1.4. Inhibition of SIRT2 Enhanced α-Synuclein Aggregate Formation. PD involves the progressive loss of DA neurones in

the SN and the presence of LB rich in α-synuclein [10, 29]. The α-synuclein aggregates in LB are generally formed because of the association of misfolded α-synuclein proteins and the levels of misfolded proteins can increase under several conditions such as oxidative stress [30], inhibition of protein degradation [31], or mitochondrial dysfunction [32]. SIRT2

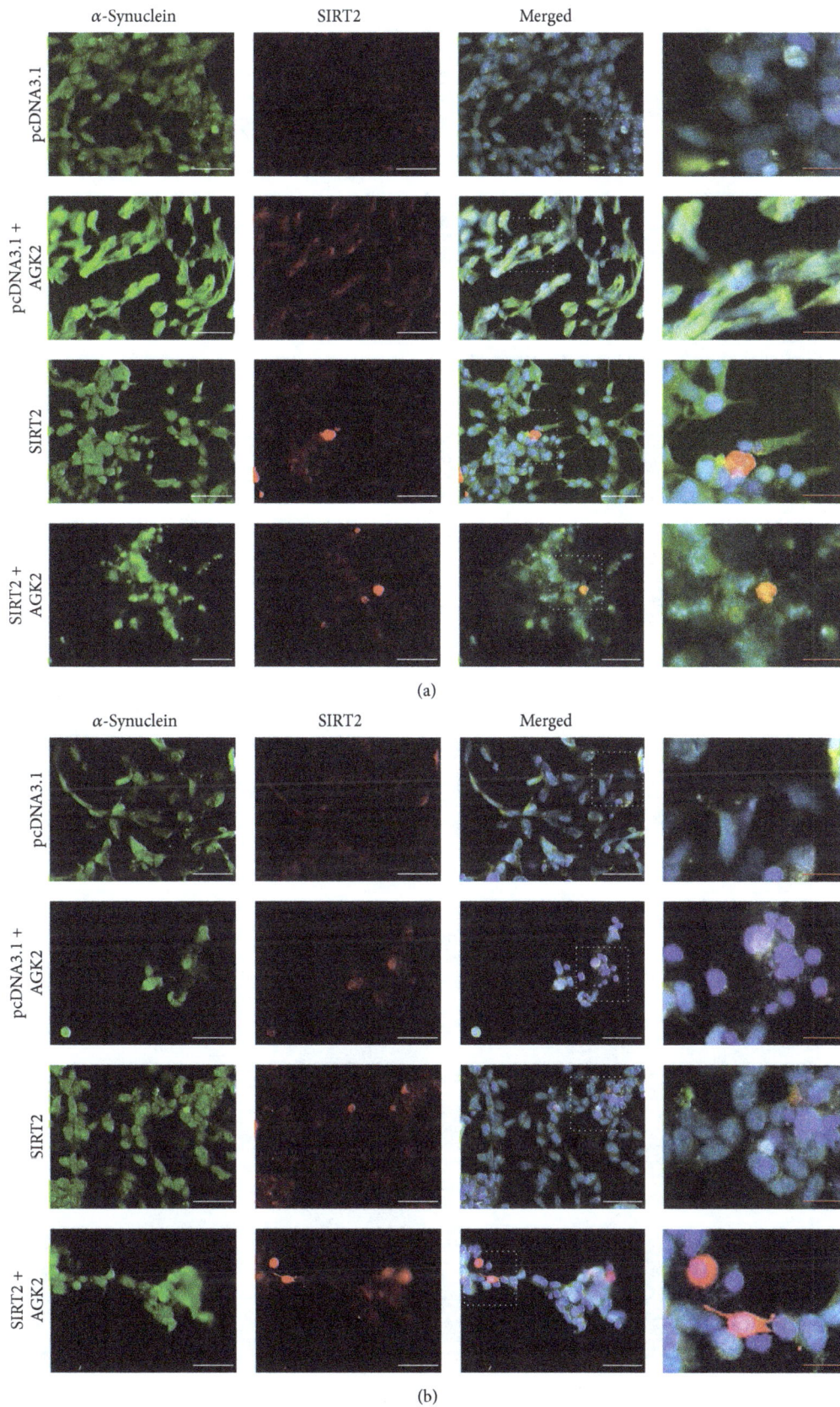

FIGURE 3: Localisation of SIRT2 and α-synuclein in diquat treated SH-SY5Y cells. Cellular distribution of SIRT2 and phospho-α-synuclein was determined using fluorescent immunocytochemistry. Images show α-synuclein immunostaining, SIRT2 immunostaining, and all staining merged including DAPI in 20 μM diquat treated cells. Scale bars, white scale bar = 50 μM and red scale bar = 20 μM; magnification: 40x. (a) represents 0.2% PBS and (b) represents 20 μM diquat treated SH-SY5Y cells.

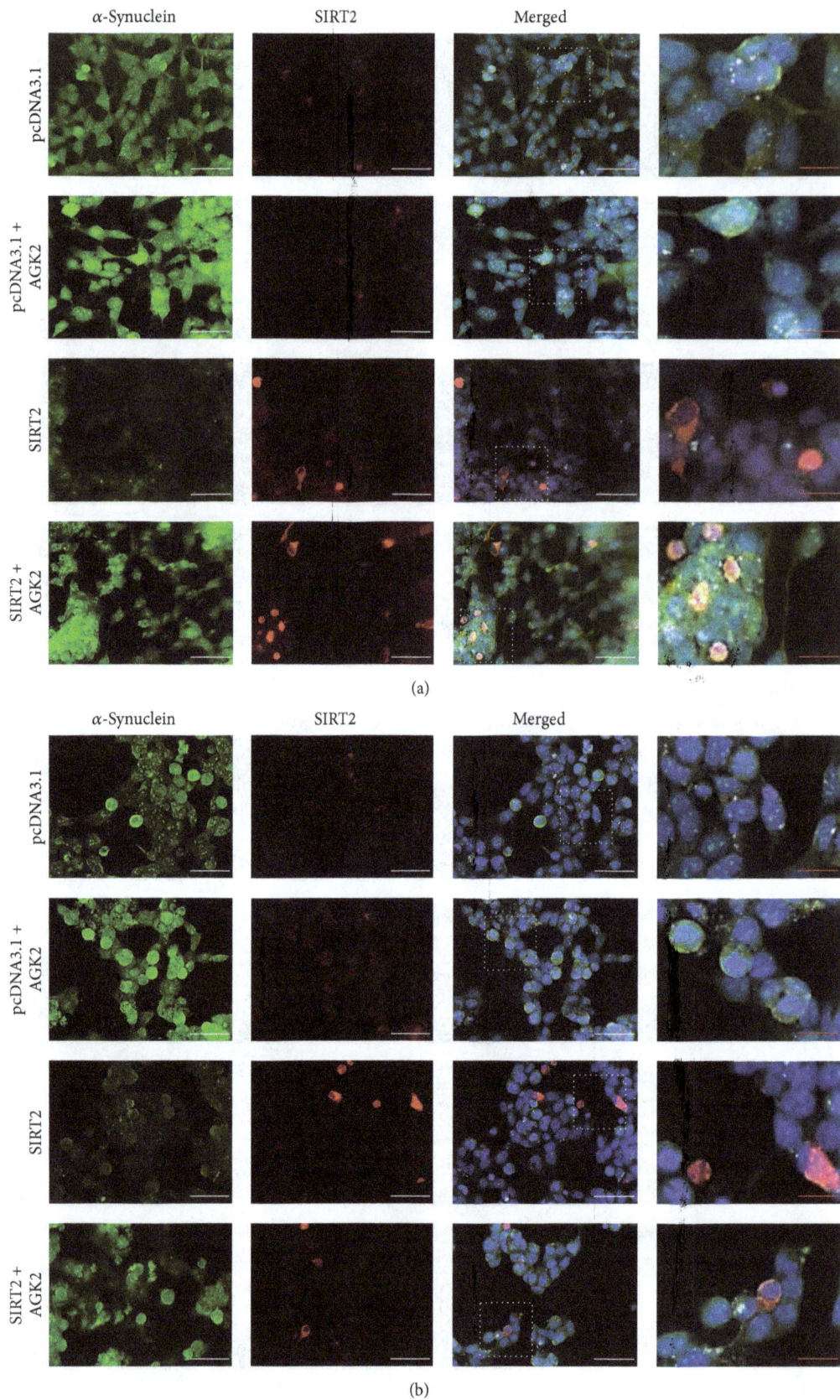

FIGURE 4: Localisation of SIRT2 and α-synuclein in rotenone treated SH-SY5Y cells. Cellular distribution of SIRT2 and phospho-α-synuclein was determined using fluorescent immunocytochemistry. Images show α-synuclein immunostaining, SIRT2 immunostaining, and all staining merged including DAPI in 20 μM rotenone treated cells. Scale bars, white scale bar = 50 μM and red scale bar = 20 μM; magnification: 40x. (a) represents 0.2% DMSO and (b) represents 20 μM rotenone treated SH-SY5Y cells.

showed minimal colocalisation with α-synuclein suggesting that SIRT2 may not physically interact with α-synuclein (Figures 3 and 4). The minimal proportion of colocalisation may potentially be attributed to the interaction of both SIRT2 and α-synuclein with α-tubulin [33, 34]. The effect of SIRT2 on α-synuclein aggregate formation was determined in toxin and AGK2 treated SH-SY5Y cells. In diquat treated cells, a significant increase in aggregate formation was seen in AGK2 treated control cells when compared to 0.2% PBS treated control cells ($p < 0.001$). In SIRT2 + AGK2 cells, aggregate formation was higher than control ($p < 0.01$) and SIRT2 cells ($p < 0.001$) but was significantly lower than control + AGK2 ($p < 0.001$) cells when treated with 20 μM diquat. Overexpression of SIRT2 inhibited α-synuclein aggregate formation in 20 μM diquat treated cells compared to control cells ($p < 0.001$; <23%). In rotenone treated cells, AGK2 treated control ($p < 0.001$) and SIRT2 ($p < 0.001$) cells showed increased aggregate formation in all treatments with SIRT2 overexpression causing reduced aggregate formation ($p < 0.001$) (Figure 5).

3.1.5. SIRT2 Protein in Neurodegeneration. In the frontal cortex of PD cases, SIRT2.3 and SIRT2.2 isoforms were detected but not isoforms 1 and 4. Levels of SIRT2 were elevated, SIRT2.3 by 25% ($p < 0.05$) and SIRT2.2 by 30% ($p < 0.01$). In the temporal cortex, no significant difference was observed in the expression of either isoforms of SIRT2 between control and PD cases ($p > 0.05$). In the putamen, there was no observable difference in the level of SIRT2.3 whereas a reduction of 23% in the expression of SIRT2.2 was observed in PD but the difference was not statistically significant ($p > 0.05$). Western blot analysis of SIRT2 detected only SIRT2.2 in the cerebellum and an increase of 57% was noticed in PD compared to controls ($p < 0.001$) (Figure 6).

In PDD, the levels of SIRT2 isoforms in the frontal cortex were not changed when compared to controls. In the temporal cortex, the levels of SIRT2.3 were reduced by 23% ($p < 0.01$) and a nonsignificant reduction of 16% was seen in SIRT2.2 levels ($p > 0.05$). In the putamen, no significant change in the levels of isoforms of SIRT2 in PDD compared to controls was observed ($p > 0.05$). Similar to PD, only SIRT2.2 was detected in cerebellar samples of PDD and no significant difference in the levels of SIRT2 was observed between PDD and control ($p > 0.05$) (Figure 7).

In DLB frontal cortex samples, no significant difference was found in the levels of SIRT2 isoforms when compared to controls. In the temporal cortex of DLB patients, the levels of both the isoforms of SIRT2 were elevated, SIRT2.3 by 24% ($p < 0.05$) and SIRT2.2 by 33% ($p < 0.01$). The level of SIRT2.3 was significantly reduced in the putamen of DLB by 13% ($p < 0.05$) but no significant difference was observed in the level SIRT2.2. The levels of SIRT2.2 in hippocampal samples of DLB were not significantly changed and in cerebellar samples of DLB, the levels of SIRT2.2 showed an increase of 25% ($p < 0.01$) compared to control (Figure 8).

In AD frontal cortex samples, no significant difference was observed in the levels of either isoforms of SIRT2

compared to controls. Similarly, no significant differences were observed in the levels of SIRT2 isoforms in the temporal cortex. The levels of SIRT2.2 in hippocampal samples were marginally reduced by 14% compared to controls but not significantly ($p > 0.05$). An increase of 14% was seen in the levels of SIRT2.2 in the cerebellum of AD compared to controls ($p < 0.05$) (Figure 9).

3.1.6. SIRT2 Activity in Neurodegeneration. In the frontal cortex, measurement of total SIRT activity did not show any significant change between the disease groups and controls ($p > 0.05$); however, compared to AD, the total SIRT activity was reduced in PD and DLB by about 20% ($p < 0.01$) (though PDD did not show any significant difference). SIRT2 activity was upregulated in PD (33%; $p < 0.001$), PDD (28%; $p < 0.05$), DLB (29%; $p < 0.01$), and AD (31%; $p < 0.01$) compared to controls ($F = 5.906$, $p < 0.001$). In the temporal cortex, there was no significant difference in total SIRT activity between the disease groups and control ($p > 0.05$); however, compared to AD there was a significant reduction of 33% in total SIRT activity in PDD ($p < 0.05$), though other groups did not show any significant change. SIRT2 activity was upregulated in PD (19%; $p < 0.01$), PDD (17%; $p < 0.05$), DLB (21%; $p < 0.001$), and AD (18%; $p < 0.01$) compared to controls whereas no significant difference was seen among the disease groups ($F = 5.593$; $p < 0.001$) (Figure 10).

3.1.7. Cellular Location of SIRT2 in Human Brain. The cellular localisation of SIRT2 was determined in the temporal cortex, hippocampus, and cerebellum in PD, PDD, DLB, AD, and an age matched control group. SIRT2 staining was weak and localised predominantly in the cytoplasm and nucleus of large pyramidal neurones in these groups whereas, in AD, SIRT2 was predominantly localised in pyramidal neurone cytoplasm. Staining was also apparent in the neuropil in all cases tested. In the temporal cortex, no apparent difference was observed within PD, PDD, DLB, and controls (Figure 11; Supplementary Figure 6). SIRT2 did not show a staining pattern that appeared to show cortical LB. These results suggest that there was no significant effect of disease conditions on the location of SIRT2 within the cell. The location of SIRT2 in different brain regions is summarised in Table 3 in supplementary files and the location of SIRT2 in other brain regions is shown in Figure 6 of supplementary files.

4. Discussion

Oxidative stress is a common general mechanism involved in cell death associated with neurodegenerative disorders [35] and has been implicated in the initiation and progression of PD [36]. Studies have reported that inhibition of SIRT2 reduces α-synuclein mediated toxicity in PD models and SIRT2 inhibition also rescued cells from mutant HTT in HD models [12, 37]. In contrast, the findings from this study suggest that reduced SIRT2 activity increased cell death following oxidative stress and increasing SIRT2 protects SH-SY5Y cells and is in agreement with other studies on SIRT2 [14, 17]. As with other SIRTs, SIRT2 is NAD$^+$ dependent

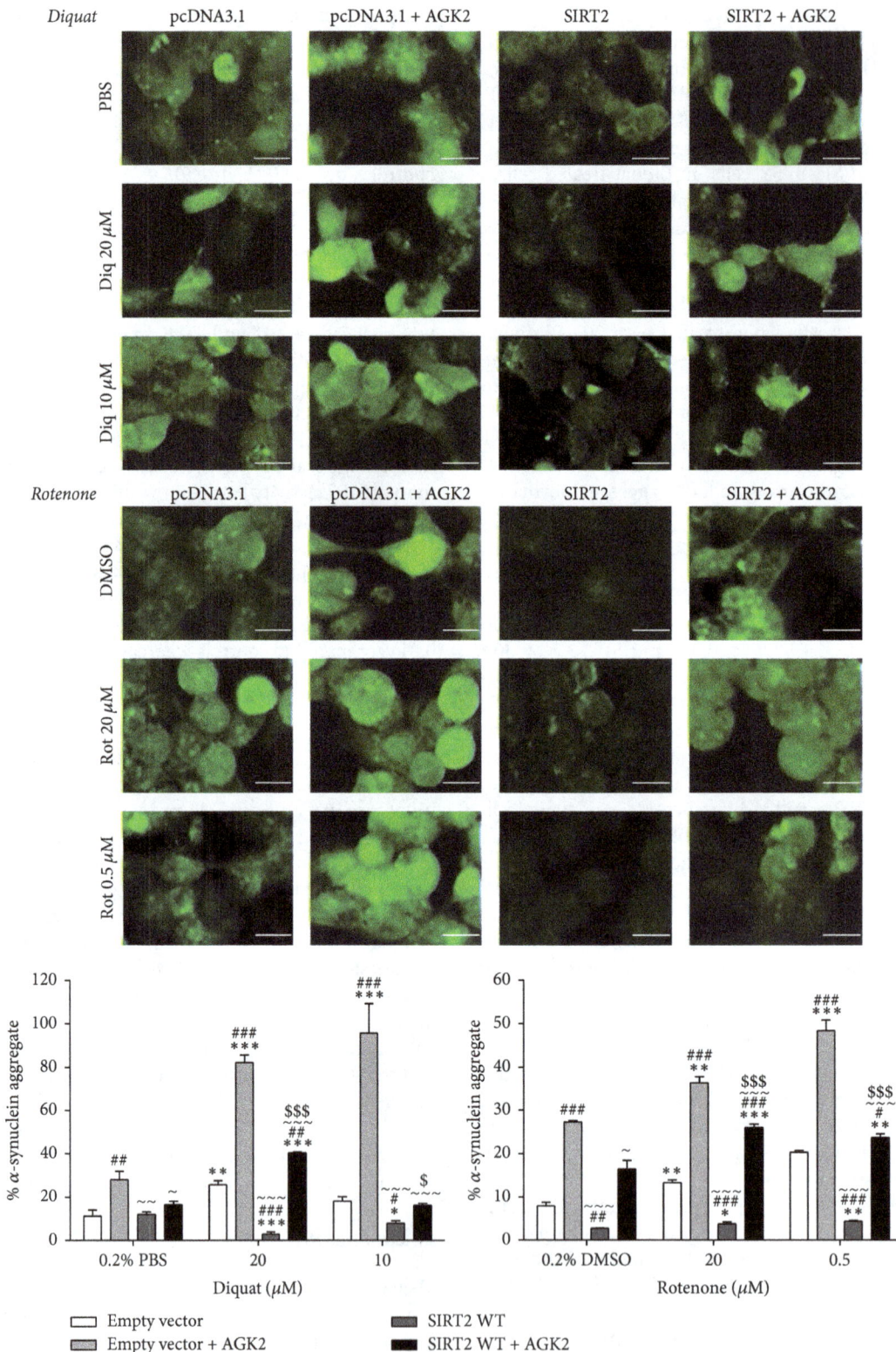

FIGURE 5: α-Synuclein aggregate formation and quantification in toxin treated SH-SY5Y cells. SIRT2 overexpressing SH-SY5Y cells were treated with toxin (20 μM or 10 μM diquat or 20 μM or 0.5 μM rotenone) and 0.2% PBS or DMSO; cells transfected with empty vector were used as a control and another set of SIRT2 and control cells was coincubated with AGK2 and toxin. Cells were immunostained with phospho-α-synuclein. Images were captured through GFP filter under 63x magnification. The captured images represent α-synuclein staining and the bar graphs represent the aggregate quantification in diquat or rotenone treated cells. Each bar represents %α-synuclein aggregates (±SD) from three independent assays ($n = 3$). $^{***}p < 0.001$, $^{**}p < 0.01$, and $^*p < 0.05$ when compared to 0.2% vehicle, one-way ANOVA (Bonferroni corrected), $^{###}p < 0.001$, $^{##}p < 0.01$, and $^#p < 0.05$ when compared to control cells, $^{\sim\sim\sim}p < 0.001$, $^{\sim\sim}p < 0.01$, and $^\sim p < 0.05$ when compared to control + AGK2 treatment, and $^{\$\$\$}p < 0.001$ and $^\$p < 0.05$ when compared to SIRT2 cells, two-way ANOVA (Bonferroni corrected). Scale bar: 20 μM.

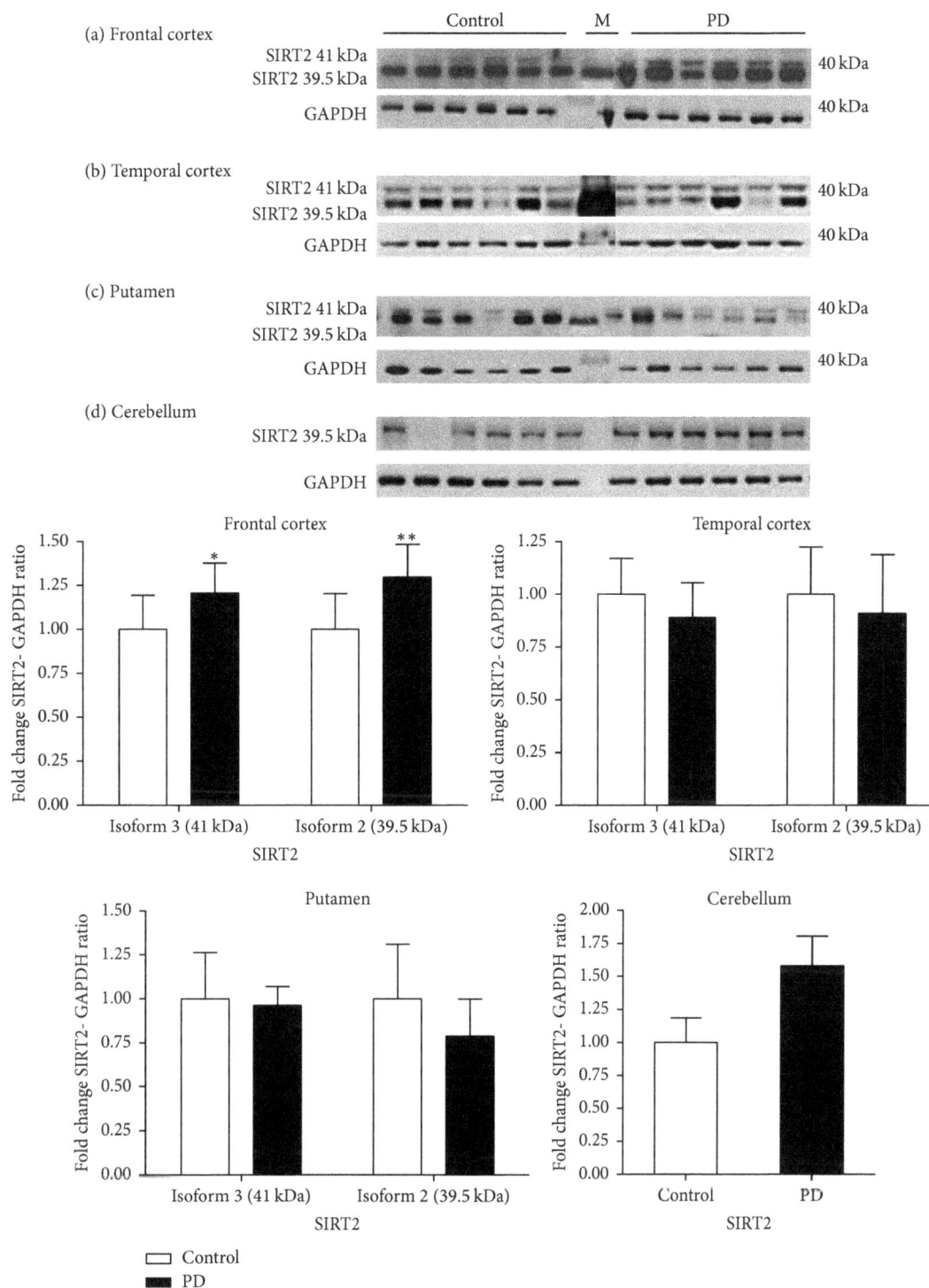

FIGURE 6: Expression of SIRT2 in different brain regions in Parkinson's disease. The levels of SIRT2 were determined in different regions of PD patients and were compared to a control-cohort. SIRT2 band intensity was normalised with GAPDH. Data are presented as fold change ($\pm$SD) with respect to control from three independent replicates. $^{**}p < 0.01$, and $^{*}p < 0.05$ when compared to control; statistical analysis was done through t-test performed on GraphPad prism. Images are representative blots of SIRT2 and GAPDH. M indicates molecular weight markers lane.

and is a potential redox sensor and studies have shown that SIRT2 enhances cell viability under oxidative stress and inhibition or knock-down of SIRT2 decreases intracellular ATP levels and enhances cell death. SIRT2 can regulate oxidative stress by deacetylating FOXO3a and increasing expression of FOXO3a targets, namely, p27^{Kip1} and SOD2, and under severe oxidative stress SIRT2 enhances the expression of the proapoptotic protein Bim [25]. Consequently, through

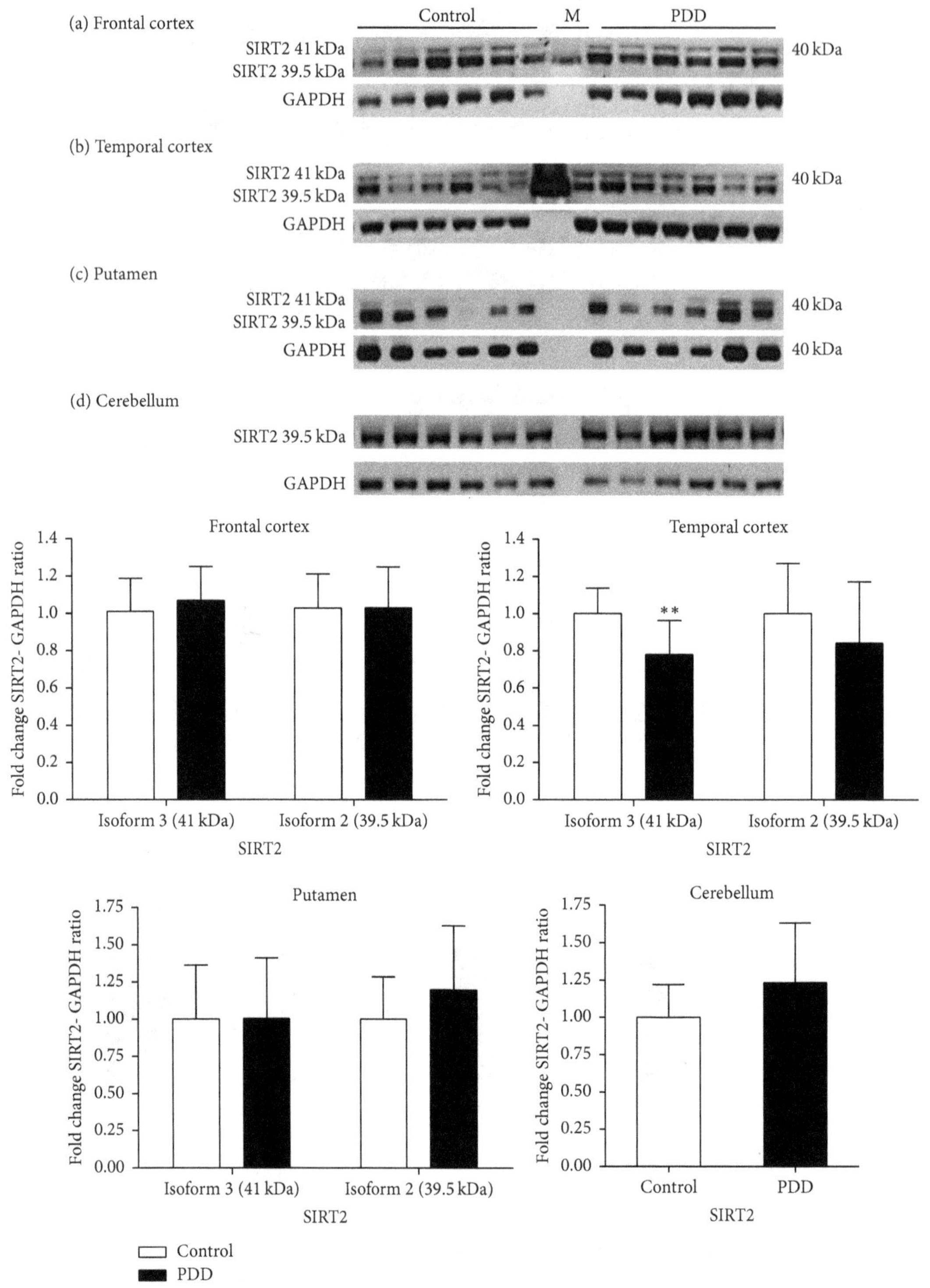

FIGURE 7: Expression of SIRT2 in different regions in Parkinson's disease with Dementia. The levels of SIRT2 were determined in different regions of PDD patients and were compared to a control-cohort. SIRT2 band intensity was normalised with GAPDH. Data are presented as fold change (±SD) with respect to control from three independent replicates. $^{**}p < 0.01$ when compared to control; statistical analysis was done through t-test performed on GraphPad prism. Images are representative blots of SIRT2 and GAPDH. M indicates molecular weight marker lane.

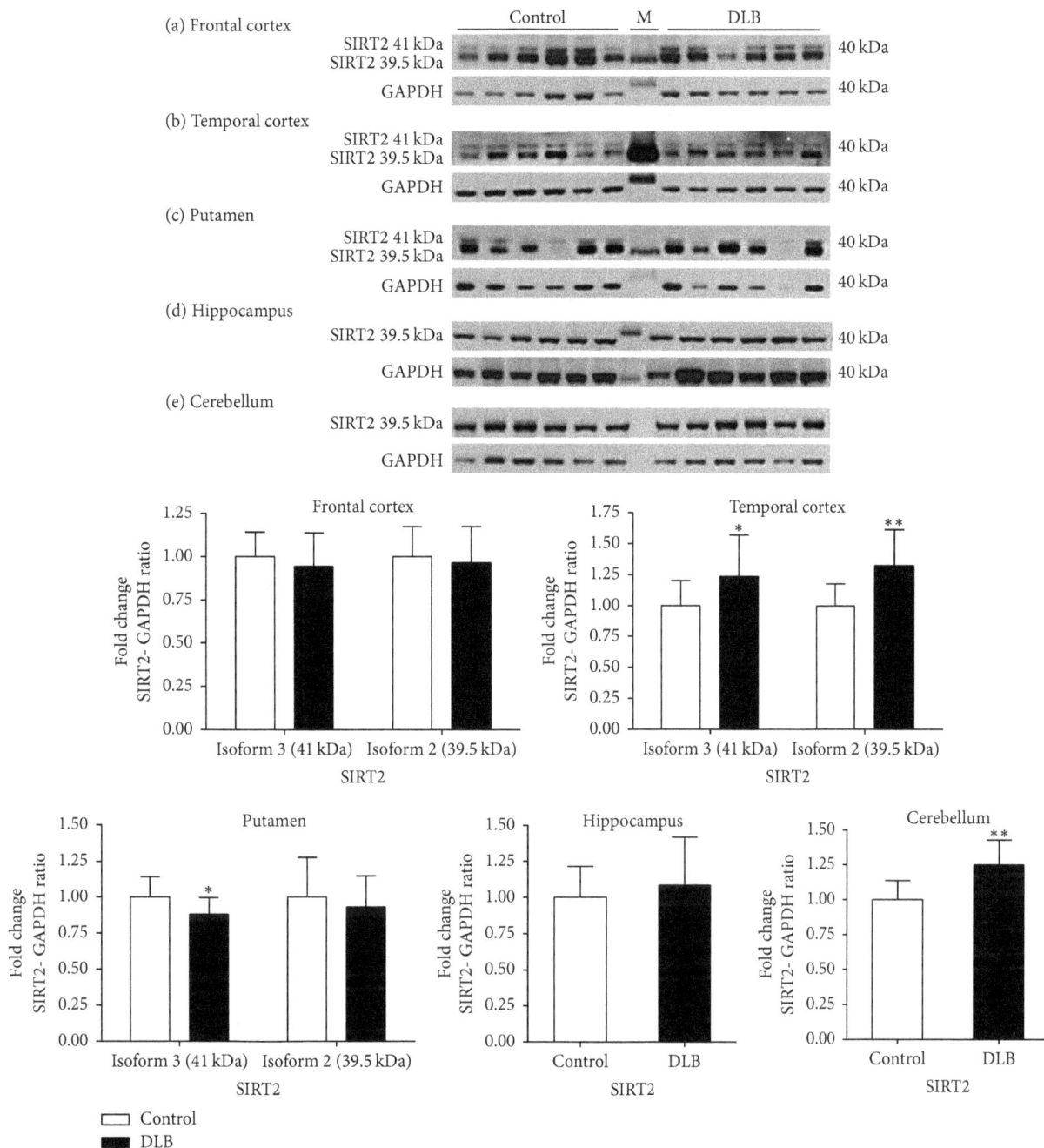

FIGURE 8: Expression of SIRT2 in different brain regions in dementia with Lewy Bodies. The levels of SIRT2 were determined in different regions of DLB patients and were compared to a control-cohort. SIRT2 band intensity was normalised with GAPDH. Data are presented as fold change ($\pm$SD) with respect to control from three independent replicates. $^{**}p < 0.01$, and $^{*}p < 0.05$ when compared to control; statistical analysis was done through t-test performed on GraphPad prism. Images are representative blots of SIRT2 and GAPDH. M indicates molecular weight marker lane.

p27^{Kip1}, SIRT2 promotes cell cycle arrest and reduces the amount of ROS via SOD2 [25]. In this study, the enhanced expression of SOD2 potentially via FOXO3a following SIRT2 overexpression may be one route by which SIRT2 confers cellular protection [25]. In PC12 cells, silencing or inhibition of SIRT2 by AGK2 led to decreased ATP levels and enhanced cell death via necrosis [14]. In contrast, Nie et al. showed that inhibition of SIRT2 rescued differentiated PC12 cells from

H$_2$O$_2$ induced toxicity and silencing of SIRT2 reduced the levels of ROS following H$_2$O$_2$ treatment [38]. These findings corroborate with results from this study and suggest that the associated upregulation of SOD2 and SIRT2 can regulate cell viability and combat oxidative stress.

Cellular stress subjects proteins to a variety of modifications which affect the stability, activity, and even the localisation of proteins [39]. In this study it was observed

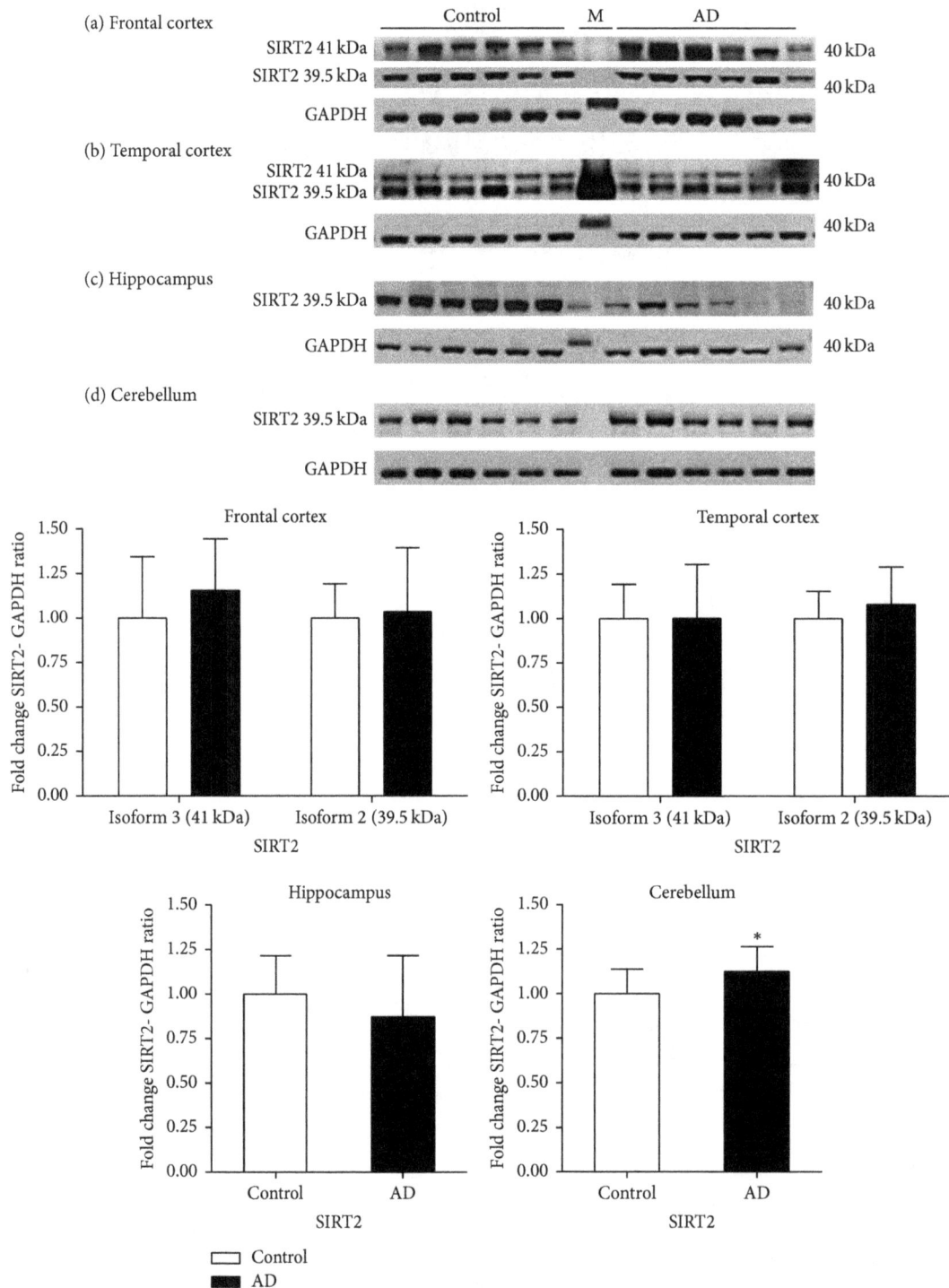

FIGURE 9: Expression of SIRT2 in different brain regions in Alzheimer's disease. The levels of SIRT2 were determined in different regions of AD patients and were compared to a control-cohort. SIRT2 band intensity was normalised with GAPDH. Data are presented as fold change (±SD) with respect to control from three independent replicates. $^*p < 0.05$ when compared to control; statistical analysis was done through t-test performed on GraphPad prism. Images are representative blots of SIRT2 and GAPDH. M indicates molecular weight marker's lane.

that under relatively high levels of oxidative stress (20 μM rotenone, 10 μM, or 20 μM diquat), SIRT2 was localised to the nucleus and cytoplasm but was prominently present in the nucleus. The absence of any effect of SIRT2 at low levels

of oxidative stress caused by 0.5 μM rotenone may be insufficient to cause major depletion of ATP and lead to activation of SIRT2 by dephosphorylation causing SIRT2 to translocate to the nucleus [7]. SIRT2 is normally a cytoplasmic protein

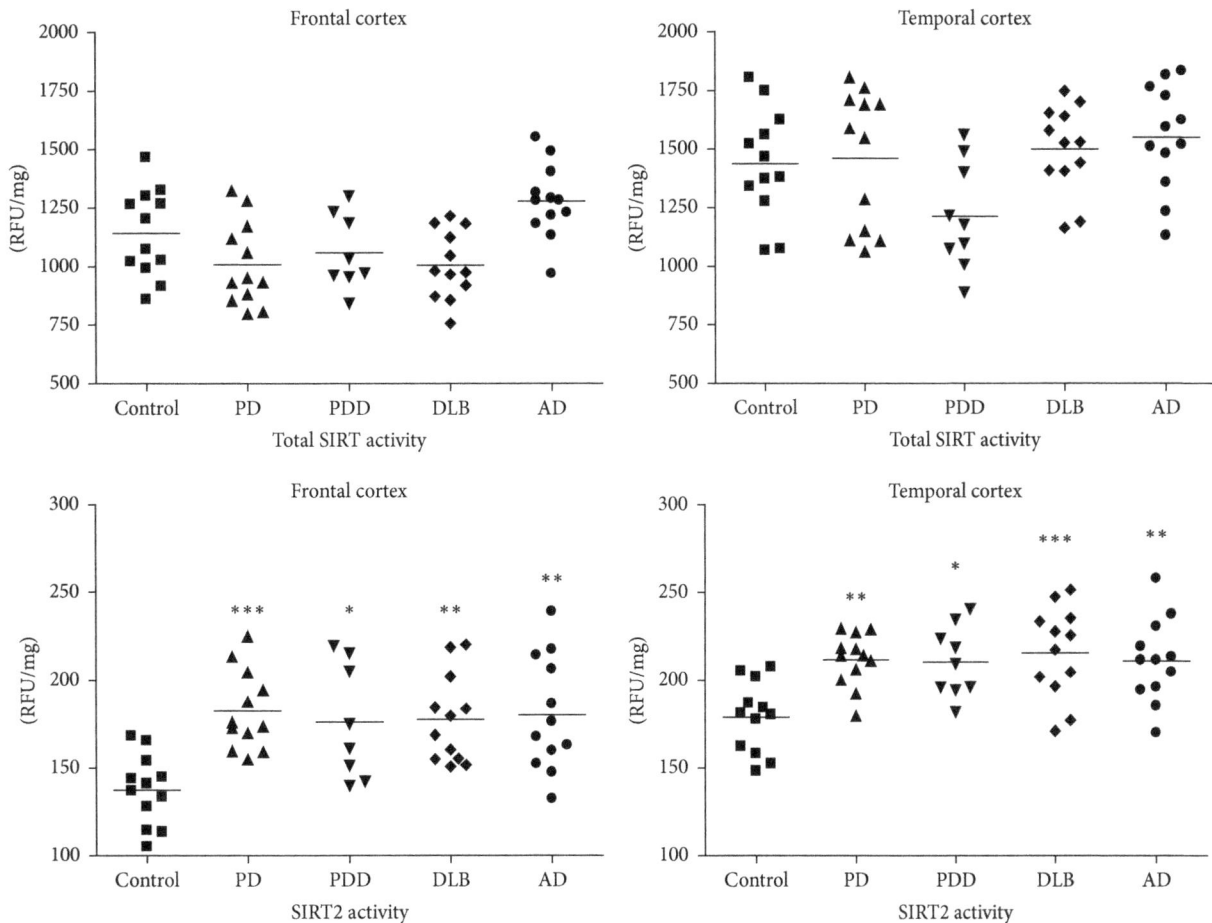

FIGURE 10: Total SIRT and SIRT2 activities in the frontal and temporal cortex in PD, PDD, DLB, AD, and controls. Total SIRT and SIRT2 activities were measured through a fluorometric enzymatic activity assay in the frontal and temporal cortices of PD, PDD, DLB, and AD patients and were compared to cohort-control group. $^{***}p < 0.001$, $^{**}p < 0.01$, and $^{*}p < 0.05$ when compared to control, one-way ANOVA (Bonferroni corrected).

but may shuttle to the nucleus based upon cell cycle stage and cellular stress [2, 26]. Under oxidative stress, the known target of SIRT2, FOXO3a, shuttles to the nucleus [40] and induces the expression of its target SOD2 and may directly activate SOD2 to counteract the effect of ROS [41]. The results from this study are consistent with previous studies that report that SIRT2 localises to the cell nucleus under stress. Our finding that there is no induction of SOD2 in cells overexpressing SIRT2 under basal conditions would indicate that, following transfer of SIRT2 to the nucleus during oxidative stress, SIRT2 may interact with nuclear transcription factors such as FOXO3a which may lead to the induced expression of protective proteins such as SOD2.

Given the role of α-synuclein aggregation in PD, we found that SIRT2 inhibition enhanced aggregate formation in diquat or rotenone treated cells with overexpression of SIRT2 reducing α-synuclein aggregate formation. This contrasts with previous studies which reported that SIRT2 inhibition rescues α-synuclein mediated toxicity [12]. This may be attributed to different treatment regimens with A53T mutant α-synuclein overexpression directly aggregating in cellular

and fly models whereas, in this study, α-synuclein aggregate formation was induced by oxidative stress. The results obtained from SH-SY5Y cells overexpressing SIRT2 under basal conditions, or from cells where SIRT2 is inhibited under basal conditions, suggest that SIRT2 does not promote de novo α-synuclein aggregate formation; rather SIRT2 impairs the formation of new or larger α-synuclein aggregates. Viability assays also corroborate the finding that SIRT2 inhibition enhances cellular death and SIRT2 overexpression promotes cell survival. All these findings suggest that SIRT2 acts as a prosurvival factor under oxidative stress.

The ageing brain shows gene expression changes specifically in the levels of stress response genes, mitochondrial genes, and genes involved in synaptic function [42]. SIRT2 plays a crucial role in antioxidant defence mechanisms [25] and in DNA damage repair [43] and elevated levels of oxidative stress and DNA damage are observed in neurodegenerative disorders such as PD and AD. In this study, the levels of SIRT2 protein did not show major or consistent changes in the disease groups compared to controls, although a tendency towards elevation in the levels

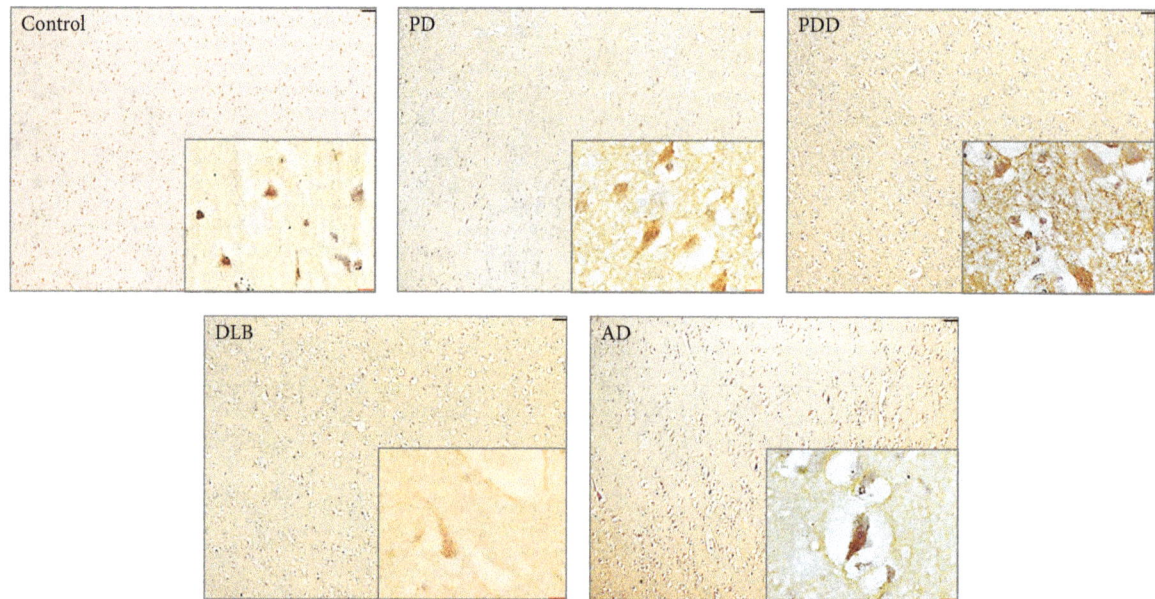

FIGURE 11: Cellular distribution of SIRT2 in the temporal cortex of disease and control groups. The images show the cellular localisation of SIRT2 in grey matter of superior temporal gyrus of temporal cortex in PD, PDD, DLB, AD, and control cases. SIRT2 was localised in both in the cytoplasm and the nucleus of the neurones in the groups, being predominantly present in the cytoplasm in AD. The picture in inset is 63x oil immersion image overlaid on 10x image. Scale bars, black scale bar = 50 μM and red scale bar = 20 μM.

of SIRT2 was observed overall. Maxwell et al. showed that SIRT2 accumulates in the ageing brain [3] and this may possibly explain why major changes were not observed in SIRT2 levels in disease groups, with age related changes masking disease related changes. While protein levels of SIRT2 were essentially unchanged, enzymatic activity for SIRT2 showed SIRT2 activity was higher in disease groups than control but no significant difference was observed between neurodegenerative disorders. The current results in induced oxidative stress in SH-SY5Y cells show SIRT2 overexpression promotes cell survival and inhibits α-synuclein aggregate formation. It is possible that elevated SIRT2 activity in neurodegenerative disorders is a compensatory mechanism to counteract the effects of oxidative stress occurring due to ageing and disease processes. SIRT1 has been shown to be neuroprotective in different neurodegenerative disorders and we found that SIRT1 activity was remarkably reduced in disease groups (unpublished data) although the total SIRT activity did not differ among the groups. SIRT1 and SIRT2 have been observed to share some targets including p53, NF-κB, histones H3, and H4 and following down-regulation of SIRT1 activity it is safe to assume that SIRT2 activity is elevated to target specific proteins such as p53 and modulate apoptosis, neuroinflammation, and genomic stability. Also, in relation to the in vitro work, it is possible that SIRT2 is upregulated in order to induce the activity of antioxidant proteins including SOD2 and catalase. Combining the in vitro and postmortem human tissue studies it is possible that SIRT2 is required to combat oxidative stress and higher SIRT2 activity in human brain tissue is a compensatory mechanism. The cellular localisation of SIRT2 showed no significant difference within the disease groups and controls. Generally, the

sections showed SIRT2 localisation to the cytoplasm but also nuclei of neurones, which may relate to the translocation of SIRT2 to the nucleus under stress, corroborating the cellular work. Future work with additional SIRT2 antibodies would be needed to determine the location of SIRT2 along with dual-immunostaining for known neurodegenerative disease biomarkers. The role of SIRT2 should be further investigated under chronic oxidative stress in additional neuronal models of PD.

5. Conclusion

In this study we have shown that, in SH-SY5Y cells, under diquat or rotenone induced oxidative stress, SIRT2 overexpression protected cells from oxidative damage and reduced α-synuclein aggregate formation. Also, the inhibition of SIRT2 by AGK2 under oxidative stress, elevated cell death and promoted α-synuclein aggregate formation. These findings suggest that SIRT2 promotes cell survival and may provide this protection through elevation of SOD2. In postmortem human brain tissue, SIRT2 protein expression did not differ between different disease groups (PD, PDD, DLB, and AD) and controls but the enzymatic activity of SIRT2 was higher in disease groups compared to controls. Based upon the findings from the in vitro work and postmortem brain tissue studies, elevated SIRT2 in neurodegenerative disorders could be a compensatory mechanism to combat oxidative stress.

Abbreviations

AD: Alzheimer's disease
DA: Dopamine
DLB: Dementia with Lewy bodies

DMSO: Dimethyl sulphoxide
FOXO: Forkhead box subgroup O
HD: Huntington disease
HDAC: Histone deacetylase
LB: Lewy bodies
NAD: Nicotinamide-adenine-dinucleotide
NAM: Nicotinamide
NF-κB: Nuclear factor kappa B
O_2^-: Superoxide anions
OL: Oligodendrocyte
PBS: Phosphate buffered saline
PD: Parkinson's disease
PDD: PD with dementia
PEI: Polyethylenimine
ROS: Reactive oxygen species
SIRT: Sirtuin
SN: Substantia nigra
SOD: Superoxide dismutase
TBS/T: Tris buffered saline/Tween
TSA: Trichostatin A.

Disclosure

The views expressed are those of the author(s) and not necessarily those of the NHS, the NIHR, or the Department of Health.

Authors' Contributions

Study concept and design were conceived by Preeti Singh, Peter S. Hanson, and Christopher M. Morris. Experimental work data collection, analysis, and interpretation were carried out by Preeti Singh. Preeti Singh drafted the manuscript with critical revisions from Peter S. Hanson and Christopher M. Morris. All authors read and approved the final manuscript.

Acknowledgments

The authors are grateful to the individuals and their families who kindly donated their tissue to the Newcastle Brain Tissue Resource. The research was funded by the National Institute for Health Research Newcastle Biomedical Research Unit and Biomedical Research Centre based at Newcastle Hospitals NHS Foundation Trust and Newcastle University. Tissue for this study was provided by the Newcastle Brain Tissue Resource, which is funded in part by a grant from the UK Medical Research Council (Grant no. G0400074) and by Brains for Dementia research, a joint venture between Alzheimer's Society and Alzheimer's Research UK.

References

[1] S. Perrod, M. M. Cockell, T. Laroche et al., "A cytosolic NAD-dependent deacetylase, Hst2p, can modulate nucleolar and telomeric silencing in yeast," *EMBO Journal*, vol. 20, no. 1-2, pp. 197–209, 2001.

[2] B. J. North and E. Verdin, "Interphase nucleo-cytoplasmic shuttling and localization of SIRT2 during mitosis," *PLoS ONE*, vol. 2, no. 8, article e784, 2007.

[3] M. M. Maxwell, E. M. Tomkinson, J. Nobles et al., "The Sirtuin 2 microtubule deacetylase is an abundant neuronal protein that accumulates in the aging CNS," *Human Molecular Genetics*, vol. 20, no. 20, pp. 3986–3996, 2011.

[4] W. Li, B. Zhang, J. Tang et al., "Sirtuin 2, a mammalian homolog of yeast silent information regulator-2 longevity regulator, is an oligodendroglial protein that decelerates cell differentiation through deacetylating α-tubulin," *The Journal of Neuroscience*, vol. 27, no. 10, pp. 2606–2616, 2007.

[5] H. Zhu, L. Zhao, E. Wang et al., "The QKI-PLP pathway controls SIRT2 abundance in CNS myelin," *Glia*, vol. 60, no. 1, pp. 69–82, 2012.

[6] B. Beirowski, J. Gustin, S. M. Armour et al., "Sir-two-homolog 2 (Sirt2) modulates peripheral myelination through polarity protein Par-3/atypical protein kinase C (aPKC) signaling," *Proceedings of the National Academy of Sciences of the United States of America*, vol. 108, no. 43, pp. E952–E961, 2011.

[7] R. Pandithage, R. Lilischkis, K. Harting et al., "The regulation of SIRT2 function by cyclin-dependent kinases affects cell motility," *Journal of Cell Biology*, vol. 180, no. 5, pp. 915–929, 2008.

[8] C. M. Tanner and S. M. Goldman, "Epidemiology of Parkinson's disease," *Neurologic Clinics*, vol. 14, no. 2, pp. 317–335, 1996.

[9] L. Bertram and R. E. Tanzi, "The genetic epidemiology of neuro-degenerative disease," *The Journal of Clinical Investigation*, vol. 115, no. 6, pp. 1449–1457, 2005.

[10] J. M. Beitz, "Parkinson's disease: a review," *Front Biosci (Schol Ed)*, vol. 6, pp. 65–74, 2014.

[11] J. Jankovic, "Parkinson's disease: Clinical features and diagnosis," *Journal of Neurology, Neurosurgery and Psychiatry*, vol. 79, no. 4, pp. 368–376, 2008.

[12] T. F. Outeiro, E. Kontopoulos, S. M. Altmann et al., "Sirtuin 2 inhibitors rescue α-synuclein-mediated toxicity in models of Parkinson's disease," *Science*, vol. 317, no. 5837, pp. 516–519, 2007.

[13] X. Wang, Q. Guan, M. Wang et al., "Aging-related rotenone-induced neurochemical and behavioral deficits: role of SIRT2 and redox imbalance, and neuroprotection by AK-7," *Drug Design, Development and Therapy*, vol. 9, pp. 2553–2563, 2015.

[14] H. Nie, H. Chen, J. Han et al., "Silencing of SIRT2 induces cell death and a decrease in the intracellular ATP level of PC12 cells," *International Journal of Physiology, Pathophysiology and Pharmacology*, vol. 3, no. 1, pp. 65–70, 2011.

[15] T. F. Pais, É. M. Szegő, O. Marques et al., "The NAD-dependent deacetylase sirtuin 2 is a suppressor of microglial activation and brain inflammation," *EMBO Journal*, vol. 32, no. 19, pp. 2603–2616, 2013.

[16] H. Nie, Y. Li, C. Wang et al., "SIRT2 plays a key role in both cell cycle regulation and cell survival of BV2 microglia," *International Journal of Physiology, Pathophysiology and Pharmacology*, vol. 6, no. 3, pp. 166–171, 2014.

[17] V. P. Patel and C. T. Chu, "Decreased SIRT2 activity leads to altered microtubule dynamics in oxidatively-stressed neuronal cells: Implications for Parkinson's disease," *Experimental Neurology*, vol. 257, pp. 170–181, 2014.

[18] A. Bobrowska, G. Donmez, A. Weiss, L. Guarente, and G. Bates, "SIRT2 ablation has no effect on tubulin acetylation in brain, cholesterol biosynthesis or the progression of huntington's disease phenotypes *in vivo*," *PLoS ONE*, vol. 7, no. 4, Article ID e34805, 2012.

[19] J. T. Greenamyre, J. R. Cannon, R. Drolet, and P.-G. Mastroberardino, "Lessons from the rotenone model of Parkinson's disease," *Trends in Pharmacological Sciences*, vol. 31, no. 4, pp. 141-142, 2010.

[20] R. Nisar et al., "Diquat causes caspase-independent cell death in SH-SY5Y cells by production of ROS independently of mitochondria," *Archives of Toxicology*, vol. 89, no. 10, pp. 1811–1825, 2015.

[21] M. M. Bradford, "A rapid and sensitive method for the quantitation of microgram quantities of protein utilizing the principle of protein dye binding," *Analytical Biochemistry*, vol. 72, no. 1-2, pp. 248–254, 1976.

[22] R. Betarbet, T. B. Sherer, G. MacKenzie, M. Garcia-Osuna, A. V. Panov, and J. T. Greenamyre, "Chronic systemic pesticide exposure reproduces features of Parkinson's disease," *Nature Neuroscience*, vol. 3, no. 12, pp. 1301–1306, 2000.

[23] J. M. Rawlings, I. Wyatt, and J. R. Heylings, "Evidence for redox cycling of diquat in rat small intestine," *Biochemical Pharmacology*, vol. 47, no. 7, pp. 1271–1274, 1994.

[24] G. M. Jones and J. A. Vale, "Mechanisms of toxicity, clinical features, and management of diquat poisoning: a review," *Journal of Toxicology—Clinical Toxicology*, vol. 38, no. 2, pp. 123–128, 2000.

[25] F. Wang, M. Nguyen, F. X. Qin, and Q. Tong, "SIRT2 deacetylates FOXO3a in response to oxidative stress and caloric restriction," *Aging Cell*, vol. 6, no. 4, pp. 505–514, 2007.

[26] L. Serrano, P. Martínez-Redondo, A. Marazuela-Duque et al., "The tumor suppressor SirT2 regulates cell cycle progression and genome stability by modulating the mitotic deposition of H4K20 methylation," *Genes and Development*, vol. 27, no. 6, pp. 639–653, 2013.

[27] R. K. Vempati, R. S. Jayani, D. Notani, A. Sengupta, S. Galande, and D. Haldar, "p300-mediated acetylation of histone H3 lysine 56 functions in DNA damage response in mammals," *Journal of Biological Chemistry*, vol. 285, no. 37, pp. 28553–28564, 2010.

[28] A. Vaquero, M. B. Scher, H. L. Dong et al., "SirT2 is a histone deacetylase with preference for histone H4 Lys 16 during mitosis," *Genes and Development*, vol. 20, no. 10, pp. 1256–1261, 2006.

[29] M. G. Spillantini, R. A. Crowther, R. Jakes, M. Hasegawa, and M. Goedert, "α-Synuclein in filamentous inclusions of Lewy bodies from Parkinson's disease and dementia with Lewy bodies," *Proceedings of the National Academy of Sciences of the United States of America*, vol. 95, no. 11, pp. 6469–6473, 1998.

[30] E. H. Norris, B. I. Giasson, H. Ischiropoulos, and V. M.-Y. Lee, "Effects of oxidative and nitrative challenges on α-synuclein fibrillogenesis involve distinct mechanisms of protein modifications," *Journal of Biological Chemistry*, vol. 278, no. 29, pp. 27230–27240, 2003.

[31] K. S. P. McNaught, C. Mytilin, R. JnoBaptiste et al., "Impairment of the ubiquitin-proteasome system causes dopaminergic cell death and inclusion body formation in ventral mesencephalic cultures," *Journal of Neurochemistry*, vol. 81, no. 2, pp. 301–306, 2002.

[32] S. Mullin and A. Schapira, "α-Synuclein and mitochondrial dysfunction in Parkinson's disease," *Molecular neurobiology*, vol. 47, no. 2, pp. 587–597, 2013.

[33] B. J. North, B. L. Marshall, M. T. Borra, J. M. Denu, and E. Verdin, "The human Sir2 ortholog, SIRT2, is an NAD^{+}-dependent tubulin deacetylase," *Molecular Cell*, vol. 11, no. 2, pp. 437–444, 2003.

[34] M. A. Alim, M. S. Hossain, K. Arima et al., "Tubulin seeds α-synuclein fibril formation," *Journal of Biological Chemistry*, vol. 277, no. 3, pp. 2112–2117, 2002.

[35] D. J. Betteridge, "What is oxidative stress?" *Metabolism*, vol. 49, no. 2 supplement 1, pp. 3–8, 2000.

[36] C. W. Olanow, "Oxidation reactions in Parkinson's disease," *Neurology*, vol. 40, no. 10 Supplement 3, pp. 37–39, 1190.

[37] R. Luthi-Carter, D. M. Taylor, J. Pallos et al., "SIRT2 inhibition achieves neuroprotection by decreasing sterol biosynthesis," *Proceedings of the National Academy of Sciences of the United States of America*, vol. 107, no. 17, pp. 7927–7932, 2010.

[38] H. Nie, Y. Hong, X. Lu et al., "SIRT2 mediates oxidative stress-induced apoptosis of differentiated PC12 cells," *NeuroReport*, vol. 25, no. 11, pp. 838–842, 2014.

[39] W. J. Welch, "Mammalian stress response: cell physiology, structure/function of stress proteins, and implications for medicine and disease," *Physiological Reviews*, vol. 72, no. 4, pp. 1063–1081, 1992.

[40] H. Huang and D. J. Tindall, "Dynamic FoxO transcription factors," *Journal of Cell Science*, vol. 120, no. 15, pp. 2479–2487, 2007.

[41] G. J. P. L. Kops, T. B. Dansen, P. E. Polderman et al., "Forkhead transcription factor FOXO3a protects quiescent cells from oxidative stress," *Nature*, vol. 419, no. 6904, pp. 316–321, 2002.

[42] B. A. Yankner, T. Lu, and P. Loerch, "The aging brain," *Annual Review of Pathology: Mechanisms of Disease*, vol. 3, pp. 41–66, 2008.

[43] K.-Y. Hsiao and C. A. Mizzen, "Histone H4 deacetylation facilitates 53BP1 DNA damage signaling and double-strand break repair," *Journal of Molecular Cell Biology*, vol. 5, no. 3, pp. 157–165, 2013.

5

Does Dopamine Depletion Trigger a Spreader Lexical-Semantic Activation in Parkinson's Disease? Evidence from a Study Based on Word Fluency Tasks

S. Zabberoni,[1,2] G. A. Carlesimo,[2,3] A. Peppe,[2] C. Caltagirone,[2,3] and A. Costa[1,2]

[1]Department of Psychology, Niccolò Cusano University, Rome, Italy
[2]IRCCS Fondazione Santa Lucia, Rome, Italy
[3]Department of Systems Medicine, Tor Vergata University, Rome, Italy

Correspondence should be addressed to S. Zabberoni; s.zabberoni@hsantalucia.it

Academic Editor: Elka Stefanova

It has been hypothesised that, in Parkinson's disease (PD), dopamine might modulate spreading activation of lexical-semantic representations. We aimed to investigate this hypothesis in individuals with PD without dementia by assessing word frequency and typicality in verbal fluency tasks. We predicted that the average values of both of these parameters would be lower in PD patients with respect to healthy controls (HC). We administered letter-cued and category-cued fluency tasks to early PD patients in two experimental conditions: the tasks were administered both after 12–18 hours of dopaminergic stimulation withdrawal ("OFF" condition) and after the first daily dose of dopaminergic therapy ("ON" condition). HC were also given the two tasks in two conditions with the same intersession delay as PD patients but without taking drugs. Results showed that in both OFF and ON treatment conditions PD patients did not differ from HC in word frequency or typicality. Moreover, in the PD group, no significant difference was found between the experimental conditions. Our results show that semantic spreading was not altered in the PD sample examined; this suggests that in early PD the functioning of the semantic system is relatively independent from the activity of dopamine brain networks.

1. Introduction

Parkinson's disease (PD) is frequently accompanied by cognitive deficits. These include dementia or mild cognitive impairment involving attention, executive functions, visual-spatial abilities, and episodic memory [1]. It has been reported that the functional and structural modifications that take place in the frontal-striatal and mesolimbic circuitries in PD are associated with these cognitive changes [2–4].

Increasing attention has been given to the functioning of the lexical-semantic system in PD. Some studies have documented reduced semantic priming in PD patients with respect to healthy controls; this suggests that these patients have delayed lexical/semantic activation [5, 6]. In this vein, there is evidence that PD patients' performance on priming tasks is affected significantly by dopamine withdrawal [7, 8]. In particular, in addition to confirming reduced priming

in PD patients when they were taking levodopa relative to healthy controls, Angwin et al. [8] also showed the lack of any priming effect when PD patients were assessed in the OFF condition. In agreement with previous studies conducted in healthy subjects [9–11], these findings underline the neuromodulatory role of dopamine within the semantic network [12] and also suggest that the speed of activation in PD patients is related to the extent of dopamine depletion [13].

According to the spreading activation theory, in the lexical-semantic network, the activation of individual nodes spreads to neighbouring concepts according to a variety of connections and nodes features [14]. In particular, the strength of association between nodes within the network might be modulated by the frequency of words. Hence, the activation of low frequency words would require greater spreading than the activation of high frequency words because the latter would have more and stronger links with other words in the network [15]. For this reason, in a word fluency task (in which subjects are required to generate as many words as possible according to some phonological or semantic constraints), healthy subjects typically produce more frequent words first. In PD patients, dopaminergic depletion could lead to an alteration of the structure of the lexical-semantic system with a reduced activation threshold difference between high and low frequency words as a manifestation of a spreader, less strategic, and seemingly random activation of the lexical units [8]. Accordingly, in a word fluency task, PD patients might generate words with lower frequency of use than healthy subjects. This issue was directly investigated in two studies which, however, reported inconsistent results. Indeed, Foster et al. [16] found that, in a phonological word fluency task, PD patients who were on dopaminergic treatment generated words with a significantly lower frequency of use compared to healthy controls. Conversely, Herrera et al. [17] found no direct effect of the manipulation of dopamine therapy on word use frequency in that PD patients produced words of comparable frequency irrespective of whether or not they were taking dopaminergic medication.

The aim of the present study was to further investigate lexical/semantic spreading activation in PD patients without dementia and its relationship to dopamine treatment. For this purpose, in addition to frequency of use computed on words generated in a letter-cued fluency task, we also assessed the typicality of the words produced in a category-cued fluency task. Indeed, the use of word typicality is underpinned by the assumption that each semantic category contains some words that are more representative than others [18]. Similar to what we discussed for high use frequency words, which should have a lower threshold of activation than low use frequency words, in a category-cued fluency task, words representing highly typical exemplars of a certain category should have a greater probability of being recalled than words representing less typical exemplars [18, 19]. To the best of our knowledge, the typicality index has never been used to investigate lexical-semantic spreading in PD patients.

Here we directly investigated the effect of dopaminergic stimulation on lexical-semantic activation in PD by contrasting the frequency of use and the typicality of words generated in fluency tasks in a sample of PD patients after withdrawal from (OFF condition) and after taking (ON condition) dopaminergic medication. Consistent with the assumption that dopamine has a significant neuromodulatory role in the strategic search and generation of words and, conversely, that dopamine depletion results in spreader, less strategic activation of units in the lexical-semantic system [16], we predicted that in the OFF condition PD patients would generate words with reduced frequency of use during the letter-cued fluency task and words less typical in the category-cued fluency task. Taking dopaminergic medication (on condition) should result in normalisation or, at the very least, in a significant increase in the average values of use frequency and typicality of the generated words.

2. Materials and Methods

2.1. Subjects. Twenty PD patients and 18 healthy controls (HC) were enrolled in the study after they gave their written informed consent. All of the patients included in the study were consecutive outpatients who had been referred by their primary care physician to the Parkinson's disease ambulatory care facilities of the IRCCS Santa Lucia Foundation in Rome. The diagnosis of idiopathic PD was made by a neurologist according to the London Brain Bank criteria [21]. Exclusion criteria for PD patients included (i) disease duration $\geq$ 5 years, (ii) diagnosis of dementia based on clinical criteria [22] and confirmed by a Mini-Mental State Examination [23] score < 26, and (iii) presence of other neurological and/or psychiatric illnesses in the patient's clinical history.

The HC participants were volunteers recruited from the patients' relatives. Exclusion criteria for the HC group included (i) cognitive impairment based on the Mini-Mental State Examination score < 26, (ii) taking medication that affects the central nervous system, and (iii) neurological and/or psychiatric illnesses, traumatic head injury, or substance abuse in the subject's history.

All PD patients were taking daily doses of dopamine or a dopamine agonist; in particular, seven patients were taking only L-Dopa, six patients were being treated with pramipexole or ropinirole only, and the remaining seven patients were taking both L-Dopa and dopamine agonists (i.e., pramipexole or ropinirole). All the patients presented bilateral akinetic-rigid form of PD and they were good and stable therapy responders. The clinical and demographic characteristics of the two experimental groups are reported in Table 1. L-Dopa equivalent doses are also reported for the patients' group.

Based on their performance on the tests included in the neuropsychological screening battery [24], 15 PD patients had only executive deficits, three patients had executive and episodic memory disorders, and the two remaining patients had visual-constructive apraxia.

2.2. Experimental Procedure

2.2.1. Tasks. PD patients and HC were given letter-cued (phonemic fluency) and category-cued (semantic fluency) tasks. The experimental procedures were administered by an expert neuropsychologist.

In the *letter-cued word fluency task*, the subject has to generate as many words as possible that begin with a specified letter in three different trials, each lasting 60 seconds. Two versions of the task were created. In one version, the letters to be used to generate words were "A," "F," and "S." In the other version, the letters to be used were "C," "E," and "L."

Word use frequency was computed for each generated word according to normative values in the COLFIS corpus of Italian words [25].

In the *category-cued word fluency task*, the subject has to say as many words as possible that belong to a specific taxonomic category in two different trials, each lasting 60 seconds. Also in this case, two versions of the task were created. In one version, the categories to be used in the two

TABLE 1: Average (SD) of anagraphic data of experimental samples and clinical features of patient's group.

	PD (n = 20)	HC (n = 18)	F (df)	p
Age	66.7 (7.6)	67.9 (5.6)	0.3 (1,37)	0.57
Years of education	11.1 (4.2)	12.4 (3.4)	1.0 (1,37)	0.31
MMSE (raw score)	26.5 (0.45)	29.4 (0.76)	5.6 (1,37)	0.23
H&Y (range) [20]	2.5–3	—	—	—
Disease duration	2.9 (1.9)	—	—	—
UPDRS "ON"	11.8 (4.3)	—	8.2 (1,19)	0.01
UPDRS "OFF"	16.3 (7.6)	—		
L-Dopa equivalents	352.1 (138.5)	—	—	—
Therapy duration (years)	1.7 (0.6)			

trials of the task were "Trees" and "Furniture" and in the second version "colours" and "animals."

The typicality value was computed for each word according to the category norms corpus for the Italian language [18].

The administration order of the two tasks was phonemic fluency followed by semantic fluency. At the beginning of each task, a training trial was given to be sure the subjects understood the instructions. Participants were told not to use proper nouns, not to use the same word with a different ending (e.g., *arancia, arancione, aranciata*), and not to conjugate verbs. In each trial, the number of legal words generated in 60 seconds was recorded. Accuracy in each task was the sum of the number of legal words generated in all trials.

In order to evaluate in more detail the pattern of words generated in the two fluency tasks (in particular, whether the participants in the two groups produced, as expected, more typical/frequent words first and less typical/frequent words later), in each subject, average word use frequency (for the letter-cued fluency task) and average typicality (for the category-cued fluency task) were computed separately for the first half and second half of the words produced in the different trials.

2.2.2. Design. PD patients were submitted to the experimental tasks after they had taken a full dose of stable dopaminergic treatment for one month. They were assessed in two experimental conditions that were performed on different days, with an intersession interval of about one month. In the "OFF" condition PD subjects performed the experimental tasks in the morning after 12/18 hours of drug withdrawal [26]. In the "ON" condition they were examined 90–120 minutes after they had taken their first morning dose of levodopa and/or dopamine agonists. To determine the efficacy of the dopamine compounds in improving extrapyramidal symptoms, in both treatment conditions, PD patients were given the UPDRS-Part III [27].

The tests of the experimental battery were administered to PD patients in both OFF and ON therapy conditions. By contrast, HC were given the tasks in two different sessions, named "blue" and "green," without any drug administration. The "blue" session was associated with the OFF condition and the "green" session with the ON condition. The order

of the experimental conditions (OFF/blue versus ON/green) was counterbalanced across subjects.

2.2.3. Statistical Analysis. Modification of the UPDRS in the PD group as a function of the treatment condition was analysed by means of a repeated measures ANOVA. The average number of words generated on the two fluency tasks was analysed by means of two-way mixed ANOVAs with Group (PD versus HCs) as between subjects variable and Treatment (ON versus OFF condition) as within subjects variable. Finally, data relative to use frequency and typicality of words generated in the letter and category word fluency tasks, respectively, were analysed by means of three-way ANOVAs with Group (PD versus HCs) as between subjects factor and Treatment (OFF/blue versus ON/green condition) and Half (first half versus second half of the generated words) as within subject factors.

3. Results

3.1. UPDRS. Confirming the beneficial effect of dopamine stimulation for extrapyramidal symptoms, the UPDRS scores of patients with PD decreased significantly (Table 1) passing from the OFF (M = 16.3; SD = 7.6) to the ON (M = 11.8; SD = 4.3) treatment condition ($F(1, 19) = 8.25$; $p = 0.01$).

3.2. Letter-Cued Word Fluency Task. The average number of words generated in the phonological word fluency task by PD patients and HC (Table 2) did not differ and it was not influenced by PD patients assuming medication as demonstrated by nonsignificant main effects of Group ($F(1, 36) = 1.70$; $p = 0.20$) and Treatment ($F(1, 36) = 0.25$; $p = 0.61$) and the Group × Treatment interaction ($F(1, 36) = .48$; $p = 0.49$).

The use frequency of words generated during the fluency task (Figure 1) also did not differ between groups and it was not influenced by dopamine stimulation. Indeed, only the main effect of Half was significant ($F(1, 36) = 8.83$; $p = 0.005$), but the main effects of Group ($F(1, 36) = 0.69$; $p = 0.40$) and Treatment ($F(1, 36) = 0.01$; $p = 0.93$) as well as all the interactions (all p consistently >0.40) were not.

TABLE 2: Average (SD) number of words generated by PD patients and HC in the letter-cued and category-cued fluency tasks. Note that PD patients performed the tasks in two distinct pharmacological conditions (ON versus OFF L-Dopa treatment), whereas HC took no drugs prior to either task session.

	Letter-cued		Category-cued	
	PD ($n = 20$)	HC ($n = 18$)	PD ($n = 20$)	HC ($n = 18$)
ON L-Dopa/green	26.7 (10.2)	31.2 (7.2)	21.9 (5.6)	21.6 (5.8)
OFF L-Dopa/blue	28.5 (10.7)	30.9 (8.6)	20.1 (8.3)	21.6 (4.5)

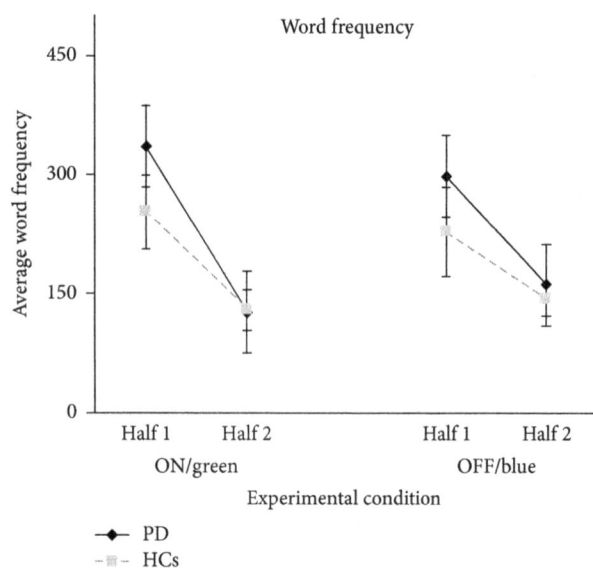

FIGURE 1: Average frequency of the words generated by PD and HC in both halves of trials of the phonemic fluency task, reported for both ON/green and OFF/blue experimental conditions.

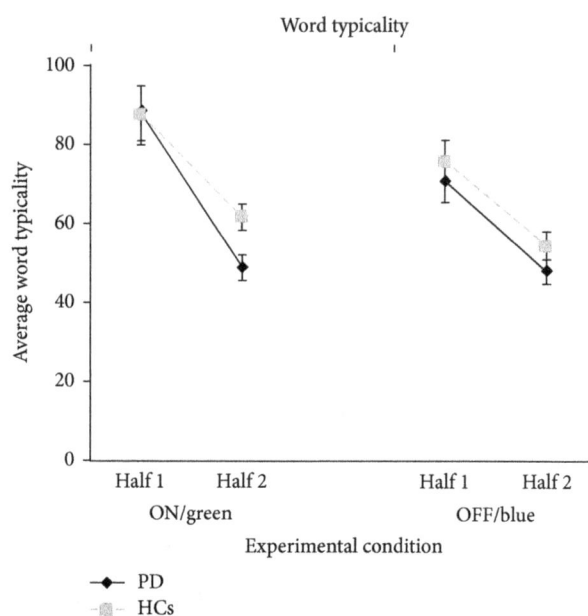

FIGURE 2: Average typicality of the words generated by PD and HC in both halves of trials of the semantic fluency task, reported for both ON/green and OFF/blue experimental conditions.

In all subjects, word use frequency was higher for the words generated in the first half of the trial (M = 280.7; SD= 669.0) than for those generated in the second half (M = 139.9; SD = 184.1). Moreover, planned comparisons documented that PD patients generated words with comparable use frequency while taking dopaminergic medication (M = 230.97; SD = 467.19) and during treatment withdrawal (M = 229.6; SD = 739.7; $F = .01$; $p = 0.97$; Cohen's $d = 0.002$) and that a comparable decrease in use frequency passing from the first half to the second half of the trial was observed in words generated while patients were in the ON (M = 209.5; SD = 578.4) and the OFF (M = 136.8; SD = 255.0; $F = .51$; $p = 0.48$) treatment conditions (Figure 1).

3.3. Category-Cued Word Fluency Task.

PD patients and HC did not differ either for the number of words generated in the two trials of the fluency task ($F(1, 36) = 0.18$; $p = 0.67$). Furthermore, neither the Treatment factor ($F(1, 36) = 0.35$; $p = 0.56$) nor the Group × Treatment interaction ($F(1, 36) = 0.35$; $p = 0.56$) revealed significant effects, thus demonstrating that the average number of words generated by the PD patients was not affected when patients took L-Dopa medication (Table 1).

The average typicality of words also did not differ between groups and was not affected by the treatment condition (Figure 2). Indeed, also in this case, the Half main effect was significant ($F(1.36) = 124.3$; $p < 0.001$), whereas the Group ($F(1.36) = 3.39$; $p = 0.07$) and Treatment ($F(1.36) = 3.20$; $p = 0.08$) main factors and the second-order and third-order interactions were not (all p consistently >0.30). These data indicate that all subjects generated more typical words (within the semantic category) in the first (M = 80.7; SD = 52.5) than in the second (M = 53.3; SD = 30.0) half of the trials. Moreover, planned comparisons showed that the typicality of the words generated by PD patients when taking dopamine medication (M = 68.8; SD = 38.7) was not different from the typicality of words generated during medication withdrawal (M = 59.7; SD = 32.0; $F = 1.64$; $p = 0.20$; Cohen's $d = 0.002$) and that the average typicality of the generated word values decreased at the same rate passing from the first half to the second half in the ON (M = 39.3; SD = 57.2) and in the OFF (M = 22.9; SD = 47.9; $F = .54$; $p = 0.46$) treatment conditions.

4. Discussion

This study was aimed at investigating whether dopaminergic stimulation has a modulatory effect on the spreading activation of lexical-semantic representations in individuals with PD. In particular, we investigated whether reduced dopamine concentration results in increased spreading activation which could potentially influence strategic organization and retrieval of internal representations [16]. For this purpose, we administered a group of PD patients letter-cued and category-cued fluency tasks in two different pharmacological treatment conditions: (a) after a dopaminergic treatment wash-out period ("OFF" treatment condition) and (b) after they took their usual dopaminergic medication dose ("ON" treatment condition). We predicted that in the OFF condition PD patients, unlike HC, would show increased spreading activation documented by the generation of less frequent words in the letter-cued task and of less typical words in the category-cued task. Moreover, we predicted that taking dopamine medication ("ON" condition) would result in significantly less spreading of lexical-semantic activation, thus resulting in the generation of more frequent and more typical words.

Results did not confirm our predictions. Indeed, neither frequency nor typicality of the generated words differed between PD patients (in both OFF and ON treatment conditions) and HC. Moreover, no significant difference in these two parameters was found in the PD group in the two treatment conditions. To the extent that frequency of use and typicality of words generated in fluency tasks are behavioural indices of spreading activation within the lexical-semantic system [16], we can conclude that our PD sample did not present any significant alteration in this lexical-semantic system property and, therefore, that dopamine stimulation has no appreciable effect on the activation level of lexical-semantic representations.

Our findings are consistent with those of Herrera et al. [17]. These authors found no difference between PD patients and matched HC for frequency of use of words generated in a letter-cued fluency task and in two category-cued fluency tasks. The same study failed to reveal any effect of medication administration/withdrawal on the same indices in the PD group. However, these authors [17] found that, in an action-cued fluency task, PD patients in the OFF condition generated action words with greater use frequency than HC. Although the finding of an effect confined to the grammatical class of words is of interest in light of previous evidence of a special role of the frontal lobes in verb generation [28] and of a significant deficit of PD patients on verbs and action words [28], it is difficult to interpret. Indeed, in their PD sample, use frequency of words was not modulated by L-Dopa intake (i.e., there was no significant difference between PD patients in the ON and OFF treatment conditions). Moreover, the average frequency values in the group of PD patients and in HC could have been confounded by the different number of words generated (with higher values in the PD group possibly related to the lower number of words generated).

Therefore, taking together the above observations and the evidence that most PD participants in our study showed dysexecutive deficits, we argue that in the early stage of PD prefrontal lobe dysfunction does not affect processes involved in the maintenance of stable representations, such as those related to semantic knowledge. Coherently, the null effect of the therapy manipulation we found could be interpreted

in the view that, in the early phases of PD, dopamine neurotransmission is mainly involved in the modulation of flexibility processes depending on the activity of the D2 dopamine receptors in the caudate nucleus [29–31] and does not affect the on-line processing of consolidated information.

However, our findings are at variance with those of Foster et al. [16]. These authors administered a letter-cued fluency task to groups of PD patients and matched controls and found that the frequency of use of words generated by PD patients was significantly lower than that generated by HC. One way of explaining these contrasting data is that the PD patients enrolled by Foster et al. [16] were in a more advanced stage of the disease compared to the PD patients who participated in our study (Foster et al.'s [16] study: mean disease duration = 6.8 years; mean UPDRS score = 32; our study: mean disease duration = 2.9 years; mean UPDRS score = 16.3). Therefore, we argue that the cortical regions responsible for the integrity of lexical-semantic processing are affected to a lesser extent in our PD sample than in the patients enrolled by Foster et al. [16]. Unfortunately, Foster et al. [16] did not manipulate dopamine treatment; thus we are unable to formulate any hypotheses about the role of dopamine stimulation on the effects they found.

Some limitations of the present study have to be discussed. First, likely because in the early stages of the disease, PD patients in the present study did not generate fewer words in the phonological and category-cued fluency tasks as compared to healthy controls, this could have reduced the possibility of finding significant effects of dopamine stimulation on the use frequency and/or typicality of produced words. Second, the PD patients were assessed while undergoing their usual dopamine therapy, which seemed to be quite heterogeneous as it includes levodopa and/or dopamine agonists. This could be another factor responsible of a lack of an effect of dopamine stimulation on spreading activation. Indeed, it is reported that the different molecules involved in dopaminergic compounds may have different effects on cognitive functions depending on their differential affinity with brain D_n receptors [32].

In conclusion, our results do not show a significant relationship between semantic spreading and dopamine stimulation in early-stage PD patients. However, also taking into account the above limitations, our findings might suggest the relative independence of the functioning of the semantic system and the activity of dopamine brain networks in the early stages of PD.

Finally, studies combining different paradigms (e.g., associative priming and verbal fluency) could be designed to further investigate the effect of dopamine treatment on lexical-semantic processing in PD.

References

[1] A. A. Kehagia, R. A. Barker, and T. W. Robbins, "Neuropsychological and clinical heterogeneity of cognitive impairment and

dementia in patients with Parkinson's disease," *The Lancet Neurology*, vol. 9, no. 12, pp. 1200–1213, 2010.

[2] G. A. Carlesimo, F. Piras, F. Assogna, F. E. Pontieri, C. Caltagirone, and G. Spalletta, "Hippocampal abnormalities and memory deficits in Parkinson disease: a multimodal imaging study," *Neurology*, vol. 78, no. 24, pp. 1939–1945, 2012.

[3] A. Brück, T. Kurki, V. Kaasinen, T. Vahlberg, and J. O. Rinne, "Hippocampal and prefrontal atrophy in patients with early non-demented Parkinson's disease is related to cognitive impairment," *Journal of Neurology, Neurosurgery & Psychiatry*, vol. 75, no. 10, pp. 1467–1469, 2004.

[4] I. Ferrer, "Early involvement of the cerebral cortex in Parkinson's disease: Convergence of multiple metabolic defects," *Progress in Neurobiology*, vol. 88, no. 2, pp. 89–103, 2009.

[5] A. J. Angwin, H. J. Chenery, D. A. Copland, B. E. Murdoch, and P. A. Silburn, "The speed of lexical activation is altered in Parkinson's disease," *Journal of Clinical and Experimental Neuropsychology*, vol. 29, no. 1, pp. 73–85, 2007.

[6] W. L. Arnott, H. J. Chenery, B. E. Murdoch, and P. A. Silburn, "Semantic priming in Parkinson's disease: Evidence for delayed spreading activation," *Journal of Clinical and Experimental Neuropsychology*, vol. 23, no. 4, pp. 502–519, 2001.

[7] A. J. Angwin, D. A. Copland, H. J. Chenery, B. E. Murdoch, and P. A. Silburn, "The influence of dopamine on semantic activation in Parkinson's disease: evidence from a multipriming task," *Neuropsychology*, vol. 20, no. 3, pp. 299–306, 2006.

[8] A. J. Angwin, W. L. Arnott, D. A. Copland et al., "Semantic activation in Parkinson's disease patients on and off levodopa," *Cortex*, vol. 45, no. 8, pp. 950–959, 2009.

[9] U. Kischka, T. H. Kammer, S. Maier, M. Weisbrod, M. Thimm, and M. Spitzer, "Dopaminergic modulation of semantic network activation," *Neuropsychologia*, vol. 34, no. 11, pp. 1107–1113, 1996.

[10] D. Roesch-Ely, S. Weiland, H. Scheffel et al., "Dopaminergic Modulation of Semantic Priming in Healthy Volunteers," *Biological Psychiatry*, vol. 60, no. 6, pp. 604–611, 2006.

[11] A. J. Angwin, H. J. Chenery, D. A. Copland, W. L. Arnott, B. E. Murdoch, and P. A. Silburn, "Dopamine and semantic activation: An investigation of masked direct and indirect priming," *Journal of the International Neuropsychological Society*, vol. 10, no. 1, pp. 15–25, 2004.

[12] A. S. Pederzolli, M. E. Tivarus, P. Agrawal, S. K. Kostyk, K. M. Thomas, and D. Q. Beversdorf, "Dopaminergic modulation of semantic priming in parkinson disease," *Cognitive and Behavioral Neurology*, vol. 21, no. 3, pp. 134–137, 2008.

[13] M. Grossman, E. Zurif, C. Lee et al., "Information processing speed and sentence comprehension in Parkinson's disease," *Neuropsychology*, vol. 16, no. 2, pp. 174–181, 2002.

[14] A. M. Collins and E. F. Loftus, "A spreading-activation theory of semantic processing," *Psychological Review*, vol. 82, no. 6, pp. 407–428, 1975.

[15] P. A. Allen, M. McNeal, and D. Kvak, "Perhaps the lexicon is coded as a function of word frequency," *Journal of Memory and Language*, vol. 31, no. 6, pp. 826–844, 1992.

[16] P. S. Foster, V. Drago, D. B. FitzGerald, B. M. Skoblar, G. P. Crucian, and K. M. Heilman, "Spreading activation of lexical-semantic networks in Parkinson's disease," *Neuropsychologia*, vol. 46, no. 7, pp. 1908–1914, 2008.

[17] E. Herrera, F. Cuetos, and R. Ribacoba, "Verbal fluency in Parkinson's disease patients on/off dopamine medication," *Neuropsychologia*, vol. 50, no. 14, pp. 3636–3640, 2012.

[18] W. F. Battig and W. E. Montague, "Category norms of verbal items in 56 categories A replication and extension of the Connecticut category norms," *Journal of Experimental Psychology*, vol. 80, no. 3, pp. 1–46, 1969.

[19] M. Boccardi and S. F. Cappa, "Normative values of categorical production for the Italian language," *Giornale Italiano di Psicologia*, vol. 24, pp. 425–436, 1997.

[20] M. M. Hoehn and M. D. Yahr, "Parkinsonism: onset, progression and mortality.," *Neurology*, vol. 17, no. 5, pp. 427–442, 1967.

[21] G. Brébion, C. Stephan-Otto, E. Huerta-Ramos et al., "Abnormal functioning of the semantic network in schizophrenia patients with thought disorganization. An exemplar production task," *Psychiatry Research*, vol. 205, no. 1-2, pp. 1–6, 2013.

[22] B. Dubois, D. Burn, C. Goetz et al., "Diagnostic procedures for Parkinson's disease dementia: recommendations from the movement disorder society task force," *Movement Disorders*, vol. 22, no. 16, pp. 2314–2324, 2007.

[23] M. F. Folstein, S. E. Folstein, and P. R. McHugh, "Mini mental state. A practical method for grading the cognitive state of patients for the clinician," *Journal of Psychiatric research*, vol. 12, no. 3, pp. 189–198, 1975.

[24] A. Laudanna, A. M. T. C. Thornton, G. Brown, C. Burani, and L. Marconi, "Un corpus dell'italiano scritto contemporaneo dalla parte del ricevente," in *II Giornate internazionali di analisi statistica dei dati testuali*, S. Bolasco, L. Lebart, and A. Salem, Eds., vol. 1, pp. 103–109, Cisu, Roma, Italy, 1995.

[25] G. A. Carlesimo, C. Caltagirone, G. Gainotti et al., "The mental deterioration battery: normative data, diagnostic reliability and qualitative analyses of cognitive impairment," *European Neurology*, vol. 36, no. 6, pp. 378–384, 1996.

[26] J. W. Langston, H. Widner, C. G. Goetz et al., "Core assessment program for intracerebral transplantations (CAPIT)," *Movement Disorders*, vol. 7, no. 1, pp. 2–13, 1992.

[27] S. Fahn, R. L. Elton, and Members of the UPDRS Committee, "Unified Parkinson's disease rating scale," in *Recent development in Parkinson's disease*, pp. 153–163, Mac Millan Health Care Information, Florham Park, NJ, USA, 1987.

[28] P. Péran, A. Cherubini, F. Assogna et al., "Magnetic resonance imaging markers of Parkinson's disease nigrostriatal signature," *Brain*, vol. 133, no. 11, pp. 3423–3433, 2010.

[29] R. Cools and M. D'Esposito, "Inverted-U-shaped dopamine actions on human working memory and cognitive control," *Biological Psychiatry*, vol. 69, no. 12, pp. e113–e125, 2011.

[30] A. Costa, A. Peppe, G. Dell'Agnello, C. Caltagirone, and G. A. Carlesimo, "Dopamine and cognitive functioning in de novo subjects with Parkinson's disease: Effects of pramipexole and pergolide on working memory," *Neuropsychologia*, vol. 47, no. 5, pp. 1374–1381, 2009.

[31] A. Costa, A. Peppe, I. Mazzù, M. Longarzo, C. Caltagirone, and G. A. Carlesimo, "Dopamine treatment and cognitive functioning in individuals with parkinson's disease: The "cognitive flexibility" hypothesis seems to work," *Behavioural Neurology*, vol. 2014, Article ID 260896, 2014.

[32] R. Cools, "Dopaminergic modulation of cognitive function-implications for L-DOPA treatment in Parkinson's disease," *Neuroscience and Biobehavioral Reviews*, vol. 30, no. 1, pp. 1–23, 2006.

6

The Effect of Hyperhomocysteinemia on Motor Symptoms, Cognitive Status, and Vascular Risk in Patients with Parkinson's Disease

Bilge Kocer,[1] Hayat Guven,[1] Isik Conkbayir,[2] Selim Selcuk Comoglu,[1] and Sennur Delibas[1]

[1]*Department of Neurology, Diskapi Yildirim Beyazit Training and Research Hospital, 06110 Ankara, Turkey*
[2]*Department of Radiology, Diskapi Yildirim Beyazit Training and Research Hospital, 06110 Ankara, Turkey*

Correspondence should be addressed to Bilge Kocer; bilge.gonenli@gmail.com

Academic Editor: Ivan Bodis-Wollner

Factors related with hyperhomocysteinemia (HHcy) and the impact of HHcy in Parkinson's disease (PD) are not well understood. We investigated the factors associated with increased levels of homocysteine (Hcy) and the relationship between HHcy and motor symptoms, cognitive status, and vascular risk in patients with Parkinson's disease. Among 60 patients (29 males, 48.3%) with PD, the stage of the disease, the severity of clinical symptoms, and the patients' cognitive status were measured using a modified Hoehn and Yahr Staging Scale (mHY), Unified Parkinson's Disease Rating Scale (UPDRS) II and III, and Mini-Mental State Examination (MMSE), respectively. Patients were also noted for having dyskinesia and hallucinations. Serum vitamin B12, folic acid, and plasma Hcy levels were measured. Furthermore, the presence of vascular risk factors was recorded. Finally, we investigated carotid artery intima-media thickening and stenosis using colour Doppler ultrasonography as well as the presence of ischemic lesions using brain imaging techniques. Plasma Hcy levels were higher with advanced age and in males. In addition, there was an inverse relationship between Hcy and vitamin B12 levels. There was no correlation between HHcy and the stage of the disease, severity of motor symptoms, cognitive status as assessed by the MMSE, vascular risk factors, carotid artery atherosclerotic findings, and ischemic brain lesions. Plasma Hcy levels may rise due to several factors in PD. However, the resulting HHcy has no significant effect on the clinical picture in terms of motor features, cognitive status, and vascular diseases.

1. Introduction

Hyperhomocysteinemia (HHcy) is an established risk factor for cardiovascular, cerebrovascular, and peripheral vascular diseases [1–3]. In Parkinson's disease (PD) patients undergoing levodopa (LD) therapy, plasma homocysteine (Hcy) levels are elevated as a result of the transmethylation of LD via catechol O-methyl transferase (COMT) [4, 5]. The effect of this HHcy on vascular diseases in PD patients is unclear; HHcy could potentially cause vascular pathologies or the worsening of motor features.

Experimental studies have demonstrated that Hcy can be neurotoxic and excitotoxic to the substantia nigra. Furthermore, Hcy may be associated with dyskinesias, which is an indicator of possible neurodegeneration due to the disruption of the balance of striatal activity [6, 7].

The prevalence of neuropsychiatric symptoms, such as depression and dementia, is increased in PD [8, 9]. Among the elderly, HHcy is a well-known risk factor for dementia [10]. HHcy has been proposed to also be a risk factor for the neuropsychiatric disorders, cognitive deterioration, dementia, and depression that are seen in PD, but some studies have not confirmed these results [11–15].

Therefore, we examined the relationship between plasma Hcy levels and the severity of PD-related motor features and cognitive status. We also determined the risk of vascular disease in PD patients by using vascular risk factors, previous vascular diseases, atherosclerotic findings detected by carotid artery colour Doppler ultrasonography, and ischemic changes in brain imaging studies.

2. Materials and Methods

2.1. Study Design. This prospective study included 60 patients (29 males, 48.3%) randomly selected from patients diagnosed with idiopathic PD according to the UK Brain Bank criteria [16]. Patients with vascular parkinsonism and severe metabolic disorders or those who used vitamin supplements were excluded from the study.

For all patients, the duration of the disease, on-going treatments, and dosage and duration of levodopa therapy were recorded. In addition, patients were also examined for the presence of vascular risk factors, such as hypertension, diabetes mellitus, and hyperlipidemia and for vascular diseases, such as coronary artery disease and stroke.

The stage of PD and the severity of disease findings were determined by the "modified Hoehn and Yahr (mHY) Staging Scale" and "Unified Parkinson's Disease Rating Scale" (UPDRS) II and III, respectively [17, 18]. The dominant motor features of PD were determined by using the subscores calculated from questions about tremor (20, 21), rigidity (22), bradykinesia (23, 24, 25, 26, 31), and balance/postural instability (27, 28, 29, and 30) in the UPDRS III. In addition, the presence of dyskinesia was also noted.

The assessment of global cognitive status was conducted with the standardised "Mini-Mental State Examination" (MMSE). We also noted the presence of visual hallucinations.

Blood samples were collected from peripheral veins into vacuum tubes containing EDTA in the early morning after 12 hours of fasting and 12-hour drug-free periods. Plasma Hcy levels were measured by high-performance liquid chromatography with fluorescence detection (HPLC-FLD). Serum vitamin B12 and folic acid levels were measured by an immunoassay.

The carotid arteries of patients and control subjects were investigated using carotid colour Doppler ultrasonography with a 6 to 11 MHz linear probe performed by the same physician in the Radiology Department who was blinded from the clinical history of 50 subjects. The common carotid arteries and extracranial internal carotid arteries were investigated on the axial and longitudinal planes using the B mode and colour Doppler methods, starting at the origin and including the bifurcation point; intimal thickening, plaques, and stenosis were noted. The frequency levels, gain adjustments, and grey scale and Doppler parameters were manually adjusted to optimise visualisation of stenosis [19].

Among 45 patients, ischemic lesions at the lacunar and specific arterial irrigation areas were recorded by brain computed tomography (CT) and magnetic resonance imaging (MRI) examinations.

The study was carried out according to the Helsinki Declaration and was approved by the Institutional Ethics Committee.

2.2. Statistical Analysis. All statistical data analyses were performed with SPSS Statistics (version 19, IBM, Chicago, IL,

TABLE 1: Demographic and clinical characteristics and values of vitamin B12 and folic acid in PD patients[*].

	PD ($n = 60$)
Age (years)	68.4 ± 8.95
Duration of disease (years)	7.0 ± 5.75
Age of PD onset (years)	61.4 ± 10.92
mHY stage	2.2 ± 0.99
UPDRS-II score	12.1 ± 6.86
UPDRS-III score	17.4 ± 8.37
UPDRS tremor subscore	2.3 ± 1.56
UPDRS rigidity subscore	1.4 ± 0.90
UPDRS bradykinesia subscore	7.1 ± 3.29
UPDRS gait/postural instability subscore	3.4 ± 2.99
MMSE score	24.2 ± 4.21
Vitamin B12 (pg/ml)	344.4 ± 206.54
Folic acid (ng/ml)	9.3 ± 3.74

[*]Data reported as the mean ± SD.
PD: Parkinson's disease; mHY: modified Hoehn and Yahr Staging Scale; UPDRS: Unified Parkinson's Disease Rating Scale; MMSE: Mini-Mental State Examination.

USA). Prior to the analysis, the normality of the distribution of Hcy levels was examined and the distribution of the 60 values was found to be consistent with the normal distribution (Kolmogorov-Smirnov: 0.066, $p < 0.05$). All analyses were conducted using parametric tests on the data from 60 patients. We established the necessary hypotheses to examine the differences between the patients with different clinical manifestations of plasma Hcy levels and to identify independent variables that affect plasma Hcy levels and tested these hypotheses using t-tests, ANOVAs, and correlation analyses.

3. Results

The mean age of 60 patients (29 males, 48.3%) with idiopathic PD was 68.4 ± 8.95 years. Demographic and clinical characteristics and serum vitamin B12 and folic acid levels of the patients are shown in Table 1.

In male and female patients, the mean plasma Hcy levels were 16.26 ± 4.57 μmol/L and 11 ± 3.76 μmol/L, respectively. Plasma Hcy levels were significantly higher in male patients ($p < 0.001$). In addition, there was a statistically significant positive relationship between plasma Hcy levels and the age of the patients ($p < 0.04$), whereas an inverse relationship was found between plasma Hcy levels and serum levels of vitamin B12 ($p < 0.01$). There was no significant correlation between plasma Hcy levels and the duration of PD, disease stage, severity of motor symptoms as determined by UPDRS II and III, clinical features, and cognitive status as assessed by standardised MMSE (Table 2).

There was also no significant correlation between plasma Hcy levels and the presence of dyskinesia. Likewise, although the patients with hallucinations had slightly higher plasma Hcy levels, this difference was not statistically significant.

We found no significant correlation between plasma Hcy levels and diabetes mellitus, hypertension, hyperlipidemia, or

TABLE 2: Correlation between plasma homocysteine levels and demographic and clinical characteristics and serum B12 and folic acid values.

	Homocysteine levels	
	r	p
Age (years)	0.27	**0.04**[*]
Duration of disease (years)	0.23	0.07
Age of PD onset (years)	0.14	0.30
mHY stage	−0.10	0.44
UPDRS-II score	0.09	0.48
UPDRS-III score	0.01	0.91
UPDRS tremor subscore	0.11	0.42
UPDRS rigidity subscore	0.18	0.16
UPDRS bradykinesia subscore	−0.01	0.92
UPDRS gait/postural instability subscore	0.02	0.90
MMSE score	0.03	0.85
Vitamin B12 (pg/ml)	−0.32	**0.01**[*]
Folic acid (ng/ml)	0.06	0.68

[*]Difference is statistically significant ($p < 0.05$).
PD: Parkinson's disease; mHY: modified Hoehn and Yahr Staging Scale; UPDRS: Unified Parkinson's Disease Rating Scale; MMSE: Mini-Mental State Examination.

coronary artery disease. Two patients had a history of strokes; their plasma Hcy levels were 15.5 and 20.4 μmol/L. Although these patients had relatively slightly higher plasma Hcy levels than the mean, this was not statistically significant.

The mean plasma Hcy levels of the patients with intima-media thickening (IMT), atherosclerotic plaques, and stenosis of greater than 50% as detected by colour Doppler ultrasonography of the carotid artery were found to be slightly higher than those of patients without these symptoms, but the difference was not statistically significant. Similarly, we found no significant relationship between plasma Hcy levels and multiple ischemic lesions detected by brain imaging studies (Table 3).

When the correlation between ongoing treatments and plasma Hcy levels was examined, the patients on only dopamine agonist therapy and on LD therapy without COMT inhibitors were found to have the lowest and highest plasma Hcy levels, respectively. However, the difference between plasma Hcy levels and treatment groups was not statistically significant.

Although the dose and duration of LD therapy in patients with plasma Hcy levels >14 μmol/L were slightly higher, this difference was not statistically significant (Table 4).

4. Discussion

In PD, motor symptoms occur as a result of dopaminergic cell loss and therefore LD replacement therapy is the most effective treatment option. Patients treated with LD have been reported to have higher plasma Hcy levels [12, 13, 20]. In addition, plasma Hcy levels were higher in PD patients using LD therapy than in patients not using LD and the control group [12, 21]. This increase in Hcy levels has largely been attributed to chronic LD use and, specifically, drug catabolism [21]. LD is subjected to O-methylation via the enzyme COMT in the brain and peripheral tissues. This reaction requires S-adenosylmethionine (SAM) as a methyl donor and, ultimately, yields methylated S-adenosylhomocysteine (SAH). SAH is hydrolysed rapidly and is eventually converted to Hcy [4]. Therefore, long-term LD treatment leads to HHcy by increasing the production of Hcy [4].

Plasma Hcy levels may also be affected by the patient's methylene tetrahydrofolate reductase (MTHFR) enzyme genotype and vitamin B status, except in cases of LD therapy [12]. The MTHFR enzyme needs folic acid and vitamin B12 to function properly. Plasma Hcy levels increase as a result of folic acid, vitamin B6, and vitamin B12 deficiencies and mutations of the enzyme encoding the MTHFR gene [21].

In elderly individuals, Hcy is an independent risk factor for vascular diseases, cognitive deterioration, and dementia [21]. *In vitro* studies have indicated a relationship between Hcy and DNA damage, apoptosis, excitotoxicity, and oxidative stress, which are of great importance in neurodegeneration [21, 22]. Neuronal degeneration in peripheral nerves as well as central nervous system during LD treatment in PD patients may also occur due to secondary metabolic changes such as HHcy and low vitamin values of folic acid and B12 [23].

Some studies have suggested a correlation between HHcy, advanced age, and male gender, but this correlation has not been demonstrated in other studies [11, 15, 21, 24]. In our study, we found a positive correlation between plasma Hcy levels, advanced age, and male gender and a negative correlation between plasma Hcy levels and serum levels of vitamin B12. In patients with HHcy on LD treatment, vitamin B12 levels may be lower or within the normal range [15]. As Hcy is generated through demethylation of methionine and hydrolisation of SAH, accumulation of Hcy inhibits methyltransferases through negative feedback mechanisms. Therefore elevated plasma Hcy is associated with reduced methylation capacity. Folic acid and vitamin B12 reduce Hcy levels by reversible metabolism of Hcy to methionine. Negative correlation between plasma Hcy and vitamin B12 levels may reflect the methyl group consuming side effect of chronic levodopa metabolism. Vitamin supplementation decreases Hcy generation by reversible degradation of Hcy to methionine [25].

In our study, as reported in the literature, we did not find a significant correlation between plasma Hcy levels and the duration of PD [13, 15, 24], whereas some authors have noted such a relationship [11]. Although plasma Hcy levels of patients using LD are generally higher than controls, the results of studies investigating the effect of the dose and duration of LD on plasma Hcy levels can be confusing. Some researchers have suggested a correlation between daily dose of LD and plasma Hcy levels, whereas others have suggested no correlation [11–13, 15, 22, 24, 26]. Likewise, there are also studies that showed or did not show a correlation between the duration of LD and plasma Hcy levels [11, 12, 15, 22, 26]. We think that the differences between these results are due to the patient selection criteria, study design, and sample size.

TABLE 3: Plasma homocysteine levels and their relationships with hallucinations, dyskinesia, vascular risk factors, carotid colour Doppler US, brain MRI findings, and anti-parkinsonian medication in patients with Parkinson's disease.

		n	Homocysteine levels (μmol/L)[*]	p
Hallucinations	Absent	46	13.34 ± 4.62	0.13
	Present	14	15.53 ± 4.99	
Dyskinesia	Absent	44	14.14 ± 5.00	0.44
	Present	16	13.05 ± 4.05	
Hypertension	Absent	33	14.15 ± 4.38	0.60
	Present	27	13.49 ± 5.25	
Diabetes mellitus	Absent	51	14.15 ± 4.83	0.24
	Present	9	12.12 ± 4.18	
Hyperlipidemia	Absent	39	13.35 ± 4.48	0.27
	Present	21	14.77 ± 5.23	
Coronary heart disease	Absent	47	13.6 ± 5.02	0.44
	Present	13	14.77 ± 3.67	
Previous stroke	Absent	58	13.71 ± 4.76	0.22
	Present	2	17.95 ±3.47	
Carotid colour Doppler US	Normal	14	12.96 ± 4.18	0.42
	Atherosclerotic findings[†]	36	14.24 ± 5.27	
Brain MRI	Normal	22	13.08 ± 4.88	0.85
	Ischemic lesions[‡]	23	13.37 ± 5.03	
Anti-parkinsonian medication	LD ± DA	31	15.06 ± 4.78	0.07
	LD ± DA ± COMTI	18	12.89 ± 5.08	
	DA	11	11.25 ± 3.26	

[*]Data reported as the mean ± SD.
[†]Atherosclerotic findings including intima-media thickness, atherosclerotic plaques, and stenosis.
[‡]Ischemic lesions including multiple lacunar and vascular territorial infarcts.
US: ultrasonography; MRI: magnetic resonance imaging; LD: levodopa; DA: dopamine agonists; COMTI: catechol O-methyl transferase inhibitors.

TABLE 4: Comparison of daily levodopa dose and duration of levodopa medication between patients with plasma homocysteine levels ≤14 and >14 μmol/L.

	Homocysteine levels (μmol/L)[*]		p
	Homocysteine ≤ 14 ($n = 18$)	Homocysteine > 14 ($n = 31$)	
Levodopa dose (mg/daily)	370.50 ± 138.20	430.65 ± 232.26	0.26
Duration of levodopa medication (years)	5.54 ± 5.68	7.65 ± 5.32	0.16

[*]Data reported as the mean ± SD.

In our study, we did not find a relationship between plasma Hcy levels and the daily dose or the duration of LD. Although we did not find a statistically significant correlation between LD dose and plasma Hcy levels, we noted that the plasma Hcy levels of patients on LD therapy tended to be higher. Furthermore, we found no relationship between plasma Hcy levels, the mHY stage of PD, and UPDRS III parameters of disease severity, including the clinical features of the disease, tremor, bradykinesia, rigidity, and gait/postural instability subscores. Absence of correlation between plasma Hcy levels and clinical outcome scores may be explained with the effect of LD treatment on clinical picture. Moreover response to LD may be different in each patient due to the impact of body weight on LD plasma appearance. Therefore, clinical outcome parameters may not always be consistent with the plasma Hcy values in clinical practice.

Following the in vitro and in vivo observations on the toxic effects of Hcy on dopaminergic neurons in the substantia nigra, some authors have suggested that HHcy associated with LD may play a role in the progression of PD and the development of motor complications and that dyskinesias and motor fluctuations may be due to the toxic effects of Hcy [7, 12].

In one study, the plasma Hcy levels of patients with dyskinesia were found to be higher, but no correlation was found between plasma Hcy levels and the duration of dyskinesia. Hence, it was suggested that plasma HHcy may play a role in the development of dyskinesias due to the toxic effects of Hcy on dopaminergic and nondopaminergic neurons [7].

Hcy is thought to affect dopamine turnover and cause dyskinesia by disrupting the balance of striatal activity.

However, some studies have not demonstrated an association between plasma Hcy levels and an increased risk of dyskinesia [12]. In our study, we found no significant difference between plasma Hcy levels of patients with and without dyskinesia.

HHcy is a major risk factor for vascular diseases and has been associated with stroke, myocardial infarction, and dementia in elderly individuals without PD [1–3, 27]. Some reports indicated that LD-induced HHcy in PD patients can lead to atherosclerosis [27]. In screening early atherosclerotic changes, intima-media thickening (IMT) is an easily measured biomarker, which in addition to showing local changes in blood vessels also provides information about generalised atherosclerosis [27, 28].

Previous studies evaluated IMT in patients with PD who were treated with long-term LD therapy and identified hypertrophic changes. Furthermore, these studies found a correlation between the duration of LD therapy and the degree of the intima-media hypertrophy [27].

In the literature, there are studies indicating no correlation between LD-related HHcy and IMT of the carotid artery or even showing a lower IMT in PD patients than in controls [11, 29]. Therefore, the patients with PD are thought to have a lower risk of preclinical atherosclerosis [29]. The autonomic dysfunction and/or hypotensive effects of LD in PD are thought to be protective against atherosclerosis [29, 30].

In our study, we compared the plasma Hcy levels of patients with and without vascular changes, including carotid artery IMT, atherosclerotic plaques, and stenosis, but we did not find any significant correlations.

The prevalence of coronary artery disease has been reported to be increased in patients with high levels of Hcy on LD therapy [31]. However, another study showed no correlation between Hcy levels and carotid artery IMT and cardiovascular morbidity [11].

Ischemic brain lesions may affect the clinical condition in PD. Nonetheless, clinically evident cerebrovascular disease is rarely seen in PD patients [28]. Because of the high incidence of cerebrovascular diseases, it has been suggested that cerebrovascular diseases can coincidentally be seen in some patients with PD [28]. In our patient group, we did not detect a correlation between the plasma Hcy levels of those with and without coronary artery disease. The mean plasma Hcy levels of two patients with a history of stroke were higher than the group mean, but this difference was not statistically significant due to the low number of patients. We suggest that an investigation should be carried out in a larger patient cohort to determine whether these higher plasma Hcy levels were the result of the LD treatment predisposing patients to stroke.

The decrease in blood pressure in PD has been thought to provide protection against stroke [30]. However, if LD-induced HHcy was the only factor that causes vascular complications, there should be data indicating that Hcy-related diseases are more common in patients with PD. However, there is still no convincing data indicating a higher incidence of cardiovascular disease and stroke in PD patients than in controls [11].

Patients with PD have a 4–6 times greater risk of developing dementia compared with the age-matched population [13, 30]. LD therapy has been thought to affect the risk of dementia and cognitive impairment because it increases Hcy levels [20, 26]. Furthermore, the correlation between HHcy and Alzheimer's disease suggests that PD patients with HHcy may be prone to dementia [30].

Dementia is a common nonmotor feature in PD. Moreover, the relationship between increased levels of Hcy and dementia in PD has not been fully clarified, although a significant proportion of PD patients develop cognitive impairment [12, 15].

In a rodent study, Lee et al. showed a decrease in dopamine levels and behavioural changes following intraventricular injection of Hcy [32]. On this basis, HHcy has been suggested to play a role in the development of cognitive impairment in PD [15].

In vitro studies suggested that Hcy can enhance oxidative stress, induce accumulation of cytosolic calcium, impair DNA repair mechanisms, and cause neuronal damage and apoptotic death by triggering excitotoxicity through stimulation of NMDA and glutamate receptors [33]. Moreover, Hcy can have cytotoxic effects on endothelial and neuronal cultures [24, 33].

Zoccolella et al. found higher Hcy levels in PD patients than in controls and in PD patients with dementia than in patients without dementia and suggested a significant association between high Hcy levels and dementia [20]. In another study, significantly higher plasma Hcy levels were found in PD patients with cognitive impairments than in those without cognitive impairments and the risk of cognitive dysfunction was found to increase with plasma Hcy levels after adjustment for age, gender, and vitamin B status [15]. Similarly, there are imaging studies indicating that white matter changes in the brain may affect cognition in PD along with the vitamin B12, folic acid, and Hcy levels [34]. However, while previous studies have shown that plasma Hcy levels of >14 μmol/L in elderly people without dementia decreased cognitive performance by 25%, a study conducted on two groups of PD patients with plasma Hcy levels greater and lower than 14 μmol/L found no difference in cognitive performance [13].

In many studies, plasma Hcy levels were correlated with cognitive function, dementia, and markers of neurodegeneration in PD patients [14, 24]. However, some studies showed no correlation between plasma Hcy levels and neuropsychiatric symptoms such as depression, cognitive impairment, and psychosis [11]. Rodriguez-Oroz et al. demonstrated no correlation between plasma Hcy levels and cognitive disorders, dementia, silent infarcts, or genetic polymorphisms [35]. Likewise, in another study, no correlation was detected between plasma Hcy levels and hallucinations [11].

The difference between the results of the studies arises from the retrospective nature of some studies, the small number of patients, and the diversity of neuropsychiatric batteries.

Degenerative brain changes associated with disease are the primary cause of cognitive and motor deterioration in PD. However, comorbid hypoperfusion can contribute to the emergence and severity of this cognitive and motor deterioration [28]. Concomitant vascular pathology aggravates the clinical condition in PD [28].

In conclusion, plasma Hcy levels may be elevated for a variety of reasons in PD, and HHcy is a well-known risk factor for vascular disease and dementia in the elderly. Because of the higher prevalence of vascular diseases and increased risk of cognitive impairment throughout the course of PD, PD patients often have coincidental vascular diseases or dementia. In addition, LD therapy is not the only cause of HHcy. Hence, given the results of our study, we conclude that HHcy has no significant effect on clinical status in PD in terms of motor deterioration, vascular disease, and dementia.

References

[1] C. J. Boushey, S. A. A. Beresford, G. S. Omenn, and A. G. Motulsky, "A quantitative assessment of plasma homocysteine as a risk factor for vascular disease probable benefits of increasing folic acid intakes," *The Journal of the American Medical Association*, vol. 274, no. 13, pp. 1049–1057, 1995.

[2] J. W. Eikelboom, E. Lonn, J. Genest Jr., G. Hankey, and S. Yusuf, "Homocysteine and cardiovascular disease: a critical review of the epidemiologic evidence," *Annals of Internal Medicine*, vol. 131, no. 5, pp. 363–375, 1999.

[3] A. G. Bostom, I. H. Rosenberg, H. Silbershatz et al., "Nonfasting plasma total homocysteine levels and stroke incidence in elderly persons: the Framingham Study," *Annals of Internal Medicine*, vol. 131, no. 5, pp. 352–355, 1999.

[4] T. Müller, D. Woitalla, B. Fowler, and W. Kuhn, "3-OMD and homocysteine plasma levels in parkinsonian patients," *Journal of Neural Transmission*, vol. 109, no. 2, pp. 175–179, 2002.

[5] T. Müller, D. Woitalla, B. Hauptmann, B. Fowler, and W. Kuhn, "Decrease of methionine and S-adenosylmethionine and increase of homocysteine in treated patients with Parkinson's disease," *Neuroscience Letters*, vol. 308, no. 1, pp. 54–56, 2001.

[6] T. Müller, H. Hefter, R. Hueber et al., "Is levodopa toxic?" *Journal of Neurology*, vol. 251, supplement 6, pp. 44–46, 2004.

[7] S. Zoccolella, P. Lamberti, G. Iliceto et al., "Elevated plasma homocysteine levels in L-dopa-treated Parkinson's disease patients with dyskinesias," *Clinical Chemistry and Laboratory Medicine*, vol. 44, no. 7, pp. 863–866, 2006.

[8] D. Aarsland, K. Andersen, J. P. Larsen, A. Lolk, and P. Kragh-Sørensen, "Prevalence and characteristics of dementia in Parkinson disease: an 8-year prospective study," *Archives of Neurology*, vol. 60, no. 3, pp. 387–392, 2003.

[9] W. Poewe and E. Luginger, "Depression in Parkinson's disease: impediments to recognition and treatment options," *Neurology*, vol. 52, supplement 3, no. 7, pp. 2–6, 1999.

[10] N. D. Prins, T. Den Heijer, A. Hofman et al., "Homocysteine and cognitive function in the elderly: the Rotterdam Scan Study," *Neurology*, vol. 59, no. 9, pp. 1375–1380, 2002.

[11] S. Hassin-Baer, O. Cohen, E. Vakil et al., "Plasma homocysteine levels and parkinson disease: disease progression, carotid intima-media thickness and neuropsychiatric complications," *Clinical Neuropharmacology*, vol. 29, no. 6, pp. 305–311, 2006.

[12] R. M. Camicioli, T. P. Bouchard, and M. J. Somerville, "Homocysteine is not associated with global motor or cognitive measures in nondemented older Parkinson's disease patients," *Movement Disorders*, vol. 24, no. 2, pp. 176–182, 2009.

[13] F. Ozer, H. Meral, L. Hanoglu et al., "Plasma homocysteine levels in patients treated with levodopa: motor and cognitive associations," *Neurological Research*, vol. 28, no. 8, pp. 853–858, 2006.

[14] S. Zoccolella, S. V. Lamberti, G. Iliceto, A. Santamato, P. Lamberti, and G. Logroscino, "Hyperhomocysteinemia in L-dopa treated patients with Parkinson's disease: potential implications in cognitive dysfunction and dementia?" *Current Medicinal Chemistry*, vol. 17, no. 28, pp. 3253–3261, 2010.

[15] S. Zoccolella, P. Lamberti, G. Iliceto et al., "Plasma homocysteine levels in L-dopa-treated Parkinson's disease patients with cognitive dysfunctions," *Clinical Chemistry and Laboratory Medicine*, vol. 43, no. 10, pp. 1107–1110, 2005.

[16] A. J. Hughes, S. E. Daniel, L. Kilford, and A. J. Lees, "Accuracy of clinical diagnosis of idiopathic Parkinson's disease: a clinico-pathological study of 100 cases," *Journal of Neurology Neurosurgery and Psychiatry*, vol. 55, no. 3, pp. 181–184, 1992.

[17] M. M. Hoehn and M. D. Yahr, "Parkinsonism: onset, progression, and mortality," *Neurology*, vol. 17, no. 5, pp. 427–442, 1967.

[18] S. Fahn, R. L. Elton, and Members of the UPDRS Development Committee, "Unified Parkinson's disease rating scale," in *Recent Developments in Parkinson's Disease*, S. Fahn, C. D. Marsden, D. B. Calne, and M. Goldstein, Eds., vol. 2, pp. 153–163, Macmillan, New York, NY, USA, 1987.

[19] E. G. Grant, C. B. Benson, G. L. Moneta et al., "Carotid artery stenosis: gray-scale and Doppler US diagnosis—Society of Radiologists in Ultrasound Consensus Conference," *Radiology*, vol. 229, no. 2, pp. 340–346, 2003.

[20] S. Zoccolella, C. dell'Aquila, G. Abruzzese et al., "Hyperhomocysteinemia in levodopa-treated patients with Parkinson's disease Dementia," *Movement Disorders*, vol. 24, no. 7, pp. 1028–1033, 2009.

[21] E. Martignoni, C. Tassorelli, G. Nappi, R. Zangaglia, C. Pacchetti, and F. Blandini, "Homocysteine and Parkinson's disease: a dangerous liaison?" *Journal of the Neurological Sciences*, vol. 257, no. 1-2, pp. 31–37, 2007.

[22] S. Zoccolella, D. Martino, G. Defazio, P. Lamberti, and P. Livrea, "Hyperhomocysteinemia in movement disorders: current evidence and hypotheses," *Current Vascular Pharmacology*, vol. 4, no. 3, pp. 237–243, 2006.

[23] T. Müller, C. Jugel, R. Ehret et al., "Elevation of total homocysteine levels in patients with Parkinson's disease treated with duodenal levodopa/carbidopa gel," *Journal of Neural Transmission*, vol. 118, no. 9, pp. 1329–1333, 2011.

[24] P. E. O'Suilleabhain, V. Sung, C. Hernandez et al., "Elevated plasma homocysteine level in patients with Parkinson disease: motor, affective, and cognitive associations," *Archives of Neurology*, vol. 61, no. 6, pp. 865–868, 2004.

[25] T. Müller, D. Woitalla, and S. Muhlack, "Inhibition of catechol-O-methyltransferase modifies acute homocysteine rise during repeated levodopa application in patients with Parkinson's disease," *Naunyn-Schmiedeberg's Archives of Pharmacology*, vol. 383, no. 6, pp. 627–633, 2011.

[26] J. J. Martín-Fernández, R. Carles-Díes, F. Cañizares et al., "Homocysteine and cognitive impairment in Parkinson's disease," *Revista de Neurologia*, vol. 50, no. 3, pp. 145–151, 2010.

[27] K. Nakaso, K. Yasui, H. Kowa et al., "Hypertrophy of IMC of carotid artery in Parkinson's disease is associated with L-DOPA, homocysteine, and MTHFR genotype," *Journal of the Neurological Sciences*, vol. 207, no. 1-2, pp. 19–23, 2003.

[28] I. Rektor, D. Goldemund, K. Sheardová, I. Rektorová, Z. Michálková, and M. Dufek, "Vascular pathology in patients with idiopathic Parkinson's disease," *Parkinsonism and Related Disorders*, vol. 15, no. 1, pp. 24–29, 2009.

[29] J.-M. Lee, K.-W. Park, W.-K. Seo et al., "Carotid intima-media thickness in Parkinson's disease," *Movement Disorders*, vol. 22, no. 16, pp. 2446–2449, 2007.

[30] R. B. Postuma and A. E. Lang, "Homocysteine and levodopa: should Parkinson disease patients receive preventative therapy?" *Neurology*, vol. 63, no. 5, pp. 886–891, 2004.

[31] J. D. Rogers, A. Sanchez-Saffon, A. B. Frol, and R. Diaz-Arrastia, "Elevated plasma homocysteine levels in patients treated with levodopa: association with vascular disease," *Archives of Neurology*, vol. 60, no. 1, pp. 59–64, 2003.

[32] E.-S. Y. Lee, H. Chen, K. F. A. Soliman, and C. G. Charlton, "Effects of homocysteine on the dopaminergic system and behavior in rodents," *NeuroToxicology*, vol. 26, no. 3, pp. 361–371, 2005.

[33] S. A. Lipton, W.-K. Kim, Y.-B. Choi et al., "Neurotoxicity associated with dual actions of homocysteine at the N- methyl-D-aspartate receptor," *Proceedings of the National Academy of Sciences of the United States of America*, vol. 94, no. 11, pp. 5923–5928, 1997.

[34] J. Sławek, A. Roszmann, P. Robowski et al., "The impact of MRI white matter hyperintensities on dementia in parkinson's disease in relation to the homocysteine level and other vascular risk factors," *Neurodegenerative Diseases*, vol. 12, no. 1, pp. 1–12, 2013.

[35] M. C. Rodriguez-Oroz, P. M. Lage, J. Sanchez-Mut et al., "Homocysteine and cognitive impairment in Parkinson's disease: a biochemical, neuroimaging, and genetic study," *Movement Disorders*, vol. 24, no. 10, pp. 1437–1444, 2009.

7

Experience Reduces Surgical and Hardware-Related Complications of Deep Brain Stimulation Surgery: A Single-Center Study of 181 Patients Operated in Six Years

Mehmet Sorar,[1] Sahin Hanalioglu,[1] Bilge Kocer (ID),[2] Muhammed Taha Eser,[1] Selim Selcuk Comoglu,[2] and Hayri Kertmen (ID)[1]

[1]Department of Neurosurgery, Diskapi Yildirim Beyazit Training and Research Hospital, Health Sciences University, Ankara, Turkey
[2]Department of Neurology, Diskapi Yildirim Beyazit Training and Research Hospital, Health Sciences University, Ankara, Turkey

Correspondence should be addressed to Hayri Kertmen; hayri_kertmen@yahoo.com

Academic Editor: Carlo Colosimo

Objective. Deep brain stimulation (DBS) surgery has increasingly been performed for the treatment of movement disorders and is associated with a wide array of complications. We aimed to present our experience and discuss strategies to minimize adverse events in light of this contemporary series and others in the literature. *Methods.* A retrospective chart review was conducted to collect data on age, sex, indication, operation date, surgical technique, and perioperative and late complications. *Results.* A total of 181 patients (113 males, 68 females) underwent DBS implantation surgery (359 leads) in the past six years. Indications and targets were as follows: Parkinson's disease (STN) ($n = 159$), dystonia (GPi) ($n = 13$), and essential tremor (Vim) ($n = 9$). Mean age was 55.2 ± 11.7 (range 9–74) years. Mean follow-up duration was 3.4 ± 1.6 years. No mortality or permanent morbidity was observed. Major perioperative complications were confusion (6.6%), intracerebral hemorrhage (2.2%), stroke (1.1%), and seizures (1.1%). Long-term adverse events included wound (7.2%), mostly infection, and hardware-related (5.5%) complications. Among several factors, only surgical experience was found to be related with overall complication rates (early period: 31% versus late period: 10%; $p = 0.001$). *Conclusion.* The rates of both early and late complications of DBS surgery are acceptably low and decrease significantly with cumulative experience.

1. Introduction

Since its introduction in 1987, deep brain stimulation (DBS) has become an effective treatment modality in the management of movement disorders [1, 2]. Clinical trials have proven its efficacy in Parkinson's disease (PD) and other hyperkinetic diseases [2–4]. In recent years, its indications have been broadened by successful applications in many other neuropsychiatric disorders [5].

As in all surgical operations, this procedure is not without complications and problems. In addition to operative complications, inherent to the technique are hardware- and stimulation-related adverse events, which have increasingly been recognized in the literature as the experience has exponentially grown in the past years [6–10]. Here, we present our experience with 181 patients undergoing DBS placement and discuss strategies to minimize complications and adverse events in the light of this contemporary series and others in the literature.

2. Materials and Methods

2.1. Patients. All patients who had undergone DBS implantation surgery at Diskapi Yildirim Beyazit Training and Research Hospital between 2012 and 2017 were included in this retrospective study. Primary diagnoses and surgical targets were as follows: Parkinson's disease (subthalamic nucleus (STN)), dystonia (globus pallidus interna (GPi)), and essential tremor (ET) (ventral intermediate nucleus of the thalamus (Vim)). All procedures were performed by the same surgical team (MS and HK). Patient data were extracted from electronic health records, patient charts, radiological images, and manufacturers' records of hardware implantations. The DBS devices were primarily St. Jude Medical neuromodulation system (n = 159, all PD patients); however, Medtronic implants were also used in some patients (n = 22, all dystonia and ET patients). All patients were referred by neurologists at the Movement Disorders Clinic, and the DBS treatment decision was made jointly by the multidisciplinary team.

Patient data were analyzed retrospectively for the demographics, operative details, and the occurrence of early postoperative and long-term adverse events. Early perioperative period was defined as the first 30 days after implantation surgery, whereas the long-term as the period beyond the first 30 postoperative days. Surgery-related complications were defined as complications that occurred during or within 30 days of surgery and directly related to the operative procedure itself (hemorrhages, seizures, etc.). Hardware-related complications were defined as adverse events due to the problems in hardware components or body parts (e.g., skin) in direct contact with them, irrespective of the time of occurrence. Complications occurring after the surgery for internal pulse generator (IPG) replacement due to depletion were excluded.

2.2. Surgical Procedure. Preoperative volumetric MR imaging is done one day prior to surgery. On the day of surgery, a stereotactic frame (ZD stereotactic system) is placed, and a patient undergoes volumetric CT imaging which is fused by preoperative volumetric MR images using Brainlab planning software (BrainLab AG). Indirect targeting is completed based on reference to the anterior commissure-posterior commissure line. The trajectory is determined to avoid cortical vessels (using TOF MRA) and, if possible, the lateral ventricle, usually choosing burr hole locations 4-5 cm lateral from the midline at the coronal suture. The surgery is performed under local anesthesia (except for dystonia). Microelectrode recording (MER) was routinely performed for all targets (the number of inserted electrodes ranging 1 to 3). Intraoperative test stimulation was performed to verify the target accuracy and the lack of sustained side effects. The placement of lead extensions and IPG was performed during the same time as lead implantation. Postoperative MRI was routinely performed to verify the location of leads. In addition, cases suspected for intracranial hemorrhage underwent head CT.

2.3. Statistical Analysis. All statistical analyses were performed using the standard statistical software (SPSS Statistics, version 22.0; SPSS Inc.). Risk factors for the occurrence of adverse effects such as patient's age, diagnosis, and date of surgery (early period: 2011–2014; late period: 2014–2017) were analyzed with logistic regression. Student's t-test with equal variances was used to compare age at implantation between patients with adverse effects and those without. Evaluation of differences between patients with adverse events depending on surgical experience was

TABLE 1: Summary of the early postoperative and long-term complications in the current series.

Complication/adverse event	Number	%
Early perioperative complications (<30 days)		
Confusion/alteration in mental status	12	6.6
Hemorrhages	5	2.8
Intracerebral hematoma	4	2.2
Asymptomatic	2	1.1
Symptomatic	2	1.1
Venous hemorrhagic infarct	1	0.6
Ischemic infarct	1	0.6
Seizure	2	1.1
Long-term complications (>30 days)		
Wound complications	13	7.2
Infection/dehiscence	11	6.1
Inflammation/allergy	2	1.1
Hardware-related complications	10	5.5
Lead malposition/migration	2	1.1
Fracture/disconnection (lead or lead extension)	8	4.4
Other complications	2	1.1
Chronic subdural hematoma	2	1.1

performed using the Fisher exact test. A p value below 0.05 was considered as statistically significant.

3. Results

3.1. Demographic Data. One hundred eighty-one patients received 359 new DBS leads in a total of 181 stereotactic procedures. Two hundred and one IPG replacement procedures were performed during the study period. Of the newly implanted leads and IPGs, a majority (85%) were manufactured by St. Jude Medical and others by Medtronic.

One hundred fifty-nine patients suffered from PD, 13 from dystonia, and 9 from essential tremor. Targets were bilateral STN in all PD, bilateral GPi in all dystonia, and bilateral Vim in all ET patients except for three cases in whom unilateral DBS implantation was done. Patients' age ranged from 9 to 74 years (mean: 55.2 ± 11.7 years), and 62.4% were male. A vast majority of the patients (87.8%) had follow-up of more than 1 year (mean: 3.4 ± 1.6 years). No patients have been lost to follow-up.

3.2. Perioperative Events. A summary of perioperative and long-term complications is presented in Table 1. No mortality or permanent morbidity was observed after surgery in this series. Perioperative complications were detected in a total of 17 patients (9.4%). The most common perioperative adverse event was postoperative confusion/delirium, which was seen in 12 patients (6.6%). All these patients had PD and underwent bilateral STN DBS implantation. Confusion resolved in all patients with medication during hospitalization approximately within a week. Two patients (1.1%) had seizures in the early postoperative period and treated with a single antiepileptic drug (AED). They were seizure-free at the 6th month after surgery, and AED was discontinued.

The most common severe complication of surgery was hemorrhage (n = 5, 2.8%), including four cases of intracerebral hematoma (ICH) (2.2%) and one case of venous hemorrhagic stroke (0.6%). In two of them (1.1%), small hematomas along the leads were detected with no or only slight transient symptoms. However, one patient developed moderate paresis in both upper extremities (with a few hours interval) due to slowly evolving hemorrhages, possibly of venous origin, around both leads. The patient was treated conservatively and recovered completely in 6 months. In another patient, an ICH was suspected intraoperatively due to development of left hemiparesis following lead implantation. Immediate postoperative CT scan showed right caudate hematoma with associated intraventricular hemorrhage (Figures 1(a) and 1(b)). Then, the IPG placement was postponed, and the patient was transferred to the ICU where he was treated conservatively. One week later, his symptoms and hematoma largely resolved and he underwent IPG placement with no further problems.

Another patient developed slight right hemiparesis and dysphasia at postoperative day 3. She underwent CT scan which showed a left frontal venous hemorrhagic stroke (Figures 1(c) and 1(d)) evidenced by a relatively large infarct area around a small hemorrhagic component surrounding the lead. This patient recovered completely with no sequelae within 3 months.

One patient with essential tremor had ischemic stroke (0.6%). He became dysphasic immediately after the DBS implantation. Diffusion-weighted MRI showed acute diffusion restriction in the left frontal cortex around the electrode. He was also treated conservatively and recovered completely within a month.

3.3. Long-Term Events. Those events were described as adverse events that occurred later than 30 days after surgery. Wound and hardware complications constituted a majority of those problems.

3.3.1. Wound Complications. Infection was the most common wound complication ($n = 11$, 6.1%) followed by allergic inflammation ($n = 2$, 1.1%). A majority of those cases were self-limiting and managed with antibiotics. Four patients (2.2%) underwent surgery for debridement and repair of wound erosion and/or dehiscence without need for system removal. Scalp reconstruction was performed in two of them. Five patients (2.8%) required removal of the IPG due to infection or recurrent allergic inflammation at the IPG site. Two of them had infections due to trauma; two had abscess formation, and another had sterile seroma around the IPG. Revision surgery was performed depending on the system components affected (either IPG only or IPG + lead extensions).

3.3.2. Hardware Complications. Lead position was found to be suboptimal (>2 mm change from the initial position) in only two patients (1.1%) as confirmed by the comparison of late CT with early postoperative MRI and CT (fused images were used to identify the exact anatomic location of the leads). However, fracture or disconnection of leads or lead extensions (including component malfunction as indicated

by high impedance in the system) was relatively common in this series ($n = 8$, 4.4%). In most cases ($n = 7$), the problem was detected in the lead extensions and only they were replaced. Twiddler's syndrome was diagnosed in one of them. In one patient, iatrogenic injury to the DBS system (during an operation for a trauma in another center) resulted in the revision of the entire system including leads and extensions and IPG revision.

3.3.3. Other Complications and Problems. Two patients suffered from chronic subdural hematomas (cSDHs). One patient presented with speech disturbance and slight right-sided weakness 6 weeks after the DBS implantation. A CT scan showed a cSDH with multiple septations over the left hemisphere (Figure 1(e)). He underwent craniotomy to evacuate hematoma with preservation of DBS hardware (Figure 1(f)). He had an uneventful postoperative course and complete recovery. Another patient had a bilateral cSDH (more on the left than the right) following a mild head trauma 3 years after initial DBS surgery. He underwent an endoscope-assisted evacuation of the cSDH through burr holes, with preservation of DBS hardware. This patient also recovered completely.

3.4. Risk Factors. Potential predictors of adverse events were analyzed. Neither age nor sex was found to be related to risk of complications. Furthermore, there was not significant difference between age of the patients with and without complications (54.9 ± 9.9 versus 56.7 ± 9.3, $p = 0.319$). The primary diagnosis/indication, anatomical target, and device manufacturer did not appear to affect complication rates (20.1% versus 22.7%, $p = 0.776$), except for confusion occurring only in PD patients who underwent bilateral STN DBS. On the contrary, surgical experience seems to be directly related to overall complication rates (early period (2012–2014): 31.0% versus late period (2015–2017): 10.6%, $p = 0.001$). A drastic reduction in complication rates is observed throughout the years (Figure 2).

4. Discussion

Deep brain stimulation surgery has been utilized for the treatment of medically intractable movement disorders for more than two decades. Various clinical series have shown that it is a safe procedure with low rates of complications and adverse events, particularly in the experienced large-volume centers [8–10]. Here, we investigated occurrences and risk factors of surgical and hardware-related complications of DBS surgery performed by a single primary surgeon in a single center.

Early adverse events within 30 days of surgery are generally attributed to surgery [11, 12]. Literature regarding surgical complications in DBS surgery is extensive [6–16]. Incidences of overall short-term or surgery-related complications vary considerably between 2 and 20% depending largely on the definition of adverse events [12–14]. In our series, 11% of the patients experienced early complications. The most common surgical adverse event was perioperative

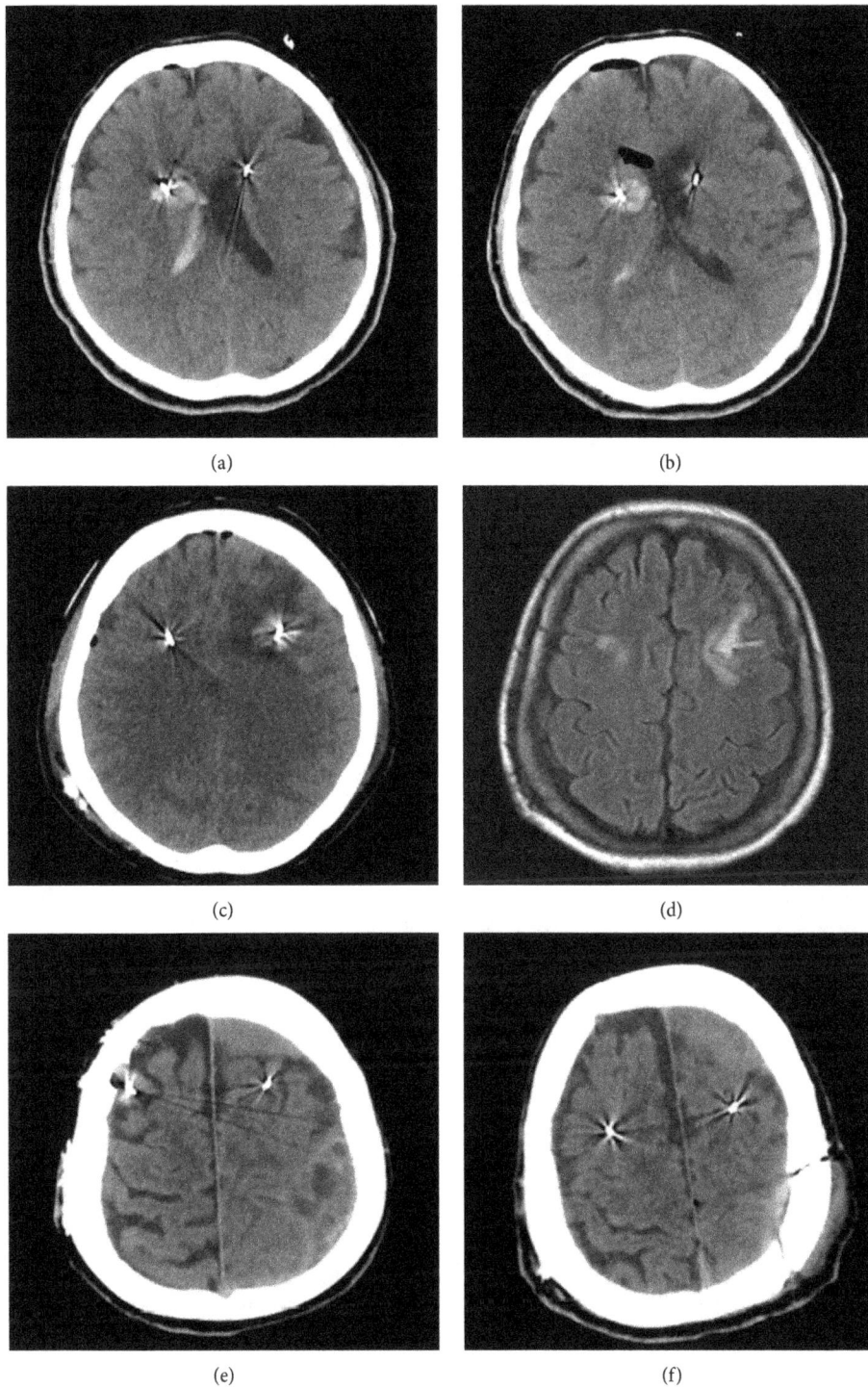

FIGURE 1: Operative complications due to deep brain stimulation surgery. (a, b) Right caudate hematoma with intraventricular hemorrhage. (c) Venous hemorrhagic infarction around the left-sided DBS lead; (d) 6-month follow-up FLAIR MRI. (e, f) Pre- and postoperative images of the left-sided chronic subdural hematoma over the parietal cortex. Note that the frontal component of the cSDH was left intact to avoid iatrogenic injury to the lead.

confusion (6.6%). Various studies have reported similar rates (3–7%) regarding postoperative mental status change, confusion, or delirium [9, 13, 15, 16]. It usually has a favorable course and resolves spontaneously or with adequate medication within a few days of hospitalization.

Seizures are also important complications of DBS surgery [17]. We had two patients (1.1%) having seizures following the hardware implantation. Their seizures were controlled with a single antiepileptic drug, which were discontinued 6 months after the operation. Some groups

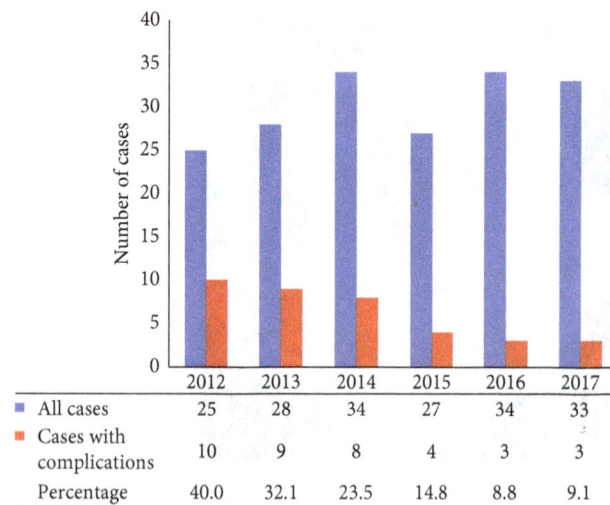

	2012	2013	2014	2015	2016	2017
■ All cases	25	28	34	27	34	33
■ Cases with complications	10	9	8	4	3	3
Percentage	40.0	32.1	23.5	14.8	8.8	9.1

FIGURE 2: Cumulative experience reduces the rate of complications following DBS surgery. The graph shows relatively constant annual caseload but remarkable reduction in the percentage of cases with complications throughout the years.

have reported higher frequencies (4–7%) of postoperative seizures, nevertheless, in virtually all series; their outcomes were quite favorable posing no serious risk for DBS hardware or chronic epilepsy [17–19].

Although it is not very common, hemorrhagic events are the most feared ones of operative complications [20, 21]. Various large series reported incidences of hemorrhagic complications, mainly in the form of intracerebral hemorrhage, between 0.5 and 5% [8, 20–24]. Immediate postoperative imaging could miss an ICH as some ICHs develop or enlarge in delayed fashion [24]. Furthermore, more than half of ICHs are asymptomatic and usually require no intervention at all [8]. However, when large and symptomatic, ICH is one of the most dreadful complications of DBS surgery. Fortunately, such a symptomatic ICH is rarely encountered (<1-2%) and usually has a relatively benign course [6, 8, 25]. In our series, we observed two such cases (1.1%), both of whom recovered fully with medical treatment and observation only. On the contrary, we had to operate on a patient who presented with chronic subdural hematoma 1.5 months after the operation. Extensive membranes within the cSDH prevented us from doing minimally invasive drainage via burr holes [26]; therefore, we had to do craniotomy to evacuate hematoma while preserving the DBS system.

Stroke, both ischemic and hemorrhagic [27], is also a rare but serious complication after DBS implantation. We encountered one ischemic and one venous hemorrhagic infarct during the postoperative course. Both patients have eventually recovered with supportive medical treatment without necessitating hardware removal. Careful planning on preoperative images is a prerequisite for avoidance of vascular injury [23]. We routinely use TOF MRI in image fusion to track vascular structures, while other groups reported successful use of CT angiography [28], contrast-enhanced MRI [25], and SWI-MR venography [29]

separately or in combination for this purpose. Whether microelectrode recording increases the risk of vascular injury is also a matter of debate [22, 23], with some groups reporting a significant drop in the rates of hemorrhagic complications after minimizing or refraining from microelectrode recording [21, 30]. Likewise, we usually perform MER with only two electrodes (between one and three), which could possibly reduce the risk of vascular injury in comparison to multiple microelectrode insertion techniques.

Late complications might be equally, or even more, problematic [31]. Wound complications, particularly infection, comprise the majority of these complications [32, 33]. A recent systematic review of hardware-related complications of DBS surgery revealed that infections (5.12%) were followed by lead migration (1.60%), fracture or failure of the lead or other parts of the implant (1.46% and 0.73%, resp.), IPG malfunctions (1.06%), and skin erosions without infections (0.48%). The authors also indicated that new indications for DBS, including Tourette's syndrome, cluster headache, and refractory partial epilepsy, were found to pose a higher risk of hardware-related infections than established indications such as Parkinson's disease [33]. In our series, slightly higher proportion (10%) of the patients suffered from the wound problems. But fortunately, most of the infections respond to antibiotherapy and/or surgical debridement. Only a fraction of these patients had intractable infection or inflammation that made removal of hardware components (mostly extension and IPG) inevitable. With the advent of new technologies, better surgical techniques, and prevention strategies [10, 34, 35], the rates of such serious wound complications have diminished considerably. Also, alternative medical and surgical strategies have been used to tackle these complications once occurred [36, 37].

Cumulative probability of hardware-related complications increases with longer follow-up durations [6, 38, 39]. In our series, we observed only two instances of lead malposition (1.1%), which represent a lower rate than that in most published series [7, 8, 16, 38, 40]. Of note, we confirm position of leads with routine immediate postoperative MRI and can check for lead migration using image fusion with CT scans during follow-up. On the contrary, fracture or disconnection of lead extensions, but not leads themselves, was more common in our series, possibly due to frequent traumatic incidents that those patients experienced. Replacement of lead extensions and IPG yielded good results in these patients.

Regarding the risk factors for surgical and hardware-related complications, many factors have been determined in previous studies such as advanced age, male sex, primary diagnosis, hypertension, obesity, and anemia [7, 12, 22]. In this series, we did not observe any effect of age, sex, or primary diagnosis on complication rates in line with findings of some other studies [14, 41]. In fact, the only factor we could determine to relate to complications was surgical experience [42, 43]. The fact that both multidisciplinary team dealing with and the protocols used for planning and execution of DBS implantation in our institute have remained unchanged for the past six years makes this series a unique one to demonstrate the impact of accumulating surgical experience in reducing complication rates over the years.

As the indications and availability of DBS expand, the number of patients suffering from its complications will also increase [33]. Therefore, our main goal should be to minimize the complication rates with the help of better technologies and more efficient surgical techniques and, most importantly, to better understand the mechanisms and cumulative experience in the field [43, 44]. This study underscores the critical role of surgical experience in reducing complications and thus shows that instead of making DBS surgery widely available, centralization at several large-volume centers could yield better results with fewer complications.

5. Conclusions

A wide range of complications and adverse events are associated with deep brain stimulation surgery. Neurosurgeons should inform patients about these potential problems and be prepared for them before, during, and after the surgery. Advances in our understanding, related technology, and surgical techniques have led to a dramatic decrease in the rates of these adverse events in the past two decades. Our study affirms the role of cumulative experience at individual centers in reducing the rate of complications. Further studies with larger cohorts are warranted to establish other risk factors and develop better strategies to tackle problems related to DBS surgery.

References

[1] A. L. Benabid, S. Chabardes, J. Mitrofanis, and P. Pollak, "Deep brain stimulation of the subthalamic nucleus for the treatment of Parkinson's disease," *The Lancet Neurology*, vol. 8, no. 1, pp. 67–81, 2009.

[2] S. Miocinovic, S. Somayajula, S. Chitnis, and J. L. Vitek, "History, applications, and mechanisms of deep brain stimulation," *JAMA Neurology*, vol. 70, no. 2, pp. 163–171, 2013.

[3] G. Deuschl, C. Schade-Brittinger, P. Krack et al., "A randomized trial of deep-brain stimulation for Parkinson's disease," *New England Journal of Medicine*, vol. 355, no. 9, pp. 896–908, 2006.

[4] F. M. Weaver, K. Follett, M. Stern et al., "Bilateral deep brain stimulation vs best medical therapy for patients with advanced Parkinson disease: a randomized controlled trial," *JAMA*, vol. 301, no. 1, pp. 63–73, 2009.

[5] N. R. Awan, A. Lozano, and C. Hamani, "Deep brain stimulation: current and future perspectives," *Neurosurgical Focus*, vol. 27, no. 1, p. E2, 2009.

[6] J. Voges, Y. Waerzeggers, M. Maarouf et al., "Deep-brain stimulation: long-term analysis of complications caused by hardware and surgery–experiences from a single centre," *Journal of Neurology, Neurosurgery & Psychiatry*, vol. 77, no. 7, pp. 868–872, 2006.

[7] J. F. Baizabal Carvallo, G. Mostile, M. Almaguer, A. Davidson, R. Simpson, and J. Jankovic, "Deep brain stimulation hardware complications in patients with movement disorders: risk factors and clinical correlations," *Stereotactic and Functional Neurosurgery*, vol. 90, no. 5, pp. 300–306, 2012.

[8] A. J. Fenoy and R. K. Simpson Jr., "Risks of common complications in deep brain stimulation surgery: management and avoidance," *Journal of Neurosurgery*, vol. 120, no. 1, pp. 132–139, 2014.

[9] D. M. Patel, H. C. Walker, R. Brooks, N. Omar, B. Ditty, and B. L. Guthrie, "Adverse events associated with deep brain stimulation for movement disorders: analysis of 510 consecutive cases," *Neurosurgery*, vol. 11, no. 1, pp. 190–199, 2015.

[10] J. Zhang, T. Wang, C. C. Zhang et al., "The safety issues and hardware-related complications of deep brain stimulation therapy: a single-center retrospective analysis of 478 patients with Parkinson's disease," *Clinical Interventions in Aging*, vol. 12, pp. 923–928, 2017.

[11] J. Voges, R. Hilker, K. Bötzel et al., "Thirty days complication rate following surgery performed for deep-brain-stimulation," *Movement Disorders*, vol. 22, no. 10, pp. 1486–1489, 2007.

[12] K. Hu, Z. B. Moses, M. M. Hutter, and Z. Williams, "Short-term adverse outcomes after deep brain stimulation treatment in patients with Parkinson disease," *World Neurosurgery*, vol. 98, pp. 365–374, 2017.

[13] X. Hu, X. Jiang, X. Zhou et al., "Avoidance and management of surgical and hardware-related complications of deep brain stimulation," *Stereotactic and Functional Neurosurgery*, vol. 88, no. 5, pp. 296–303, 2010.

[14] V. Levi, G. Carrabba, P. Rampini, and M. Locatelli, "Short term surgical complications after subthalamic deep brain stimulation for Parkinson's disease: does old age matter?," *BMC Geriatrics*, vol. 15, p. 116, 2015.

[15] E. J. Boviatsis, L. C. Stavrinou, M. Themistocleous, A. T. Kouyialis, and D. E. Sakas, "Surgical and hardware complications of deep brain stimulation. A seven-year experience and review of the literature," *Acta Neurochirurgica*, vol. 152, no. 12, pp. 2053–2062, 2010.

[16] P. K. Doshi, "Long-term surgical and hardware-related complications of deep brain stimulation," *Stereotactic and Functional Neurosurgery*, vol. 89, no. 2, pp. 89–95, 2011.

[17] E. Coley, R. Farhadi, S. Lewis, and I. R. Whittle, "The incidence of seizures following deep brain stimulating electrode implantation for movement disorders, pain and psychiatric conditions," *British Journal of Neurosurgery*, vol. 23, no. 2, pp. 179–183, 2009.

[18] N. Pouratian, D. L. Reames, R. Frysinger, and W. J. Elias, "Comprehensive analysis of risk factors for seizures after deep brain stimulation surgery," *Journal of Neurosurgery*, vol. 115, no. 2, pp. 310–315, 2011.

[19] F. Seijo, S. Alvarez de Eulate Beramendi, E. Santamarta Liébana et al., "Surgical adverse events of deep brain stimulation in the subthalamic nucleus of patients with Parkinson's disease. The learning curve and the pitfalls," *Acta Neurochirurgica*, vol. 156, no. 8, pp. 1505–1512, 2014.

[20] D. K. Binder, G. Rau, and P. A. Starr, "Hemorrhagic complications of microelectrode-guided deep brain stimulation," *Stereotactic and Functional Neurosurgery*, vol. 80, no. 1–4, pp. 28–31, 2003.

[21] J. H. Park, S. J. Chung, C. S. Lee, and S. R. Jeon, "Analysis of hemorrhagic risk factors during deep brain stimulation surgery for movement disorders: comparison of the circumferential paired and multiple electrode insertion methods," *Acta Neurochirurgica*, vol. 153, no. 8, pp. 1573–1578, 2011.

[22] C. A. Sansur, R. C. Frysinger, N. Pouratian et al., "Incidence of symptomatic hemorrhage after stereotactic electrode placement," *Journal of Neurosurgery*, vol. 107, no. 5, pp. 998–1003, 2007.

[23] L. Zrinzo, T. Foltynie, P. Limousin, and M. I. Hariz, "Reducing hemorrhagic complications in functional neurosurgery: a large case series and systematic literature review," *Journal of Neurosurgery*, vol. 116, no. 1, pp. 84–94, 2012.

[24] C. K. Park, N. Y. Jung, M. Kim, and J. W. Chang, "Analysis of delayed intracerebral hemorrhage associated with deep brain stimulation surgery," *World Neurosurgery*, vol. 104, pp. 537–544, 2017.

[25] M. Tonge, L. Ackermans, E. Kocabicak et al., "A detailed analysis of intracerebral hemorrhages in DBS surgeries," *Clinical Neurology and Neurosurgery*, vol. 139, pp. 183–187, 2015.

[26] G. Oyama, M. S. Okun, T. A. Zesiewicz et al., "Delayed clinical improvement after deep brain stimulation-related subdural hematoma. Report of 4 cases," *Journal of Neurosurgery*, vol. 115, no. 2, pp. 289–294, 2011.

[27] T. Morishita, M. S. Okun, A. Burdick, C. E. Jacobson, and K. D. Foote, "Cerebral venous infarction: a potentially avoidable complication of deep brain stimulation surgery," *Neuromodulation: Technology at the Neural Interface*, vol. 16, no. 5, pp. 407–413, 2013.

[28] M. Piacentino, G. Zambon, M. Pilleri, and L. Bartolomei, "Comparison of the incidence of intracranial hemorrhage in two different planning techniques for stereotactic electrode placement in the deep brain stimulation," *Journal of Neurosurgical Sciences*, vol. 57, no. 1, pp. 63–67, 2013.

[29] S. Bériault, A. F. Sadikot, F. Alsubaie, S. Drouin, D. L. Collins, and G. B. Pike, "Neuronavigation using susceptibility-weighted venography: application to deep brain stimulation and comparison with gadolinium contrast," *Journal of Neurosurgery*, vol. 121, no. 1, pp. 131–141, 2014.

[30] I. L. Maldonado, T. Roujeau, L. Cif et al., "Magnetic resonance-based deep brain stimulation technique: a series of 478 consecutive implanted electrodes with no perioperative intracerebral hemorrhage," *Operative Neurosurgery*, vol. 65, no. S6, pp. 196–201, 2009.

[31] G. Fernández-Pajarín, A. Sesar, B. Ares et al., "Delayed complications of deep brain stimulation: 16-year experience in 249 patients," *Acta Neurochirurgica*, vol. 159, no. 9, pp. 1713–1719, 2017.

[32] S. Bjerknes, I. M. Skogseid, T. Sæhle, E. Dietrichs, and M. Toft, "Surgical site infections after deep brain stimulation surgery: frequency, characteristics and management in a 10-year period," *PLoS One*, vol. 9, no. 8, Article ID e105288, 2014.

[33] O. Jitkritsadakul, R. Bhidayasiri, S. K. Kalia, M. Hodaie, A. M. Lozano, and A. Fasano, "Systematic review of hardware-related complications of deep brain stimulation: do new indications pose an increased risk?," *Brain Stimulation*, vol. 10, no. 5, pp. 967–976, 2017.

[34] R. Bhatia, A. Dalton, M. Richards, C. Hopkins, T. Aziz, and D. Nandi, "The incidence of deep brain stimulator hardware infection: the effect of change in antibiotic prophylaxis regimen and review of the literature," *British Journal of Neurosurgery*, vol. 25, no. 5, pp. 625–631, 2011.

[35] J. D. Hilliard, A. Bona, S. Vaziri, R. Walz, M. S. Okun, and K. D. Foote, "Delayed scalp erosion after deep brain stimulation surgery: incidence, treatment, outcomes, and prevention," *Neurosurgery*, vol. 63, no. S1, p. 156, 2016.

[36] M. Lanotte, G. Verna, P. P. Panciani et al., "Management of skin erosion following deep brain stimulation," *Neurosurgical Review*, vol. 32, no. 1, pp. 111–115, 2009.

[37] A. J. Fenoy and R. K. Simpson Jr., "Management of device-related wound complications in deep brain stimulation surgery," *Journal of Neurosurgery*, vol. 116, no. 6, pp. 1324–1332, 2012.

[38] M. Y. Oh, A. Abosch, S. H. Kim, A. E. Lang, and A. M. Lozano, "Long-term hardware-related complications of deep brain stimulation," *Neurosurgery*, vol. 50, no. 6, pp. 1268–1274, 2002.

[39] K. E. Lyons, S. B. Wilkinson, J. Overman, and R. Pahwa, "Surgical and hardware complications of subthalamic stimulation: a series of 160 procedures," *Neurology*, vol. 63, no. 4, pp. 612–616, 2004.

[40] C. Hamani and A. M. Lozano, "Hardware-related complications of deep brain stimulation: a review of the published literature," *Stereotactic and Functional Neurosurgery*, vol. 84, no. 5-6, pp. 248–251, 2006.

[41] M. R. DeLong, K. T. Huang, J. Gallis et al., "Effect of advancing age on outcomes of deep brain stimulation for Parkinson disease," *JAMA Neurology*, vol. 71, no. 10, pp. 1290–1295, 2014.

[42] S. Bhatia, M. Oh, T. Whiting, M. Quigley, and D. Whiting, "Surgical complications of deep brain stimulation. A longitudinal single surgeon, single institution study," *Stereotactic and Functional Neurosurgery*, vol. 86, no. 6, pp. 367–372, 2008.

[43] S. M. Falowski, Y. C. Ooi, and R. A. Bakay, "Long-term evaluation of changes in operative technique and hardware-related complications with deep brain stimulation," *Neuromodulation: Technology at the Neural Interface*, vol. 18, no. 8, pp. 670–677, 2015.

[44] J. F. Baizabal Carvallo, R. Simpson, and J. Jankovic, "Diagnosis and treatment of complications related to deep brain stimulation hardware," *Movement Disorders*, vol. 26, no. 8, pp. 1398–1406, 2011.

8

Impact of Mézières Rehabilitative Method in Patients with Parkinson's Disease: A Randomized Controlled Trial

Teresa Paolucci,[1] Federico Zangrando,[1] Giulia Piccinini,[1] Laura Deidda,[2]
Rossella Basile,[1] Enrico Bruno,[1] Emigen Buzi,[1] Alice Mannocci,[3] Franca Tirinelli,[4]
Shalom Haggiag,[5] Ludovico Lispi,[5] Ciro Villani,[6] and Vincenzo M. Saraceni[1]

[1]Complex Unit of Physical Medicine and Rehabilitation, Policlinico Umberto I Hospital, "Sapienza" University of Rome,
  Piazzale Aldo Moro 5, 00185 Rome, Italy
[2]Department of Physical Medicine and Rehabilitation, San Camillo-Forlanini Hospital, Circonvallazione Gianicolense 87,
  00151 Rome, Italy
[3]Department of Public Health and Infectious Diseases, "Sapienza" University of Rome, Piazzale Aldo Moro 5, 00185 Rome, Italy
[4]Department of Physical Medicine and Rehabilitation, A.C.I.S.M.O.M., San Giovanni Battista Hospital, Via Luigi Ercole Morselli 13,
  00148 Rome, Italy
[5]Department of Neurology, San Camillo-Forlanini Hospital, Circonvallazione Gianicolense 87, 00151 Rome, Italy
[6]University Department of Anatomic, Histologic, Forensic and Locomotor Apparatus Sciences, Section of Locomotor Apparatus
  Sciences, Policlinico Umberto I Hospital, "Sapienza" University of Rome, Piazzale Aldo Moro 5, 00185 Rome, Italy

Correspondence should be addressed to Teresa Paolucci; teresapaolucci@hotmail.com

Academic Editor: Matej Skorvanek

The aim of this study was to assess the efficacy of Mézières method in improving trunk flexibility of the back muscles and balance in patients with Parkinson's disease (PD). *Materials and Methods.* Thirty-six patients were randomized into 2 groups: the Mézières treatment group and the control group (home exercise group). The primary outcome was the improvement in balance per the Berg Balance Scale (BBS) and the trunk flexibility of the back for the anterior flexion trunk test. Also, we evaluated pain, gait balance for the Functional Gait Assessment (FGA), disease-related disability for the Modified Parkinson's Activity Scale and the Unified Parkinson's Disease Rating Scale (UPDRS), the quality of life, and the functional exercise capacity. All the measures were evaluated at baseline ($T0$), at the end of the rehabilitative program ($T1$), and at the 12-week follow-up ($T2$). *Results.* In the Mézières group, the BBS ($p < .001$) and trunk flexion test ($p < .001$) improved significantly at $T1$ and remained the same at $T2$. Between groups, significant changes were reported in FGA ($p = .027$) and UPDRS Total ($p = .007$) at $T1$ and in FGA ($p = .03$) at $T2$. *Conclusion.* The Mézières approach is efficacious in improving the flexibility of the trunk and balance in PD patients.

1. Introduction

The Mézières method was created and is used to restore global mobility of joints and muscles, allowing posture reharmonizing, particularly by changing the alignment of the curves of the spine in the sagittal plane [1–3].

In Parkinson's disease, a tendency to bend or flex forward is the most common change in posture linked to a shortening of the muscular back kinetic chain [4].

It is not known why this occurs, but it may be due to many factors including muscle rigidity, brain changes that control posture, or dystonia. Muscle rigidity and imbalance of bigger muscles overpowering the smaller muscles can cause the patient to bend over [5].

Also, patients with PD usually present with impairments in motor control and sensory integration, causing static and dynamic postural control deficits: balance and gait limitations are not fully addressed by pharmacological agents in PD necessitating a nonpharmacological approach as rehabilitation. The existence of a biased representation of verticality in PD, resulting in severe retropulsion and recurrent falls, has prompted interest in a novel rehabilitation method that is dedicated to the sense of verticality [6, 7]. Most conventional and innovative exercises in PD are focused on the motor features of posture and gait, ignoring the perceptive aspects of balance. Introducing perceptive training to the exercises that are proposed for patients with PD is necessary to reduce their static and dynamic balance limitations and increase the efficacy of rehabilitative programs [8].

PD patients have to rethink their individual motor and cognitive resources to perceive, which is highly challenging in maintaining balance; thus, balance training needs to be specific and progressive [9]. Also, patients with PD have greater postural sway versus healthy subjects, which is significantly associated with a major risk of falls [10].

There is limited evidence about the efficacy of a specific physiotherapy treatment program over another in improving balance in PD. For example, there is weak evidence that freely coordinated resistance training is more effective than balance training [11], whereas complementary physical therapies, such as dancing and martial arts, hydrotherapy, virtual reality and exergaming, motor imagery, action observation, and robotic gait training, appear to have therapeutic benefits, increasing mobility and quality of life in certain patients with PD [12].

A rehabilitative program for PD should be "goal-based" (targeted towards practicing and learning specific activities), but several practice variables (intensity, specificity, and complexity) must be identified, and the program should be tailored to individual patient's characteristics [13].

On this basis, between various postural rehabilitation approaches, the Mézières method [1–3] embodies the characteristics that are useful for balance rehabilitation in patients with PD: establishing alignment according to a vertical reference and reminding the patient of motor imagery in perceiving and imagining body posture. Mézières's concept is a radical shift in therapeutic approaches, valuing relaxation, tonic inhibition, and global and progressive stretching of the muscular regions with imbalances [1–3].

Also, one of the most common nonmotor symptoms of PD is chronic pain. Pain perception is altered in PD, for example, manifesting as elevations in sensory threshold, wherein the interaction between sensory input and motor output modulates pain perception [14]. In particular, lower limb pain is a variant of central pain and merits recognition as a specific nonmotor phenotype in PD [15]. Mézières physiotherapy is effective in other chronic pain conditions, such as low back pain [16], like other muscle stretching programs, such as the Global Postural Reeducation (GPR) approach; both rehabilitation methods have various levels of progression and advocate stretching the antigravity muscle chains with parallel enhancement of the basal tone of antagonistic muscles to improve static and dynamic stability [16]. To date, there is no published article evaluating the Mézières method alone for people with PD. A few studies utilized this technique as part of a rehabilitation program for individuals with PD [17, 18].

Thus, the aim of this research is to determine the efficacy of the Mézières method in trunk flexibility of the back muscles and balance in patients with Parkinson's disease (PD).

2. Materials and Methods

2.1. Design. We conducted a single-blinded, randomized, controlled trial with a 3-month follow-up to determine the efficacy of a rehabilitative protocol, based on the Mézières method, with regard to balance and posture in patients with PD.

Patients of either gender who had been diagnosed with idiopathic PD for at least 1 year were enrolled from the physical medicine and rehabilitation outpatient clinic of Policlinico Umberto I Hospital, Sapienza University of Rome (Italy), and the neurological outpatient clinics of S. Camillo-Forlanini Hospital and S. Giovanni Battista Hospital of Rome (Italy) from July 2015 to January 2016. Eligible patients were referred to a physiatrist who was uninvolved in the study, who provided them with detailed information on the experimental protocol and performed a standardized, blinded assessment at baseline and at the follow-up to minimize potential bias when performing the clinical examination and recording the data. To maintain the blinding and limit the risk of biased observations, the examiner did not have access to the clinical examination results.

To ensure that participants were assessed under similar conditions during each examination session, all procedures were completed within 1-2 h after the patients took their medications, allowing the participants to feel comfortable and safe during the examination and the results to be representative of how a subject performed a similar task in everyday life. All tests were performed during the "on" phase.

Forty-six patients were screened, 36 of whom were enrolled and randomized into 2 groups: the Mézières treatment group (MTG: $N = 17$, median age 66.00 and IQR 18.50) and the home exercise group, or control group (CG: $N = 17$, median age 67.00 and IQR 11.00). A statistician provided a computer-generated randomization list at a ratio of 1 : 1 (MATLAB R2007b®, MathWorks Inc., USA). Sealed envelopes were prepared for each group. Participants received their randomization letter after the first neurological visit was completed.

2.2. Participants. Patients were recruited after a neurological examination and then subjected to a physiatrist visit. The inclusion criteria were a diagnosis of idiopathic PD with a level on the Hoehn and Yahr scale ≤ 3 (in the "on" phase) [19], age between 40 and 80 years, Mini-Mental State Examination score > or = 27 [20, 21], other disabling diseases that affected movement and gait, and steady pharmacological treatment with anti-Parkinson agents for at least 1 month.

The exclusion criteria were cognitive and visual impairments that could prevent the understanding and execution of the tasks; engagement in other rehabilitative study protocols; participation in a conflicting research study; previous treatment with deep-brain stimulation for symptom management; significant neck, shoulder, or back injuries; and uncontrolled hypertension or heart failure, rheumatic diseases, tumors, and other neurological pathologies associated.

This study was approved by the ethical committee of Sapienza University of Rome (registration number 2519/15, ClinicalTrials.gov identifier NCT02891473). All participants signed informed consent forms after receiving detailed information about the study's aims and procedures as per the Declaration of Helsinki. The rights of human subjects involved in the study were protected. This study protocol was developed in accordance with the Consolidated Standards of Reporting Trials (CONSORT) guidelines [22].

2.3. Measures. Sociodemographic and clinical data were collected at baseline. The following outcome measures were assessed at baseline, 1 day before starting the treatment (*T*0), at the end of the rehabilitative program (10 sessions for 5 weeks) (*T*1), and at the 12-week follow-up (*T*2).

The primary outcome was the improvement in balance per the Berg Balance Scale (BBS). The BBS is a widely used instrument that measures static and dynamic balance by assessing performance on functional tasks. It includes a series of 14 simple tasks, each of which is scored from 0 (lowest level of function) to 4 (highest level of function). The maximum score is 56 (41–56 = low risk of falls; 21–40 = medium risk; 0–20 = high risk) [23].

Pain was evaluated using the Visual Analog Scale (VAS). The VAS is a simple and sensitive instrument that enables patients to express their pain intensity as a numerical value. Patients were asked to mark the point that corresponded to their perceived pain intensity on a 10 cm line (0 = absence of pain, 10 = most severe pain) [24].

Balance and posture were evaluated using the Functional Gait Assessment (FGA) scale, which measures walking balance activity and was developed from the Dynamic Gait Index (DGI) to improve reliability and decrease the ceiling effect. The FGA consists of 10 items, each of which is scored on a 3-point scale from 0 (severe impairment) to 3 (normal deambulation). The highest possible score is 30 (normal gait function) [25].

Parkinson's disease symptoms and disease-related disability were recorded using the Modified Parkinson's Activity Scale (MPAS) and Unified Parkinson's Disease Rating Scale (UPDRS). The MPAS comprises 14 items in 3 domains: chair transfer, gait akinesia, and bed mobility. Scores range from 0 (dependent) to 4 (normal), and the highest possible score is 56 [26, 27].

The UPDRS is the most commonly used scale for monitoring the course of the disease in PD patients. It consists of 6 parts, with questions on mental state, behavior and mood, ADL, motor functions, complications of advanced disease, stage of disease per the Hoehn and Yahr scale, and abilities in everyday life activities per the Schwab and England scale. The UPDRS is based on a metric scale, ranging from 0 (no disability) to 147 (severe disability) points [28].

In this study, we measured scores for UPDRS Part I: Mentation, Behaviour, and Mood; UPDRS Part II: Activities in Daily Living; UPDRS Part III: Motor Examination; and UPDRS Part IV: Complications of Therapy and Total.

Trunk flexibility was analyzed by evaluating the anterior flexion of the trunk, measuring the finger-to-floor distance.

Functional exercise capacity was measured through the six-minute walking test (SMWT). It is a practical simple test that measures the distance that a patient can quickly walk on a flat, hard surface in a period of 6 minutes. The individual is requested to walk as far as possible in six minutes [29].

The Short Form 36 Health Survey (SF-36) was administered to collect information about health status and quality of life. The SF-36 is a generic multidimensional health questionnaire that collects practical, reliable, and valid information about patients' functional health and well-being [26]. It comprises 36 items and two overall indices that summarize the physical and mental health. Physical health includes 4 domains: physical functioning (PF), physical role functioning (PR), bodily pain (BP), and general health perceptions (GH). Emotional health, instead, includes the domains of mental health (MH), social role functioning (SF), emotional role functioning (RE), and vitality (VT). Each scale ranges from 0 to 100 (worst and best health state, resp.). The questionnaire has already been validated in Italian [30, 31].

2.4. Rehabilitative Intervention. For both groups, the treatment program aimed to prevent and reduce pain; the exercise was not performed if it increased pain or put the patient's safety at risk. In both programs, the level of the exercises could be adjusted step by step, based on the observations of the physician and physical therapist and the patient's needs.

2.4.1. Mézières Treatment Group. The Mézières treatment regimen consisted of 3 postures that could be adapted to each patient, depending on his/her needs to correct variations in the dorsal curve and promote diaphragmatic breathing. The first objective was to recover extensibility of the hypertonic muscle groups and, in particular, those in the low back muscular chain: the paravertebral muscles and latissimus dorsi.

During execution of the postures, the physiotherapist always required the patient to follow the rhythm of his breathing, perceive the alignment of his trunk, and imagine the posture that was instructed before executing it (to promote motor imagery and attention with respect to the movement) to constantly raise awareness of the posture that was requested. All postures obligatorily passed the alignment in the same plane of 3 levels: the occipital bone, the scapula (7th thoracic vertebra), and the sacrum. Each session comprised a sequence of postures that were held to maintain rigorous and prolonged tension of the muscle groups that were considered to be responsible for the lordosis, internal rotations, and inspiratory thoracic block.

The treatment was administered over sessions twice per week for 5 weeks. Each session lasted for 1 hour and was performed by a trained physical therapist on this method. The Mézières method is usually performed for 1 or 2 sessions per week in adults, with often more than 60 minutes per session, and always twice for children. In this study, we administered 2 sessions per week, also considering that the rehabilitation guidelines for PD recommend more than one session per week [32, 33].

First Posture. The patient was placed in the supine position and aligned, based on his vertical line (occipital bone, 7th dorsal vertebra, and sacrum), to recreate the correct curves according to the lordosis of the spine. Then, the patient was

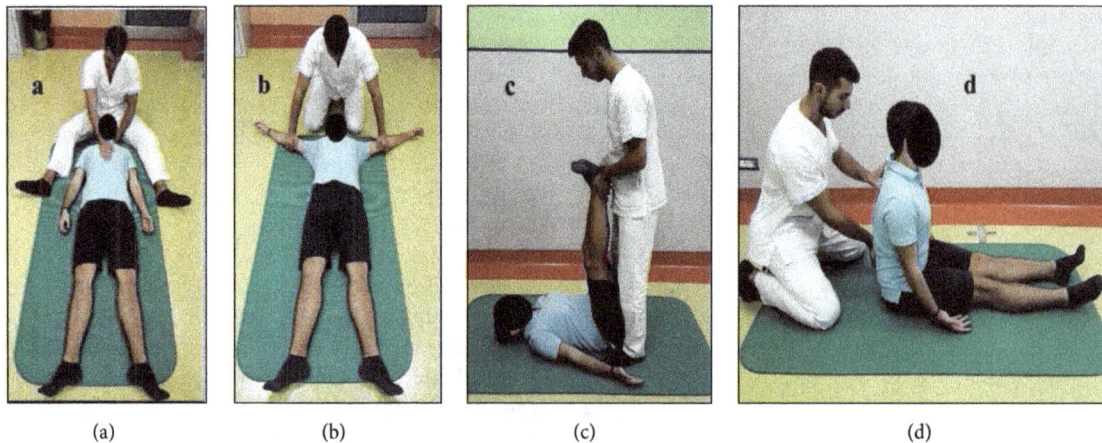

FIGURE 1: Mézières rehabilitative method: (a) the first posture, (b) the second posture, (c) the third posture, and (d) variation of the third posture. Source of pictures: UOC Physical Medicine and Rehabilitation Unit, Policlinico Umberto I Hospital, Rome, Italy.

asked to first breathe normally and then perform diaphragmatic breathing, focusing on the use of the rectus abdominis to lower the last thoracic ribs.

Second Posture. The patient was placed in the supine position, with the upper limbs abducted to 120° (to obtain maximum elongation of the latissimus dorsi). This posture aims to achieve bilateral passive stretching of the latissimus dorsi. The patient was also requested to change this position by performing isometric contraction of the latissimus dorsi in the maximum elongation permitted. The physical therapist corrected the patient's raising of the last thoracic ribs on expiration.

Third Posture. The patient was placed in the supine position, with the lower extremities elevated at more than 90° of flexion of the hips and the knees extended or flexed, resting on a wall or supported by the physiotherapist, if the patient was unable to reach this position with the knees extended. This exercise aimed to stretch the posterior muscle chain and especially the latissimus dorsi. Extreme care was taken to prevent inspiratory block.

The patient was sitting with his back leaning against the floor and aligned to his vertical line (occipital bone, 7th dorsal vertebra, and sacrum) to recreate the correct curves according to the lordosis of the spine. Then, the patient was asked to perform normal breathing and then diaphragmatic breathing to activate the rectus femoris (physiological position of the pelvis) and rectus abdominis (lumbar lordosis control). In some patients, it was possible to progress and vary the third posture in the sitting position, but this position was tiring for many patients and difficult to maintain properly (Figure 1).

At the end of the 10 Mézières treatment sessions, the patients kept their normal activities and then were assessed again in the 12-week follow-up.

For ethical reasons, we did not consider a third group in the waiting list without any rehabilitation treatment.

2.5. Home Exercise Group. The home exercises consisted of simple exercises that were performed by the patients at home,

accompanied by spontaneous or diaphragmatic breathing, if necessary, based on the PD guidelines [32, 33].

While performing each exercise, the patient was allowed to use a support if he felt insecure. No exercise had to exacerbate or cause pain during its execution. The exercise program progressed in difficulty. The treatment was administered over 10 sessions, twice per week for 5 weeks. Each session lasted for 1 hour. The patients kept their normal activities and then were assessed again in the 12-week follow-up.

First, each patient attended two single 1-hour educational sessions with the physical therapist to learn how to perform the exercises at home well. Each patient was contacted by telephone every 2 weeks to monitor his/her adherence to the rehabilitation program. A booklet with an explanation and pictures of the exercises was given to the patients: each exercise was proposed for 3 sets of 10 repetitions with a rest period of at least 2 minutes between sets.

  (i) *From Weeks 1 to 2.* Supine position: (i) spontaneous and diaphragmatic breathing, (ii) rolling on the side, (iii) bridge exercise, by lifting the legs alternately, (iv) prone position: exercise of the greeting from a crouching position, (v) in quadruped position, pelvic tilt exercises, and (vi) in crawling position for cross-pattern exercise.

 (ii) *From Weeks 2 to 3 (Add Exercises with respect to the First Few Weeks).* (vii) In the cavalier servant position: moving the legs alternately, (viii) in sitting position: hands-knees cross-pattern, (ix) upright: legs slightly apart, semilateral squats, and (x) sitting position: rotation of the trunk to the right and left.

(iii) *From Weeks 3 to 5 (Add Exercises).* (xi) From sitting to standing position without support: postural step exercises, (xii) upright, semifront squats, moving the legs alternately, (xiii) upright position: back semisquat exercises, moving the legs alternately, (xiv) upright, semisquat exercises with the trunk leaning against the wall and interposition of a soft ball, both legs together, and (xv) upright, exercises with a stick for rotation and flexion-extension movements of the shoulder.

In the treatment program, the number of repetitions was allowed to increase. When possible, it was recommended that the exercises be performed in open spaces. Each rehabilitation session was preceded by a preparation phase of 15 minutes of low-intensity aerobic impact exercises (as walking) with adequate rest phases if necessary.

2.6. Sample Size Calculation. Given that there are no similar studies in the literature that used the Mézières method in PD, data from our preliminary pilot study of 10 patients with PD, considering the same inclusion and exclusion criteria previously described in the Materials and Methods, was used to determine the sample size, based on the following assumptions: (i) average risk of falling in patients with Parkinson's disease > 40 on the Berg Balance Scale and specifically a medium score of 45 for BBS with a standard deviation (SD) = 4 and (ii) an increase of 4 points after Mézières treatment on the Berg Balance Scale for minimal clinically important change per the literature [34]. A significance level of 95% was considered for a power of 80% by two-tailed t-test. The sample size was increased by 10% to account for eventual dropouts. The number of patients enrolled in each group was thus 17 (http://www.statisticalsolutions.net/pssTtest_calc.php). We did not publish the data of this preliminary study.

2.7. Data Analysis. A nonparametric approach was used, based on the low number of patients and assessing the normality using Shapiro-Wilk's test. The descriptive statistics were expressed as median with interquartile range (IQR) for quantitative variables according to the nonparametric approach and as percentage and tables of frequencies for qualitative ones. To compare the control versus treatment groups at the 3 times ($T0$, $T1$, and $T2$), nonparametric Mann–Whitney test was performed. To determine the significance difference in each group between $T0$, $T1$, and $T2$, we applied the nonparametric Friedman test for intragroup assessment and Wilcoxon test with Bonferroni correction (0.017 is the critical level of significance of Bonferroni correction, i.e., 0.05/3). The effect size for the post hoc significant comparisons was calculated. The chi-squared test was used to determine whether there is a significant difference between the categorical variables. If the expected counts were below 5, Fisher's Exact Test was applied as an alternative to a chi-square test for 2×2 tables.

SPSS version 20.0 (Chicago, IL, USA) was used for the statistical analyses. All tests were two-tailed with a level of significance of $p < .05$.

3. Results

3.1. Sample Characteristics. Forty-six patients were assessed for eligibility ($N = 46$), of whom 10 were excluded for not meeting the inclusion criteria ($N = 6$) or refusal to participate ($N = 4$). Ultimately, 36 patients ($N = 36$) were enrolled and randomly assigned into 2 groups: $n = 17$ in the Mézières group (Group A) and $n = 19$ in the control

TABLE 1: Characteristics of the groups with regard to gender, age, and BMI (body mass index) at baseline (median and IQR, frequencies, and percentages).

Characteristics	Control group ($N = 17$)		Mézières group ($N = 17$)		
Qualitative variables	N	%	N	%	p
Gender					
Female	8	47	7	41	
Male	9	53	10	59	.95
Continuous variables	Median	IQR	Median	IQR	p
Age	67.00	11.00	66.00	18.50	.65
BMI	25.00	5.50	25.80	2.90	.99

IQR: interquartile range; BMI: body mass index.

group (Group B). Two subjects left the control group during the treatment between $T0$ and $T1$ due to family issues; their data were not included in the statistical analysis because the evaluation scales had not been completed in whole parts (flowchart, Figure 2). Thus, the data for 17 patients per group were analyzed.

Baseline scores ($T0$) did not differ significantly with regard to age, BMI, gender, or evaluation scale scores, except for UPDRS Total. The patient characteristics at baseline are listed in Table 1, with a median age of 66 years (IQR = 18.50) for Group A and 67 (IQR = 11.00) for Group B; the median UPDRS Total scores were 44 (IQR: 0.00) and 44 (IQR: 7.50), respectively ($p = .04$). The mean of the duration of the disease was 3 ± 1.2 years with a Hoehn and Yahr score of 1.5 ± 0.8 for all the sample without statistically significant differences if we consider the two groups separately.

3.2. Between Groups. By Mann–Whitney test, there were nonsignificant differences between Groups A and B except for FGA ($p = .027$ at $T1$ and $p = .03$ at $T2$) and for UPDRS Total ($p = .007$ at $T1$) (Figures 3, 4, and 5 and Tables 2 and 3).

3.3. In the Mézières Group. By Wilcoxon signed-rank test with Bonferroni correction, we observed significant changes in the Mézières-treated group between $T0$ and $T1$ for VAS ($p < .001$, $p = .004$), RP-SF36 ($p = .019$), Berg Balance Scale ($p = .004$), trunk flexion test ($p < .001$), FGA ($p < .001$), SMWT ($p = .002$), MPAS ($p < .001$), and UPDRS Total ($p < .001$) (UPDRS Part I, $p =< .001$; Part II, $p = .001$; and Part III, $p \leq .001$). In addition, these statistically significant results were maintained at the follow-up ($T2$) except for RP-SF36 (Table 4).

3.4. In the Control Group. In the control group (Table 5), we noted significant changes between $T0$ and $T1$ for trunk flexion test ($p = .013$), FGA ($p = .001$), SMWT ($p = .012$), MPAS ($p = .001$), and UPDRS Total ($p < .001$) (UPDRS Part II, $p = .028$; Part IV, $p = .010$). At the follow-up ($T0$ versus $T2$), the results were significant for FGA, MPAS, and UPDRS Total (Part IV) and trunk flexibility. No adverse events or side effects in each intervention group were observed.

TABLE 2: Quality of life: comparison between groups at $T1$ (end of treatment) and $T2$ (follow-up) for SF-36 and subscales.

SF-36	Group B (N = 17) T1		Group A (N = 17) T1		p^*	Group B (N = 17) T2		Group A (N = 17) T2		p^*
	Median	IQR	Median	IQR		Median	IQR	Median	IQR	
PF	75.00	35.00	75.00	15.00	.40	85.00	45.00	85.00	25.00	.90
PR	100.00	50.00	100.00	50.00	.50	100.00	45.00	100.00	37.50	.60
BD	61.00	31.00	62.00	30.00	.20	61.00	50.00	72.00	43.50	.20
GH	47.00	25.00	47.00	24.80	.60	45.00	33.00	42.00	37.50	.90
VT	50.00	15.00	57.50	15.00	.10	50.00	23.00	55.00	27.50	.50
SF	75.00	25.00	87.30	25.00	.60	87.50	23.00	87.50	25.00	.75
RE	66.70	34.00	100.00	33.80	.20	100.00	50.00	100.00	33.40	.40
MH	64.00	28.00	70.00	28.00	.30	60.00	28.00	76.00	22.00	.10

$^*p$ value by Mann–Whitney test. Group A: Mézières treatment group; Group B: control group. IQR: interquartile range; SF-36: Short Form 36 Health Survey; PF: physical functioning; PR: physical role functioning; BD: bodily pain; GH: general health perceptions; VT: vitality; SF: social role functioning; RE: emotional role functioning; MH: mental health.

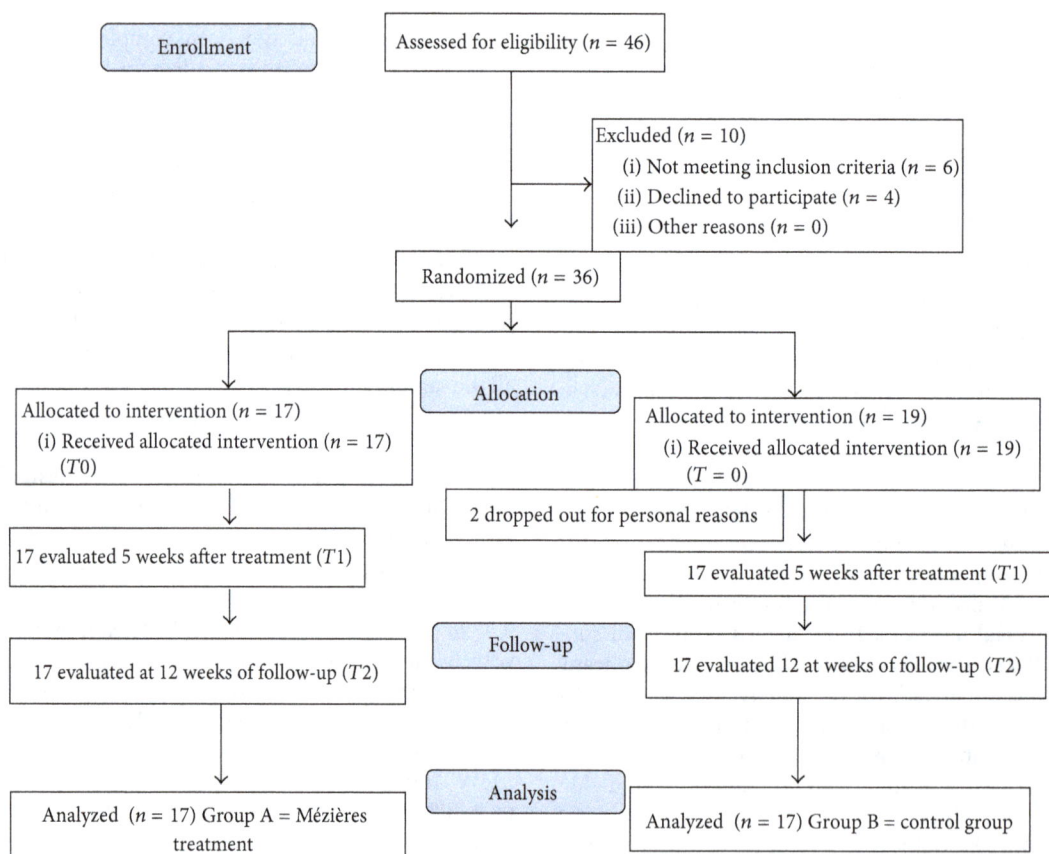

FIGURE 2: CONSORT flow diagram.

4. Discussion

The primary aim of our study was to determine the efficacy of the Mézières method in improving trunk flexibility of the back muscles and balance in patients with Parkinson's disease (PD). With regard to the risk of falls per the BBS and dynamic balance per the FGA, the Mézières approach resulted to be effective as the control group rehabilitative program. In particular, the Mézières treatment effected greater improvements on the BBS, which were stable at the follow-up, versus the control group. Even in the early stages of PD, alignment of the spine curves in the sagittal plane is lost, and the perception [31] of the body midline [32] adversely affects postural control, increasing postural instability and the risk of falls.

TABLE 3: Scales and clinical evaluation: comparison between groups at $T1$ (end of treatment) and $T2$ (follow-up) for pain, mobility (balance and posture), and disability (median and IQR, $p < .05$).

Scales and clinical evaluations	Group B (N = 17) T1		Group A (N = 17) T1		p^*	Group B (N = 17) T2		Group A (N = 17) T2		p^*
	Median	IQR	Median	IQR		Median	IQR	Median	IQR	
VAS (cm)	2.50	4.00	2.00	4.00	.20	3.00	4.00	1.50	4.00	.80
BBS	50.00	8.00	54.50	8.00	.10	50.00	5.00	51.50	7.50	.28
Trunk flexion test (cm)	10,00	10.00	10.00	11.80	.60	10.00	10.00	8.00	12.00	.50
FGA	11.00	6.00	9.00	6.00	**.027**	11.00	5.00	8.00	6.00	**.03**
MPAS	40.00	10.00	47.00	13.50	.30	40.00	10.00	47.00	14.00	.11
SMWT (min)	500.00	145.00	510.00	171.30	.90	500.00	130.00	480.00	277.50	.80
UPDRS Part I	7.00	7.00	7.50	7.00	.3	8.00	8.00	5.00	7.00	.05
UPDRS Part II	7.00	6.00	6.00	5.80	.40	6.00	8.00	6.00	5.50	.90
UPDRS Part III	11.00	8.00	10.00	8.50	.50	13.00	10.00	10.00	9.00	.20
UPDRS Part IV	2.00	5.00	2.50	4.80	.98	0.99	5.00	3.00	4.50	.95
UPDRS Total	49.00	0.00	49.00	12.50	**.007**	37.00	0.00	38.00	20.00	.80

* p value by Mann–Whitney test. Group A: Mézières treatment group; Group B: control group. IQR: interquartile range. VAS: Visual Analog Scale; BBS: Berg Balance Scale; FGA: Functional Gait Assessment; MPAS: Modified Parkinson's Activity Scale; SMWT: six-minute walking test; UPDRS: Unified Parkinson's Disease Rating Scale.

TABLE 4: Scales and clinical evaluation: comparison for Mézières group at 3 evaluation times.

Scales and clinical evaluations for Mézières group	T0		T1		T2		p^a	WB[b]	Effect size[c]
	Median	IQR	Median	IQR	Median	IQR			
VAS (cm)	3.0	4.0	2.0	4.0	1.5	4.0	**<0.001**	1; 2	0.24; 0.25
SF-36 PF	72.5	33.8	75.0	15.0	85.0	25.0	0.014	—	
SF-36 RP	75.0	72.5	100.0	50.0	100.0	37.5	**0.002**	1	0.24
SF-36 BP	62.0	22.3	62.0	30.0	72.0	43.5	0.598	—	
SF-36 GH	42.0	29.0	47.0	25.0	42.0	37.5	0.198	—	
SF-36 VT	50.0	15.0	57.5	15.0	55.0	27.5	0.018	—	
SF-36 SF	75.0	34.8	87.3	25.0	87.5	25.0	**0.002**	—	
SF-36 RE	100.0	66.7	100.0	33.8	100.0	33.0	0.368	—	
BBS	48.0	6.5	54.5	8.0	51.5	7.5	**<0.001**	1; 2	0.25; 0.25
Trunk flexion test (cm)	10.5	10.0	10.0	11.8	8.0	12.0	**<0.001**	1; 2	0.24; 0.24
FGA	15.0	5.0	9.0	6.0	8.0	6.0	**<0.001**	1; 2	0.24; 0.24
MPAS	37.0	16.0	47.0	13.5	47.0	14.0	**<0.001**	1; 2	0.24; 0.24
SMWT (min)	467.5	157.5	510.0	171.3	480.0	277.5	0.081	—	
UPDRS Part I	10.0	9.0	7.5	7.0	5.0	7.0	**<0.001**	1; 2	0.24; 0.24
UPDRS Part II	9.0	6.8	6.0	5.8	6.0	5.5	**<0.001**	1; 2	0.24; 0.24
UPDRS Part III	15.5	10.8	10.0	8.5	10.0	9.0	**<0.001**	1; 2	0.24; 0.24
UPDRS Total	38.0	20	27.0	12.5	23.0	16.5	**<0.001**	1; 2	0.24; 0.24

Group A: Mézières treatment group; IQR: interquartile range; VAS: Visual Analog Scale; SF-36: Short Form 36 Health Survey; PF: physical functioning; PR: physical role functioning; BD: bodily pain; GH: general health perceptions; VT: vitality; SF: social role functioning; RE: emotional role functioning; MH: mental health; BBS: Berg Balance Scale; FGA: Functional Gait Assessment; MPAS: Modified Parkinson's Activity Scale; SMWT: six-minute walking test; UPDRS: Unified Parkinson's Disease Rating Scale. [a]p value obtained by Friedman test. [b]Significant comparisons obtained by Wilcoxon test with Bonferroni correction (0.017 is the critical level of significance of Bonferroni correction, i.e., 0.05/3: 1 → $T0$ versus $T1$; 2 → $T0$ versus $T2$; 3 → $T1$ versus $T2$; not significant comparisons). [c]Effect size for the post hoc comparison. Bold font indicates statistical significance.

TABLE 5: Scales and clinical evaluation: comparison for the control group at 3 evaluation times.

Scales and clinical evaluations for the control group	T0		T1		T2		p^a	WB[b]	Effect size[c]
	Median	IQR	Median	IQR	Median	IQR			
VAS (cm)	3.0	3.5	2.5	4.0	3.0	4.0	0.226	—	
SF36-PF	75.0	45.0	75.0	35.0	85.0	45.0	0.108	—	
SF36-RP	50.0	75.0	100.0	50.00	100.0	45.0	0.054	—	
SF-36 BP	61.0	20.0	61.0	31.00	61.0	50.0	0.497	—	
SF-36 GH	42.0	13.0	47.0	25.00	45.0	33.0	0.627	—	
SF-36 VT	50.0	10.0	50.0	15.00	50.0	23.0	0.412	—	
SF-36 SF	75.0	38.0	75.0	25.00	87.5	23.3	0.575	—	
SF-36 RE	66.7	66.7	66.7	34.00	100.0	50.0	0.430	—	
SF-36 MH	68.0	16.0	64.0	28.00	60.0	28.0			
BBS	48.00	7.0	50.0	8.00	50.0	5.0	0.360	—	
Trunk flexion test (cm)	11.00	10.0	10.0	10.00	10.0	10.0	0.012	1; 2	0.26; 0.26
FGA	14.00	6.0	11.0	6.00	11.0		**<0.001**	1; 2	0.26; 0.26
MPAS	37.00	13.0	40.0	10.00	40.0	10.0	**<0.001**	1; 2	0.26; 0.26
SMWT (min)	480.00	120.0	500.0	145.00	500.0	130.0	**0.005**	1	0.26
UPDRS Part I	10.00	8.0	7.0	7.00	8.0	8.0	0.262	—	
UPDRS Part II	9.00	9.0	7.0	6.00	6.0	8.0	0.050	—	
UPDRS Part III	14.00	10.0	11.0	8.00	13.0	10.0	0.064	—	
UPDRS Part IV	4.00	6.0	2.0	5.00	0.9	5.0	**<0.001**	1; 2	0.26; 0.26
UPDRS Total	44.00	0.0	49.0	0.00	37.0	0.0	**0.015**	2	

Group B: control group; IQR: interquartile range; SF-36: Short Form 36 Health Survey; PF: physical functioning; PR: physical role functioning; BD: bodily pain; GH: general health perceptions; VT: vitality; SF: social role functioning; RE: emotional role functioning; MH: mental health; VAS: Visual Analog Scale; BBS: Berg Balance Scale; FGA: Functional Gait Assessment; MPAS: Modified Parkinson's Activity Scale; SMWT: six-minute walking test; UPDRS: Unified Parkinson's Disease Rating Scale. [a]p value obtained by Friedman test. [b]Significant comparisons obtained by Wilcoxon test with Bonferroni correction (0.017 is the critical level of significance of Bonferroni correction, i.e., 0.05/3: 1 → T0 versus T1; 2 → T0 versus T2; 3 → T1 versus T2; not significant comparisons). [c]Effect size for the post hoc comparison. Bold font indicates statistical significance.

Some authors proposed that proprioceptive training, based on the association of many intensive perceptive stimuli during cognitive tasks that are focused on improving proprioception and sensory integration, helps patients with PD restore correct midline perception and, in turn, improves postural control in realigning the body midline to the gravitational axis [33].

The Mézières approach focuses on "awareness" of the trunk, alignment of the sagittal curves of the column, and alignment of the trunk, even with respect to the midline of the body. Thus, proprioception rehabilitation [3] approaches that solely target kinesthetic awareness [32] are recommended for patients with PD.

The Mézières method appears to synthesize both of these rehabilitative aspects to improve the kinesthetic and proprioceptive awareness of the trunk. When a patient adopts his posture during the progression of the Mézières regimen, the physical therapist always asks him to feel the stretch and recognize the position of the body and focus on the tactile sensations of the body surface. In our research, we have directed Mézières realignment towards the stretching of the latissimus dorsi, which is considered primarily to be a muscle with actions at the shoulder but also potentially makes contributions to lumbar spine function. Other data have demonstrated how this muscle affects spine-stabilizing

ability to generate force and change length throughout the spine and ranges of motion in the shoulder [34].

Jobst et al. reported that patients learn to generate internal adaptive strategies with a combination of active posture correction strategies [35]; thus, working on the representation of the midline and motor imagery of the trunk to bridge perception and movement can yield new functional strategies for patients with PD to generate an internal cue reference. Further, in our study, dynamic balance and gait, as assessed with the FGA, improved significantly in the treatment group at T1 and T2.

Conversely, external cues might require less effort and attention by the patient, and their use during more complex activities could facilitate walking [36]. The Global Postural Reeducation (GPR), as a physical therapy approach that is based on the stretching of antigravity muscle chains with parallel enhancement of the basal tone of antagonistic muscles, improves the kinematic gait pattern, as evidenced by the recovery of the flexion amplitude of the knee and thigh [37]. Further, in the Mézières group, we observed significant differences in FGA, with good improvement in walking balance activity.

A secondary goal of our study was to determine the impact of Mézières rehabilitation exercises on pain, but we found no significant differences between the groups at

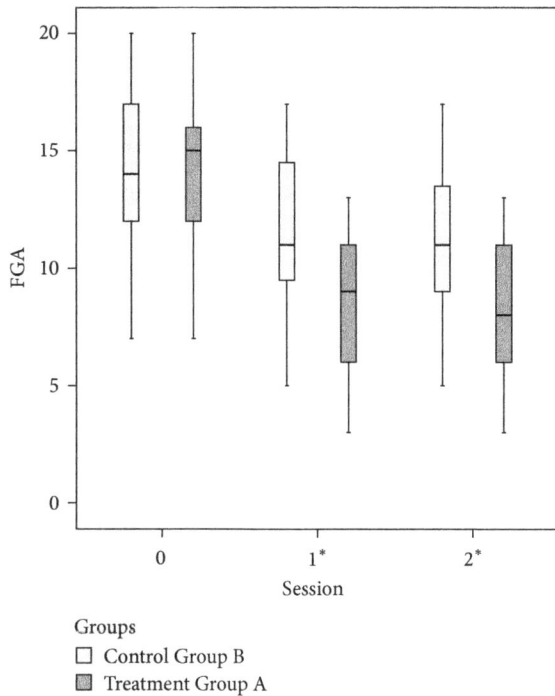

FIGURE 3: Functional Gait Assessment (FGA) at baseline (=T0) and at the end of treatment (=T1) and follow-up (=T2) for the two groups. The symbol "*" indicates $p < .05$.

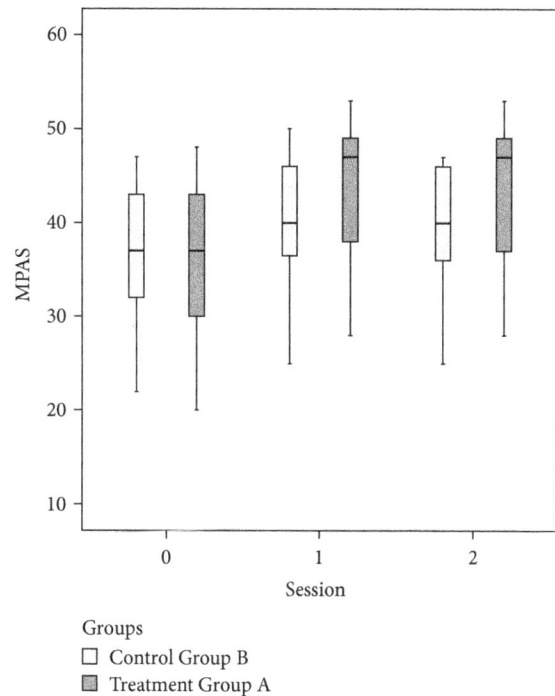

FIGURE 5: Modified Parkinson's Activity Scale (MPAS) at baseline (=T0) and at the end of the treatment (=T1) and follow-up (=T2) for the two groups.

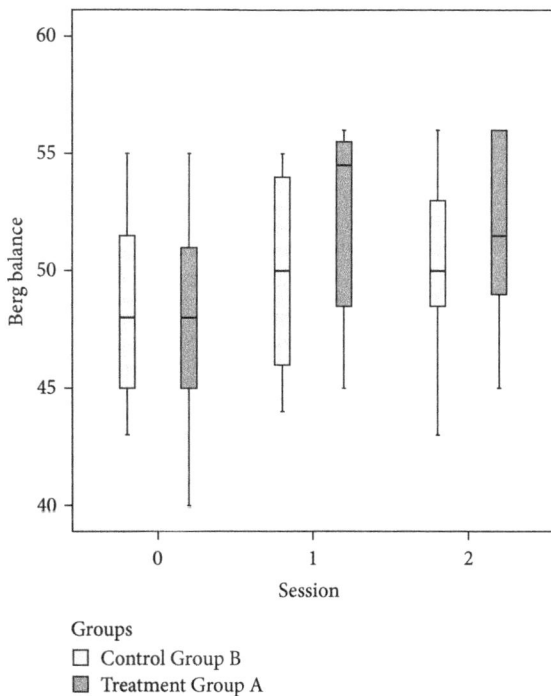

FIGURE 4: Berg Balance Scale (BBS) at baseline (=T0) and at the end of the treatment (=T1) and follow-up (=T2) for the two groups.

the three observation times; thus, both approaches were efficacious with respect to pain relief.

Chronic pain, a distressing nonmotor symptom that is experienced by up to 85% of people with PD, is correlated with disease-related factors, such as rigidity, and daily living activities, such as coexisting musculoskeletal and neuropathic pain conditions. Moreover, exercise can activate the dopaminergic and nondopaminergic pain inhibitory pathways, suggesting that exercise helps modulate the experience of pain in PD [38]. Thus, the Mézières approach, through generating awareness of the body, could introduce the patient to a new experience without pain through exercise.

Chronic pain can negatively affect the HRQoL of patients with PD [17], necessitating additional rehabilitation focused on non-motor-associated pain. In our study, the control group did not experience any improvement in the quality of life, whereas in the Mézières group, RP and VT scores improved, Thus, we hypothesize that the presence of a physical therapist who guided the session has a positive impact on the perception of quality of life, leading the patient to feel more cared for and with a higher takeover of the patient together with the improvement in physical functioning and improvement in UPDRS.

Another important factor in the treatment group was the sequence of exercises. We first proposed a more postural and global approach to the body, closely related to control of the body midline and the recovery of the extensibility of the hypertonic muscle groups, in particular those of the low back muscular chain, such as the latissimus dorsi. Then, the subsequent steps were based on more dynamic exercises to ensure patient safety and autonomy in his motor habits.

Exercising consistently and beginning regular exercise were associated with small but significant positive effects on HRQoL and mobility over 2 years [39].

Strengths. This study was designed as a randomized controlled trial, which is considered the ideal methodological approach for evaluating the efficacy of a specific intervention. This study is the first trial to assess the efficacy of the Mézières approach in improving balance stability and trunk flexibility in PD.

Limits. The findings might be applicable only to patients who experience mild-to-moderate symptoms and are healthy enough to perform the exercises. Thus, alternative interventions might be necessary for patients who present with more advanced symptoms. All evaluations and rehabilitation treatments were performed during the "on" phase.

5. Conclusions

Outcomes of the present study suggest that the Mézières approach is efficacious in improving balance in patients with PD and is also a good exercise program with a focus on increasing flexibility in the stronger muscles; strengthening of back muscles can help keep the spine erect in PD patients. It would be desirable in the future to include the Mézières method in multidisciplinary rehabilitation protocols for patients with Parkinson's disease with longer rehabilitation sessions.

Acknowledgments

The authors would like to thank the Physiotherapy School of San Camillo-Forlanini Hospital, "Sapienza" University of Rome, in particular Dr. Carla Siccardi (FT) and Dr. Cecilia Pizzi (FT). The authors would also like to thank all the patients who participated in this study.

References

[1] F. Mézières, *La Révolution en Gymnastique Orthopédique*, Vuibert, Paris, France, 1949.

[2] L. O. Coelho, "Anti-fitness ou o Manifesto Anti-Desportivo," Introdução ao Conceito de Reeducação Postural, Quinta do Conde: Editora Contra Margem, 2008.

[3] F. Mézières, *Originalité de la Méthode Mézières*, Maloine, Paris, France, 1984.

[4] E. Melamed and R. Djaldetti, "Camptocormia in Parkinson's disease," *Journal of Neurology*, vol. 253, no. 7, p. VII/16, 2006.

[5] S. Wunderlich, I. Csoti, K. Reiners et al., "Camptocormia in Parkinson's disease mimicked by focal myositis of the paraspinal muscles," *Movement Disorders*, vol. 17, no. 3, pp. 598–600, 2002.

[6] C. Curtze, J. G. Nutt, P. Carlson-Kuhta, M. Mancini, and F. B. Horak, "Objective gait and balance impairments relate to balance confidence and perceived mobility in people with parkinson disease," *Physical Therapy in Sport*, vol. 96, no. 11, pp. 1734–1743, 2016.

[7] L. Mathevon, N. Leroux, C. Piscicelli et al., "Sustainable reduction in the occurrence of falls in a Parkinson's patient who followed an intensive and specific rehabilitation program to recalibrate verticality perception," *Annals of Physical and Rehabilitation Medicine*, vol. 59, supplement e65, 2016.

[8] T. Paolucci, G. Morone, A. Fusco et al., "Effects of perceptive rehabilitation on balance control in patients with Parkinson's disease," *NeuroRehabilitation*, vol. 34, no. 1, pp. 113–120, 2014.

[9] B. Leavy, K. S. Roaldsen, K. Nylund, M. Hagströmer, and E. Franzén, ""Pushing the limits": Rethinking motor and cognitive resources after a highly challenging balance training program for parkinson disease," *Physical Therapy in Sport*, vol. 97, no. 1, pp. 81–89, 2017.

[10] F. Doná, C. C. Aquino, J. M. Gazzola et al., "Changes in postural control in patients with Parkinson's disease: a posturographic study," *Physiotherapy (United Kingdom)*, vol. 102, no. 3, pp. 272–279, 2016.

[11] C. Schlenstedt, S. Paschen, A. Kruse, J. Raethjen, B. Weisser, and G. Deuschl, "Resistance versus balance training to improve postural control in Parkinson's disease: a randomized rater blinded controlled study," *PLoS ONE*, vol. 10, no. 10, Article ID e0140584, 2015.

[12] P. Alves Da Rocha, J. McClelland, and M. E. Morris, "Complementary physical therapies for movement disorders in parkinson's disease: a systematic review," *European Journal of Physical and Rehabilitation Medicine*, vol. 51, no. 6, pp. 693–704, 2015.

[13] G. Abbruzzese, R. Marchese, L. Avanzino, and E. Pelosin, "Rehabilitation for Parkinson's disease: current outlook and future challenges," *Parkinsonism & Related Disorders*, vol. 22, supplement 1, pp. S60–S64, 2016.

[14] A. Fil, R. Cano-de-la-Cuerda, E. Muñoz-Hellín, L. Vela, M. Ramiro-González, and C. Fernández-de-las-Peñas, "Pain in Parkinson disease: a review of the literature," *Parkinsonism & Related Disorders*, vol. 19, no. 3, pp. 285–294, 2013.

[15] V. C. J. Wallace and K. R. Chaudhuri, "Unexplained lower limb pain in Parkinson's disease: A phenotypic variant of "painful Parkinson's disease"," *Parkinsonism & Related Disorders*, vol. 20, no. 1, pp. 122–124, 2014.

[16] P. Lawand, I. Lombardi Júnior, A. Jones, C. Sardim, L. H. Ribeiro, and J. Natour, "Effect of a muscle stretching program using the global postural reeducation method for patients with chronic low back pain: A randomized controlled trial," *Joint Bone Spine*, vol. 82, no. 4, pp. 272–277, 2015.

[17] M. Capecci, C. Serpicelli, L. Fiorentini et al., "Postural rehabilitation and kinesio taping for axial postural disorders in Parkinson's disease," *Archives of Physical Medicine and Rehabilitation*, vol. 95, no. 6, pp. 1067–1075, 2014.

[18] V. Agosti, C. Vitale, D. Avella et al., "Effects of Global Postural Reeducation on gait kinematics in parkinsonian patients: a pilot randomized three-dimensional motion analysis study," *Neurological Sciences*, vol. 37, no. 4, pp. 515–522, 2016.

[19] M. M. Hoehn and M. D. Yahr, "Parkinsonism: onset, progression and mortality.," *Neurology*, vol. 17, no. 5, pp. 427–442, 1967.

[20] M. F. Folstein, S. E. Folstein, and P. R. McHugh, ""Mini mental state". A practical method for grading the cognitive state of patients for the clinician," *Journal of Psychiatric Research*, vol. 12, no. 3, pp. 189–198, 1975.

[21] D. Ferrazzoli, P. Ortelli, R. Maestri et al., "Does cognitive impairment affect rehabilitation outcome in Parkinson's disease?" *Frontiers in Aging Neuroscience*, vol. 8, article no. 192, 2016.

[22] D. Moher, S. Hopewell, K. F. Schulz et al., "CONSORT 2010 explanation and elaboration: updated guidelines for reporting parallel group randomised trials," *International Journal of Surgery*, vol. 10, no. 1, pp. 28–55, 2012.

[23] K. O. Berg, S. L. Wood-Dauphinee, and J. L. Williams, "Measuring balance in the elderly: validation of an instrument," *Canadian Journal of Public Health*, vol. 83, supplement 2, pp. S7–S11, 1992.

[24] E. C. Huskisson, "Measurement of pain," *The Lancet*, vol. 2, no. 7889, pp. 1127–1131, 1974.

[25] D. M. Wrisley, G. F. Marchetti, D. K. Kuharsky, and S. L. Whitney, "Reliability, internal consistency, and validity of data obtained with the functional gait assessment," *Physical Therapy in Sport*, vol. 84, no. 10, pp. 906–918, 2004.

[26] A. Nieuwboer, W. De Weerdt, R. Dom, K. Bogaerts, and G. Nuyens, "Development of an activity scale for individuals with advanced Parkinson disease: Reliability and 'on-off' variability," *Physical Therapy in Sport*, vol. 80, no. 11, pp. 1087–1096, 2000.

[27] S. H. J. Keus, A. Nieuwboer, B. R. Bloem, G. F. Borm, and M. Munneke, "Clinimetric analyses of the Modified Parkinson Activity Scale," *Parkinsonism & Related Disorders*, vol. 15, no. 4, pp. 263–269, 2009.

[28] S. Fahn, R. L. Elton, and Members of the UPDRS Development Committee, "Unified Parkinson's disease rating scale," in *Recent Developments in Parkinson's Disease*, S. Fahn, C. D. Marsden, D. B. Calne, and M. Goldstein, Eds., pp. 153–163, Macmillan Healthcare Information, Florham Park, NJ, USA, 1987.

[29] R. J. A. Butland, J. Pang, E. R. Gross, A. A. Woodcock, and D. M. Geddes, "Two-, six-, and 12-minute walking tests in respiratory disease," *British Medical Journal*, vol. 284, no. 6329, pp. 1607-1608, 1982.

[30] J. E. Ware, "SF-36 health survey update," *The Spine Journal*, vol. 25, no. 24, pp. 3130–3139, 2000.

[31] G. Apolone and P. Mosconi, "The Italian SF-36 Health Survey: translation, validation and norming," *Journal of Clinical Epidemiology*, vol. 51, no. 11, pp. 1025–1036, 1998.

[32] W. J. Weiner, "An algorithm (decision tree) for the management of Parkinson's disease (2001): treatment guidelines," *Neurology*, vol. 58, no. 1, article 8, pp. 156-157, 2002.

[33] S. Keus, M. Munneke, M. Graziano et al., "European Physiotherapy Guideline for Parkinson's Disease," Parkinson Net and the Royal Dutch Society for Physical Therapy (KNGF), 2014.

[34] D. Donoghue and E. K. Stokes, "How much change is true change? The minimum detectable change of the Berg Balance Scale in elderly people," *Journal of Rehabilitation Medicine*, vol. 41, no. 5, pp. 343–346, 2009.

[35] E. E. Jobst, M. E. Melnick, N. N. Byl, G. A. Dowling, and M. J. Aminoff, "Sensory perception in Parkinson disease," *JAMA Neurology*, vol. 54, no. 4, pp. 450–454, 1997.

[36] T. Manzoni, P. Barbaresi, F. Conti, and M. Fabri, "The callosal connections of the primary somatosensory cortex and the neural bases of midline fusion," *Experimental Brain Research*, vol. 76, no. 2, pp. 251–266, 1989.

[37] M. Morrone, S. Miccinilli, M. Bravi et al., "Perceptive rehabilitation and trunk posture alignment in patients with Parkinson disease: a single blind randomized controlled trial," *European Journal of Physical and Rehabilitation Medicine*, vol. 52, no. 6, pp. 799–809, 2016.

[38] M. E. Gerling and S. H. M. Brown, "Architectural analysis and predicted functional capability of the human latissimus dorsi muscle," *Journal of Anatomy*, vol. 223, no. 2, pp. 112–122, 2013.

[39] M. G. Ceravolo, "Rehabilitation goals and strategies in Parkinson's disease," *European Journal of Physical and Rehabilitation Medicine*, vol. 45, pp. 205–208, 2009.

9

Cognitive Impact of Deep Brain Stimulation on Parkinson's Disease Patients

Raja Mehanna,[1] Jawad A. Bajwa,[2] Hubert Fernandez,[3] and Aparna Ashutosh Wagle Shukla[4]

[1]University of Texas Health Science Center, Houston, TX, USA
[2]Parkinson's, Movement Disorders and Neurorestoration Program, National Neuroscience Institute, King Fahad Medical City, Riyadh, Saudi Arabia
[3]Center for Neurological Restoration, Cleveland Clinic, Cleveland, OH, USA
[4]University of Florida, Gainesville, FL, USA

Correspondence should be addressed to Raja Mehanna; raja.mehanna@uth.tmc.edu

Academic Editor: Carlo Colosimo

Subthalamic nucleus (STN) or globus pallidus interna (GPi) deep brain stimulation (DBS) is considered a robust therapeutic tool in the treatment of Parkinson's disease (PD) patients, although it has been reported to potentially cause cognitive decline in some cases. We here provide an in-depth and critical review of the current literature regarding cognition after DBS in PD, summarizing the available data on the impact of STN and GPi DBS as monotherapies and also comparative data across these two therapies on 7 cognitive domains. We provide evidence that, in appropriately screened PD patients, worsening of one or more cognitive functions is rare and subtle after DBS, without negative impact on quality of life, and that there is very little data supporting that STN DBS has a worse cognitive outcome than GPi DBS.

1. Introduction

Parkinsonism is defined as bradykinesia with rest tremor or rigidity. Parkinson's disease (PD) is the most frequent cause of parkinsonism and defined by the presence of parkinsonism in the absence of exclusion criteria [1]. With a prevalence of 1 to 2% above the age of 60 years [2], it typically develops between the ages of 55 and 65 years. Pathologically, PD is associated predominantly with the loss of dopaminergic neurons in the substantia nigra. However other brainstem neurons also degenerate in PD, likely contributing to nonmotor impairment [3]. Indeed, PD is a complex syndrome with motor, dermatological, autonomic, neurobehavioral, sensory, and special sense disorders [4]. Many studies have also reported cognitive changes, including impairments in executive functions, language, memory, vision, and psychomotor speed [5–8]. In a cohort comparing 115 patients with newly diagnosed PD to 70 healthy controls, for example, Muslimović et al. [8] reported statistically worse performance in PD patients in most cognitive measures, particularly attention/concentration and executive functions, with 24% of newly diagnosed PD patients (versus 4% of controls) meeting the criteria for cognitive impairment.

Deep brain stimulation (DBS) of the subthalamic nucleus (STN) or the globus pallidus pars interna (GPi) improves quality of life and decreases motor complications in PD and has been approved as such by the Food and Drug Administration in the USA since 2002 [9]. Ablative surgery or DBS of the ventral intermediate (Vim) nucleus of the thalamus is being used for essential and other secondary causes of tremor. However, because it does not address the other cardinal motor symptoms of PD, Vim DBS is rarely used for that disorder [10]. Patients considered for DBS should undergo a thorough multidisciplinary preoperative screening, including a neuropsychological test to rule out dementia or psychiatric comorbidities that could be a contraindication to surgery, in order to avoid implanting poor candidates that will either not benefit enough from DBS or poorly tolerate it [11–15]. However, the cognitive impact of DBS in appropriately selected PD patients is unclear, with various studies producing conflicting results as we will see below. We here endeavor to review the available literature on this subject.

We will first review the available studies on the impact of STN and GPi DBS on each of the following cognitive domains: language, executive function, attention and concentration, memory, visual function, psychomotor and processing speed, and global cognition. We will then review more specifically controlled studies as well as studies directly comparing the cognitive impacts of STN and GPi DBS.

2. Methods

Preliminary literature search was conducted through PubMed. Keywords used were "deep brain stimulation", "parkinson", and "cognition". The reference lists of relevant articles were also inspected to locate any potential cited articles that address cognition following STN or GPi DBS. Since Vim DBS is rarely used for PD, and with most of the data on DBS in PD patients stemming from studies on the STN and GPi, studies on Vim DBS in PD patients were not included in our search.

The research terms were intentionally broad to capture as many studies as possible. Studies were reviewed if they were published in the English language and met our minimum inclusion criteria: (1) patients with idiopathic PD who underwent STN or GPi DBS, (2) reporting neuropsychological data after DBS surgery, (3) using at least one standardized neuropsychological instrument, and (4) including at least five subjects followed for a mean of at least 3 months postoperatively.

3. Results

3.1. Cognitive Changes after DBS. 72 studies totaling 2,410 STN DBS patients and 702 GPi DBS patients were reviewed (Tables 1 and 2). Among these, only 20 included statistical correction for multiple analyses or did not require correction because of the statistical method used [16–35], 20 had a control arm formed by PD patients who did not undergo DBS (nonsurgically treated PD patients) [16, 17, 21, 24, 32, 33, 36–49], and 9 compared outcomes between GPi and STN DBS patients [26, 34, 47, 50–55]. All these studies were reviewed with post hoc corrections for multiple analyses when required.

We will first briefly summarize studies that investigated the cognitive outcomes related to STN and GPi and were not designed to directly compare the two targets. There were 62 such studies, totaling 1,913 STN DBS patients and 165 GPi DBS patients.

Our findings are summarized below (Tables 1 and 2).

3.1.1. Language. In the reviewed studies, language was most often assessed using the Boston Naming Test and the subtest Similarities of the Wechsler Adult Intelligence Scale III (WAIS-III), phonemic fluency, and sematic fluency.

(1) STN. Statistically significant worsening in one or more language functions was reported in 27 studies, most often a decrease in fluency, while 3 studies [24, 29, 46] reported improvement in at least one measure of language. There was no significant change in at least one assessed measure of language in 38 studies (Table 1), 21 of which reported no change in any measure of language.

Among the studies reporting worsening, it is unclear if one [56] was corrected for multiple analyses by its authors and, if not, whether such a correction would change the conclusions. Another study [57] was not corrected for multiple analyses, and a post hoc correction was not possible due to the lack of reported *p* value, making it unclear if such a correction would have made the reported worsening statistically not significant.

In all these studies, cognitive outcomes after surgery were compared to baseline preoperative performance (Table 1). In addition, 9 studies compared language performance ON and OFF stimulation [29, 31, 38, 49, 58–62]. After correcting for multiple analyses, a study from Daniele et al. [58] reported worsening of letter verbal fluency compared to the preoperative assessment only at 3 months, when the stimulation was OFF, but not at 6 or 12 months, when the stimulation was ON. This might suggest that a decline in verbal fluency was either more pronounced in the early postoperative stages or attenuated by stimulation. On the other hand, after correction for multiple analyses, Pillon et al. [60] reported no worsening of fluency at 3 months but worsening at 12 months after implant with stimulation ON or OFF. Since patients were assessed ON medications in the study earlier study [58] and, and OFF medication in latter [60], this might suggest a positive synergistic effect of medication and stimulation on fluency. Castner et al. [31] assessed 8 patients ON and OFF stimulation at least 4 months after STN DBS and found that stimulation increased errors in word generation suggesting that STN stimulation might affect the ability to select from many competing lexical alternatives during word generation. In contrast, Silveri et al. [29] studied 12 patients 8 years after STN DBS implant and found an improvement in performance (accuracy and response time) when STN DBS was ON compared to OFF, with less semantic errors, suggesting STN DBS might improve lexical search. The 5 other studies [38, 49, 59, 61, 62] could not elicit any statistical difference between ON and OFF stimulation states.

Most recently, Tröster et al. [35] reported on a total of 136 STN DBS patients followed for 12 months after surgery, divided between 101 receiving constant current stimulation immediately after surgery and 35 starting activation 3 months after surgery. The cognitive assessment at 3 months did indicate some decrease in attention and language even before the device was turned on, with additional deterioration from stimulation. However, the study showed an overall good safety profile of constant current STN DBS.

With regard to the timing of a potential decline in language, Funkiewiez et al. [22] reported worsening of category fluency and total score of fluency at 1 and 3 years compared to baseline, without any further worsening between the two time points.

A parasagittal trajectory for electrode implantation was suggested as a cause of language worsening in some studies [60, 63], as activation of the paracingulate and cingulate sulci

TABLE 1: Studies assessing cognitive change in PD patients after STN DBS.

Author, year	N	F/u (mo)	Controlled	Status of stimulation/medication at cognitive assessment	Improved cognitive measure(s)	Worsened cognitive measure(s)	Unchanged cognitive measure(s)
Alberts et al., 2008 [18]	8	N/A	No	UL, BL, ON, OFF/ON	None	E	None
Alegret et al., 2001 [75]	15	3	No	ON/OFF	None	None	E, PS, L, M, V
Ardouin et al., 1999 [25]	49	3–6	No	ON/inconstant	E	L	GC, E, PS
Asahi et al., 2014 [27]	11	12	No	Unspecified	None	None	GC, A/C, M, L, V
Castelli et al., 2006 [56]	72	15	No	ON/-	E	L	E, L, M
Castelli et al., 2007 [90]	19	17	No	ON/ON	None	L	E, V, M, L,
Castelli et al., 2010 [39]	27	12	Yes	ON/ON	None	L	E, A/C, M, L
Castner et al., 2007 [30]	18	At least 4	No	ON and OFF/ON	A/C	None	A/C
Castner et al., 2008 [31]	8	At least 4	No	ON and OFF/ON	None	L	L
Cilia et al., 2007 [16]	20	12	Yes	ON/ON	None	L	GC, L, E, A/C
Contarino et al., 2007 [91]	11	60	No	ON/ON	None	None	L, V, M, E
Daniele et al., 2003 [58]	20	12	No	ON or OFF/ON	None	L	GC, L, E, A/C, M
De Gaspari et al., 2006 [21]	12	12	Yes	ON/ON	None	L	L, GC, E
Dujardin et al., 2001 [92]	9	3	No	ON/ON	None	None	GC, E, M, PS, L
Erola et al., 2006 [93]	19	12	No	ON/ON	None	L	GC, E, PS
Fasano et al., 2010 [57]	16	96	No	ON/ON	None	E, L, M	GC, M, E, L
Fraraccio et al., 2008 [62]	15	16	No	ON and OFF/ON	None	A/C	E, A/C, M, L, V, CG
Funkiewiez et al., 2003 [94]	50	12[a]	No	ON/OFF	None	None	GC, E
Funkiewiez et al., 2004 [22]	70	36	No	ON/69% OFF	None	L	GC, E, M, PS
Gironell et al., 2003 [36]	8	6	Yes	ON/ON	None	None	L, E, A/C, M, V, PS
Hälbig et al., 2004 [59]	12	16	No	ON and OFF/ON	None	None	PS, M, GC, E, L
Heo et al., 2008 [95]	46	12	No	ON/ON	None	None	GC, A/C, M, L, E
Hershey et al., 2004 [67]	24	7[b]	No	ON and OFF/OFF	None	E	None
Hilker et al., 2004 [37]	8	4	Yes	ON/-	M	None	GC, E, L, A/C, M, V
Jahanshahi et al., 2000 [63]	7	12	No	ON and OFF/OFF	E, A/C, PS	M	None
Kim et al., 2014 [78]	103	42[b]	No	ON/ON	None	GC, but similar incidence to incidence of PDD	None
Krack et al., 2003 [20]	42	60	No	ON/ON	None	None	GC, E

TABLE 1: Continued.

Author, year	N	F/u (mo)	Controlled	Status of stimulation/medication at cognitive assessment	Improved cognitive measure(s)	Worsened cognitive measure(s)	Unchanged cognitive measure(s)
Krugel et al., 2014 [96]	14	N/A	No	ON/ON	None	None	L
Lhommée et al., 2012 [97]	63	3	No	ON/ON	None	L	GC, E
Limousin et al., 1998 [70]	24	12	No	ON/OFF	None	None	E, L, V, PS
Moretti et al., 2003 [46]	9	12	Yes	ON/ON	L	L, E	E, L, A/C, M, V
Moro et al., 1999 [98]	7	9	No	ON/ON	None	None	GC, E, L, M
Morrison et al., 2004 [38]	17	3	Yes	ON and OFF/OFF	None	None	L, A/C, M, E, V
Rukmini Mridula et al., 2015 [48]	50	23[b]	Yes	ON/ON	None	None	GC, A/C
Page and Jahanshahi, 2007 [68]	12	N/A	No	ON and OFF/ON	PS, A/C	None	PS, A/C, E
Perozzo et al., 2001 [69]	20	6	No	ON/ON and OFF	None	None	E, A/C, M, PS
Phillips et al., 2012 [49]	11	13.8[b]	Yes	ON and OFF/ON and OFF	None	None	L
Pillon et al., 2000 [60]	63	12	No	ON and OFF/75% OFF	None	L	E, PS, L, M
Rothlind et al., 2007 [50]	15	21	No	ON/ON	None	L	A/C, E, L, V, M
Rothlind et al., 2015 [47]	84	6	Yes	ON/ON	None	E, A/C, PS (see text)	E, M, A/C, L, PS
Sáez-Zea et al., 2012 [44]	9	6	Yes	ON/ON	None	L, A/C	A, M, V, E, L
Saint-Cyr et al., 2000 [99]	11	12	No	ON/ON	None	L	E, L, M, A/C, V
Saint-Cyr and Albanese, 2006 [82]	99	6	No	ON/ON	None	L, E	E, L, A/C, M, PS
Schüpbach et al., 2005 [23]	37	60	No	ON/ON	None	CG, E	None
Silveri et al., 2012 [29]	12	96	No	ON and OFF/ON	L	None	None
Smeding et al., 2011 [33]	105	12	Yes	ON/ON	None	GC, E, L, V, M, A/C	L, A/C
Smeding et al., 2006 [43]	99	6	Yes	ON/ON	None	L, A/C	L, M, V, A/C
Tang et al., 2015 [73]	27	12	No	ON/ON	M	L	GC, M, V, A/C, E, L
Tremblay et al., 2015 [28]	8	At least 7 wks	No	OFF DBS and then ON DBS/unspecified med status	None	L	L
Trepanier et al., 2000 [87]	9	6	No	ON/ON	None	None	A/C, M, V, L, E
Whelan et al., 2003 [24]	5	3	No	ON/ON	L	L	None

TABLE 1: Continued.

Author, year	N	F/u (mo)	Controlled	Status of stimulation/medication at cognitive assessment	Improved cognitive measure(s)	Worsened cognitive measure(s)	Unchanged cognitive measure(s)
Williams et al., 2011 [40]	19	24	Yes	ON/ON	None	None	GC, M, E, A/C, L, V, PS
Witt et al., 2004 [61]	23	12	No	ON and OFF/ON	None	None	L, E, GC
Witt et al., 2008 [42]	60	6	Yes	ON/ON	None	A/C	GC, E, L, A/C
Witt et al., 2013 [41]	31	6	Yes	ON/ON	None	None	GC, A/C, L
Yágüez et al., 2014 [100]	30	9	No	ON/ON	None	L, M	GC, M, L, V, E
York et al., 2008 [17]	23	6	Yes	ON/ON	None	M	GC, E, A/C, M, L, V, PS
Zangaglia et al., 2009 [45]	32	36	Yes	ON/ON	None	L	GC, M, E, A/C
Zangaglia et al., 2012 [32]	30	96	Yes	ON/ON	None	L	GC, M, E, A/C

PD: Parkinson's disease; STN: subthalamic nucleus; N: number of patients; mo: months; A/C: attention/concentration; E: executive; GC: global cognition; L: language; M: memory; PS: psychomotor/processing speed; V: visual. [a]Median; [b]mean. *Note.* Multiple tests were performed for each domain in each study, and often a few of these showed a difference while other tests assessing the same domain did not. This explains why the same domain might appear more than once and under different results for the same study. Adapted from Mehanna [101] with permission from the author.

TABLE 2: Studies assessing cognitive change in PD patients after GPi DBS.

Author, year	N	F/u (mo)	Controlled	Status of stimulation/medication at cognitive assessment	Improved cognitive measure(s)	Worsened cognitive measure(s)	Unchanged cognitive measure(s)
Ardouin et al., 1999 [25]	13	3–6	No	ON/inconsistent	E	L	GC, E, PS
Jahanshahi et al., 2000 [63]	6	12	No	ON and OFF/OFF	None	None	E, A/C, PS, M,
Pillon et al., 2000 [60]	13	12	No	ON and OFF/75% OFF	None	None	E, PS, L, M
Trépanier et al., 2000 [87]	4	6	No	ON/ON	None	None	A/C, M, V, L, E
Rothlind et al., 2007 [50]	14	21	No	ON/ON	None	L	A/C, E, L, V, M
Fields et al., 1999 [74]	6	5	No	ON/ON	M	None	GC, E, A/C, V, L, M
Tröster et al., 1997 [66]	9	3	No	ON/ON	None	V, L	GC, E, A/C, V, M, L
Tröster et al., 2017 [35]	136	12	No	ON/not specified	None	L, A/C	GC, A/C, E, M
Vingerhoets et al., 1999 [76]	20	3	No	ON/ON	None	None	M, V, E, PS
Rothlind et al., 2015 [47]	80	6	Yes	ON/ON	None	E, A/C	E, M, A/C, L, PS

PD: Parkinson's disease; GPi: globus pallidus interna; N: number of patients; mo: months; A/C: attention/concentration; E: executive; GC: global cognition; L: language; M: memory; PS: psychomotor/processing speed; V: visual. *Note.* Multiple tests were performed for each domain in each study, and often a few of these showed a difference while other tests assessing the same domain did not. This explains why the same domain might appear more than once and under different results for the same study. Adapted from Mehanna [101] with permission from the author.

was visible on fMRI during word generation [64]. On the other hand, STN DBS might impact the cognitive circuit involved in language as decreased perfusion in the ventral caudate nucleus, anterior cingulate cortex, and left dorsolateral prefrontal cortex (DLPFC) is visible on single photon emission computed tomography (SPECT) in patients with decreased fluency after STN DBS [16]. A more recent study comparing brain positron emission tomographies (PET) in STN DBS patients with and without decreased fluency reported metabolism change in the right middle occipital gyrus, right fusiform gyrus, and right superior temporal gyrus when deficit in phonemic fluency was detected. Decline in semantic fluency however was associated with metabolic changes in the left inferior precentral/postcentral gyrus and the left inferior parietal lobule. Thus, different brain areas were involved in post-DBS deficits in phonemic or semantic fluency in this study, and none of them were frontal areas involved in cognitive functions [65].

On the other hand, Silveri et al. [29] hypothesized that the observed improvement in response time was secondary to improvement of motor components and increased accuracy was due to restoration of the corticostriatal circuits involved in selection processes of a target word among different alternatives.

(2) GPi. Decline in one or more measures of language, most often fluency, was reported in 3 studies totaling 36 patients followed up to 21 months after GPi DBS [25, 50, 66]. While one of these [66] reported this deterioration in both DBS and ablation of GPi, suggesting a consequence of the procedure itself rather than stimulation, this study was not corrected for multiple analyses, and a post hoc correction was not possible due to the lack of reported *p* value, making it unclear if such a correction would have made the reported worsening statistically not significant. In addition, fluency was the only worsened measure of language in 2 of these studies [50, 66].

Three other studies totaling 97 patients followed up to 12 months reported no change in any measure of language (Table 2).

3.1.2. Executive Function. Executive functions were most often assessed using the Wisconsin Card Sorting Test, Trail Making Test Part (Trails B), and Stroop Color-Word Test (Stroop Color-Word).

(1) STN. Worsening in at least one measure of executive function was reported in 8 studies. However, one [57] of these was not corrected for multiple analyses, and a post hoc correction was not possible due to the lack of reported *p* value, making it unclear if such a correction would have made the reported worsening statistically not significant. On the other hand, improvement was reported in 3 studies and no statistical difference in any assessed measures of executive function was reported in 36 studies (Table 1).

Executive function ON and OFF stimulations were compared in 10 studies [18, 38, 58–63, 67, 68]. Spatial delayed response was worse with stimulation ON under a high but not low memory load condition in 2 studies [18, 67]. In particular, Alberts et al. [18] reported further worsening in

executive functions when multitasking in bilateral compared to unilateral stimulation. On the other hand, one study [63] reported improvement of frontal executive functions with stimulation ON, and the 7 other studies reported no statistically significant change in the assessed measures of executive functions. Additionally, no change in executive function 6 months after surgery with DBS ON, whether ON or OFF medications, was reported in another study [69].

Improvement in executive functions and attention/concentration after STN DBS might be secondary to a decrease in the excessive inhibitory output from the basal ganglia to the frontal cortex [63], and increased activation of the DLPFC on PET scan was reported after STN DBS [70].

(2) GPi. No statistically significant change in any measure of executive function up to 21 months after GPi DBS was reported in 7 studies, while one study reported improvement of at least one measure of executive function at 6 months [25] (Table 2). One study by Rothlind et al. [47] showed worsening on some measure of executive functions and attention 6 months after GPi DBS, visible at a population level but unlikely to affect individual patients as we will detail in the controlled studies section below.

3.1.3. Attention and Concentration. Attention and working memory were most often assessed using the Stroop Word Test, Trail Making Test part A, the subtests Letter and Number Sequencing and Digit Span of the Wechsler Adult Intelligence Scale III (WAIS-III), the Vienna Test System's simple and choice reaction speed tests, and the Symbol Digit Modalities administration.

(1) STN. All reported measures of attention and concentration (A/C) were improved with stimulation ON compared to OFF in 7 patients [63]. Another series of 12 patients reported similar improvement in some of the reported measures [68]. Comparing 18 patients ON and OFF stimulation at least 4 months after DBS, Castner et al. [30] reported improvement in one measure of attention and no change in another one with ON stimulation. It must be noted that there was no comparison to the pre-DBS level of A/C in these 3 studies to assess if DBS implant, rather than stimulation alone, might be the cause of these changes. Conversely, 8 studies with assessments up to 16 months after STN DBS follow-up reported worsening of at least one measure of A/C, one of which reported no difference between ON and OFF stimulation [62]. Finally, no statistically significant impact of STN DBS implant and/or stimulation on A/C was reported in 21 other series (Table 1), including 2 evaluating patients ON and OFF stimulation [38, 58] and one evaluating patient ON DBS and ON and OFF medications [69].

The missing digit task, used by some studies, specifically activates the posterior premotor cortex and the DLPFC on PET [71], giving a substratum for the observed improvement since the STN projects to these cortical sites [72].

(2) GPi. Five studies assessing attention and concentration up to 21 months after GPi DBS reported no statistically significant change (Table 2), including no change with DBS

ON versus OFF in one study [63]. However, Rothlind et al. [47] reported worsening in some, but not all, measures of A/C 6 months after GPi DBS.

3.1.4. Memory. Memory was most often assessed by the Rey Auditory Verbal Learning Test (RAVLT), the Brief Visuospatial Memory Test, and the Hopkins Verbal Learning Test.

(1) STN. Memory improvement 4 months after STN DBS was reported in a series of 8 patients [37]. However, the study was not corrected for multiple analyses, and a post hoc correction was not possible due to the lack of reported p value, making it unclear if such a correction would have made the reported improvement statistically not significant. Tang et al. did report such improvement, in a series of 27 patients followed for 12 months [73], in a study corrected for multiple analyses. Conversely, worsening in at least one measure of memory was reported in 5 studies, up to 16 months after DBS (Table 1). However, one of these [57] was not corrected for multiple analyses and a post hoc correction was not possible due to the lack of reported p value, making it unclear if such a correction would have made the reported worsening statistically not significant. In addition, there was no difference in memory assessment ON and OFF stimulation in 2 of these studies after correction for multiple analyses [59, 63].

Finally, no statistically significant impact of DBS implant and/or stimulation on memory was reported in 30 other studies (Table 1), including one evaluating patients ON DBS and ON and OFF medications [69].

(2) GPi. Worsening in one but not all measures of memory was reported in one series of 6 bilateral GPi DBS patients followed for 5 months [74]. However, this study was not corrected for multiple analyses and a post hoc correction was not possible due to the lack of reported p value, making it unclear if such a correction would have made the reported worsening statistically not significant. Conversely, no significant change in any measure of memory was detected in 7 other studies totaling 146 patients followed for up to 21 months (Table 2), including 2 studies comparing patients ON and OFF stimulations [60, 63].

3.1.5. Visual Function. Visual function was most often assessed by the subtest Matrix Reasoning of the WAIS-III and Clock Drawing.

(1) STN. Alegret et al. [75] first reported worsening of visuospatial function after STN DBS that was not statistically significant after correction for multiple analyses. However, Smeding et al. [33] reported decrease in visual function in a controlled study of 105 STN DBS patients followed for 12 months. Conversely, 18 other studies, including 2 assessing patients ON and OFF stimulation [38, 62], reported no impact on visual function (Table 1).

(2) GPi. Worsening of one but not all measures of visual function was reported in one series of 9 patients followed for 3 months after bilateral GPi DBS [66]. However, this study was not corrected for multiple analyses and a post

hoc correction was not possible due to the lack of reported p value, making it unclear if such a correction would have made the reported worsening statistically not significant. Conversely, no significant change in any used measure of visual function was detected in 4 studies totaling 44 patients followed up to 21 months (Table 2).

3.1.6. Psychomotor and Processing Speed. The assessment of psychomotor and processing speed is usually included in the assessment of executive and A/C. In some studies though, it was assessed separately, most often assessed using the Stroop Word Test, Trail Making Test part A, the subtest Digit Span of the WAIS-III, and the Symbol Digit Modalities Test oral administration.

(1) STN. Improvement in processing and psychomotor speed with STN stimulation ON compared to OFF was reported in 2 studies [63, 68], while another [47] reported worsening of some measures of psychomotor and processing speed when compared to PD patients controls in the medication ON state [47]. Conversely, 13 other studies, including 2 evaluating patients with stimulation ON and OFF [59, 63] and one evaluating patients ON and OFF medications with stimulation ON [69], could not detect significant change after STN DBS (Table 1).

(2) GPi. No significant change in psychomotor and processing speed from GPi implant with or without stimulation could be detected in 5 studies totaling 132 patients [25, 47, 60, 63, 76] (Table 2).

3.1.7. Global Cognition. General cognition was most often assessed by the Mini Mental Status Exam and the Mattis Dementia Rating Scale.

(1) STN. Two series totaling 140 patients evaluating ON stimulation and ON medications reported significant worsening of global cognition 5 years after surgery [23, 76]. However, the reported worsening might have been secondary to the natural evolution of PD [77] since none of these studies had a control arm. On the other hand, a controlled study with 105 STN DBS patients [33] reported worsening of all cognitive domains 12 months after surgery (global cognition, memory, executive function, visual function, attention/concentration, and language).

No significant change was reported in 27 other studies up to 8 years after surgery, including 7 controlled studies comparing a total of 265 STN DBS patients to nonsurgically treated PD patients [16, 17, 32, 40–42, 45, 48] (Table 1). In addition, the incidence of dementia 3 years after bilateral STN DBS in 50 PD patients was estimated at 89 per 1000 by Aybek et al. [19], while Kim et al. [78] had an incidence rate of 35.7 per 1000 person-years in their cohort of 103 STN DBS patients followed for 42 months. Both rates were comparable to the reported incidence in medically managed PD (42.6 to 112 per 1,000) [79].

(2) GPi. No statistically significant change in global cognition up to 6 months after surgery could be detected in 3 studies totaling 28 patients [25, 66, 74] (Table 2).

TABLE 3: Controlled studies assessing cognitive change in PD patients after DBS.

Author, year	N of DBS patients	F/u (mo)	Lead location	Status of stimulation/medication at cognitive assessment	Cognitive performance(s) improved in DBS group	Cognitive performance(s) worsened in DBS group	Cognitive performance(s) not different between DBS and control group
Castelli et al., 2010 [39]	27	12	STN	ON/ON	None	L	E, A/C, M, L
Cilia et al., 2007 [16]	20	12	STN	ON/ON	None	L	GC, L, E, A/C
De Gaspari et al., 2006 [21]	12	12	STN	ON/ON	None	L	GC, E, L
Gironell et al., 2003 [36]	8	6	STN	ON/ON	None	None	L, E, A/C, M, V, PS
Hilker et al., 2004 [37]	8	4	STN	ON/-	M	None	GC, E, L, A/C, M, V
Moretti et al., 2003 [46]	9	12	STN	ON/ON	L	L, E	E, L, A/C, M, V
Morrison et al., 2004 [38]	17	3	STN	ON and OFF/OFF	None	None	L, A/C, M, E, V
Rukmini Mridula et al., 2015 [48]	50	23[a]	STN	ON/ON	None	None	GC, A/C
Phillips et al., 2012 [49]	11	13.8[a]	STN	ON and OFF/ON and OFF	None	None	L
Rothlind et al., 2015 [47]	281	6	STN $n = 84$ and GPI $n = 80$	ON/ON	None	A/C, E, PS, see text	A/C, E, L, M, PS
Sáez-Zea et al., 2012 [44]	9	6	STN	ON/ON	None	None	A, M, V, E, L, A/C
Smeding et al., 2011 [33]	105	12	STN	ON/ON	None	GC, E, L, V, M, A/C	L, A/C
Smeding et al., 2006 [43]	99	6	STN	ON/ON	None	L, A/C	L, M, V, A/C
Whelan et al., 2003 [24]	5	3	STN	ON/ON	L	L	None
Williams et al., 2011 [40]	19	24	STN	ON/ON	None	None	GC, M, E, A/C, L, V, PS
Witt et al., 2008 [42]	60	6	STN	ON/ON	None	A/C	GC, E, L, A/C
Witt et al., 2013 [41]	31	6	STN	ON/ON	None	None	GC, A/C, L
York et al., 2008 [17]	23	6	STN	ON/ON	None	M	GC, E, A/C, M, L, V, PS
Zangaglia et al., 2009 [45]	32	36	STN	ON/ON	None	L	GC, M, E, A/C
Zangaglia et al., 2012 [32]	30	96	STN	ON/ON	None	L	GC, M, E, A/C

PD: Parkinson's disease; STN: subthalamic nucleus; N: number; mo: months; A/C: attention/concentration; E: executive; GC: global cognition; L: language; M: memory; PS: psychomotor/processing speed; V: visual. [a]mean. *Note.* Multiple tests were performed for each domain in each study, and often a few of these showed a difference while other tests assessing the same domain did not. This explains why the same domain might appear more than once and under different results for the same study. Adapted from Mehanna [11] with permission from the author.

3.2. Controlled Studies. Because most of the available information is provided by open label uncontrolled series, a major concern is that Parkinson's' disease natural history, rather than DBS, might be the cause of any detected cognitive worsening. It is thus important to consider more attentively the 20 controlled studies available (Table 3).

Among these, seven reported no difference between DBS and non-DBS PD patients. Gironell et al. [36] reported worse semantic verbal fluency in the DBS group when comparing 8 bilateral STN DBS patients 6 months after surgery to 8 age- and stage-matched PD patients who refused surgery. However, this difference was not statistically significant when corrected for multiple analyses, and there was no difference in the other cognitive tasks assessed. A year later, Morrison et al. [38] reported no statistically significant difference at 3 months after surgery between 17 bilateral STN DBS patients and 11 nonsurgically treated PD patients. In addition, within the DBS group, there was no difference between the preoperative assessment and stimulation ON at 3 months, or between stimulation ON and stimulation OFF at 3 months. York et al. [17] reported worse verbal memory in 23 STN DBS patients at 6 months compared to 27 medically managed PD patients. There was no difference in visual memory or other cognitive measures. However, in a follow-up to this study including 19 STN DBS patients and 18 controls 2 years after surgery, Williams et al. [40] reported worsening of some measures of memory, processing, and fluency, but these differences were not significant after correction for multiple analyses. More recently, Sáez-Zea et al. [44] reported no difference 6 months after surgery between 9 bilateral STN DBS patients and 12 nonsurgical PD patients, with worsening of 4 measures of language and attention in each group, out of the 18 cognitive measures assessed. In addition, STN DBS patients had a nonstatistically significant trend to worse phonemic verbal fluency that was significantly correlated with reductions in the L-dopa-equivalent daily dose, suggesting that a decrease in the antiparkinsonian medication might be the actual cause of worse fluency observed after STN DBS. Witt et al. [41] also reported worsening of semantic fluency, but not of letter fluency or other cognitive measures assessed, 6 months after surgery in 31 bilateral STN DBS patients compared to 31 nonsurgical PD patients. However, this difference was not statistically significant after correction for multiple analyses. In a prospective study comparing 11 BL STN DBS and 11 PD controls and 18 healthy controls, Phillips et al. [49] reported improvement in some aspects of language with STN DBS but worsening of others. However, after correction for multiple analyses, these differences were not statistically significant except for a longer reaction time with DBS ON and medication ON compared to DBS OFF and medication OFF, for regular verbs in past tense only, through indirect comparison. However, a direct comparison of these results did not show a statistical significance. Finally, Rukmini Mridula et al. [48] prospectively compared 56 patients who underwent bilateral STN DBS to 53 PD controls in the ON state with a mean follow-up of 23 months, showing no difference in any of the cognitive measures assessed.

In contrast, worsening of some cognitive measures after DBS, sometimes mitigated by improvement of others, was reported in 11 controlled studies. Moretti et al. [46] reported worsening of semantic and syllabic fluency as well as some executive functions, but with an increase in control of linguistic production, 12 months after surgery in 9 bilateral STN DBS patients compared to 9 nonsurgical PD patients. Zangaglia et al. [45] reported worsening of verbal fluency but none of other cognitive measures assessed, 3 years after surgery in 32 STN DBS patients compared to 33 nonsurgical PD patients. In a follow-up publication on that cohort, the authors reported a similar cognitive status 8 years after surgery, concluding that STN DBS was safe from a cognitive standpoint and did not modify the cognitive evolution along

the course of the disease [32]. Witt et al. [42] reported worse scores on 2 measures of attention but none of other cognitive measures assessed, 6 months after surgery in 60 bilateral STN DBS patients compared to 63 nonsurgical PD patients, but without comparison to the preoperative baseline. Smeding et al. [43] reported a significantly worse decline in fluency and attention/concentration but none of the other cognitive measures assessed, 6 months after surgery in 99 STN DBS patients compared to 39 nonsurgical PD patients. Cilia et al. [16] reported statistically significant worsening of category fluency but not of phonemic fluency or other cognitive measures assessed, 12 months after surgery in 20 STN DBS patients compared to 12 nonsurgical PD patients. De Gaspari et al. similarly reported decrease in category fluency 12 months after surgery in 12 STN DBS patients compared to 13 nonsurgical PD patients [21]. Last, Castelli et al. [39] reported worsening of phonemic fluency but not of semantic fluency or other cognitive measures assessed, 12 months after surgery in 27 STN DBS patients compared to 31 matched nonsurgical PD patients. In a study comparing 105 STN DBS patients with 40 non-DBS PD controls 12 months after surgery, Smeding et al. [33] reported worsening of all cognitive domains (global cognition, memory, executive function, visual function, attention/concentration, and language) with no worsening in one or more measures of attention/concentration and language. However, disease duration was statistically longer in the STN group, so the possibility of cognitive decline related to the disease rather than DBS cannot completely be ruled out. Regardless, quality of life was significantly better in STN group than in the control group. Whelan et al. [24] compared language 3 months after surgery in 5 bilateral STN PD patients, 16 nonsurgical PD patients, and 16 healthy aged matched subjects. Compared to the nonsurgical PD patients, DBS patients had improvement on the word test-revised but worsening in the accuracy of lexical decisions about words with many meanings and a high degree of relatedness between meanings. The impact of these detailed differential results on the patients' daily life is unclear. More recently, in a prospective unblinded randomized controlled study comparing neuropsychological outcomes between patients treated with bilateral DBS ON stimulation and ON medication (164 patients, 84 implanted in the STN and 80 in the GPi) and patients treated with optimal medication management ON medication (n = 116), Rothlind et al. [47] reported significantly greater mean reductions at 6 months in performance on multiple measures of processing speed and working memory in the combined DBS group, as well as higher rates of decline in neuropsychological test performance in this group [47]. Decline by multiple indicators in two or more cognitive domains was seen in 11% of the DBS patients and 3% of the medically managed patients. This multidomain cognitive decline was associated with less beneficial change in subjective ratings of everyday functioning and quality of life. However, the authors noted that the majority of individual patients receiving DBS did not display changes on individual measures or combinations of measures that would clearly distinguish them from patients treated with optimal medication management and in fact showed, for most of them, a balance of isolated declines and improvements in test performance similar to the pattern observed in the optimal medication management arm. In other words, worsening of some neuropsychological tests after DBS was observed at a population level but was unlikely to affect individual patients in the majority of the cases.

However, Hilker et al. [37] reported significant improvement in verbal and nonverbal long-term memory 4 months after surgery in 8 bilateral STN DBS PD patients compared to 10 healthy matched controls suggesting STN DBS might in fact improve memory circuits. The study was not corrected for multiple analyses and a post hoc correction was not possible due to the lack of reported p value, making it unclear if such a correction would have made the reported improvement statistically not significant.

In summary, 10 of the 20 available controlled studies reported statistically significant worsening on some cognitive measures after bilateral STN DBS and 2 reported improvement in some and worsening in other cognitive measures. Different subtypes of fluency (semantic, phonemic, and category) worsened in some studies but not others. Worsening of attention was also reported in more than one controlled study. On the other hand, one controlled study reported improvement and 7 did not detect any cognitive difference between STN DBS and non-DBS PD patients.

3.3. Target Selection. Currently, most DBS centers prefer to implant in the GPi in PD patients with mild cognitive impairment, out of fear that STN DBS would cause more cognitive side effects. There is indeed more data in the literature reporting cognitive worsening after STN DBS than GPi DBS, but this data is markedly imbalanced as the studies detailed above have evaluated 1,777 STN DBS patients but only 165 GPi patients. It is important therefore to look more attentively at head-to-head comparison between the 2 targets.

Head-to-head comparison of the cognitive impact of STN and GPi DBS was reported in 9 studies to our knowledge, with a total of 581 STN and 617 GPi patients [26, 34, 47, 50–55] (Table 4). Only one of these [51] reported correction for multiple analyses. After corrections were applied when needed, the following studies revealed a difference between the 2 groups.

Weaver et al. [53] followed 159 patients for 3 years after surgery and reported worsening of one out of 4 memory measures after STN DBS compared to GPi DBS. The authors suggested that this difference might be secondary to a larger decrease in dopamine replacement doses in the STN group. Although Rothlind et al. [47] reported slightly greater reductions in some aspects of processing speed in the STN group and greater reductions in verbal learning and recall in participants in the GPi group, the 2 groups were deemed similar overall. Odekerken et al. [54] reported a bigger negative change in the STN group 12 months after surgery, in 4 out of 11 measures of attention, out of the 24 cognitive measures assessed. However, the frequency of cognitive decline and the quality of life were similar between the 2 groups. Of note, the authors also reported that an older age at surgery was associated with a higher risk of cognitive

decline (62.4 versus 58.4 years). On the other hand, in a 36-month follow-up to this study, Odekerken et al. [34] reported no difference between the 2 groups on a composite score for cognition, mood, and behavior but reported better OFF drug motor symptoms and functioning in the STN group, as well as bigger medication reduction in that group and a higher rate of repeat surgery in the GPi group.

In summary, and after correction for multiple analyses, only 2 out of 9 studies [53, 54], totaling 126 STN and 145 GPi patients, reported worse outcome in the STN group in some measures of attention or memory. However, quality of life was similar in the 2 groups. Interestingly, these studies did not report any worse decline in language, fluency, or executive function in the STN group, as would have been expected from the open label and controlled studies. Overall, these data do not support favoring GPi over STN for fear of cognitive complications from the latter [80] in properly screened PD patients.

4. Discussion

Studies on cognitive changes after DBS in PD patients have reported different and sometimes opposite results. However, any change revealed by cognitive tests is likely subtle as detected cognitive worsening on specialized tests was usually not reported by patients, caregivers, or healthcare providers [25, 81]. In addition, quality of life measures in these patients showed improvement, even when cognitive worsening was detected [33, 53, 54, 58, 82].

Our findings confirm results from a recently published meta-analysis by Combs et al. [81] including 38 articles with an aggregated sample size of 1622 patients. The authors searched keywords and had selection criteria similar to ours, with the exception of needing sufficient report of study results to allow for an effect size to be calculated. These additional criteria might explain the lower number of studies included in the meta-analysis compared to our current review. Among the articles reviewed, 30 included STN DBS patients only, 5 reported on GPi DBS only, and 3 compared GPi and STN DBS. Combs et al. reported a small decline in psychomotor speed, learning and memory, fluency, attention/concentration, executive functions, and general cognition after STN DBS. GPi DBS patients had small changes in attention/concentration and fluency. The authors warned against concluding that GPi DBS would be cognitively safer than STN DBS, because of the small number of GPi DBS studies included.

Kumar et al. [83] suggested that variability in lead placement inside the target might explain the variation in the results of different studies. Tsai et al. [84] suggested that an active contact anteriorly located within the ventral STN could cause the neuropsychological effects reported in chronic STN DBS. York et al. [85] suggested that, in addition to the precise location of the active electrode inside the STN, a surgical trajectory through the frontal lobe might also influence the cognitive outcome. Indeed, Witt et al. [41] reported a higher risk of decline in working memory performance and global cognition associated with a trajectory intersecting the caudate nucleus. On the other hand, Smith et al. [86] could

TABLE 4: Studies comparing cognitive outcomes between GPi and STN DBS in PD patients.

Author, year	N STN/GPi	Laterality	F/u (mo)	Status of stimulation/medication at cognitive assessment	Cognitive measures assessed	Differences between GPI and STN
Boel et al., 2016 [55]	63/65	BL	36	ON/ON	GC, A/C, E, M, L	None
Follett et al., 2010 [52]	147/152	BL	24	ON/OFF	GC, L, V, E, M	None
Odekerken et al., 2013 [26]	63/65	BL	12	ON/integrated ON and OFF	Composite test	None
Odekerken et al., 2015 [54]	56/58	BL	12	ON/ON	A/C, E, M, L, V	4/11 measures of A/C worse with STN
Odekerken et al., 2016 [34]	43/47	BL	36	ON/ON	A/C, E, M, composite score	None
Okun et al., 2009 [51]	22/23	UL	7	ON/OFF	L	None
Rothlind et al., 2007 [50]	19/23	UL	6	ON/ON	A/C, E, L, V, M	None
Rothlind et al., 2007 [50]	14/15	BL	21	ON/ON	A/C, E, L, V, M	None
Rothlind et al., 2015 [47]	84/80	BL	6	ON/ON	A/C, E, GC, L, M	None overall, E worse with STN, M worse with Gpi
Weaver et al., 2012 [53]	70/89	BL	36	ON/OFF	GC, L, V, E, M	M worse with STN

PD: Parkinson's disease; GPi: globus pallidus interna; STN: subthalamic nucleus; N: number of patients; mo: months; UL: unilateral; BL: bilateral; A/C: attention/concentration; E: executive; GC: global cognition; L: language; M: memory; V: visual. Adapted from Mehanna [101] with permission from the author.

not find any correlation between decline in verbal fluency and any of age at surgery, number of intraoperative microelectrode penetrations, coordinates of the lead tip, or active stimulation site in a series of 28 STN DBS patients. Larger series have yet to duplicate these results. Trépanier et al. [87] also suspected variations in the characteristics of the patients selected for surgery between different centers (age, preoperative cognitive status, and comorbidity with other conditions such as psychiatric disorders) to explain conflicting conclusions from different studies.

In addition, outcome can also be influenced by stimulation parameters. Wojtecki et al. [88] reported a frequency-dependent modulation of cognitive circuits involving the STN, with low frequency (10 Hz) STN DBS improving verbal fluency compared to no stimulation and high frequency (130 Hz) STN DBS causing a nonsignificant trend towards worsening of fluency compared to no stimulation. Schoenberg et al. [89] reported improvement in cognitive test scores with increased amplitude and pulse width of the stimulation in 20 bilateral STN PD patients.

The respective contribution of lead implant and stimulation to post-DBS cognitive change is difficult to ascertain. The COMPARE trial [51] reported worsening of letter verbal fluency that persisted even when DBS was turned OFF, suggestive of a surgical rather than a stimulation-induced effect. On the other hand, Tröster et al. [35] reported worsening of measures of language and attention even before DBS was tuned ON, with further worsening after activation.

Studies assessing cognitive change after DBS for PD can have the following limitations. First, most the available studies lack a control arm of non-DBS treated PD patients, and a reported cognitive decline might thus be caused by the natural evolution of PD rather than DBS. Second, a reported cognitive improvement may stem from practice effect in the case of repeated cognitive assessment [58]. Using parallel forms of cognitive tasks might mitigate this practice effect, but it may be logistically difficult. Alternatively, cognitive assessments could be repeated at relatively long intervals [58]. Third, all studies did not assess patients in the same pharmacological condition, with most studies assessing patients ON antiparkinsonian medications, some studies assessing them OFF antiparkinsonian medications [38, 51–53, 63, 67, 75], and some other studies assessing them in a nonhomogeneous way [25]. Some authors did not specify the medication and/or stimulation status of the patients at the time of cognitive evaluation [27, 28, 35]. Finally, cognitive worsening after DBS might be at least partially secondary to a postoperative reduction in antiparkinsonian medications, which is seen more after STN DBS than GPi DBS [9, 34]. A uniform assessment ON stimulation and OFF medications could minimize this confounding factor. However, severity of symptoms OFF medications might render such a preoperative assessment impossible in some patients.

5. Conclusion

After reviewing the available studies assessing cognitive changes after STN and GPi DBS in PD patients, we arrive at the following suggestions. (1) In PD patients who are adequately screened for surgery, worsening of one or more cognitive functions is rare after DBS, with available studies reporting conflicting results. (2) Any change revealed by cognitive tests is likely subtle as a detected cognitive worsening on specialized tests is usually not reported by patients, caregivers, or healthcare providers. Furthermore, there is an improvement in quality of life after DBS, even when cognitive worsening is detected. (3) Worse cognitive outcome after STN DBS compared to GPi DBS was reported only in 2 out of 9 randomized trials. As such, fear of cognitive worsening should not systematically exclude STN as a potential DBS target. (4) Ideally, future studies on this topic should include controls for the natural evolution of PD. This can be done by using nonsurgically treated PD patients matched for all clinical and demographic variables. In addition, DBS patients should be assessed ON and OFF stimulation, thus providing direct comparison of the stimulatory effects while controlling for the effects of surgery. (5) Additional reports on anatomo-clinical correlation of cognitive worsening after DBS would help improve surgical planning to avoid sensitive structures.

Abbreviations

DBS: Deep brain stimulation
STN: Subthalamic nucleus
GPi: Globus pallidus interna
PD: Parkinson's disease
LID: Levodopa induced dyskinesias
DLPFC: Dorsolateral prefrontal cortex.

References

[1] R. B. Postuma, D. Berg, M. Stern et al., "MDS clinical diagnostic criteria for Parkinson's disease," *Movement Disorders*, vol. 30, no. 12, pp. 1591–1601, 2015.

[2] C. M. Tanner and D. A. Aston, "Epidemiology of Parkinson's disease and akinetic syndromes," *Current Opinion in Neurology*, vol. 13, no. 4, pp. 427–430, 2000.

[3] R. Mehanna and J. Jankovic, "Respiratory problems in neurologic movement disorders," *Parkinsonism & Related Disorders*, vol. 16, no. 10, pp. 628–638, 2010.

[4] R. Mehanna and J. Jankovic, "Movement disorders in cerebrovascular disease," *The Lancet Neurology*, vol. 12, no. 6, pp. 597–608, 2013.

[5] M. Grossman, C. Lee, J. Morris, M. B. Stern, and H. I. Hurtig, "Assessing resource demands during sentence processing in Parkinson's disease," *Brain and Language*, vol. 80, no. 3, pp. 603–616, 2002.

[6] C. Lee, M. Grossman, J. Morris, M. B. Stern, and H. I. Hurtig, "Attentional resource and processing speed limitations during sentence processing in Parkinson's disease," *Brain and Language*, vol. 85, no. 3, pp. 347–356, 2003.

[7] B. Pillon, V. Czernecki, and B. Dubois, "Dopamine and cognitive function," *Current Opinion in Neurology*, vol. 16, no. 2, pp. S17–S22, 2003.

[8] D. Muslimović, B. Post, J. D. Speelman, and B. Schmand, "Cognitive profile of patients with newly diagnosed Parkinson disease," *Neurology*, vol. 65, no. 8, pp. 1239–1245, 2005.

[9] R. Mehanna and E. C. Lai, "Deep brain stimulation in Parkinson's disease," *Translational Neurodegeneration*, vol. 2, no. 1, article 22, 2013.

[10] D. J. Pedrosa and L. Timmermann, "Review: management of Parkinson's disease," *Neuropsychiatric Disease and Treatment*, vol. 9, pp. 321–340, 2013.

[11] R. Mehanna, "Deep brain stimulation for parkinson's disease," in *Deep Brain Stimulation*, R. Mehanna, Ed., pp. 107–146, Nova Science Publishers, 2015.

[12] J. L. Houeto, V. Mesnage, L. Mallet et al., "Behavioural disorders, Parkinson's disease and subthalamic stimulation," *Journal of Neurology, Neurosurgery & Psychiatry*, vol. 72, no. 6, pp. 701–707, 2002.

[13] M. S. Okun, H. H. Fernandez, O. Pedraza et al., "Development and initial validation of a screening tool for Parkinson disease surgical candidates," *Neurology*, vol. 63, no. 1, pp. 161–163, 2004.

[14] M. S. Okun and K. D. Foote, "Parkinson's disease DBS: What, when, who and why? The time has come to tailor DBS targets," *Expert Review of Neurotherapeutics*, vol. 10, no. 12, pp. 1847–1857, 2010.

[15] H. Abboud, R. Mehanna, A. Machado et al., "Comprehensive, Multidisciplinary Deep Brain Stimulation Screening for Parkinson Patients: No Room for "Short Cuts"," *Movement Disorders Clinical Practice*, vol. 1, no. 4, pp. 336–341, 2014.

[16] R. Cilia, C. Siri, G. Marotta et al., "Brain networks underlining verbal fluency decline during STN-DBS in Parkinson's disease: an ECD-SPECT study," *Parkinsonism & Related Disorders*, vol. 13, no. 5, pp. 290–294, 2007.

[17] M. K. York, M. Dulay, A. Macias et al., "Cognitive declines following bilateral subthalamic nucleus deep brain stimulation for the treatment of Parkinson's disease," *Journal of Neurology, Neurosurgery & Psychiatry*, vol. 79, no. 7, pp. 789–795, 2008.

[18] J. L. Alberts, C. Voelcker-Rehage, K. Hallahan, M. Vitek, R. Bamzai, and J. L. Vitek, "Bilateral subthalamic stimulation impairs cognitive - Motor performance in Parkinson's disease patients," *Brain*, vol. 131, no. 12, pp. 3348–3360, 2008.

[19] S. Aybek, A. Gronchi-Perrin, A. Berney et al., "Long-term cognitive profile and incidence of dementia after STN-DBS in Parkinson's disease," *Movement Disorders*, vol. 22, no. 7, pp. 974–981, 2007.

[20] P. Krack, A. Batir, N. van Blercom et al., "Five-year follow-up of bilateral stimulation of the subthalamic nucleus in advanced Parkinson's disease," *The New England Journal of Medicine*, vol. 349, no. 20, pp. 1925–1934, 2003.

[21] D. De Gaspari, C. Siri, A. Landi et al., "Clinical and neuropsychological follow up at 12 months in patients with complicated Parkinson's disease treated with subcutaneous apomorphine infusion or deep brain stimulation of the subthalamic nucleus," *Journal of Neurology, Neurosurgery & Psychiatry*, vol. 77, no. 4, pp. 450–453, 2006.

[22] A. Funkiewiez, C. Ardouin, E. Caputo et al., "Long term effects of bilateral subthalamic nucleus stimulation on cognitive function, mood, and behaviour in Parkinson's disease," *Journal of Neurology, Neurosurgery & Psychiatry*, vol. 75, no. 6, pp. 834–839, 2004.

[23] W. M. M. Schüpbach, N. Chastan, M. L. Welter et al., "Stimulation of the subthalamic nucleus in Parkinson's disease: a 5 year follow up," *Journal of Neurology, Neurosurgery & Psychiatry*, vol. 76, no. 12, pp. 1640–1644, 2005.

[24] B.-M. Whelan, B. E. Murdoch, D. G. Theodoros, B. Hall, and P. Silburn, "Defining a role for the subthalamic nucleus within

operative theoretical models of subcortical participation in language," *Journal of Neurology, Neurosurgery & Psychiatry*, vol. 74, no. 11, pp. 1543–1550, 2003.

[25] C. Ardouin, B. Pillon, E. Peiffer et al., "Bilateral subthalamic or pallidal stimulation for Parkinson's disease affects neither memory nor executive functions: A consecutive series of 62 patients," *Annals of Neurology*, vol. 46, no. 2, pp. 217–223, 1999.

[26] V. J. Odekerken, T. van Laar, and M. J. Staal, "Subthalamic nucleus versus globus pallidus bilateral deep brain stimulation for advanced Parkinson's disease (NSTAPS study): a randomised controlled trial," *Lancet Neurol*, vol. 12, no. 1, pp. 37–44, 2013.

[27] T. Asahi, N. Nakamichi, A. Takaiwa et al., "Impact of bilateral subthalamic stimulation on motor/cognitive functions in Parkinson's disease," *Neurologia Medico-Chirurgica*, vol. 54, no. 7, pp. 529–536, 2014.

[28] C. Tremblay, J. Macoir, M. Langlois, L. Cantin, M. Prud'homme, and L. Monetta, "The effects of subthalamic deep brain stimulation on metaphor comprehension and language abilities in Parkinson's disease," *Brain and Language*, vol. 141, pp. 103–109, 2015.

[29] M. C. Silveri, N. Ciccarelli, E. Baldonero et al., "Effects of stimulation of the subthalamic nucleus on naming and reading nouns and verbs in Parkinson's disease," *Neuropsychologia*, vol. 50, no. 8, pp. 1980–1989, 2012.

[30] J. E. Castner, D. A. Copland, P. A. Silburn, T. J. Coyne, F. Sinclair, and H. J. Chenery, "Lexical-semantic inhibitory mechanisms in Parkinson's disease as a function of subthalamic stimulation," *Neuropsychologia*, vol. 45, no. 14, pp. 3167–3177, 2007.

[31] J. E. Castner, H. J. Chenery, P. A. Silburn et al., "Effects of subthalamic deep brain stimulation on noun/verb generation and selection from competing alternatives in Parkinson's disease," *Journal of Neurology, Neurosurgery & Psychiatry*, vol. 79, no. 6, pp. 700–705, 2008.

[32] R. Zangaglia, C. Pasotti, F. Mancini, D. Servello, E. Sinforiani, and C. Pacchetti, "Deep brain stimulation and cognition in Parkinson's disease: An eight-year follow-up study," *Movement Disorders*, vol. 27, no. 9, pp. 1192–1194, 2012.

[33] H. M. M. Smeding, J. D. Speelman, H. M. Huizenga, P. R. Schuurman, and B. Schmand, "Predictors of cognitive and psychosocial outcome after STN DBS in Parkinson's disease," *Journal of Neurology, Neurosurgery & Psychiatry*, vol. 82, no. 7, pp. 754–760, 2011.

[34] V. J. J. Odekerken, J. A. Boel, B. A. Schmand et al., "GPi vs STN deep brain stimulation for Parkinson disease," *Neurology*, vol. 86, no. 8, pp. 755–761, 2016.

[35] A. I. Tröster, J. Jankovic, M. Tagliati, D. Peichel, and M. S. Okun, "Neuropsychological outcomes from constant current deep brain stimulation for Parkinson's disease," *Movement Disorders*, vol. 32, no. 3, pp. 433–440, 2017.

[36] A. Gironell, J. Kulisevsky, L. Rami, N. Fortuny, C. García-Sánchez, and B. Pascual-Sedano, "Effects of pallidotomy and bilateral subthalamic stimulation on cognitive function in Parkinson disease: a controlled comparative study," *Journal of Neurology*, vol. 250, no. 8, pp. 917–923, 2003.

[37] R. Hilker, J. Voges, S. Weisenbach et al., "Subthalamic Nucleus Stimulation Restores Glucose Metabolism in Associative and Limbic Cortices and in Cerebellum: Evidence from a FDG-PET Study in Advanced Parkinson's Disease," *Journal of Cerebral Blood Flow & Metabolism*, vol. 24, no. 1, pp. 7–16, 2004.

[38] C. E. Morrison, J. C. Borod, K. Perrine et al., "Neuropsychological functioning following bilateral subthalamic nucleus

stimulation in Parkinson's disease," *Archives of Clinical Neuropsychology*, vol. 19, no. 2, pp. 165–181, 2004.

[39] L. Castelli, L. Rizzi, M. Zibetti, S. Angrisano, M. Lanotte, and L. Lopiano, "Neuropsychological changes 1-year after subthalamic DBS in PD patients: a prospective controlled study," *Parkinsonism & Related Disorders*, vol. 16, no. 2, pp. 115–118, 2010.

[40] A. E. Williams, G. M. Arzola, A. M. Strutt, R. Simpson, J. Jankovic, and M. K. York, "Cognitive outcome and reliable change indices two years following bilateral subthalamic nucleus deep brain stimulation," *Parkinsonism & Related Disorders*, vol. 17, no. 5, pp. 321–327, 2011.

[41] K. Witt, O. Granert, C. Daniels et al., "Relation of lead trajectory and electrode position to neuropsychological outcomes of subthalamic neurostimulation in Parkinson's disease: results from a randomized trial," *Brain*, vol. 136, no. 7, pp. 2109–2119, 2013.

[42] K. Witt, C. Daniels, J. Reiff et al., "Neuropsychological and psychiatric changes after deep brain stimulation for Parkinson's disease: a randomised, multicentre study," *The Lancet Neurology*, vol. 7, no. 7, pp. 605–614, 2008.

[43] H. M. M. Smeding, J. D. Speelman, M. Koning-Haanstra et al., "Neuropsychological effects of bilateral STN stimulation in Parkinson disease: a controlled study," *Neurology*, vol. 66, no. 12, pp. 1830–1836, 2006.

[44] C. Sáez-Zea, F. Escamilla-Sevilla, M. J. Katati, and A. Mínguez-Castellanos, "Cognitive effects of subthalamic nucleus stimulation in Parkinson's disease: A controlled study," *European Neurology*, vol. 68, no. 6, pp. 361–366, 2012.

[45] R. Zangaglia, C. Pacchetti, C. Pasotti et al., "Deep brain stimulation and cognitive functions in Parkinson's disease: a three-year controlled study," *Movement Disorders*, vol. 24, no. 11, pp. 1621–1628, 2009.

[46] R. Moretti, P. Torre, R. M. Antonello et al., "Neuropsychological changes after subthalamic nucleus stimulation: A 12 month follow-up in nine patients with Parkinson's disease," *Parkinsonism & Related Disorders*, vol. 10, no. 2, pp. 73–79, 2003.

[47] J. C. Rothlind, M. K. York, K. Carlson et al., "Neuropsychological changes following deep brain stimulation surgery for Parkinson's disease: comparisons of treatment at pallidal and subthalamic targets versus best medical therapy," *Journal of Neurology, Neurosurgery & Psychiatry*, vol. 86, no. 6, pp. 622–629, 2015.

[48] K. Rukmini Mridula, R. Borgohain, SA. Jabeen et al., "Comparison of frequencies of non motor symptoms in Indian Parkinson's disease patients on medical management versus deep brain stimulation: A case-control study," *Iranian Journal of Neurology*, vol. 14, pp. 86–93, 2015.

[49] L. Phillips, K. A. Litcofsky, M. Pelster, M. Gelfand, M. T. Ullman, and P. D. Charles, "Subthalamic nucleus deep brain stimulation impacts language in early parkinson's disease," *PLoS ONE*, vol. 7, no. 8, Article ID e42829, 2012.

[50] J. C. Rothlind, R. W. Cockshott, P. A. Starr, and W. J. Marks Jr., "Neuropsychological performance following staged bilateral pallidal or subthalamic nucleus deep brain stimulation for Parkinson's disease," *Journal of the International Neuropsychological Society*, vol. 13, no. 1, pp. 68–79, 2007.

[51] M. S. Okun, H. H. Fernandez, S. S. Wu et al., "Cognition and mood in Parkinson's disease in subthalamic nucleus versus globus pallidus interna deep brain stimulation: the COMPARE trial," *Annals of Neurology*, vol. 65, no. 5, pp. 586–595, 2009.

[52] K. A. Follett, F. M. Weaver, M. Stern et al., "Pallidal versus subthalamic deep-brain stimulation for Parkinson's disease,"

The New England Journal of Medicine, vol. 362, no. 22, pp. 2077–2091, 2010.

[53] F. M. Weaver, K. A. Follett, M. Stern et al., "Randomized trial of deep brain stimulation for Parkinson disease: thirty-six month outcomes," *Neurology*, vol. 79, no. 1, pp. 55–65, 2012.

[54] V. J. J. Odekerken, J. A. Boel, G. J. Geurtsen et al., "Neuropsychological outcome after deep brain stimulation for Parkinson disease," *Neurology*, vol. 84, no. 13, pp. 1355–1361, 2015.

[55] J. A. Boel, V. J. J. Odekerken, B. A. Schmand et al., "Cognitive and psychiatric outcome 3 years after globus pallidus pars interna or subthalamic nucleus deep brain stimulation for Parkinson's disease," *Parkinsonism & Related Disorders*, vol. 33, pp. 90–95, 2016.

[56] L. Castelli, P. Perozzo, M. Zibetti et al., "Chronic deep brain stimulation of the subthalamic nucleus for Parkinson's disease: Effects on cognition, mood, anxiety and personality traits," *European Neurology*, vol. 55, no. 3, pp. 136–144, 2006.

[57] A. Fasano, L. M. Romito, A. Daniele et al., "Motor and cognitive outcome in patients with Parkinson's disease 8 years after subthalamic implants," *Brain*, vol. 133, no. 9, pp. 2664–2676, 2010.

[58] A. Daniele, A. Albanese, M. F. Contarino et al., "Cognitive and behavioural effects of chronic stimulation of the subthalamic nucleus in patients with Parkinson's disease," *Journal of Neurology, Neurosurgery & Psychiatry*, vol. 74, no. 2, pp. 175–182, 2003.

[59] T. D. Hälbig, D. Gruber, U. A. Kopp et al., "Subthalamic stimulation differentially modulates declarative and nondeclarative memory," *NeuroReport*, vol. 15, no. 3, pp. 539–543, 2004.

[60] B. Pillon, C. Ardouin, P. Damier et al., "Neuropsychological changes between 'off' and 'on' STN or GPi stimulation in Parkinson's disease," *Neurology*, vol. 55, no. 3, pp. 411–418, 2000.

[61] K. Witt, U. Pulkowski, J. Herzog et al., "Deep Brain Stimulation of the Subthalamic Nucleus Improves Cognitive Flexibility but Impairs Response Inhibition in Parkinson Disease," *JAMA Neurology*, vol. 61, no. 5, pp. 697–700, 2004.

[62] M. Fraraccio, A. Ptito, A. Sadikot, M. Panisset, and A. Dagher, "Absence of cognitive deficits following deep brain stimulation of the subthalamic nucleus for the treatment of Parkinson's disease," *Archives of Clinical Neuropsychology*, vol. 23, no. 4, pp. 399–408, 2008.

[63] M. Jahanshahi, C. M. Ardouin, and R. G. Brown, "The impact of deep brain stimulation on executive function in Parkinson's disease," *Brain*, vol. 123, no. 6, pp. 1142–1154, 2000.

[64] B. Crosson, J. R. Saclek, J. A. Bobholz et al., "Activity in the paracingulate and cingulate sulci during word generation: An fMRI study of functional anatomy," *Cerebral Cortex*, vol. 9, no. 1, pp. 307–316, 1999.

[65] J.-F. Houvenaghel, F. L. Jeune, T. Dondaine et al., "Reduced verbal fluency following subthalamic deep brain stimulation: A frontal-related cognitive deficit?" *PLoS ONE*, vol. 10, no. 10, Article ID e0140083, 2015.

[66] A. I. Tröster, J. A. Fields, S. B. Wilkinson et al., "Unilateral pallidal stimulation for Parkinson's disease: neurobehavioral functioning before and 3 months after electrode implantation," *Neurology*, vol. 49, no. 4, pp. 1078–1083, 1997.

[67] T. Hershey, F. J. Revilla, A. Wernle, P. S. Gibson, J. L. Dowling, and J. S. Perlmutter, "Stimulation of STN impairs aspects of cognitive control in PD," *Neurology*, vol. 62, no. 7, pp. 1110–1114, 2004.

[68] D. Page and M. Jahanshahi, "Deep brain stimulation of the subthalamic nucleus improves set shifting but does not affect dual task performance in Parkinson's disease," *IEEE Transactions on Neural Systems and Rehabilitation Engineering*, vol. 15, no. 1, pp. 198–206, 2007.

[69] P. Perozzo, M. Rizzone, B. Bergamasco et al., "Deep brain stimulation of the subthalamic nucleus in Parkinson's disease: Comparison of pre- and postoperative neuropsychological evaluation," *Journal of the Neurological Sciences*, vol. 192, no. 1-2, pp. 9–15, 2001.

[70] P. Limousin, P. Krack, P. Pollak et al., "Electrical stimulation of the subthalamic nucleus in advanced Parkinsonian's disease," *The New England Journal of Medicine*, vol. 339, no. 16, pp. 1105–1111, 1998.

[71] M. Petrides, B. Alivisatos, E. Meyer, and A. C. Evans, "Functional activation of the human frontal cortex during the performance of verbal working memory tasks," *Proceedings of the National Acadamy of Sciences of the United States of America*, vol. 90, no. 3, pp. 878–882, 1993.

[72] C. H. Halpen, J. H. Rick, S. F. Danish, M. Grossman, and G. H. Baltuch, "Cognition following bilateral deep brain stimulation surgery of the subthalamic nuclear for Parkinson's disease," *International Journal of Geriatric Psychiatry*, vol. 24, no. 5, pp. 443–451, 2009.

[73] V. Tang, C. X. L. Zhu, D. Chan et al., "Evidence of improved immediate verbal memory and diminished category fluency following STN-DBS in Chinese-Cantonese patients with idiopathic Parkinson's disease," *Neurological Sciences*, vol. 36, no. 8, pp. 1371–1377, 2015.

[74] J. A. Fields, A. I. Tröster, S. B. Wilkinson, R. Pahwa, and W. C. Koller, "Cognitive outcome following staged bilateral pallidal stimulation for the treatment of Parkinson's disease," *Clinical Neurology and Neurosurgery*, vol. 101, no. 3, pp. 182–188, 1999.

[75] M. Alegret, C. Junqué, F. Valldeoriola et al., "Effects of bilateral subthalamic stimulation on cognitive function in Parkinson disease," *JAMA Neurology*, vol. 58, no. 8, pp. 1223–1227, 2001.

[76] G. Vingerhoets, C. Van Der Linden, E. Lannoo et al., "Cognitive outcome after unilateral pallidal stimulation in Parkinson's disease," *Journal of Neurology, Neurosurgery & Psychiatry*, vol. 66, no. 3, pp. 297–304, 1999.

[77] M. A. Hely, W. G. J. Reid, M. A. Adena, G. M. Halliday, and J. G. L. Morris, "The Sydney multicenter study of Parkinson's disease: the inevitability of dementia at 20 years," *Movement Disorders*, vol. 23, no. 6, pp. 837–844, 2008.

[78] H.-J. Kim, B. S. Jeon, S. H. Paek et al., "Long-term cognitive outcome of bilateral subthalamic deep brain stimulation in Parkinson's disease," *Journal of Neurology*, vol. 261, no. 6, pp. 1090–1096, 2014.

[79] D. Aarsland, K. Andersen, J. P. Larsen, A. Lolk, H. Nielsen, and P. Kragh-Sørensen, "Risk of dementia in Parkinson's disease: a community-based, prospective study," *Neurology*, vol. 56, no. 6, pp. 730–736, 2001.

[80] J. Massano, "Comment: New insights on cognition after deep brain stimulation in Parkinson Disease," *Neurology*, vol. 84, no. 13, p. 1360, 2015.

[81] H. L. Combs, B. S. Folley, and D. T. R. Berry, "Cognition and depression following deep brain stimulation of the subthalamic nucleus and globus pallidus pars internus in parkinson's disease: a meta-analysis," *Neuropsychology Review*, vol. 25, no. 4, pp. 439–454, 2015.

[82] J. A. Saint-Cyr and A. Albanese, "STN DBS in PD: Selection criteria for surgery should include cognitive and psychiatric factors," *Neurology*, vol. 66, no. 12, pp. 1799-1800, 2006.

[83] R. Kumar, A. E. Lang, M. C. Rodriguez-Oroz et al., "Deep brain stimulation of the globus pallidus pars interna in advanced Parkinson's disease," *Neurology*, vol. 55, pp. S34–S39, 2000.

[84] S.-T. Tsai, S.-H. Lin, S.-Z. Lin, J.-Y. Chen, C.-W. Lee, and S.-Y. Chen, "Neuropsychological effects after chronic subthalamic stimulation and the topography of the nucleus in Parkinson's disease," *Neurosurgery*, vol. 61, no. 5, pp. E1024–E1029, 2007.

[85] M. K. York, E. A. Wilde, R. Simpson, and J. Jankovic, "Relationship between neuropsychological outcome and DBS surgical trajectory and electrode location," *Journal of the Neurological Sciences*, vol. 287, no. 1-2, pp. 159–171, 2009.

[86] K. M. Smith, M. O'Connor, E. Papavassiliou, D. Tarsy, and L. C. Shih, "Phonemic verbal fluency decline after subthalamic nucleus deep brain stimulation does not depend on number of microelectrode recordings or lead tip placement," *Parkinsonism & Related Disorders*, vol. 20, no. 4, pp. 400–404, 2014.

[87] L. L. Trépanier, R. Kumar, A. M. Lozano, A. E. Lang, and J. A. Saint-Cyr, "Neuropsychological outcome of GPi pallidotomy and GPi or STN deep brain stimulation in Parkinson's disease," *Brain and Cognition*, vol. 42, no. 3, pp. 324–347, 2000.

[88] L. Wojtecki, L. Timmermann, S. Jörgens et al., "Frequency-dependent reciprocal modulation of verbal fluency and motor functions in subthalamic deep brain stimulation," *JAMA Neurology*, vol. 63, no. 9, pp. 1273–1276, 2006.

[89] M. R. Schoenberg, K. M. Mash, K. J. Bharucha, P. C. Francel, and J. G. Scott, "Deep brain stimulation parameters associated with neuropsychological changes in subthalamic nucleus stimulation for refractory Parkinson's disease," *Stereotactic and Functional Neurosurgery*, vol. 86, no. 6, pp. 337–344, 2008.

[90] L. Castelli, M. Lanotte, M. Zibetti et al., "Apathy and verbal fluency in STN-stimulated PD patients: An Observational Follow-up Study," *Journal of Neurology*, vol. 254, no. 9, pp. 1238–1243, 2007.

[91] M. F. Contarino, A. Daniele, A. H. Sibilia et al., "Cognitive outcome 5 years after bilateral chronic stimulation of subthalamic nucleus in patients with Parkinson's disease," *Journal of Neurology, Neurosurgery & Psychiatry*, vol. 78, no. 3, pp. 248–252, 2007.

[92] K. Dujardin, L. Defebvre, P. Krystkowiak, S. Blond, and A. Destée, "Influence of chronic bilateral stimulation of the subthalamic nucleus on cognitive function in Parkinson's disease," *Journal of Neurology*, vol. 248, no. 7, pp. 603–611, 2001.

[93] T. Erola, E. R. Heikkinen, T. Haapaniemi, J. Tuominen, A. Juolasmaa, and V. V. Myllylä, "Efficacy of bilateral subthalamic nucleus (STN) stimulation in Parkinson's disease," *Acta Neurochirurgica*, vol. 148, no. 4, pp. 389–393, 2006.

[94] A. Funkiewiez, C. Ardouin, P. Krack et al., "Acute psychotropic effects of bilateral subthalamic nucleus stimulation and Levodopa in Parkinson's disease," *Movement Disorders*, vol. 18, no. 5, pp. 524–530, 2003.

[95] J.-H. Heo, K.-M. Lee, S. H. Paek et al., "The effects of bilateral Subthalamic Nucleus Deep Brain Stimulation (STN DBS) on cognition in Parkinson disease," *Journal of the Neurological Sciences*, vol. 273, no. 1-2, pp. 19–24, 2008.

[96] L. K. Krugel, F. Ehlen, H. O. Tiedt, A. A. Kühn, and F. Klostermann, "Differential impact of thalamic versus subthalamic deep brain stimulation on lexical processing," *Neuropsychologia*, vol. 63, pp. 175–184, 2014.

[97] E. Lhommée, H. Klinger, S. Thobois et al., "Subthalamic stimulation in Parkinson's disease: restoring the balance of motivated behaviours," *Brain*, vol. 135, no. 5, pp. 1463–1477, 2012.

[98] E. Moro, M. Scerrati, L. M. A. Romito, R. Roselli, P. Tonali, and A. Albanese, "Chronic subthalamic nucleus stimulation reduces medication requirements in Parkinson's disease," *Neurology*, vol. 53, no. 1, pp. 85–90, 1999.

[99] J. A. Saint-Cyr, L. L. Trépanier, R. Kumar, A. M. Lozano, and A. E. Lang, "Neuropsychological consequences of chronic bilateral stimulation of the subthalamic nucleus in Parkinson's disease," *Brain*, vol. 123, no. 10, pp. 2091–2108, 2000.

[100] L. Yágüez, A. Costello, J. Moriarty et al., "Cognitive predictors of cognitive change following bilateral subthalamic nucleus deep brain stimulation in Parkinson's disease," *Journal of Clinical Neuroscience*, vol. 21, no. 3, pp. 445–450, 2014.

[101] R. Mehanna, "Cognitive Changes after Deep Brain Stimulation in Parkinson's Disease: A Critical Review," *Brain Disorders & Therapy*, vol. 03, no. 2, 2014.

10

Are Patients Ready for "EARLYSTIM"? Attitudes towards Deep Brain Stimulation among Female and Male Patients with Moderately Advanced Parkinson's Disease

Maria Sperens,[1] Katarina Hamberg,[2] and Gun-Marie Hariz[1,3]

[1]*Department of Community Medicine and Rehabilitation, Occupational Therapy, Umeå University, 901 87 Umeå, Sweden*
[2]*Department of Public Health and Clinical Medicine, Family Medicine, Umeå University, 901 87 Umeå, Sweden*
[3]*Department of Pharmacology and Clinical Neuroscience, Umeå University, 90 187 Umeå, Sweden*

Correspondence should be addressed to Gun-Marie Hariz; gun.marie.hariz@umu.se

Academic Editor: Hubert H. Fernandez

Objective. To explore, in female and male patients with medically treated, moderately advanced Parkinson's disease (PD), their knowledge and reasoning about Deep Brain Stimulation (DBS). *Methods.* 23 patients with PD (10 women), aged 46–70, were interviewed at a mean of 8 years after diagnosis, with open-ended questions concerning their reflections and considerations about DBS. The interviews were transcribed verbatim and analysed according to the difference and similarity technique in Grounded Theory. *Results.* From the patients' narratives, the core category "Processing DBS: balancing symptoms, fears and hopes" was established. The patients were knowledgeable about DBS and expressed cautious and well considered attitudes towards its outcome but did not consider themselves ill enough to undergo DBS. They were aware of its potential side-effects. They considered DBS as the last option when oral medication is no longer sufficient. There was no difference between men and women in their reasoning and attitudes towards DBS. *Conclusion.* This study suggests that knowledge about the pros and cons of DBS exists among PD patients and that they have a cautious attitude towards DBS. Our patients did not seem to endorse an earlier implementation of DBS, and they considered that it should be the last resort when really needed.

1. Introduction

Deep Brain Stimulation (DBS) of mainly the subthalamic nucleus (STN) has become an established surgical procedure for patients with advanced Parkinson's disease (PD) [1–3].

Nevertheless, it is not unusual that the beneficial effect of DBS is mitigated by various side-effects such as dysarthria, decrease in verbal fluency, and changes in behaviour, fatigue, and depression [4–6]. Careful selection criteria of patients considered for DBS have been established, including Levodopa response, age, normal brain MRI, good cognition, and realistic expectations [3, 7]. Following adequate information about the pros and cons of the procedure [8], the final decision to undergo surgery will be taken by the patient.

Research on the decision-making process of patients having already undergone DBS for PD had shown in retrospect that the individual patient's knowledge about (and attitude towards) DBS had been crucial for their final decision to undergo DBS [9]. However, non-operated upon patients' own thoughts, considerations, and apprehensions concerning advanced therapy for PD have received scarce attention in the literature [10, 11]. This issue is all the more interesting in light of existing gender differences, with more men than women undergoing DBS for PD [12–15] and given the current trend of suggesting DBS earlier in the disease progress [16–18].

The aim of this qualitative study was to explore, in female and male patients with medically treated, moderately advanced PD, their knowledge, feelings, and reasoning about DBS.

2. Material and Methods

2.1. Participants. In order to enroll in this study patients who may have had reason to consider DBS as a treatment alternative, a strategic selection was used: a nurse specialized in PD at Umeå University Hospital helped us to identify patients with

TABLE 1: Sociodemographic and clinical characteristics of 23 participants (10 women) with Parkinson's disease.

	Whole group	Men (%)	Women (%)	P
Number of Participants	23	13/(56.5)	10 (43.5)	
Age	Mean ± SD (range)	Mean ± SD (range)	Mean ± SD (range)	
Age at diagnosis	52.4 ± 7.15 (40–63)	53.7 ± 7.5 (41–63)	50.7 ± 6.7 (40–61)	ns
Years since diagnosis	7.8 ± 4.7 (1–19)	8.0 ± 4.3 (3–17)	7.6 ± 5.5 (1–19)	ns
Age at interview	60.2 ± 6.8 (46–70)	61.6 ± 7.2 (46–70)	58.3 ± 6.1 (47–67)	ns
LEDD (mg)[€]	1185.5 ± 555.4 (525–2322)[€]	1356.7 ± 618.9 (525–2322)[€]	889.6 ± 250.4 (600–1310)[€]	ns
Number of daily doses[¥]	5.3 ± 1.8 (3–9)	5.9 ± 1.9 (3–9)	4.3 ± 1.2 (3–6)	0.045
Number (%) of patients who needed assistance in some daily activities	13 (56.5)	9 (69.2)	4 (40)	
Civil status	N (%)	N (%)	N (%)	
Cohabitant/single	19 (83)/4 (17)	11 (85)/2 (14)	8 (80)/2 (20)	
Level of education	N (%)	N (%)	N (%)	
Primary school	5 (21.7)	3 (23.1)	2 (20.0)	
High school	7 (30.4)	4 (30.8)	3 (30.0)	
University	11 (47.8)	6 (46.2)	5 (50.0)	
Employment status at time of interview	N (%)	N (%)	N (%)	
Working full time	1 (4.3)	1 (7.7)	0	
Working part time & sick-leave part time	7 (30.4)	2 (15.4)	5 (50.0)	
Sick-leave full time	8 (34.8)	4 (30.8)	4 (40.0)	
Retired	7 (30.4)	6 (46.2)	1 (10.0)	
Perceived general health at time of interview[#]	N (%)[#]	N (%)[#]	N (%)	
Excellent	1 (4.5)	0 (0.0)	1 (10.0)	
Very good	5 (22.7)	3 (25.0)	2 (20.0)	
Good	5 (22.7)	2 (16.7)	3 (30.0)	
Fair	10 (45.5)	7 (58.3)	3 (30.0)	
Bad	1 (4.5)	0 (0.0)	1 (10.0)	
Overall impact of PD on life at time of interview	N (%)	N (%)	N (%)	
Mild	1 (4.3)	1 (7.7)	0	
Moderate	22 (95.7)	12 (92.3)	10 (100.0)	
Severe	0	0	0	
Number of members of PD society (%)	19 (82.6)	11 (84.6)	8 (80.0)	

L-dopa = Levodopa.
LEDD = Levodopa equivalent daily doses.
[€]Missing data in 4 (1 male) patients.
[¥]Missing data in 2 female patients.
[#]Missing data in 1 male patient.

PD who despite high and/or frequent doses of dopaminergic medication experienced difficult symptoms and problems in daily life. There were 36 patients (23 males, 13 females) who fulfilled these criteria. Information about the study was sent to them and they were asked if they agreed to participate in an interview. One reminder was sent to those who did not answer. Twenty-one patients (14 men) accepted to be interviewed. One 80-year-old patient was excluded since he would not have been eligible for DBS due to high age. Three additional women were recruited along the same criteria after contact with Parkinson's Disease Society. Table 1 shows the description of the 23 enrolled patients.

The local ethical board at Umeå University approved the study, and all patients gave written informed consent before the interview (D.No: 2012-36-32M).

2.2. Data Collection. Data were collected through qualitative interviews [19, 20]. The majority of the interviews were conducted face to face by one interviewer (MS, GMH, or KH) in a setting chosen by the patient, usually in the patient's home. Due to practical difficulties (e.g., long distances) four patients were interviewed by telephone. The interviews were semistructured, with open-ended questions concerning broad areas, such as how the patients felt and reacted when they received the diagnosis, their experiences of PD and its treatments over time, how it has been and how it is now to live with PD, their knowledge about treatments other than oral medication, especially DBS, and how they felt and thought about future treatment. In this paper, we focus on the patients' knowledge, feelings, and reasoning about DBS. Sample questions related to this focus included the following: *"Can you tell about the treatment that you currently have for Parkinson's disease?"; "Do you know of other treatments than oral medications?"; "How did you learn about these other treatments?";* and *"What do you think and feel about DBS as a treatment for PD?"* The interviewer tried to facilitate the narrative by follow-up questions such as, *"Please, can you explain further"; "What do you mean?"; "Please, could you give me an example?"*

Each interview lasted 60–140 minutes and was digitally recorded and transcribed verbatim.

In addition to the interview, each participant completed a short questionnaire about sociodemographic information. The patients were also asked to assess the overall impact of PD on their health by answering the questions *"In general, how do you perceive your overall health on a five-point scale (excellent, very good, good, fair, bad)?"* and *"How do you experience the overall impact of your Parkinson's disease (mild, moderate, severe)?"*

The patients' Levodopa equivalent daily doses (LEDD) at time of the interview were obtained from the patients' medical record.

2.3. Data Analysis

2.3.1. Qualitative Analysis of the Interviews. According to qualitative research design [19], preliminary analyses of the transcriptions were conducted in parallel with the interview process. The authors could thereby learn and reflect during the interview process, refine interview questions, and be alert when new aspects were described.

The main analysis of the interviews was made according to the constant comparison technique in Grounded Theory [19, 20]. The analysis contained the following phases:

(1) In a first phase all researchers separately read and coded three interviews and then met to compare codes and discuss content and meaning of the participants' experiences. Case narratives summarizing the essentials of each interview were written down. Another three interviews were then coded, compared, and summarized, and this process of sorting the data continued until all interviews were worked through and summarized in case narratives.

(2) In a second phase all interviews were reread by the first author and passages that concerned the participants' thoughts, reflections, and utterances about future treatment and DBS were identified, cut out, and organized in separate *"considerations-about-treatment"* files, one for each participant. These files were read and systematically coded and compared for similarities and differences by all researchers separately. In joint sessions the codes were compared and discussed, and categories and subcategories were elaborated. A core category embracing the content and meaning in the participants' narratives was also established.

(3) Thereafter the *"considerations-about-treatment"* files were analysed specifically for similarities and differences between men and women.

(4) Finally the whole interviews were reread to ensure that the categories and interpretations could be recontextualized into the interviews, that is, that the results were grounded in the data.

2.4. Statistical Analysis. Descriptive continuous variables were presented as average ± standard deviation and range by use of the SPSS for Mac 21.0. A p value < 0.05 was considered significant.

3. Results

3.1. Demographic Data and Clinical Outcome. Table 1 shows the sociodemographic and clinical characteristics of the participants, their self-assessed general health, and the overall impact of PD on life as a whole, as well as the Levodopa equivalent daily dose (LEDD). The mean disease duration was 7.8 years and the mean LEDD was 1186 mg. One patient was treated with Duodopa pump. Thirteen patients (4 women and 9 men) reported that they needed help in some of the daily activities. All but one patient considered that PD had a moderate overall impact on their life (Table 1).

3.2. Interviews. The participants displayed interest and engagement in the interview. They described in detail their symptoms and how these impacted on their everyday life. The most common symptoms reported by the patients were in various combinations: shaking, stiffness, wear-off and fluctuations, involuntary movements, cramps, fatigue, gait problems, low mood, and sensitivity to stress. There were no differences in symptom profile between men and women.

With respect to DBS, all participants were knowledgeable about it, and shared their views and reflections about DBS as a potential additional treatment. The sources of their knowledge were information from (and discussions with) medical staff, as well as information from the Internet, from watching TV-programs and by reading newsletters published by the patients' society. Several participants had also met other people who had undergone DBS for PD.

The analysis of the interviews resulted in the core category "Processing DBS: balancing symptoms, fears and hopes." This core category was underpinned by two main categories: *"Neurosurgical treatment requires careful consideration"* and *"Timing of concurrent issues of importance for DBS."* Each of these two categories was supported by three and four subcategories, respectively (see Table 2). In the following, the categories and subcategories are presented and illustrated with quotes from the participants. The participants are given fictitious numbers from Mr. 1 to Ms. 23.

3.2.1. Processing DBS: Balancing Symptoms, Fears and Hopes. The participants' main opinion about DBS as a treatment

TABLE 2: A core category underpinned by two main categories. Each main category is supported by three and four subcategories, respectively.

Core category	Processing DBS: balancing symptoms, fears and hopes	
Main categories	Neurosurgical treatment requires careful consideration	Timing of concurrent issues of importance for DBS
Subcategories	(1) *Worries related to the neurosurgical procedure* (2) *Cautious attitudes towards outcome after DBS* (3) *Concerns about suitability of DBS for one's own symptoms*	(1) *Bringing up the issue of DBS* (2) *Utilizing the treatment alternatives gradually, step by step* (3) *Considering disease progression and life situation* (4) *Hoping for future breakthrough in PD research*

alternative was that DBS was not on their agenda for the time being. However, most of our interviewees considered that DBS might become an alternative later due to progress of the disease or to drawbacks and inefficacy of medication. Their current situation and the degree of difficulties that they experienced in daily life, as well as their hopes for research and discoveries of new and better treatment options for PD, also impacted on the way women and men reasoned about eventual DBS treatment.

Neurosurgical Treatment Requires Careful Consideration

(1) Worries Related to the Neurosurgical Procedure. Both men and women expressed worries about undergoing a neurosurgical intervention and the potential risk of damaging a very important and sensitive organ. Mr. 1 described his fascination about the capacity of the brain and at the same time his fear of being damaged during surgery: "*I remember a fishing tour, it is twenty-five years ago, I can spot it in a split second. . .*" and he continued "*they* (the electrodes) *are very close to the memory centre.*"

Some of the participants' considerations consisted of more general expressions about surgery being something that always could pose a risk, whereas other concerns were more specifically related to the surgical procedure per se, such as being attached to the surgical equipment. Such thoughts implied feelings of uneasiness, as phrased by Mr. 10, "*would you like to be strapped up?*" The participants expressed both positive and negative concerns about the new routine of having DBS under general anaesthesia: on one hand, they felt relief at being asleep during drilling of the skull, and on the other hand they expressed fear of being totally without control during the course of surgery.

(2) Cautious Attitudes towards Outcome after DBS. Both men and women were concerned about what they perceived to be an inconsistent outcome after DBS. They had noticed that some friends and acquaintances who had DBS felt very well while others seemed to have deteriorated to a state worse than before surgery. Mr. 1 referred to the following observation of a friend: "*I know a person who was convinced DBS would turn out well and that was also the case initially, but then he encountered complications and now he is not that well anymore.*" The participants' thoughts and considerations were mainly related to a potential negative outcome after DBS rather than

to possible positive effects, and the risk of impaired balance after DBS was frequently mentioned as a concern.

Another common perception among the interviewed patients was that after DBS some patients seemed to need higher and more frequent doses of medication. The participants regarded this as a negative outcome of DBS. Ms. 14 said, "*I think that they* (fellow people with PD after DBS) *are in need of lots of medications.*" Further, some of the participants had met people who after DBS did not seem to be their "*usual self*" any more. They were more low-spirited and nearly depressed, as told by Ms. 16, who stated, "*I must say that they became low, I would say depressed and their reasoning was in a different way, as well*"; and Mr. 3 stated, "*I think they have become more quiet, one might say a bit less positive.*" These participants implied thus that there is a possible risk that DBS may induce personality changes.

(3) Concerns about Suitability of DBS for One's Own Symptoms. The participants expressed concerns about whether they themselves would be suitable candidates for DBS surgery. The interviewees whose tremor was their main symptom considered that the shaking was difficult to treat only with oral medication, and they also knew that DBS might be efficient for alleviating tremor, "*I would probably be a good candidate for DBS because I am shaking. . .*" (Ms. 18). On the other hand, participants with impaired balance explained that they were less likely to be ideal candidates for DBS and Mr. 7 said that his neurologist considered that "*to offer me surgery would not be a good idea because it can lead to worsening of gait and some patients may get poorer balance.*"

Timing of Concurrent Issues of Importance for DBS

(1) Bringing Up the Issue of DBS. The participants considered that they had enough knowledge about DBS as a treatment alternative, and the majority of them expressed no wish or need for more discussion about DBS for the time being.

Three women reported that they had found it difficult to consider DBS surgery when their clinician suggested it early in the course of the disease, and when one of them was referred to the DBS team, she declined to undergo the presurgical evaluation. Six of the men had been offered DBS and two of them declined to undergo presurgical screening. Among the four men who were assessed in view of DBS, two were not found to be ill enough, while the two others eventually understood that they were not considered suitable due to early signs of cognitive decline. Both of them expressed that it would have been easier to accept the denial of DBS had they received a careful explanation of the reasons, as exemplified by Mr. 1: *"yes, my understanding perhaps would have been better if I had had a proper explanation as to why they instead recommended pump to me."*

Still, bringing up the issues about DBS was considered highly relevant for two of the male participants and they were awaiting the right moment to bring it up themselves, as Mr. 12 put it: *"well, absolutely, I can bring up DBS myself, but today I do not feel it is the right time."*

(2) Utilizing the Treatment Alternatives Gradually, Step by Step. The participants considered oral medication as the basic treatment, and they were hoping to be able to keep their current treatment stable for as long as possible. They considered advanced treatment alternatives, such as infusions and injections and DBS as a limited treatment resource. These different treatment alternatives were described as something linear, to be taken step by step. The typical description was that medication was followed by an increase of oral medication, thereafter apomorphine injection pens, and then pumps and finally ending with DBS. This can be illustrated by Mr. 8 in the following: *"I have to put up with certain things because I know that the more medications I 'waste' the more I tear on future resources"* and Ms. 19 stated that *"DBS is the last* (treatment alternative)." To utilize the last step, that is, DBS, was something unwanted, and, for the participants, it implied having nothing left to turn to if needed after surgery. Mr. 13 explained, *"So I'm still acting cowardly. You also need to have some treatment alternative left."* Thus, the majority described DBS as a step they rather would postpone as long as possible. For a few patients though, DBS was more of a natural treatment step when medication no longer efficiently could control the symptoms of the disease, as described by Ms. 20, *"if the impact of medication ceases, then there is more (DBS), like a continuum."*

(3) Considering Disease Progression and Life Situation. Even if most participants did not consider DBS in their current situation, they envisaged it as an alternative later on, if, or when, the symptoms became even worse. Both women and men expressed that when the disease had progressed to a level when they would have great difficulties managing their lives, DBS might be an additional treatment option. At a certain point of disease progression, any treatment that may provide a better life could be considered. This reasoning was put forward by Ms. 23 in the following: *"When I no longer am able to brush my teeth, then I might consider DBS"* and by Mr. 6: *"I would keep away from it (DBS) as long as possible. But it is hard to say, if you are struck by these difficulties you might feel that you would do anything…."*

(4) Hoping for Future Breakthrough in PD Research. The participants were aware of the importance of research for improved life conditions for persons with PD, and they expressed hope that research would open up for totally new treatments. Some conveyed a hope for a real cure of

the disease, rather than only better or newer pills to keep the symptoms at a manageable level, as uttered by Ms. 20, *"and then some researcher will find something marvelous."* The patients' wishes for research-driven new and better treatments were particularly focused on nonsurgical options rather than new surgical procedures. They hoped for more efficacious oral medication, for reducing the numbers of daily doses to only one intake a day and for an easier handling of equipment when using pumps. Expectations and hope related to DBS were expressed in more general terms, such as wishes for even better surgical skills and techniques. There was awareness about stem cells research and also about alternative nonmedical treatment such as dietary advice, for example, eating blueberries.

However, even if most participants hoped for breakthroughs in research they underlined that research takes time and Mr. 4 confessed that he nowadays had low expectations: *"I've been interested but I have sort of given up on that now. It takes so long before it becomes available, stem cells and so on."*

4. Discussion

The aim of this interview study was to explore attitudes towards (and perceptions of) DBS, among women and men with medically treated, moderately advanced Parkinson's disease, who could have had reasons to consider DBS as a treatment option. The most interesting findings were that both women and men were quite knowledgeable about DBS but they did not feel that DBS was an option for them for the time being. They had respect for DBS as being a serious surgical procedure done on the brain, and they considered that it should be kept as a last resort. They were also aware of its side-effects such as impaired balance and personality changes. In contrast to what has been reported in the literature [21–26] and what is commonly depicted in the lay press [27], our patients kept low expectations from DBS. However, the patients were also aware of the symptom profiles that are commonly considered to benefit from DBS (such as tremor) as well as the contraindications, such as balance problems and cognitive decline. There were no differences in those respects between male and female participants. On the whole, despite having had the disease for several years and despite the myriad of symptoms that they described, there was an agreement among patients that DBS should be utilized as a last treatment, when all other options were exhausted. This approach, conveyed by the patients themselves, is at odds with the recent "EARLYSTIM" trend in the literature in favor of proposing DBS for patients earlier in the disease progression [16–18].

4.1. Patients' Considerations about DBS. How come that our patients showed more reserved and less enthusiastic attitudes towards DBS than what one can commonly find in the literature? [16–18]. There may be several explanations to this: our patients had in general a high level of education with 78% of them having a high school or university degrees (Table 1), which could imply that they were able to better judge information conveyed by the lay media and health care professionals. Additionally, 83% of our patients were members of a Parkinson's disease organization (Table 1) and hence may be well knowledgeable about the disease and its various treatments modalities, including their side-effects, as shown in other studies [8, 28]. Another factor to consider is that several of our patients had friends and acquaintances who had had DBS and they could thus see that the reality of DBS was sometimes different from the glamour, in particular concerning the side-effects. Patients who were on DBS may have conveyed to our participants a sense of disappointment despite the motor improvement [29]. The fact that our patients rated the impact of PD on their life as moderate (Table 1) and did not have a very long disease duration did not motivate them to consider a surgical procedure that may harbor complications and side-effects: they felt that for the time being they may have more to lose than to gain from DBS. In this respect, it is important to underline that it may be difficult for patients to admit that a chronic progressive illness is "severe" such that it may lead to seeking a treatment that they consider as a "last resort." Hence, our patients would most probably not have submitted themselves to an "EARLYSTIM" procedure [16, 30]. Three of the 13 men and five of the 10 women who were interviewed were still professionally active and this could also be a factor that influenced their attitude to DBS especially in relation to the possible side-effects from surgery that all patients were aware of. Finally, our patients expressed hope that research would bring about other nonsurgical treatments that they would benefit from, enabling them thus to avoid a surgical procedure on their brains.

4.2. Gender Differences in Perceptions of DBS? Earlier studies have shown that, in relation to the gender prevalence of PD, women are underrepresented among those treated with DBS [12, 14, 15, 31]. The reason for this is unknown but it has been suggested that women might be more "afraid" of (and hesitant towards) neurosurgery compared to men [32]. Our results here showed that the narratives and ways of reasoning about DBS were similar in men and women. Both men and women contributed to all subcategories and categories. Both expressed some worries for surgery and its risks and had modest expectations on the positive effects of DBS. Likewise, both men and women considered DBS to be a treatment modality to postpone until the symptoms were too difficult to cope with and to consider when no other treatment option was left. Consequently, our results do not give evidence for any differences in perceptions and attitudes towards DBS among men and women that could explain the male predominance among patients treated with DBS for Parkinson's disease [12, 15, 16]. Additionally, it seems that our patients may not endorse an "EARLYSTIM strategy" for treatment of their PD, such as has been advocated recently in the literature [16, 17].

5. Limitations of This Study

For this study, near half of the patients who were invited to participate either declined the invitation or did not reply. This may have introduced a selection bias in favor of patients who are more outgoing and willing to discuss their disease and attitudes to DBS. Additionally, our participants are all living in Sweden and the results may not be applicable elsewhere.

6. Conclusions

In conclusion, our study showed that patients with moderately advanced PD who would be potential candidates for DBS had indeed good knowledge about the pros and cons of this treatment modality and expressed a realistic view about its potential limitations. They were not ready yet to submit to "early" DBS; they perceived DBS as a last resort that should be carefully considered only if absolutely needed. There were no differences between men and women concerning their reasoning and attitude towards DBS.

Acknowledgments

The authors thank the participants for giving them of their time to conduct the interviews. This study was supported by The Swedish Research Council and The Parkinson Foundation in Sweden.

References

[1] G. Deuschl, C. Schade-Brittinger, P. Krack et al., "A randomized trial of deep-brain stimulation for Parkinson's disease," *New England Journal of Medicine*, vol. 355, no. 9, pp. 896–908, 2006.

[2] F. M. Weaver, K. Follett, M. Stern et al., "Bilateral deep brain stimulation vs best medical therapy for patients with advanced parkinson disease: a randomized controlled trial," *JAMA*, vol. 301, no. 1, pp. 63–73, 2009.

[3] J. M. Bronstein, M. Tagliati, R. L. Alterman et al., "Deep brain stimulation for Parkinson disease—an expert consensus and review of key issues," *Archives of Neurology*, vol. 68, no. 2, pp. 165–171, 2011.

[4] K. Witt, C. Daniels, and J. Volkmann, "Factors associated with neuropsychiatric side effects after STN-DBS in Parkinson's disease," *Parkinsonism and Related Disorders*, vol. 18, supplement 1, pp. S168–S170, 2012.

[5] A.-S. Moldovan, S. J. Groiss, S. Elben, M. Südmeyer, A. Schnitzler, and L. Wojtecki, "The treatment of Parkinson's disease with deep brain stimulation: current issues," *Neural Regeneration Research*, vol. 10, no. 7, pp. 1018–1022, 2015.

[6] V. J. J. Odekerken, J. A. Boel, G. J. Geurtsen et al., "Neuropsychological outcome after deep brain stimulation for Parkinson disease," *Neurology*, vol. 84, no. 13, pp. 1355–1361, 2015.

[7] T. Foltynie and M. I. Hariz, "Surgical management of Parkinson's disease," *Expert Review of Neurotherapeutics*, vol. 10, no. 6, pp. 903–914, 2010.

[8] R. Erasmi, G. Deuschl, and K. Witt, "Tiefe Hirnstimulation bei Morbus Parkinson: wann und für wen?" *Der Nervenarzt*, vol. 85, no. 2, pp. 137–146, 2014.

[9] K. Hamberg and G.-M. Hariz, "The decision-making process leading to deep brain stimulation in men and women with parkinson's disease—an interview study," *BMC Neurology*, vol. 14, no. 1, article 89, 2014.

[10] F. A. P. Nijhuis, J. Van Heek, B. R. Bloem, B. Post, and M. J. Faber, "Choosing an advanced therapy in Parkinson's disease; is it an evidence-based decision in current practice?" *Journal of Parkinson's Disease*, vol. 6, no. 3, pp. 533–543, 2016.

[11] M. G. Weernink, J. A. van Til, J. P. van Vugt et al., "Involving patients in weighting benefits and harms of treatment in Parkinson's disease," *PLoS ONE*, vol. 11, no. 8, Article ID e0160771, 2016.

[12] M. Setiawan, S. Kraft, K. Doig et al., "Referrals for movement disorder surgery: under-representation of females and reasons for refusal," *Canadian Journal of Neurological Sciences*, vol. 33, no. 1, pp. 53–57, 2006.

[13] E. Accolla, E. Caputo, F. Cogiamanian et al., "Gender differences in patients with Parkinson's disease treated with subthalamic deep brain stimulation," *Movement Disorders*, vol. 22, no. 8, pp. 1150–1156, 2007.

[14] G.-M. Hariz, T. Nakajima, P. Limousin et al., "Gender distribution of patients with Parkinson's disease treated with subthalamic deep brain stimulation; a review of the 2000–2009 literature," *Parkinsonism and Related Disorders*, vol. 17, no. 3, pp. 146–149, 2011.

[15] G.-M. Hariz, P. Limousin, L. Zrinzo et al., "Gender differences in quality of life following subthalamic stimulation for Parkinson's disease," *Acta Neurologica Scandinavica*, vol. 128, no. 4, pp. 281–285, 2013.

[16] V. M. M Schuepbach, J. Rau, K. Knudsen et al., "Neurostimulation for Parkinson's disease with early motor complications," *The New England Journal of Medicine*, vol. 368, no. 7, pp. 610–622, 2013.

[17] W. M. M. Schüpbach, J. Rau, J.-L. Houeto et al., "Myths and facts about the EARLYSTIM study," *Movement Disorders*, vol. 29, no. 14, pp. 1742–1750, 2014.

[18] G. Deuschl, M. Schüpbach, K. Knudsen et al., "Stimulation of the subthalamic nucleus at an earlier disease stage of Parkinson's disease: concept and standards of the EARLYSTIM-study," *Parkinsonism and Related Disorders*, vol. 19, no. 1, pp. 56–61, 2013.

[19] J. Corbin and A. Strauss, *Basics of Qualitative Research: Techniques and Procedures for Developing Grounded Theory*, SAGE, Thousand Oaks, Calif, USA, 3rd edition, 2008.

[20] K. Charmaz, *Constructing Grounded Theory*, SAGE Publications, Thousand Oaks, Calif, USA, 2nd edition, 2014.

[21] M. I. Hariz, "What is deep brain stimulation 'failure' and how do we manage our own failures?" *Archives of Neurology*, vol. 62, no. 12, p. 1938, 2005.

[22] R. L. Rodriguez, H. H. Fernandez, I. Haq, and M. S. Okun, "Pearls in patient selection for deep brain stimulation," *The Neurologist*, vol. 13, no. 5, pp. 253–260, 2007.

[23] M. S. Okun, R. L. Rodriguez, K. D. Foote et al., "A case-based review of troubleshooting deep brain stimulator issues in movement and neuropsychiatric disorders," *Parkinsonism and Related Disorders*, vol. 14, no. 7, pp. 532–538, 2008.

[24] E. Bell, B. Maxwell, M. P. McAndrews, A. Sadikot, and E. Racine, "Hope and patients' expectations in deep brain stimulation: healthcare providers' perspectives and approaches," *The Journal of Clinical Ethics*, vol. 21, no. 2, pp. 112–124, 2010.

[25] P. Reddy, P. Martinez-Martin, R. G. Brown et al., "Perceptions of symptoms and expectations of advanced therapy for Parkinson's disease: preliminary report of a Patient-Reported Outcome tool for Advanced Parkinson's disease (PRO-APD)," *Health and Quality of Life Outcomes*, vol. 12, article 11, 2014.

[26] H. Hasegawa, M. Samuel, A. Douiri, and K. Ashkan, "Patients' expectations in subthalamic nucleus deep brain stimulation surgery for Parkinson disease," *World Neurosurgery*, vol. 82, no. 6, pp. 1295–1299.E2, 2014.

[27] E. Racine, S. Waldman, N. Palmour, D. Risse, and J. Illes, ""Currents of hope": neurostimulation techniques in U.S. and U.K. print media," *Cambridge Quarterly of Healthcare Ethics*, vol. 16, no. 3, pp. 312–316, 2007.

[28] M. Südmeyer, J. Volkmann, L. Wojtecki, G. Deuschl, A. Schnitzler, and B. Möller, "Tiefe Hirnstimulation—Erwartungen und Bedenken—Bundesweite Fragebogenstudie mit Parkinson-Patienten und deren Angehörigen," *Der Nervenarzt*, vol. 83, no. 4, pp. 481–486, 2012.

[29] F. Maier, C. J. Lewis, N. Horstkoetter et al., "Subjective perceived outcome of subthalamic deep brain stimulation in Parkinson's disease one year after surgery," *Parkinsonism and Related Disorders*, vol. 24, pp. 41–47, 2016.

[30] T. A. Mestre, A. J. Espay, C. Marras, M. H. Eckman, P. Pollak, and A. E. Lang, "Subthalamic nucleus-deep brain stimulation for early motor complications in Parkinson's disease—the EARLYSTIM trial: Early is not always better," *Movement Disorders*, vol. 29, no. 14, pp. 1751–1756, 2014.

[31] E. N. Eskandar, A. Flaherty, G. R. Cosgrove, L. A. Shinobu, and F. G. Barker II, "Surgery for Parkinson disease in the United States, 1996 to 2000: practice patterns, short-term outcomes, and hospital charges in a nationwide sample," *Journal of Neurosurgery*, vol. 99, no. 5, pp. 863–871, 2003.

[32] G.-M. Hariz and M. I. Hariz, "Gender distribution in surgery for Parkinson's disease," *Parkinsonism and Related Disorders*, vol. 6, no. 3, pp. 155–157, 2000.

11

Physical Activity, Fatigue, and Sleep in People with Parkinson's Disease: A Secondary per Protocol Analysis from an Intervention Trial

S. Coe [ID],[1] M. Franssen,[2] J. Collett,[1] D. Boyle,[1] A. Meaney,[1] R. Chantry,[1] P. Esser,[1] H. Izadi,[3] and H. Dawes[1]

[1]*Department of Sport, Health Sciences and Social Work, Oxford Brookes University, Headington Rd., Oxford OX3 0BP, UK*
[2]*Nuffield Department of Primary Care Health Sciences, University of Oxford, Radcliffe Primary Care Building, Oxford OX2 6GG, UK*
[3]*School of Engineering, Computing and Mathematics, Oxford Brookes University, Wheatley, Oxford OX33 1HX, UK*

Correspondence should be addressed to S. Coe; scoe@brookes.ac.uk

Academic Editor: Seyed-Mohammad Fereshtehnejad

Symptoms of Parkinson's can result in low physical activity and poor sleep patterns which can have a detrimental effect on a person's quality of life. To date, studies looking into exercise interventions for people with Parkinson's (PwP) for symptom management are promising but inconclusive. The aim of this study is to estimate the effect of a clearly defined exercise prescription on general physical activity levels, fatigue, sleep, and quality of life in PwP. *Method.* PwP randomised into either an exercise group (29; 16 males, 13 females; mean age 67 years (7.12)) or a control handwriting group (36; 19 males, 17 females; mean age 67 years (5.88)) as part of a larger trial were included in this substudy if they had completed a 6-month weekly exercise programme (intervention group) and had complete objective physical activity data (intervention and control group). Sleep and fatigue were recorded from self-reported measures, and physical activity levels measured through the use of accelerometers worn 24 hours/day over a seven-day testing period at baseline and following the 24-week intervention. A Wilcoxon's test followed by a Mann–Whitney post hoc analysis was used, and effect sizes were calculated. *Results.* Participants showed a significant increase in time spent in sedentary and light activities during the overnight period postintervention in both exercise and handwriting groups ($p < 0.05$) with a moderate effect found for the change in sedentary and light activities in the overnight hours for both groups, over time (0.32 and 0.37-0.38, resp.). There was no impact on self-reported fatigue or sleep. *Conclusion.* The observed moderate effect on sedentary and light activities overnight could suggest an objective improvement in sleep patterns for individuals participating in both exercise and handwriting interventions. This supports the need for further studies to investigate the role of behavioural interventions for nonmotor symptoms.

1. Introduction

Parkinson's is a progressive neurological condition, and it is estimated that one in every 350 people in the UK are diagnosed with the condition. Although pharmaceutical interventions are the primary treatment option, exercise is becoming increasingly recognised as an effective addition to commonly used drug treatments for the control of both motor and nonmotor symptoms [1]. There is strong evidence supporting beneficial effects of exercise programs on disease progression, motor and nonmotor symptom management, and health and wellbeing in PwP [2–8]. Exercise interventions and a dose of 30 minutes or more a week of moderate to vigorous physical activity have been suggested to positively impact on the global nonmotor symptom burden including depression, apathy, fatigue, daytime sleepiness, sleep, and cognition [2–7, 9]. However, the evidence supporting a positive benefit of exercise to physical activity, fatigue, daytime sleepiness, and sleep is not strong [9].

PwP report sleep problems, daytime sleepiness, and fatigue as significant nonmotor symptoms [10–12]. When considering the mechanism of potential effects of exercise on these symptoms, there are a number of possible positive interactions of a physically active lifestyle including its impact to provide cognitive stimulation, meaningful social interactions, and improvement in healthy eating which may induce better sleep and reduce fatigue [13]. The interaction is complex and not well understood, with these factors interacting together in a formative and reflective manner [9, 13–16]. It is interesting that PwP are observed to have reduced motor symptoms in the morning following sleep, referred to as "sleep benefit" and that fatigue levels are lower in the morning after sleep [17]. Importantly, sleep-related symptoms in Parkinson's have been shown to relate to disease disability and worsening of motor symptoms [18]. In the general population, exercise is known to improve sleep and resulting fatigue [19].

Therefore, there is a benefit of understanding the sleep, exercise, fatigue interaction, and the limited evidence to date to support the impact of exercise on physical activity, fatigue, and sleep in PwP [20–23] and the underpinning mechanism. This study set out to estimate the potential effect of an exercise programme that combined aerobic and strength exercises on sleep patterns, activity levels, and fatigue in a group of PwP who had adhered to a prescribed aerobic and strength training exercise program and had at least three out of seven days of objective activity data collected pre- and postintervention. Therefore, the aim of this study is to estimate the potential effect of a clearly defined exercise prescription compared to an active control condition of a handwriting intervention matched for social contact on objective measures of physical activity levels and self-reported measures of fatigue, quality of life, and sleep in PwP.

2. Methods

2.1. Design. This research was carried out on a subset of data collected as part of an interventional study of exercise training in PwP in which data for PwP were obtained from a two-arm parallel single-blind phase II randomised controlled trial (RCT) of community-delivered exercise for PwP [8]. The current study included all participants from the RCT who were randomised, who adhered to the exercise group in the RCT (≥ one session a week), and who provided comprehensive objective physical activity data in the exercise group and in the handwriting group. The trial was registered with ClinicalTrials.Gov (NCT01439022).

2.2. Setting. Parkinson's assessments were carried out at the Movement Science Laboratory, Oxford Brookes University, Oxford, UK, the intervention took place at community leisure facilities throughout Oxfordshire and Berkshire, and the handwriting sessions took place in the home of the participants.

2.3. Participants. The study received National Health Service ethical approval (NRES Committee South Central–Southampton A: 11/SC/0267) and was conducted in accordance with the declaration of Helsinki.

People with idiopathic Parkinson's were recruited from neurology clinics and GP practices in the Thames Valley, UK, and through local Parkinson's UK group meetings. Inclusion criteria for PwP were as follows: (i) diagnosis of idiopathic Parkinson's (as defined by the UK Parkinson's Disease Society Brain Bank clinical diagnostic criteria [24]) and (ii) ability to walk ≥100 meters. Exclusion criteria were as follows: (i) dementia; (ii) history of additional prior neurological condition; (iii) severe depression or psychosis or a mental state that would preclude consistent active involvement with the study over its duration; (iv) cardiac precautions that would prevent the subject from participating in the intervention; (v) any known contraindication to exercise; (vi) reduced cognitive function of any cause (Mini-Mental State Examination <23); and (vii) an orthopaedic condition that limited independent walking. Participants' medication was continued as normal and was recorded.

2.4. Intervention. The intervention for PwP was a prescribed exercise program consisting of sessions lasting 60 minutes or a handwriting control intervention, twice a week over a period of six months; a detailed description can be found elsewhere [8]. Demographics were recorded before and after the intervention and included fatigue using the Fatigue Severity Scale (FSS) [25] and quality of life using the EQ5D-5L [26]. Selected questions from the Unified Parkinson's Disease Rating Scale, Parts 1 and 2 subsections were recorded including the following: (1) *Over the past week, have you had trouble going to sleep at night or staying asleep through the night? Consider how rested you felt after waking up in the morning;* (2) *Over the past week, have you had trouble staying awake during the daytime?* (3) *Over the past week, do you usually have trouble turning over in bed?* Only PwP who adhered (did not discontinue intervention) to the exercise program and had at least three full days of objective activity data out of total seven days for both the pre- and postassessment were included in the training response analysis. Physical activity in PwP was measured using the wrist-worn activity monitor (GENEActiv, UK). The activity monitor was worn around the wrist for seven consecutive days following an assessment. The activity monitor consisted out of a triaxial accelerometer, sampling at 100 Hz for the duration of seven days. The data were downloaded from the device onto a computer and exported as a 60-second epoch comma delimited file. A bespoke Excel macro using adjusted activity cutoff levels derived minutes per day and relevant percentages spent sedentary, performing light, moderate, or vigorous activities [27]. The physical activity data was analysed in three ways: one 24-hour period, two 12-hour periods involving a daytime section from 08.00 to 20.00, and an overnight section from 20.00 to 08.00, and an 8-hour and a 4-hour evening section from 24.00 to 08.00 and 20.00 to 24.00, respectively. Matthews et al. [28] observed that a minimum of three days was required to accurately calculate average physical activity levels; therefore, files with less than three days of recorded data were excluded from analysis.

2.5. Data Analysis. Descriptive statistics were calculated for demographic characteristics. For activity data, the thresholds were based on amplitude of the single vector magnitude as assessed by the triaxial accelerometer within the periods outlined above. Data was presented as median physical activity levels over a 24-hour period. Due to nonnormality, for outcome data, a Wilcoxon's test followed by a Mann–Whitney post hoc test was used to determine the changes over time and according to two intervention regimes (exercise and handwriting). Further and based on the differences, effect sizes ($r = Z/\sqrt{N}$) were calculated.

3. Results

3.1. Participants. Participant flow for the PwP recruited to the RCT can be found elsewhere [8]. Between December 2011 and August 2013 105 participants were recruited, 37 people adhered to the exercise intervention, and accelerometer data were complete on 29 of these participants (16 males, 13 females; mean age 67 years (7.12)) and 36 in the control handwriting group (19 males; 17 females; mean age 67 years (5.88)) and therefore were included in this secondary analysis. Demographic information is provided in supplementary (available here). Changes in health measures can be seen in Table 1. There were no significant differences pre- and postintervention ($p > 0.05$) or between groups at each time point.

3.2. Accelerometer. The majority of subjects wore the accelerometer for the entire seven days of each of the testing period, and although a small minority of subjects did not achieve this target, inclusion criteria for at least three days out of each seven day period were met. Tables 2–4 show physical activity measurement results. During 20:00–08:00 hours, sedentary time increased while light activity decreased in both groups with the addition of moderate activity decreasing in the control group ($p < 0.05$; Table 3). When the overnight period was considered, from 20:00 to 24:00 and 24:00 to 08:00, again sedentary time increased in both groups with a resulting reduction in time spent in light activity in the intervention group ($p < 0.05$; Table 4). Effect sizes for the same time points showed a moderate effect in the intervention and control groups (0.32 and 0.37-0.38, resp.).

4. Discussion

These findings support the potential use of combined aerobic and strength exercise as a moderator of general physical activity for PwP and as a potential aid for improving sleep as evidenced by reduced activity during the nighttime hours. Importantly, there was a similar effect in the active control group suggesting that behavioural exercise interventions may benefit sleep in PwP.

To examine how participants' physical activity levels changed over the course of the intervention in greater depth, the physical activity data were broken down into 12-hour, 8-hour, and 4-hour time slots. No significant differences were observed at any physical activity level during daytime; however, during the overnight period, there was a significant

TABLE 1: Measures of health before and after the 24-week exercise intervention.

	Exercise		Handwriting	
	Before	After	Before	After
FSS	3 ± 1.38	3 ± 1.35	4 ± 1.46	3 ± 1.56
EQ5D-5L	79.21 ± 12.22	78.48 ± 17.89	76.58 ± 16.29	74.75 ± 17.94
Sleep problems[a]	1.5 ± 1.43	1.3 ± 1.26	1.4 ± 1.33	1.5 ± 1.38
Daytime sleepiness[a]	1.5 ± 0.78	1.5 ± 0.87	1.2 ± 0.94	1.3 ± 0.91
Turning in bed[a]	0.5 ± 0.69	0.7 ± 0.65	0.7 ± 0.62	0.8 ± 0.84

Values are means ± standard deviations. A Wilcoxon signed rank test was used to determine differences between pre- and postintervention followed by a Mann–Whitney test for between-group differences, with *$p < 0.05$ and **$p > 0.05$, respectively. FSS: fatigue severity scale; [a]from UPDRS, Unified Parkinson's Disease Rating Scale Parts 1 and 2 subscores.

TABLE 2: Objective physical activity levels of participants following a 24-week exercise intervention averaged over a 24-hour period.

	Exercise				Handwriting			
	Before	After	Z	ES	Before	After	Z	ES
SED	0.70	0.75	−0.832	0.11	0.68	0.73*	3.488	0.41
LIGHT	0.26	0.23	−0.789	0.10	0.28	0.24*	−3.126	0.37
MOD	0.04	0.03	−0.335	0.04	0.03	0.03*	−2.388	0.28
VIG	0	0	−0.355	0.05	0	0*	−2.293	0.27

The exercise intervention consisted of both aerobic and anaerobic exercise training for 60 minutes, twice a week for 24 weeks. Values are medians of fraction of time spent at each level of activity using an accelerometer. A Wilcoxon signed rank test was used to determine differences between pre- and postintervention followed by a Mann–Whitney test for between-group differences, with *$p < 0.05$ and **$p < 0.05$, respectively. Effect sizes (ES) were calculated using the equation $r = Z/\sqrt{N}$ and were over time in each group. SED, sedentary activity level; LIGHT, light activity level; MOD, moderate activity level; VIG, vigorous activity level.

increase in time spent in sedentary and a significant decrease in time spent in light activity observed in both groups. The increase in sedentary activity overnight might suggest an improvement in the participants' sleep quality, and a good quality of sleep in PwP has been linked to a greater control over motor symptoms the following morning [17]. van Gilst et al. [17] suggest that the beneficial effect of sleep on motor symptoms in Parkinson's is due to improved dopaminergic function during sleep, which increases dopamine levels in the brain, a phenomenon known as "sleep benefit." Symptoms found in Parkinson's, such as tremors and rigidity can make the initiation and maintenance of sleep more difficult than in people without the condition, and therefore any methods or techniques to help improve sleep quality in PwP would be of use [29]. The concept of subjective sleep benefit in the absence of actual objective sleep benefit may also be of clinical relevance to PwP and has been associated with nonmotor improvements [30]. Between 24.00 and 08.00, sedentary activity increased whilst time spent in light activity decreased. Participants spent significantly more time sedentary following both interventions between 20.00 and 24.00 whilst significantly less time was also observed at the light activity level during this time period. This could suggest that PwP who took part in the

TABLE 3: Objective physical activity levels of participants following a 24-week exercise intervention averaged over two 12-hour periods.

	Exercise				Handwriting			
	Before	After	Z	ES	Before	After	Z	ES
08.00–20.00								
SED	0.65	0.63	−0.422	0.06	0.64	0.66	0.927	0.11
LIGHT	0.30	0.32	−0.638	0.08	0.31	0.27	−0.597	0.07
MOD	0.03	0.05	−0.919	0.12	0.03	0.02	−0.408	0.05
VIG	0	0	−0.118	0.02	0	0	−1.719	0.20
20.00–08.00								
SED	**0.75**	**0.87***	−2.411	**0.32**	**0.69**	**0.86***	3.236	**0.38**
LIGHT	**0.22**	**0.12***	−2.411	**0.32**	**0.26**	**0.13***	3.111	**0.37**
MOD	0.01	0.01	−1.344	0.18	0.02	0.01*	−2.662	0.31
VIG	0	0	−1.099	0.14	0	0	−1.112	0.13

The exercise intervention consisted of both aerobic and anaerobic exercise training for 60 minutes, twice a week for 24 weeks. Values are medians of fraction of time spent at each level of activity using an accelerometer. A Wilcoxon signed rank test was used to determine differences between pre- and postintervention followed by a Mann–Whitney test for between-group differences, with $*p < 0.05$ and $**p < 0.05$, respectively. Effect sizes (ES) were calculated using the equation $r = Z/\sqrt{N}$. SED, sedentary activity level; LIGHT, light activity level; MOD, moderate activity level; VIG, vigorous activity level.

TABLE 4: Objective physical activity levels of participants following a 24-week exercise intervention averaged over one eight-hour overnight and one four-hour periods.

	Exercise				Handwriting			
	Before	After	Z	ES	Before	After	Z	ES
24.00–08.00								
SED	0.76	0.89*	−2.000	0.26	0.67	*0.89	2.906	0.34
LIGHT	0.20	0.09*	−2.108	0.28	0.28	*0.09	−2.828	0.33
MOD	0.01	0	−1.658	0.22	0.01	*0	−2.080	0.25
VIG	0	0	−1.734	0.23	0	0	−1.821	0.21
20.00–24.00								
SED	0.63	0.71*	−2.389	0.31	0.68	*0.73	2.121	0.25
LIGHT	0.24	0.18*	−2.433	0.32	0.21	0.14	−1.579	0.19
MOD	0	0.01	−1.622	0.21	0.01	0.01	−0.688	0.08
VIG	0	0	0	0	0	0	−0.307	0.04

The exercise intervention consisted of both aerobic and anaerobic exercise training for 60 minutes, twice a week for 24 weeks. Values are medians of fraction of time spent at each level of activity using an accelerometer. A Wilcoxon signed rank test was used to determine differences between pre- and postintervention followed by a Mann–Whitney test for between-group differences, with $*p < 0.05$ and $**p < 0.05$, respectively. Effect sizes (ES) were calculated using the equation $r = Z/\sqrt{N}$. SED, sedentary activity level; LIGHT, light activity level; MOD, moderate activity level; VIG, vigorous activity level.

exercise intervention went to sleep earlier, or were just less active in the evenings to compensate for the increased activity as a result of the intervention. The effect of this increased daytime activity could therefore have a resulting impact on sleep quantity and quality, reducing daytime tiredness and potentially leading to beneficial changes in both motor and nonmotor symptoms [31]. Engagement with cognitive and fine motor skill tasks may reduce daytime sleepiness and increase nighttime sleep and therefore the active control group may have been receiving cognitive stimulation which may have improved sleep time [32].

Interestingly, in the current study there was no impact on fatigue as shown in previous research [33]. To date, there is limited evidence to support the impact of exercise on physical activity, fatigue, or sleep in PwP [20–23]. Variations of resistance exercise training have been shown to specifically improve subjective sleep quality whilst being safe and feasible for PwP [34]. The combination of aerobic and resistance exercise interventions may be optimal for reducing fatigue, increasing physical activity, and improving sleep quality in PwP, as this was shown in healthy elderly people

who often experience disturbed sleep [35]. In addition, the handwriting control group had engagement with cognitive and fine motor tasks which were also shown to improve sleep. However, mechanisms underlying improved sleeping habits differ and more robust research needs to be conducted in PwP. Demographic data were collected pre- and postintervention, and although there were no significant changes, sleep problems and daytime sleepiness (as recorded via the UPDRS subsections) tended to improve over the 6-month period and should be evaluated in a full trial.

There were some limitations to the current study in that the actual timings of sleep or sleep patterns were not recorded throughout the study, with sleep times being estimated through increased sedentary behaviour. It would be worth performing a subanalysis for those who experience sleep issues or daytime sleepiness at baseline; however, if this was performed in the current trial, the sample size would be small and therefore the findings of limited relevance. Lack of administration of more valid scales and tools (e.g., objective assessment of sleep with polysomnography and Pittsburg Sleep Quality Index) to assess sleep quality is an important limitation of this study. However, the results from this trial add to the current evidence for exercise interventions as a mean to improve symptom management and physical and psychological functioning in PwP [3–8].

5. Conclusion

Evidence has shown that physical activity is beneficial for PwP, yet with little research showing its potential to improve motor and nonmotor symptoms, quality of life, and sleep patterns [36]. The current study looked at the effect of an exercise intervention programme and an active handwriting control group on general physical activity levels in PwP, and it was found that participants experienced a significant increase in time spent sedentary overnight which may have been linked to an improvement in sleep. Future studies should explore the role of physical activity and behavioural interventions to determine the effect on nonmotor symptoms including sleep and fatigue in Parkinson's.

Acknowledgments

The authors thank Martin Tims, Charlotte Winward, Marko Bogdanovic, and Andrew Farmer. This research was supported by the National Institute for Health Research (NIHR) and Research for Patient Benefit Programme (PB-PG-0110-20250). Helen Dawes was supported by the Elizabeth Casson Trust, and she received support from the NIHR Oxford Biomedical Research Centre. Helen Dawes and Johnny Collett were both supported by Higher Education England Thames Valley.

References

[1] National Collaborating Centre for Chronic Conditions, *Parkinson's Disease: National Clinical Guideline for Diagnosis and Management in Primary and Secondary Care*, Royal College of Physicians, London, UK, 2006.

[2] G. M. Petzinger, B. E. Fisher, S. McEwen, J. A. Beeler, J. P. Walsh, and M. W. Jakowec, "Exercise-enhanced neuroplasticity targeting motor and cognitive circuitry in Parkinson's disease," *The Lancet Neurology*, vol. 12, no. 7, pp. 716–726, 2013.

[3] P. L. Wu, M. Lee, and T. T. Huang, "Effectiveness of physical activity on patients with depression and Parkinson's disease: a systematic review," *PLoS One*, vol. 12, no. 7, Article ID e0181515, 2017.

[4] A. Uhrbrand, E. Stenager, M. Sloth Pedersen, and U. Dalgas, "Parkinson's disease and intensive exercise therapy–a systematic review and meta-analysis of randomized controlled trials," *Journal of the Neurological Sciences*, vol. 353, no. 1-2, pp. 9–19, 2015.

[5] R. Sumec, P. Filip, K. Sheardová, and M. Bareš, "Psychological benefits of nonpharmacological methods aimed for improving balance in parkinson's disease: a systematic review," *Behavioural Neurology*, vol. 2015, Article ID 620674, 16 pages, 2015.

[6] L. Roeder, J. T. Costello, S. S. Smith, I. B. Stewart, and G. K. Kerr, "Effects of resistance training on measures of muscular strength in people with Parkinson's disease: a systematic review and meta-analysis," *PLoS One*, vol. 10, no. 7, Article ID e0132135, 2015.

[7] M. R. Rafferty, P. N. Schmidt, S. T. Luo et al., "Regular exercise, quality of life, and mobility in Parkinson's disease: a longitudinal analysis of national Parkinson foundation quality improvement initiative data," *Journal of Parkinson's Disease*, vol. 7, no. 1, pp. 193–202, 2017.

[8] J. Collett, M. Franssen, A. Meaney et al., "Phase II randomised controlled trial of a 6-month self-managed community exercise programme for people with Parkinson's disease," *Journal of Neurology, Neurosurgery & Psychiatry*, vol. 88, no. 3, pp. 204–211, 2016.

[9] M. E. Cusso, K. J. Donald, and T. K. Khoo, "The impact of physical activity on non-motor symptoms in parkinson's disease: a systematic review," *Frontiers in Medicine*, vol. 3, p. 35, 2016.

[10] B. M. Kluger, K. F. Pedersen, O.-B. Tysnes, S. O. Ongre, B. Øygarden, and K. Herlofson, "Is fatigue associated with cognitive dysfunction in early Parkinson's disease?," *Parkinsonism & Related Disorders*, vol. 37, pp. 87–91, 2017.

[11] S. O. Ongre, J. P. Larsen, O. B. Tysnes, and K. Herlofson, "Fatigue in early Parkinson's disease: the Norwegian ParkWest study," *European Journal of Neurology*, vol. 24, no. 1, pp. 105–111, 2017.

[12] B. M. Kluger, K. Herlofson, K. L. Chou et al., "Parkinson's disease-related fatigue: a case definition and recommendations for clinical research," *Movement Disorders*, vol. 31, no. 5, pp. 625–631, 2016.

[13] N. Parletta, Y. Aljeesh, and B. T. Baune, "Health behaviors, knowledge, life satisfaction, and wellbeing in people with mental illness across four countries and comparisons with normative sample," *Frontiers in Psychiatry*, vol. 7, p. 145, 2016.

[14] J. Strahler and U. M. Nater, "Differential effects of eating and drinking on wellbeing-An ecological ambulatory assessment study," *Biological Psychology*, vol. 131, pp. 72–88, 2017.

[15] K. B. Prendergast, L. M. Mackay, and G. M. Schofield, "The clustering of lifestyle behaviours in new zealand and their relationship with optimal wellbeing," *International Journal of Behavioral Medicine*, vol. 23, no. 5, pp. 571–579, 2016.

[16] H. Orpana, J. Vachon, C. Pearson, K. Elliott, M. Smith, and B. Branchard, "Correlates of well-being among Canadians with mood and/or anxiety disorders," *Health Promotion and Chronic Disease Prevention in Canada*, vol. 36, no. 12, pp. 302–313, 2016.

[17] M. M. van Gilst, B. R. Bloem, and S. Overeem, ""Sleep benefit" in Parkinson's disease: a systematic review," *Parkinsonism & Related Disorders*, vol. 19, no. 7, pp. 654–659, 2013.

[18] K. Suzuki, Y. Okuma, T. Uchiyama et al., "Impact of sleep-related symptoms on clinical motor subtypes and disability in Parkinson's disease: a multicentre cross-sectional study," *Journal of Neurology, Neurosurgery & Psychiatry*, vol. 88, no. 11, pp. 953–959, 2017.

[19] G. A. Kelley and K. S. Kelley, "Aerobic exercise and cancer-related fatigue in adults: a reexamination using the IVhet model for meta-analysis," *Cancer Epidemiology Biomarkers & Prevention*, vol. 26, no. 2, pp. 281–283, 2017.

[20] K. M. Prakash, N. V. Nadkarni, W.-K. Lye, M.-H. Yong, L.-M. Chew, and E.-K. Tan, "A longitudinal study of non-motor symptom burden in Parkinson's disease after a transition to expert care," *Parkinsonism & Related Disorders*, vol. 21, no. 8, pp. 843–847, 2015.

[21] G. Lamotte, M. R. Rafferty, J. Prodoehl et al., "Effects of endurance exercise training on the motor and non-motor features of Parkinson's disease: a review," *Journal of Parkinson's Disease*, vol. 5, no. 3, p. 621, 2015.

[22] R. G. Elbers, J. Verhoef, E. E. H. van Wegen, H. W. Berendse, and G. Kwakkel, "Interventions for fatigue in Parkinson's disease," *Cochrane Database of Systematic Reviews*, no. 10, article CD010925, 2015.

[23] M. Franssen, C. Winward, J. Collett, D. Wade, and H. Dawes, "Interventions for fatigue in Parkinson's disease: a systematic review and meta-analysis," *Movement Disorders*, vol. 29, no. 13, pp. 1675–1678, 2014.

[24] C. G. Goetz, B. C. Tilley, S. R. Shaftman et al., "Movement disorder society-sponsored revision of the unified Parkinson's disease rating scale (MDS-UPDRS): scale presentation and clinimetric testing results," *Movement Disorders*, vol. 23, no. 15, pp. 2129–2170, 2008.

[25] K. Herlofson, S. O. Ongre, L. K. Enger, O. B. Tysnes, and J. P. Larsen, "Fatigue in early Parkinson's disease. Minor inconvenience or major distress?," *European Journal of Neurology*, vol. 19, no. 7, pp. 963–968, 2012.

[26] N. J. Devlin, K. K. Shah, Y. Feng, B. Mulhern, and B. van Hout, "Valuing health-related quality of life: an EQ-5D-5L value set for England," *Health Economics*, vol. 27, no. 1, pp. 7–22, 2018.

[27] P. J. Eslinger, P. Moore, C. Anderson, and M. Grossman, "Social cognition, executive functioning, and neuroimaging correlates of empathic deficits in frontotemporal dementia," *Journal of Neuropsychiatry*, vol. 23, no. 1, pp. 74–82, 2011.

[28] C. E. Matthews, B. E. Ainsworth, R. W. Thompson, and D. R. Bassett, "Sources of variance in daily physical activity levels as measured by an accelerometer," *Medicine & Science in Sports & Exercise*, vol. 34, no. 8, pp. 1376–1381, 2002.

[29] C. L. Deschenes and S. M. McCurry, "Current treatments for sleep disturbances in individuals with dementia," *Current Psychiatry Reports*, vol. 11, no. 1, pp. 20–26, 2009.

[30] W. Lee, A. Evans, and D. R. Williams, "Subjective perception of sleep benefit in Parkinson's disease: valid or irrelevant?," *Parkinsonism & Related Disorders*, vol. 42, pp. 90–94, 2017.

[31] A. C. King, L. A. Pruitt, S. Woo et al., "Effects of moderate-intensity exercise on polysomnographic and subjective sleep quality in older adults with mild to moderate sleep complaints," *Journals of Gerontology Series A: Biological Sciences and Medical Sciences*, vol. 63, no. 9, pp. 997–1004, 2008.

[32] K. C. Richards, C. Beck, P. S. O'Sullivan, and V. M. Shue, "Effect of individualized social activity on sleep in nursing home residents with dementia," *Journal of the American Geriatrics Society*, vol. 53, no. 9, pp. 1510–1517, 2005.

[33] F. Mavrommati, J. Collett, M. Franssen et al., "Exercise response in Parkinson's disease: insights from a cross-sectional comparison with sedentary controls and a per-protocol analysis of a randomised controlled trial," *BMJ Open*, vol. 7, no. 12, article e017194, 2017.

[34] C. Silva-Batista, L. C. de Brito, D. M. Corcos et al., "Resistance training improves sleep quality in subjects with moderate parkinson's disease," *Journal of Strength and Conditioning Research*, vol. 31, no. 8, pp. 2270–2277, 2017.

[35] J. M. T. Bonardi, L. G. Lima, G. O. Campos et al., "Effect of different types of exercise on sleep quality of elderly subjects," *Sleep Medicine*, vol. 25, pp. 122–129, 2016.

[36] A. S. Mather, C. Rodriguez, M. F. Guthrie, A. M. McHarg, I. C. Reid, and M. E. T. McMurdo, "Effects of exercise on depressive symptoms in older adults with poorly responsive depressive disorder: randomised controlled trial," *British Journal of Psychiatry*, vol. 180, no. 5, pp. 411–415, 2002.

12

Meta-Analysis of Visual Evoked Potential and Parkinson's Disease

Song-bin He ⓘ,[1] Chun-yan Liu,[2] Lin-di Chen,[1] Zhi-nan Ye,[3] Ya-ping Zhang,[3] Wei-guo Tang,[1] Bin-da Wang,[1] and Xiang Gao ⓘ[4]

[1]*Department of Neurology, Zhoushan Hospital, Wenzhou Medical University, Zhoushan 316021, China*
[2]*Department of Critical Care Medicine, Huzhou Central Hospital, Huzhou 313000, China*
[3]*Department of Neurology, Taizhou Municipal Hospital, Taizhou 318000, China*
[4]*Department of Nutritional Sciences, The Pennsylvania State University, USA*

Correspondence should be addressed to Xiang Gao; xxg14@psu.edu

Academic Editor: Antonio Pisani

Background. Previous studies suggested that visual evoked potential (VEP) was impaired in patients with Parkinson's disease (PD), but the results were inconsistent. *Methods.* We conducted a systematic review and meta-analysis to explore whether the VEP was significantly different between PD patients and healthy controls. Case-control studies of PD were selected through an electronic search of the databases PubMed, Embase, and the Cochrane Central Register of Controlled Trials. We calculated the pooled weighted mean differences (WMDs) and 95% confidence intervals (CIs) between individuals with PD and controls using the random-effects model. *Results.* Twenty case-control studies which met our inclusion criteria were included in the final meta-analysis. We found that the P100 latency in PD was significantly higher compared with healthy controls (pooled WMD = 6.04, 95% CI: 2.73 to 9.35, $P = 0.0003$, $n = 20$). However, the difference in the mean amplitude of P100 was not significant between the two groups (pooled WMD = 0.64, 95% CI: −0.06 to 1.33, $P = 0.07$) based on 10 studies with the P100 amplitude values available. *Conclusions.* The higher P100 latency of VEP was observed in PD patients, relative to healthy controls. Our findings suggest that electrophysiological changes and functional defect in the visual pathway of PD patients are important to our understanding of the pathophysiology of visual involvement in PD.

1. Background

Parkinson's disease (PD) is one of the most common neurodegenerative disorders in the world. The prevalence of PD is expected to rise steadily in the future as the human population ages [1]. Visual dysfunction is a common nonmotor symptom in individuals with PD, including abnormal contrast sensitivity, motion perception abnormalities, and impaired visual acuity and color vision [2, 3]. Visual dysfunction that occurs in PD is subtle and could be easily demonstrated through electrophysiologic testing, such as the visual evoked potential (VEP). VEP is a potential change recorded in the visual cortex after retinal received light stimulation, which reflects the functional status of the entire visual pathway. VEP latency is less likely to be affected by dopaminergic drugs and seems to be a more sensitive measure of foveal electrical activity than VEP amplitude. It is thought that abnormal latency is due to delayed

conduction in visual pathways affected by the process of demyelination and/or plaque formation [2]. The P100 latency of VEP is usually used to determine the abnormalities of the visual pathway due to the relatively small individual difference.

As the pathological hallmark of PD is progressive loss of dopaminergic neurons in the substantia nigra, the human retina also contains dopaminergic amacrine and interplexiform cells, which play a regulatory role. Several observations support the concept that dopamine has a specific function in the retina of primates [4, 5]. The chemical protoxin MPTP (1-methyl-4-phenyl-1-2-3-6-tetrahydropyridine), which produces a clinical parkinsonian syndrome, significantly lowers retinal dopamine. Similarly, intravitreal injection of the neurotoxin 6-hydroxydopamine into aphakic monkeys resulted in abnormalities in both the phase and amplitude of the pattern VEP [6].

Visual dysfunction was observed in some early PD patients not yet undergoing L-dopa therapy, indicating that visual deficiency could be one of the prodromal symptoms of PD [3, 7, 8]. However, previous studies regarding visual dysfunction, as assessed by the VEP, in PD patients versus general populations generated mixed results [8–10], which could be due to small sample sizes of these individual studies (PD case numbers < 50 for all studies). We thus performed a systematic review and meta-analysis to comprehensively assess whether the pattern reversal VEP latency, as the primary exposure, was different between PD patients and controls. However, we also examined other visual indices, including pattern reversal VEP amplitude, intraocular difference of P100 latency, and N75 latency.

2. Materials and Methods

This meta-analysis was performed according to the Preferred Reporting Items for Systematic Reviews and Meta-Analyses (PRISMA) statement (PRISMA Checklist in supplementary materials (available here)) [11].

2.1. Search Strategy, Study Inclusion Criteria, and Data Extraction. Two of the coauthors (Chun-yan Liu and Ya-ping Zhang) independently searched the literature and extracted the relevant information from the eligible studies. A systematic review of the literature was conducted using the databases PubMed, Embase, and the Cochrane Central Register of Controlled Trials from 1 January 1978 up to 10 May 2016 to identify the relevant studies. We searched the medical subject heading (MeSH) terms "Parkinson's disease" and "visual evoked potentials" in PubMed, respectively, and found out their entry terms. We only included English papers. Retrieved studies were imported into Mendeley Desktop (version 1.16; PDFTron^{TM} Systems Inc.), where duplicate articles were deleted. Titles and abstracts of the remaining studies were independently scanned by Chun-yan Liu and Ya-ping Zhang. The full texts of the potentially relevant reports were then read to determine whether they met the inclusion criteria. The reference lists from all included studies were also examined.

Studies fulfilling the following inclusion criteria were included in the present meta-analysis: (1) participants were adult; (2) study design was a case-control study including a group of diagnosed idiopathic PD; (3) all participants underwent pattern reversal VEP examination, and both visual acuity test and ophthalmologic evaluation showed normal results; (4) information on peak latency of the P100 component was provided; and (5) sample size was greater than 10 in each group. Exclusion criteria were as follows: (1) participants were PD patients with dementia or undergoing deep brain stimulation; (2) authors did not make pattern reversal VEP examination; (3) studies without healthy control group; (4) studies did not provide the P100 data of pattern reversal VEP; (5) review papers; (6) reports published only in the abstract form; and (7) papers were not written in English.

A standardized data extraction form was used to collect relevant information including the name of the first author, publication year, study country, PD diagnosis criteria, mean disease duration, scales used for evaluating motor and cognitive function, number of eyes, mean age, sex, and latency of P100.

Two reviewers (Chun-yan Liu and Ya-ping Zhang) separately evaluated studies, and discrepancies were resolved by discussion. If disagreements existed, in very few cases, two reviewers consulted a third party (e.g., Xiang Gao) until both reviewers reached an agreement.

2.2. Study Quality Assessment. We assessed the methodologic quality of included studies based on the Newcastle-Ottawa Scale (NOS) [12] for quality of the case-control study. The NOS uses a star rating system to judge the quality based on 3 dimensions of the study: selection, comparability, and exposure. A study could be scored a maximum of one star for each item numbered within the categories of selection and exposure, while at most two stars could be allocated to comparability. A higher score represented better quality of the study methodology. The maximum score was 4 for selection dimension, 2 for comparability, and 3 for outcome/exposure. A study with a score equal to or higher than 6 was considered of high quality.

2.3. Statistical Analysis. Statistical analysis was performed using RevMan (version 5.3; Cochrane Collaboration, Oxford, United Kingdom) and STATA statistical software (version 12.0; StataCorp, College Station, TX, USA). Data that could not be obtained were to be calculated when necessary. For example, when standard deviation (SD) was not available, it was calculated using the sample sizes and standard error. For continuous outcome, means and standard deviations were used to calculate the pooled weighted mean differences (WMDs) and their 95% confidence intervals (CIs). The chi-square test, tau^2, and the Higgins I^2 test were used to assess heterogeneity [12]. The I^2 test is a method for quantifying inconsistency across studies and describes the percentage of variability in effect estimates due to heterogeneity. A value greater than 50% was considered substantial heterogeneity. A fixed-effects model was adopted for the analysis if the P value was >0.1 and the I^2 index was <50%, as these results would indicate no between-study heterogeneity. Otherwise, a random-effects model was applied [13].

Potential publication bias was examined using funnel plots [14]. To evaluate the influence of each individual study on the stability of the overall pooled estimate, we conducted sensitivity analyses by removing each study and observing whether the result changed. Metaregression analysis and subgroup analyses were conducted according to the sample size, publication year, age, sex ratio, and mean PD duration of the cases to explore the potential inherent heterogeneity across the included studies.

3. Results

A total of 214 articles were initially identified, and 20 case-control studies which met our inclusion criteria were included in the final meta-analysis (Figure 1; Table 1)

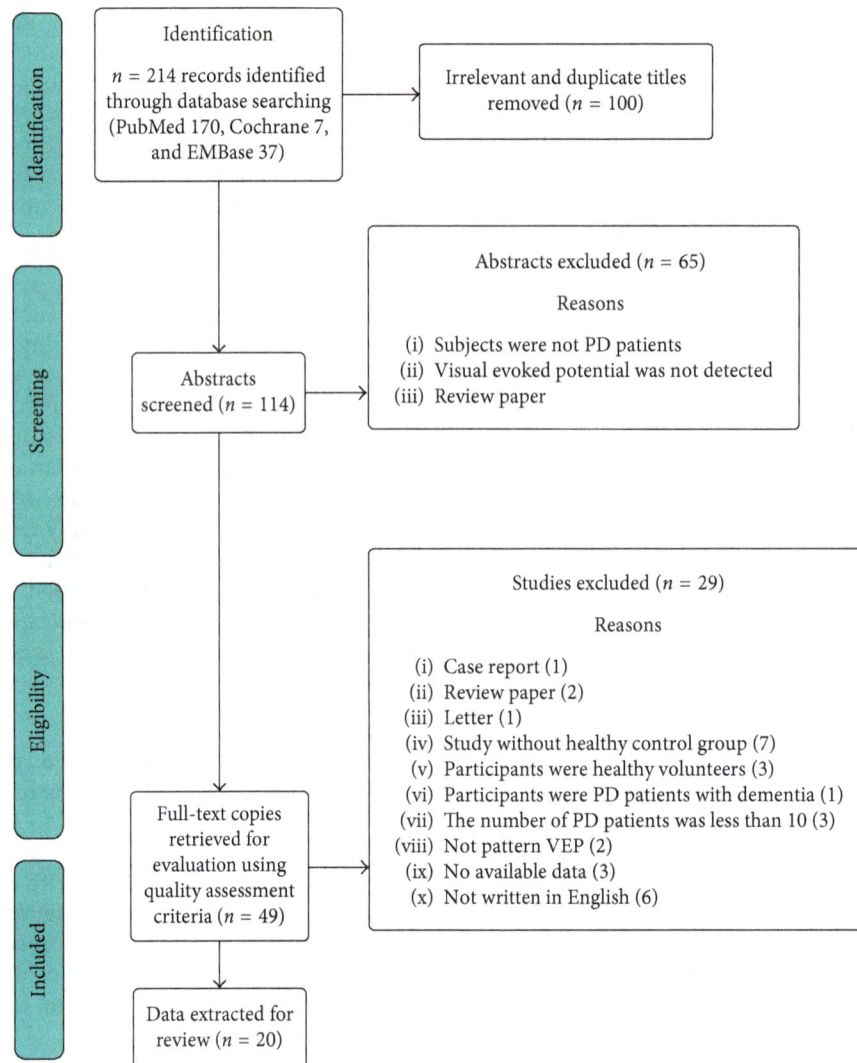

FIGURE 1: Search and study selection process.

[2, 3, 7–10, 15–28]. Seven out of the 20 studies had the NOS score equal to or more than 6, and the mean score was 6.3.

Because of significant heterogeneity ($I^2 = 93\%$) across the included studies, we used the random-effects model to calculate the WMDs. The P100 latency (WMD = 6.04, 95 % CI: 2.73 to 9.35, $P = 0.0003$, $n = 20$), but not amplitude of P100, was significantly higher in PD patients compared with healthy controls (Figures 2(a) and 2(b)).

Metaregression analysis and subgroup analyses revealed that different sample sizes, sex ratios, and disease durations across studies (all $P < 0.05$), but not publication year and age (both $P > 0.05$), were possible sources of heterogeneity observed in the current meta-analysis (Table 2). The difference in P100 latency between PD patients and controls was more pronounced in the studies with a large proportion of men and long PD duration patients (P-difference < 0.05) than the studies with a small proportion of men and short PD duration patients (P-difference > 0.05) (Table 2).

Sensitivity analyses showed no significant changes in the pooled WMD or 95% CI upon the exclusion of any study, indicating that the overall pooled estimates were stable.

The funnel plot did not support existence of publication bias (Figure 3).

4. Discussion

In this meta-analysis based on 20 case-control studies, we observed that there is a significant delay in the VEP, as assessed by P100 latency, in individuals with PD, relative to controls. PD is a disorder of the motor system in which there is no obvious clinical involvement of the visual system and with no pathological lesions (e.g., demyelination), that are considered major determinants of the delays in conduction in visual pathways [2]. Our findings could lead to a better understanding of the physiology of human and primate vision: how and where dopamine acts in the elementary retinal processing of signals related to spatial contrast.

The changes in VEP reflect functional damage in the visual pathway of PD patients. Someone also found structural damage in the retina by using optical coherence tomography which revealed thinning of the retinal nerve fiber layer and macula [29] in PD. The deficit is most evident in

TABLE 1: Characteristics and quality of studies included in the meta-analysis.

Author(s) year	Country	Diagnostic criteria	Mean duration (months)	Motor and cognitive function	Number of eyes PD	Number of eyes HC	Mean age (years) PD	Mean age (years) HC	Sex (men/women) PD	Sex (men/women) HC	NOS Selection	NOS Comparability	NOS Exposure	NOS Total score
Altintaş 2008 [15]	Turkey	UKBB	54.96	UPDRS	34	22	59.29	58.09	9/8	6/5	3	1	3	7
Antal 2000 [16]	Austria	NR	58.1	UPDRS, H&Y, ADL, MMSE	40	40	65.3	59.8	13/7	13/7	2	2	3	7
Bodis-Wollner 1978 [2]	USA	NR	97.8	NR	70	52	62	60	NR	NR	2	1	2	5
Buttner 1996 [18]	Germany	NR	64.8	UPDRS, H&Y	78	86	64.0	62.8	20/19	18/25	2	1	3	6
Cubo 2014 [19]	Spain	UKBB	98.4	SPES/SCOPA, H&Y, MMSE	60	60	65.4	62.9	18/12	15/15	3	1	3	7
Daniels 1994 [9]	UK	NR	NR	NR	32	40	64.36	66.95	NR	NR	2	1	3	6
Deng 2006 [25]	China	CMA	NR	NR	64	60	64	64	20/12	19/11	2	1	2	5
Ehle 1982 [8]	USA	NR	65	H&Y	50	36	64	56	NR	NR	2	1	3	6
Garcia-Martin, Elena 2014 [20]	Spain	UKBB	92.4	H&Y, SE-ADL	46	33	70.72	69.67	29/17	21/12	3	2	3	8
Gawel 1981 [7]	England	NR	NR	NR	94	52	67	63	30/17	11/15	2	1	3	6
Kaur, Marpreet 2015 [21]	India	UK3B	69.6	H&Y, UPDRS	40	40	58.6	58.4	NR	NR	3	1	3	7
Kuporsmith 1982 [23]	USA	NR	NR	H&Y	28	28	62	58	NR	NR	2	1	2	5
Li 2004 [26]	China	CNCESD	56.4	UPDRS, H&Y, HDS	140	120	62.2	59.9	32/38	28/32	3	1	3	7
Miri 2016 [22]	USA	UKBB	NR	MMSE	20	16	66.3	66.5	NR	NR	3	2	3	8
Okuda 1995 [10]	Japan	NR	52.4	H&Y, MMSE	42	44	67.4	70.3	8/14	11/11	2	1	3	6
Okuda 1996 [24]	Japan	NR	52.9	H&Y, MMSE	36	24	65.7	67.3	NR	NR	2	1	3	6
Peppe 1995 [27]	Italy	NR	13.3	UPDRS, H&Y	36	16	62.5	61.2	NR	NR	2	1	3	6
Quagliato 2014 [28]	Brazil	UKBB	83.76	UPDRS, H&Y	86	76	63.1	62.4	27/16	17/21	3	1	3	7
Sagliocco 1997 [17]	Austria	NR	31.25	H&Y, MMSE	34	33	61.94	54.53	8/9	9/8	2	1	3	6
Sartucci 2006 [3]	USA	UKBB	26.4	UPDRS, H&Y	21	24	60.1	46.8	6/6	6/6	3	1	3	7

PD = Parkinson's disease; HC = healthy controls; NR = not reported; UKBB = United Kingdom Brain Bank clinical diagnostic criteria; UPDRS = Unified Parkinson's Disease Rating Scale; H&Y = Hoehn and Yahr Scale; SE-ADL = Schwab and England Activities of Daily Living Scale; MMSE = Mini-Mental State Examination; SPES/SCOPA = Short Parkinson's Evaluation Scale/Scales for Outcomes in Parkinson's disease; CMA = Chinese Medical Association clinical diagnostic criteria; CNCESD = Chinese National Conference on Extra-Pyramidal System Disease diagnostic criteria; HDS = Hasegawa Dementia Scale.

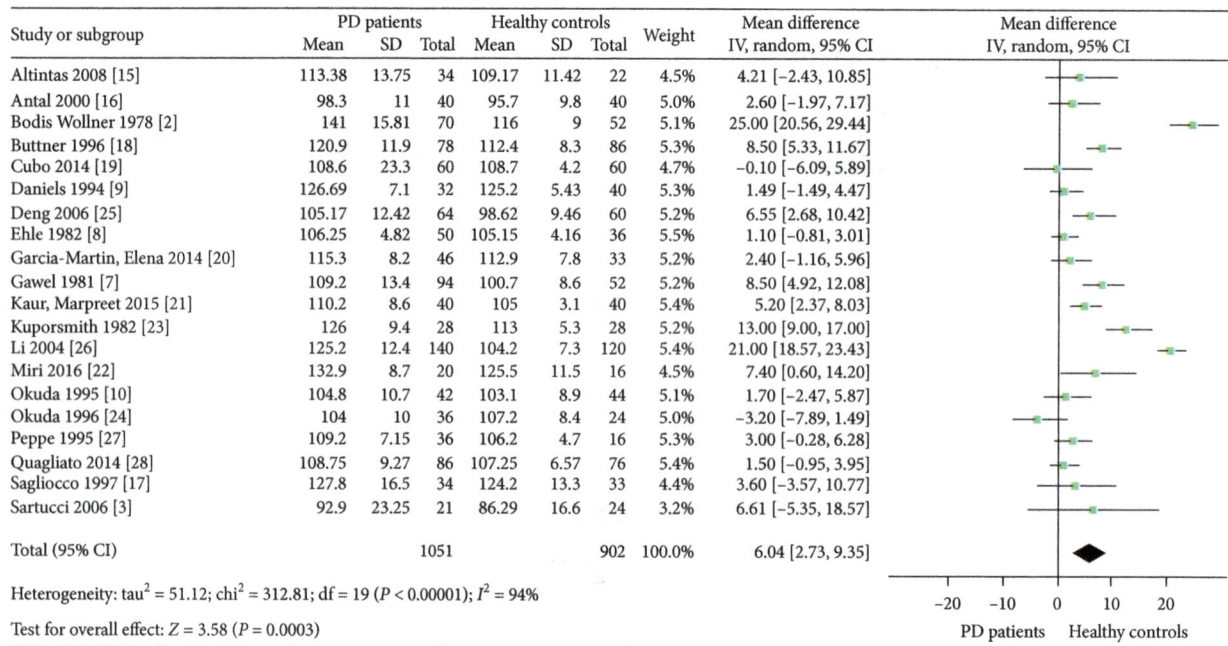

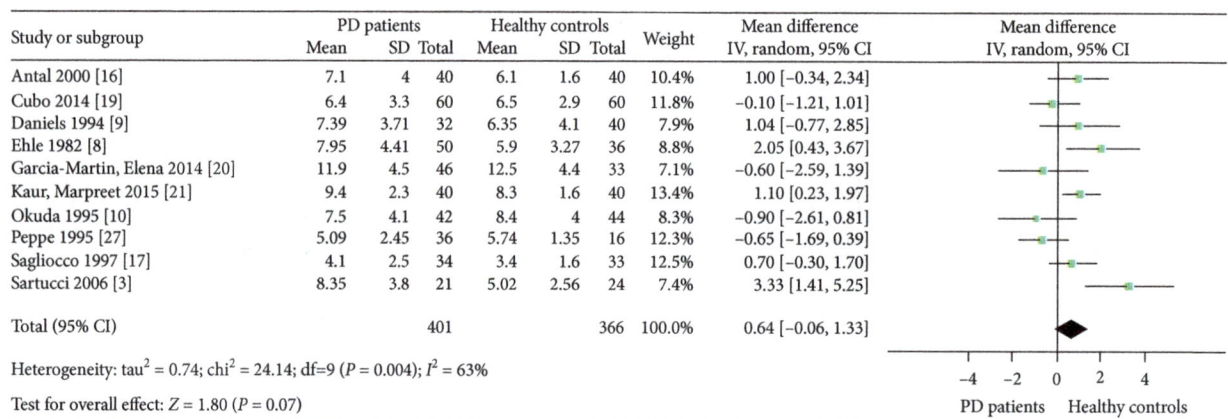

FIGURE 2: Pooled weighted mean differences in visual evoked potential: (a) P100 latency and (b) P100 amplitude.

TABLE 2: Metaregression analysis and subgroup analysis.

Subgroup factor	Assign criteria	Number of studies	WMD (95% CI)	P-difference between groups[*]
Sample size	≤20	10	4.20 (1.38, 7.02)	0.001
	>20	10	7.64 (2.21, 13.1)	
Publication year	Before 2000	10	6.25 (1.91, 10.6)	0.12
	2000 or later	10	5.79 (0.49, 11.1)	
Age (years)	<64	9	9.39 (3.04, 15.7)	0.08
	≥64	11	3.38 (1.18, 5.58)	
Proportion of men	>50%	8	4.47 (2.03, 6.91)	0.03
	≤50%	4	8.44 (−3.98, 20.9)	
Duration (months)	≤56.4	8	4.82 (−2.31, 12.0)	0.01
	>56.4	7	6.38 (1.08, 11.6)	

[*]Adjusted for all factors in this table.

the annular zone surrounding the fovea, where anatomical studies [30] demonstrated the highest concentration of dopaminergic amacrine cells. Dopaminergic deficiency is related to a VEP delay. The postmortem study of PD's retina observed a decrease in retinal dopamine concentration [31]. The thinned inner retina [32] suggests involvement of the

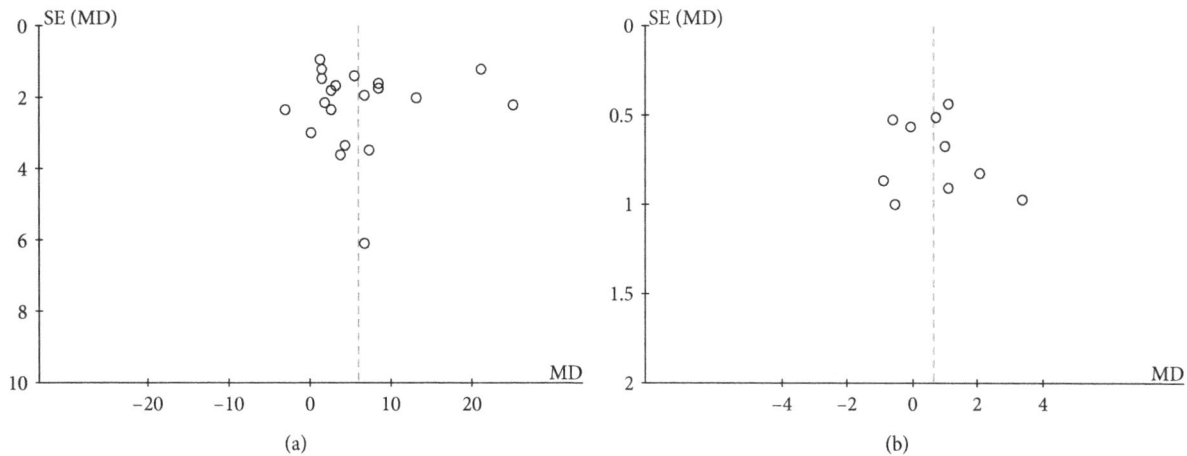

FIGURE 3: Funnel plots for evaluating the publication bias for visual evoked potential: (a) P100 latency and (b) P100 amplitude.

ganglion cell layer and dopaminergic neurons and the inner plexiform layer in PD. Importantly, previous studies suggested that the structural changes correlated significantly with functional changes [15, 19, 21, 22].

We found a significant delay in the average P100 latency in PD patients compared with the healthy controls, and this difference could be modified by different sample sizes, PD durations, and sex ratios across studies. Disease duration and sex difference may be associated with electrophysiologic changes in the visual pathway of patients with PD. Previous studies reported that the functional changes correlated significantly with disease duration and severity of PD [21, 22]. Furthermore, a prolonged mean VEP latency in PD patients was shown to be dependent on the sex of the participants (more evident in men than women) [33]. The difference in the thickness of the skull and the brain volume between men and women could also explain, at least in part, the gender difference in VEP for PD patients.

The mechanism of visual defect in PD may act as follows: pathological changes in PD are not only found in the nigra-striatum system but also in the caudal nuclei, putamen nuclei, hypothalamus, and pontine nucleus ceruleus [30]. This could result in cholinergic system dysfunction that diffusely affects the brainstem auditory pathway. The injuries to these regions cause dopaminergic neuron degeneration and decrease in dopamine production and secretion, which may affect the function of the interplexiform cells and horizontal cells in the retina to undermine the transmission of the visual signals, contributing to the abnormal changes of VEP [18]. Then, dopamine exists in the lateral geniculate body and visual cortex, and the visual cortex also contains acetylcholine and its receptors [34]. Long-term dopamine deficiency could trigger a compensatory decrement of acetylcholine and lead to changes in the VEP latency. A retinal dopaminergic deficiency could also underlie some visual changes in PD. However, the relationship between the decrement of dopamine in the nigra-striatum of PD patients and dopamine dysfunction in the visual pathway needs further study. Alpha-synuclein (α-syn) is also expressed widely in the vertebrate retina including humans [35], and it

is likely that loss or dysfunction of α-syn at this site is responsible for visual symptoms [36].

It is worth noting that VEP measures the integrity of the entire visual pathway. The changes in these potentials in PD may reflect the widespread nature of the biochemical disorder affecting both the retina and central nervous system. Thus, the VEP is a relatively poor method for assessing the anterior visual pathway dysfunction because it is incapable of differentiating impaired macular function from impaired ganglion cell function. Although all the patients were normal on ophthalmological examination, we cannot exclude involvement of the direct visual pathway in PD as a cause of delayed VEP. The pattern electroretinogram (PERG) measures the electrical activity generated by neural and non-neuronal cells in the retina in response to a light stimulus and reflects functional changes in the retina. The PERG would differentiate whether the retinal abnormalities were the cause of the VEP changes. As we expected, some studies reported impaired PERG in PD patients and confirmed the retinal functional defect [20, 21]. However, they still cannot exclude the disorder in the upper visual pathway. Furthermore, both PERG and VEP improve with therapy, but there is an apparent difference: levodopa therapy improves PERG abnormalities to a higher degree than it does VEP deficits [27, 37, 38]. One possible interpretation is that VEP changes in PD represent secondary nondopaminergic, and therefore more chronic, alterations in visual processing. It seems that additional pathology beyond the retina affects visual responses, including VEPs. Although the role of retinal dysfunction seems certain, the contribution of cortical and lateral geniculate impairment to these visual symptoms remains unknown.

This meta-analysis has some limitations, which are as follows: (1) We did not include unpublished studies and those which were not written in English. The current study thus may lose some high-quality evidences. (2) Because most studies did not provide data regarding PD severity, we failed to explore the potential impacts of disease severity on the VEP-PD relation. (3) We cannot address the potential impact of dopaminergic drugs because most PD cases were treated. Previous studies suggested that these treatments could improve contrast sensitivity and reverse VEP delays in PD patients [2, 39, 40]. Failure to control the use of dopaminergic drugs thus would underestimate the true difference in VEP latency between PD patients and controls. (4) Some participants with other neurodegenerative diseases were probably included in control groups, as screenings are not fully stringent so as to exclude early dementias.

5. Conclusion

This meta-analysis showed that the P100 latency was significantly longer in PD patients than healthy controls. The application of VEP provides an approach for a more comprehensive evaluation of the visual pathway and a better understanding of the pathophysiology of visual involvement in PD. However, further researches with longitudinal study design and incorporating the pattern electroretinogram assessment are warranted.

Authors' Contributions

Song-bin He and Xiang Gao conceived and designed the experiments. Chun-yan Liu, Ya-ping Zhang, and Zhi-nan Ye performed the experiments. Chun-yan Liu, Lin-di Chen, and Bin-da Wang analyzed the data. Wei-guo Tang, Song-bin He, and Xiang Gao contributed reagents/materials/analysis tools. Chun-yan Liu, Lin-di Chen, and Xiang Gao wrote the paper. All authors read and approved the final manuscript.

Acknowledgments

This work was supported by the project of the Department of Health and Family Planning Bureau of Zhoushan City, Zhejiang Province, China (no. 2014A17 to Song-bin He), and the NIH/NINDS R21-NS087235-02 (to Xiang Gao).

References

[1] A. Rossi, K. Berger, H. Chen, D. Leslie, R. B. Mailman, and X. Huang, "Projection of the prevalence of Parkinson's disease in the coming decades: revisited," *Movement Disorders*, 2017.

[2] I. Bodis-Wollner and M. D. Yahr, "Measurements of visual evoked potentials in Parkinson's disease," *Brain*, vol. 101, no. 4, pp. 661–671, 1978.

[3] F. Sartucci and V. Porciatti, "Visual-evoked potentials to onset of chromatic red-green and blue-yellow gratings in Parkinson's disease never treated with L-dopa," *Journal of Clinical Neurophysiology*, vol. 23, no. 5, pp. 431–436, 2006.

[4] M. F. Ghilardi, E. Chung, I. Bodis-Wollner, M. Dvorzniak, A. Glover, and M. Onofrj, "Systemic 1-methyl,4-phenyl,1-2-3-6-tetrahydropyridine (MPTP) administration decreases

retinal dopamine content in primates," *Life Sciences*, vol. 43, no. 3, pp. 255–262, 1988.

[5] J. D. Elsworth, J. R. Taylor, J. R. Sladek Jr., T. J. Collier, D. E. Redmond Jr., and R. H. Roth, "Striatal dopaminergic correlates of stable parkinsonism and degree of recovery in old-world primates one year after MPTP treatment," *Neuroscience*, vol. 95, no. 2, p. 399, 2000.

[6] M. F. Ghilardi, M. S. Marx, I. Bodiswollner, C. B. Camras, and A. A. Glover, "The effect of intraocular 6-hydroxydopamine on retinal processing of primates," *Annals of Neurology*, vol. 25, no. 4, pp. 357–364, 1989.

[7] M. J. Gawel, P. Das, S. Vincent, and F. C. Rose, "Visual and auditory evoked responses in patients with Parkinson's disease," *Journal of Neurology Neurosurgery and Psychiatry*, vol. 44, no. 3, pp. 227–232, 1981.

[8] A. L. Ehle, R. M. Stewart, N. E. Lellelid, and N. A. Leventhal, "Normal checkerboard pattern reversal evoked potentials in parkinsonism," *Electroencephalography and Clinical Neurophysiology*, vol. 54, no. 3, pp. 336–338, 1982.

[9] R. Daniels, G. F. Harding, and S. J. Anderson, "Effect of dopamine and acetylcholine on the visual evoked potential," *International Journal of Psychophysiology*, vol. 16, no. 2-3, pp. 251–261, 1994.

[10] B. Okuda, H. Tachibana, K. Kawabata, M. Takeda, and M. Sugita, "Visual evoked potentials (VEPs) in Parkinson's disease: correlation of pattern VEPs abnormality with dementia," *Alzheimer Disease and Associated Disorders*, vol. 9, no. 2, pp. 68–72, 1995.

[11] A. Liberati, D. G. Altman, J. Tetzlaff et al., "The PRISMA statement for reporting systematic reviews and meta-analyses of studies that evaluate healthcare interventions: explanation and elaboration," *Epidemiology Biostatistics and Public Health*, vol. 6, no. 4, pp. e1–e34, 2009.

[12] A. V. Margulis, M. Pladevall, N. Riera-Guardia et al., "Quality assessment of observational studies in a drug-safety systematic review, comparison of two tools: the Newcastle–Ottawa Scale and the RTI item bank," *Clinical Epidemiology*, vol. 6, no. 8, p. 359, 2014.

[13] J. P. T. Higgins and S. G. Thompson, "Quantifying heterogeneity in a meta-analysis," *Statistics in Medicine*, vol. 21, no. 11, pp. 1539–1558, 2010.

[14] J. P. Vandenbroucke, "Bias in meta-analysis detected by a simple, graphical test," *BMJ*, vol. 315, no. 7109, pp. 629–634, 1997.

[15] Ö. Altintaş, P. Işeri, B. Özkan, and Y. Cağlar, "Correlation between retinal morphological and functional findings and clinical severity in Parkinson's disease," *Documenta Ophthalmologica*, vol. 116, no. 2, pp. 137–146, 2008.

[16] A. Antal, G. Dibó, S. Kéri et al., "P300 component of visual event-related potentials distinguishes patients with idiopathic Parkinson's disease from patients with essential tremor," *Journal of Neural Transmission*, vol. 107, no. 7, pp. 787–797, 2000.

[17] L. Sagliocco, F. Bandini, M. Pierantozzi et al., "Electrophysiological evidence for visuocognitive dysfunction in younger non Caucasian patients with Parkinson's disease," *Journal of Neural Transmission*, vol. 104, no. 4-5, pp. 427–439, 1997.

[18] T. Buttner, W. Kuhn, T. Muller, T. Heinze, C. Puhl, and H. Przuntek, "Chromatic and achromatic visual evoked potentials in Parkinson's disease," *Electroencephalography and Clinical Neurophysiology*, vol. 100, no. 5, p. 443, 1996.

[19] E. Cubo, M. J. López Peña, E. Diez-Feijo Varela et al., "Lack of association of morphologic and functional retinal changes with motor and non-motor symptoms severity in Parkinson's

disease," *Journal of Neural Transmission*, vol. 121, no. 2, pp. 139–145, 2014.

[20] E. Garcia-Martin, D. Rodriguez-Mena, M. Satue et al., "Electrophysiology and optical coherence tomography to evaluate Parkinson disease severity," *Investigative Ophthalmology and Visual Science*, vol. 55, no. 2, p. 696, 2014.

[21] M. Kaur, R. Saxena, D. Singh, M. Behari, P. Sharma, and V. Menon, "Correlation between structural and functional retinal changes in Parkinson disease," *Journal of neuro-ophthalmology: the official journal of the North American Neuro-Ophthalmology Society*, vol. 35, no. 3, p. 254, 2015.

[22] S. Miri, S. Glazman, L. Mylin, and I. Bodis-Wollner, "A combination of retinal morphology and visual electrophysiology testing increases diagnostic yield in Parkinson's disease," *Parkinsonism and Related Disorders*, vol. 1, no. 5, pp. 134–137, 2016.

[23] M. J. Kupersmith, E. Shakin, I. M. Siegel, and A. Lieberman, "Visual system abnormalities in patients with Parkinson's disease," *Archives of Neurology*, vol. 39, no. 5, pp. 284–286, 1982.

[24] B. Okuda, H. Tachibana, M. Takeda, K. Kawabata, and M. Sugita, "Visual and somatosensory evoked potentials in Parkinson's and Binswanger's disease," *Dementia*, vol. 7, no. 1, pp. 53–58, 1996.

[25] Q. Deng, J. Deng, Y. Zhao, X. Yan, and P. Chen, "Analysis of brain-stem auditory evoked potential and visual evoked potential in patients with Parkinson disease," *Neural Regeneration Research*, vol. 1, no. 5, pp. 449–452, 2006.

[26] F. Li, D. X. Gu, and Y. J. Li, "Correlation of brainstem auditory evoked potential and visual evoked potential with disturbance of intelligence in patients with Parkinson disease," *Chinese Journal of Clinical Rehabilitation*, vol. 8, pp. 7002–7004, 2004.

[27] A. Peppe, P. Stanzione, F. Pierelli, A. D. De, M. Pierantozzi, and G Bernardi, "Visual alterations in de novo Parkinson's disease: pattern electroretinogram latencies are more delayed and more reversible by levodopa than are visual evoked potentials," *Neurology*, vol. 45, no. 6, pp. 1144–1148, 1995.

[28] L. B. Quagliato, C. Domingues, E. M. Quagliato, E. B. Abreu, and N. Karajunior, "Applications of visual evoked potentials and Fourier-domain optical coherence tomography in Parkinson's disease: a controlled study," *Arquivos Brasileiros de Oftalmologia*, vol. 77, no. 4, pp. 238–242, 2014.

[29] R. Inzelberg, J A. Ramirez, P. Nisipeanu, and A. Ophir, "Retinal nerve fiber layer thinning in Parkinson disease," *Vision Research*, vol. 44, no. 24, p. 2793, 2004.

[30] C. Savy, A. Simon, and J. Nguyenlegros, "Spatial geometry of the dopamine innervation in the avascular area of the human fovea," *Visual Neuroscience*, vol. 7, no 5, pp. 487–498, 1991.

[31] C. Harnois and P. T. Di, "Decreased dopamine in the retinas of patients with Parkinson's disease," *Investigative Ophthalmology and Visual Science*, vol. 31, no. 11, pp. 2473–2475, 1990.

[32] M. E. Hajee, W. F. March, D. R. Lazzaro et al., "Inner retinal layer thinning in Parkinson disease," *Archives of Ophthalmology*, vol. 127, no. 6, p. 737, 2009.

[33] S. Nightingale, K. W. Mitchell, and J. W. Howe, "Visual evoked cortical potentials and pattern electroretinograms in Parkinson's disease and control subjects," *Journal of Neurology, Neurosurgery, and Psychiatry*, vol. 49, no. 11, pp. 1280–1287, 1986.

[34] H. Tachibana, M. Takeda, M. Sugita, J. Kondo, M. Miyauchi, and A. Matsuoka, "Brainstem auditory evoked potentials in patients with multi-infarct dementia and dementia of the

Alzheimer type," *International Journal of Neuroscience*, vol. 37, no. 2, pp. 325–331, 2009.

[35] G. C. Martíneznavarrete, J. Martínnieto, J. Esteverudd, A. Angulo, and N. Cuenca, "Alpha synuclein gene expression profile in the retina of vertebrates," *Molecular Vision*, vol. 13, pp. 949–961, 2007.

[36] H. A. Lashuel, C. R. Overk, A. Oueslati, and E. Masliah, "The many faces of α-synuclein: from structure and toxicity to therapeutic target," *Nature Reviews Neuroscience*, vol. 14, no. 1, pp. 38–48, 2013.

[37] P. A. Bhaskar, S. Vanchilingam, E. A. Bhaskar, A. Devaprabhu, and R. Ganesan, "Effect of L-dopa on visual evoked potential in patients with Parkinson's disease," *Neurology*, vol. 36, no. 8, pp. 1119–1121, 1986.

[38] A. Peppe, P. Stanzione, M. Pierantozzi et al., "Does pattern electroretinogram spatial tuning alteration in Parkinson's disease depend on motor disturbances or retinal dopaminergic loss?," *Electroencephalography and Clinical Neurophysiology*, vol. 106, no. 4, pp. 374–382, 1998.

[39] L. Barbato, S. Rinalduzzi, M. Laurenti, S. Ruggieri, and N. Accornero, "Color VEPs in Parkinson's disease," *Electroencephalography and Clinical Neurophysiology/Evoked Potentials Section*, vol. 92, no. 2, pp. 169–172, 1994.

[40] M. Onofrj, M. F. Ghilardi, M. Basciani, and D. Gambi, "Visual evoked potentials in parkinsonism and dopamine blockade reveal a stimulus-dependent dopamine function in humans," *Journal of Neurology Neurosurgery, and Psychiatry*, vol. 49, no. 10, pp. 1150–1159, 1986.

13

LRRK2 G2019S Mutation: Prevalence and Clinical Features in Moroccans with Parkinson's Disease

Ahmed Bouhouche,[1,2] **Houyam Tibar,**[2] **Rafiqua Ben El Haj,**[1] **Khalil El Bayad,**[2] **Rachid Razine,**[3] **Sanaa Tazrout,**[2] **Asmae Skalli,**[1] **Naima Bouslam,**[2] **Loubna Elouardi,**[2] **Ali Benomar,**[1,2] **Mohammed Yahyaoui,**[1,2] **and Wafa Regragui**[1,2]

[1]*Research Team in Neurology and Neurogenetics, Medical School and Pharmacy, Mohammed V University, Rabat, Morocco*
[2]*Department of Neurology and Neurogenetics, Specialties Hospital, Rabat, Morocco*
[3]*Laboratory of Public Health, Medical School and Pharmacy, Mohammed V University, Rabat, Morocco*

Correspondence should be addressed to Ahmed Bouhouche; a.bouhouche@um5s.net.ma

Academic Editor: Daniel Berwick

Background. The *LRRK2* G2019S mutation is the most common genetic determinant of Parkinson's disease (PD) identified to date. This mutation, reported in both familial and sporadic PD, occurs at elevated frequencies in Maghreb population. In the present study, we examined the prevalence of the G2019S mutation in the Moroccan population and we compared the motor and nonmotor phenotype of G2019S carriers to patients with idiopathic Parkinson's disease. *Methods.* 100 PD patients were assessed for motor and nonmotor symptoms, current medication, and motor complication including motor fluctuations and dyskinesia. The *LRRK2* G2019S mutation was investigated by direct sequencing in patients and ethnically matched controls, all of Moroccan origin. *Results.* Among the 100 PD Moroccan patients, 41 (41%) were carriers of the G2019S mutation. The mutation frequency was higher among probands with autosomal dominant inheritance (76%) than among sporadic ones (28%). Interestingly, G2019S mutation was also found in 5% of control individuals. Clinically, patients carrying the G2019S mutation have more dystonia (OR = 4.6, $p = 0.042$) and more sleep disorders (OR = 2.4, $p = 0.045$) than noncarriers. *Conclusions.* The *LRRK2* G2019S prevalence in Morocco is the highest in the world reported to date. Some clinical features in G2019S carriers such as dystonia and sleep disturbances are worth noting.

1. Introduction

Parkinson's disease (PD) is the second most common neurodegenerative disorder after Alzheimer's disease affecting approximately 1-2% of the population over 60 years and 4% above 85 years [1]. It is clinically characterized by rigidity, bradykinesia, tremor, and postural instability. Other clinical features as dementia and depression can be added to this clinical array [2, 3]. Pathologically it is identified by a selective degeneration of dopaminergic neurons in the substantia nigra in the midbrain and eventually the presence of Lewy bodies in the surviving neurons [4, 5]. The etiology of PD is likely to be multifactorial involving complex interactions between genetic and environmental factors, but the exact molecular mechanism underlying the pathogenesis of the disease remains obscure. In the past 17 years, genetic studies

of PD families consolidate the hypothesis that PD has a significant genetic component. Indeed, 14 genes have been described for Mendelian PD so far [6, 7]. Among them, there are at least three confirmed genes responsible for the autosomal dominant form of PD: *SNCA* (PARK1/4), *LRRK2* (PARK8), and *VPS35* (PARK17).

Mutations in *LRRK2* gene are the most frequently reported monogenic cause of PD and are common in both early and late-onset PD, occurring in both familial and sporadic PD patients with a wide variety of clinical and pathological features and a variable frequency depending on ethnic origin [8]. Among these mutations, the glycine to serine substitution (G2019S), located within the protein kinase domain encoded by exon 41, is the most common and was estimated by the international *LRRK2* consortium to represent 1% of sporadic and 4% of familial PD patients worldwide [9]. Intriguingly, the frequency of this mutation varies greatly among ethnic groups and geographic origins. In fact, the highest frequencies were observed in North African countries with 30–40% and Ashkenazi Jews with 10–30% [10, 11]. In Europe, the frequency of G2019S mutation appears to be relatively higher in southern countries particularly in Portugal and Spain with 2–14% of PD cases, than in northern countries with 0–3% [9–13] suggesting a European north-south gradient. The presence of G2019S in PD patients is very rare in Asian populations with a frequency less than 0.1% in China, Japan, Korea, and India, whereas it can reach 1–3% in white North American population [8, 10, 11, 14]. However, none of black PD patients from Nigeria and South Africa seems to carry the G2019S mutation [15, 16]. Among apparently healthy controls, the highest frequency of the G2019S mutation has been reported in North Africa with 3.3% in Berbers of Morocco, 2.13% in Algerians, 1.57% in Tunisians, and 1.32% in Libyans [17]. This frequency is estimated at 2% in Ashkenazi Jews [18] and is reported as very rare or absent in other populations [9]. Occurrence of the G2019S mutation in patients with PD and healthy subjects suggests reduced penetrance, which has been shown to vary according to ethnic origin [12, 19–22]. This variability in penetrance suggests that other genetic or environmental factors are involved in the pathogenesis of the disease.

Clinically, G2019S mutation carriers develop a very similar PD disease to noncarriers, including the development of motor symptoms and cognitive impairment [9, 23], but some differences could be observed even within the same family [24]. Homozygous carriers of G2019S mutation are rare, mostly reported in North African populations where the rate of consanguineous marriages is high. These patients do not show differences in clinical features compared with heterozygous carriers [25–30].

The present study aims to estimate the prevalence of the G2019S mutation of the *LRRK2* gene in the Moroccan population and to assess the motor and nonmotor phenotype of G2019S mutation carriers and noncarriers.

2. Subjects and Methods

A total of 100 unrelated PD patients were recruited consecutively from the outpatient clinic of the Neurological Department at University Hospital Ibn Sina of Rabat from October 2013 to June 2015. One hundred healthy individuals were recruited from the National Blood Transfusion Institute of Rabat and were used as controls. Their mean age was 58.59 (±8.65) and 51 of them were males. Patients and controls provided a written informed consent and the study was approved by the ethic committee of the Medical School of Rabat (CERB).

2.1. Clinical Evaluation. Diagnosis of PD was made by the same neurologist using the United Kingdom Parkinson's Disease Society Brain Bank criteria [31]. Patients were submitted to a structured clinical interview including demographic data, date of onset, disease duration, motor phenotype subtype, the presence of dystonia in the early disease course,

motor fluctuations and dyskinesia, nonmotor symptoms, and current medication. Motor symptoms were assessed using the Unified Parkinson's Disease Rating Scale part III and Hoehn and Yahr stage during ON condition. The LEDD (levodopa Equivalent Daily Dose) was calculated based on a previously published algorithm combining dopamine agonist daily dose with levodopa daily dose [32]. We classified the motor phenotype as tremor-dominant, akinetic-rigid, or mixed, and for the purposes of analysis owing to low figures, we included akinetic-rigid phenotype in mixed group. Nonmotor symptoms scales used are the Pittsburgh sleep QI for sleep disturbances, the Epworth Sleepiness Scale for excessive daytime sleepiness, the SCOPA autonomic questionnaire for dysautonomia, the DN4 questionnaire for neuropathic pain, the Hamilton and the Montgomery and Asberg Depression Rating Scale (MADRS) for depressive complaints, and the Arab version of the MMSE for cognitive impairment (patients with scores below 21 were excluded to avoid reliability concerns in their answers relative to the scales of the questionnaire). For simplification, we recorded nonmotor symptoms as absent or present for constipation, urinary urgency, orthostatic vertigo, pain, hallucinations, memory complaints, and sleep disturbances.

Otherwise, all control individuals have no family history of neurological disease but have not been clinically assessed for the presence of PD.

2.2. Genetic Analysis. A pedigree was established for all patients and the mode of inheritance was classified as "familial" if at least one relative was reported with a diagnosis of PD (FPD) and as autosomal recessive or dominant based on the presence or absence of consanguinity. The remaining patients were classified as "sporadic" (SPD).

Genomic DNA was extracted from peripheral blood leukocytes using Isolate II Genomic DNA kit from Bioline. The G2019S mutation of the *LRRK2* gene was performed by direct sequencing. Briefly, a 378 bp *LRRK2* exon 41 fragment was PCR amplified as described previously [33]. The PCR products were sequenced using Big Dye Terminator Cycle Ready Reaction 3.1 Kits and an ABI 3130xl automated sequencer, and sequence chromatograms were analyzed using SeqScape 2.1 software (Applied Biosystems, Foster City, CA).

2.3. Statistical Analysis. Demographic and clinical variables between G2019S-carriers and noncarriers were compared using parametric and nonparametric tests as appropriate using SPSS 13.0 software. Quantitative data were expressed in mean ± standard deviation (SD) or median and interquartile range and were compared using t-test or Mann–Whitney test. Categorical variables were expressed as numbers and percentages and were compared using Chi-square test. The relationship between G2109S mutation and the clinical symptoms was analyzed by means of logistic regression adjusting for age, sex, and disease duration on univariate and multivariate analysis. In the multivariate analysis model, we introduced variables that had a $p \leq 0.3$ and we forced this analysis for Hoehn and Yahr score for its importance in the disease evolution. p value < 0.05 was considered as statistically

TABLE 1: Demographic features of LRRK2 G2019S carrier and noncarrier patients.

Variables	All patients (n = 100)	G2109S carriers (n = 41)	G2019S noncarriers (n = 59)	p value
Age at exam (years)[a]	60.93 ± 11.07	60.32 ± 11.83	61.35 ± 10.59	0.649
Age at onset (years)[a]	53.9 ± 11.54	52.15 ± 11.28	55.12 ± 11.65	0.207
Disease duration (years)[b]	6 [2.25–10]	7 [4–13]	5 [2–7]	0.035
Gender (male)[c]	56	19 (46.3)	37 (62.7)	0.105

Data are [a]mean ± standard deviation, [b]median [interquartile range], and [c]numbers (percentage).

TABLE 2: Prevalence of G2019S mutations among 100 Moroccan PD patients.

Form	Familial				Sporadic cases		
Inheritance	DFPD	RFPD	ND	Total	Inbred	Not inbred	Total
Patients	29 (29)	2 (2)	2 (2)	33 (33)	10 (10)	57 (57)	67 (67)
G2019S carriers	22 (76)	0 (0)	0 (0)	22 (67)	1 (10)	18 (32)	19 (28)

Data are number (percentage). DFPD = dominant familial Parkinson's disease, RFPD = recessive familial Parkinson's disease, and ND = inheritance not determined.

significant. For multiple testing, we corrected the p value by the Bonferroni method.

3. Results

We examined 100 patients with PD, 56 of whom were males and 44 were females (Table 1). The mean age at exam was 60.93 (±11.07) and the mean age at onset was 53.9 years (±11.54). Comparison of demographic features between the G2019S carriers and noncarriers (Table 1) showed no significant difference except for the disease duration; G2019S carriers have the longest disease duration (p = 0.03).

3.1. Genetic Aspects. Sixty-seven out of 100 patients were sporadic cases (67%) and 33 had a positive family history of PD (33%). Ten of the 67 SPD patients were from consanguineous marriages (Table 2). Among the 33 FPD patients, 29 had dominant inheritance (DFPD), 2 had recessive inheritance (RFPD), and in 2 patients the mode of inheritance could not be specified (parents were consanguineous and one of them is with PD). The *LRRK2* G2019S substitution was found in 41 of 100 (41%, 95% CI 31.4–50.3) PD patients, 37 of whom were heterozygous and 4 were homozygous. The G2019S prevalence increased to 67% (95% CI 48.11–81.45) for FPD patients, with 76% of patients (95% CI 56.07–88.98) having a DFPD, 0% of patients (0 of 2) having RFPD, and 0% of patients (0 of 2) having an unspecified mode of inheritance. The prevalence reaches only 28% (95% CI 18.35–40.88) for SPD patients with 32% of patients (95% CI 20.27–45.38) without consanguinity and 10% of patients (95% CI 1.79–40.41) with consanguinity (Table 2). Interestingly, there were five control individuals heterozygous for the G2019S mutation among the 100 tested (5%, 95% CI 1–10).

3.2. Clinical Features. Motor and nonmotor symptoms of all patients are given in Table 3. The initial symptom of the disease and the clinical phenotype were significantly different between LRRK2 G2019S carriers and noncarriers

(p = 0.019 and p = 0.012, resp.). LRRK2 G2019S carriers have less tremor than noncarriers do as first symptom (26.8% versus 52.5%, corrected-p = 0.03) and exhibited less of the tremor-dominant phenotype than noncarriers (corrected-p = 0.009). They also have more dystonia (p = 0.011) and more dyskinesia (p = 0.002) and take a higher dose (up to 200 mg) of dopaminergic drugs (p = 0.002). Gait disturbances, postural instability, motor fluctuations, UPDRS III score, and H&Y scale during ON state are similar between both groups. Concerning nonmotor symptoms, *LRRK2* G2019S carriers have more sleep complaints than noncarriers do (p = 0.046), while they show the same rates of psychiatric symptoms, constipation, urinary urgency, and orthostatic vertigo. There is a trend to more cognitive impairment in *LRRK2* G2019S carriers than noncarriers but the difference is not significant (p = 0.059).

The relationship between G2109S mutation and the clinical symptoms using logistic regression by adjusting for age, sex, and disease duration is shown in Table 4. *LRRK2* G2019S mutation is associated with more dystonia (OR = 4.655, p = 0.042) and sleep complaints (OR = 2.4, p = 0.045) but less tremor (OR = 0.3, p = 0.011). Nonetheless, while *LRRK2* G2019S carriers have more levodopa-induced dyskinesia (p = 0.002), the statistical significance lacked on multivariate analysis (OR = 1.965, p = 0.217).

4. Discussion

The international *LRRK2* consortium reported a worldwide frequency of *LRRK2* G2019S mutation of 1% in sporadic PD and 4% in familial PD [9]. Although the highest frequency of the G2019S mutation has been recorded in North Africa, no study on the prevalence of this mutation in the Moroccan population has been conducted until now. Previous studies have used small sample size of Moroccan patients, the majority of whom were living outside Morocco. In our cohort of 100 PD patients of Moroccan origin, the overall mutation frequency of G2019S is 41% (95% CI 31.4–50.3). Among probands with autosomal dominant mode of inheritance, this

TABLE 3: Clinical features of G2019S carrier and noncarrier patients.

	G2109S carriers (n = 41)	G2019S noncarriers (n = 59)	p value
Initial symptom			**0.019**
Akinesia[a]	14 (34.1)	9 (15.3)	
Tremor[a]	11 (26.8)	31 (52.5)	
Tremor and akinesia[a]	16 (39)	19 (32.2)	
Clinical phenotype			**0.012**
Akinetic-rigid[a]	10 (24.4)	10 (16.9)	
Tremor-dominant[a]	7 (17.1)	27 (45.8)	
Mixed[a]	24 (58.5)	22 (37.3)	
Dystonia[a]	9 (21.9)	3 (5.1)	**0.011**
Gait impairment[a]	21 (51.2)	23 (39)	0.225
Postural instability[a]	17 (41.5)	29 (49.2)	0.448
UPDRS III ON[b]	11 [6.5–19]	11 [6–21]	0.858
H-Y score[b]	2 [1–4]	3 [1–4]	0.875
LEDD[b]	727.9 [500–1100]	500 [300–800]	**0.002**
Fluctuations[a]	25 (61)	29 (49.2)	0.243
Dyskinesia[a]	23 (56.1)	15 (25.4)	**0.002**
Urinary dysfunction[a]	30 (73.2)	48 (82.8)	0.253
Constipation[a]	21 (51.2)	31 (52.5)	0.896
Orthostatic hypotension[a]	16 (39.0)	29 (49.2)	0.318
Pain[a]	22 (53.7)	31 (52.5)	0.912
Psychiatric disorders[a]	25 (61.0)	28 (47.5)	0.184
Cognitive disorders[a]	26 (63.4)	26 (44.1)	0.059
Sleep disorders[a]	22 (53.7)	19 (33.3)	**0.046**

Data are [a]number (percentage) and [b]median [interquartile range]. Significant p values are in bold.

TABLE 4: Logistic regression model of the association between G2019S mutation and PD clinical features adjusted for gender, age, and disease duration.

	OR/β	CI 95%	p value
Initial symptom	0.305	0.123–0.758	0.011
Tremor[a]			
Akinesia + mixed[a]			
Clinical phenotype	0.261	0.096–0.708	**0.008**
Tremor-dominant[a]			
Akinetic-rigid + mixed[a]			
Dystonia[a]	4.655	1.058–20.48	**0.042**
H-Y score[b]	−0.104	−0.666–458	0.717
LEDD[b]	52.57	−103.6–208.7	0.509
Fluctuations[a]	0.606	0.206–1.782	0.363
Dyskinesia[a]	1.965	0.673–5.739	0.217
Urinary dysfunction[a]	0.566	0.207–1.550	0.268
Psychiatric disorders[a]	2.023	0.856–4.782	0.109
Cognitive disorders[a]	1.892	0.812–4.409	0.140
Sleep disorders[a]	2.409	1.021–5.685	**0.045**

Data are [a]numbers (percentages) and [b]median [interquartile range]. OR = odds ratio and CI = confident interval. Significant p values are in bold.

value rises to about 76% (95% CI 56.07–88.98) and 28% (95% CI 18.35–40.88) among sporadic cases. Unexpectedly, these frequencies were higher than observed in PD patients from neighboring Maghreb countries such as Algeria and Tunisia [10, 11], representing the highest prevalence in the world reported to date for the G2019S mutation.

Among the 41 patients with G2019S mutation, four were homozygous carriers with different mode of inheritance, including two with autosomal dominant inheritance and two sporadic cases of which one comes from a consanguineous marriage. This could be due to the high prevalence of the mutation in the general population. Indeed, there were five heterozygous G2019S carriers among the 100 control individuals (5%).

Clinically, most authors reported a similar phenotype between *LRRK2* G2019S carriers and noncarriers [34, 35]. In our series, the phenotypes are overlapping but the *LRRK2* subjects have less tremor. This finding is in line with some series [34] whereas others reported the tremor as a more common presenting feature in *LRRK2* carriers [30, 36, 37]. Contrariwise, we found a nonsignificant increase of dyskinesia frequency as reported earlier [38], which can be explained by the higher LEDD recorded in this group. Moreover, *LRRK2* G2019S carriers had a similar UPDRS III and H&Y scores for longest disease duration (7 [4–13] versus 5 [2–7], $p = 0.035$) compared to noncarriers. It can reflect in some extent a slower disease evolution in LRRK2 G2019S patients. In the same line, Healy et al. [9] reported longer latency between disease onset and first fall among carriers compared to noncarriers. However, longitudinal follow-up is needed to compare disease course between the two groups.

Furthermore, dystonia is the most specific feature that characterizes *LRRK2* G2019S carriers in our series with an ODDS ratio of 4.65. Dystonia is a well-defined symptom in early onset Parkinson's disease (EOPD) as reported by Kilarski et al. [39] in their systematic review and UK-based study of EOPD. The high frequency in our study can be explained somehow by the overall young age of onset of Parkinson's disease in Moroccan patients [40], but there was no statistically difference in age of onset between *LRRK2* G2019S carriers and noncarriers ($p = 0.207$).

Otherwise, *LRRK2* G2019S patients exhibited more sleep complaints in our series. This feature is in line with other series that reported more sleep onset insomnia, few or no rapid eye behavior disorders, and less nocturia in *LRRK2* G2019S carriers [41–43].

Other reports described more specific clinical features in *LRRK2* carriers such as a lower limb onset [34], more hallucinations, behavioral disorders, and dopaminergic dysregulation syndrome [36, 38, 44] but less cognitive impairment [34, 36, 45]. Kalia et al. [46] explained this phenomenon by the lack of Lewy bodies in some cases with *LRRK2* G2019S mutation; the presence of Lewy bodies is strongly correlated to some nonmotor symptoms especially cognitive impairment and dementia. In our study, *LRRK2* carriers have a trend to more cognitive impairment that was not confirmed in the logistic regression model. Future studies with wider cohorts are required to determine the cognitive profile of *LRRK2* carriers.

5. Conclusions

Our study showed that Morocco has the highest reported prevalence of the G2019S mutation in the world, with a mutation frequency of 41% overall and 76% for patients with autosomal dominant mode of inheritance. Furthermore, G2019S carrier patients exhibit clinical features quite similar to noncarriers with some mild differences in particular more dystonia and more sleep complaints.

Acknowledgments

The authors are grateful to the patients for their participation in this study. They also gratefully acknowledge the National Center of Blood Transfusion of Rabat for providing the control samples. The study was supported by Novartis Pharma Maroc SA and the "Centre National de Recherche Scientifique et Technique" (CNRST) of "Ministère de l'Enseignement Supérieur, de la Recherche Scientifique et de la Formation des Cadres" (MESRSFC) of Morocco.

References

[1] F. Copped, "Genetics and epigenetics of Parkinson's disease," *The Scientific World Journal*, vol. 2012, Article ID 489830, 2012.

[2] B. Thomas and M. Flint Beal, "Parkinson's disease," *Human Molecular Genetics*, vol. 16, no. 2, pp. R183–R194, 2007.

[3] J. Jankovic, "Parkinson's disease: clinical features and diagnosis," *Journal of Neurology, Neurosurgery and Psychiatry*, vol. 79, no. 4, pp. 368–376, 2008.

[4] M. C. J. Dekker, V. Bonifati, and C. M. Van Duijn, "Parkinson's disease: piecing together a genetic jigsaw," *Brain*, vol. 126, no. 8, pp. 1722–1733, 2003.

[5] D. J. Moore, A. B. West, V. L. Dawson, and T. M. Dawson, "Molecular pathophysiology of Parkinson's disease," *Annual Review of Neuroscience*, vol. 28, pp. 57–87, 2005.

[6] V. Bonifati, "Genetics of Parkinson's disease—state of the art, 2013," *Parkinsonism and Related Disorders*, vol. 20, no. 1, pp. S23–S28, 2014.

[7] M. K. Lin and M. J. Farrer, "Genetics and genomics of Parkinson's disease," *Genome Medicine*, vol. 6, no. 6, article 48, 2014.

[8] P. Gómez-Garre, F. Carrillo, and P. Mir, "Prevalence and clinical features of LRRK2 mutations in patients with Parkinson disease," *European Neurology Journal*, vol. 2, pp. 1–7, 2010.

[9] D. G. Healy, M. Falchi, S. S. O'Sullivan et al., "Phenotype, genotype, and worldwide genetic penetrance of LRRK2-associated Parkinson's disease: a case-control study," *The Lancet Neurology*, vol. 7, no. 7, pp. 583–590, 2008.

[10] H. T. S. Benamer and R. De Silva, "LRRK2 G2019S in the North African population: a review," *European Neurology*, vol. 63, no. 6, pp. 321–325, 2010.

[11] S. Lesage, E. Patin, C. Condroyer et al., "Parkinson's disease-related LRRK2 G2019S mutation results from independent mutational events in humans," *Human Molecular Genetics*, vol. 19, no. 10, Article ID ddq081, pp. 1998–2004, 2010.

[12] J. Kachergus, I. F. Mata, M. Hulihan et al., "Identification of a novel LRRK2 mutation linked to autosomal dominant

parkinsonism: evidence of a common founder across European populations," *American Journal of Human Genetics*, vol. 76, no. 4, pp. 672–680, 2005.

[13] M. Sierra, I. González-Aramburu, P. Sánchez-Juan et al., "High frequency and reduced penetrance of lRRK2 g2019S mutation among Parkinson's disease patients in Cantabria (Spain)," *Movement Disorders*, vol. 26, no. 13, pp. 2343–2346, 2011.

[14] H. F. Chien, T. R. Figueiredo, M. A. Hollaender et al., "Frequency of the LRRK2 G2019S mutation in late-onset sporadic patients with Parkinson's disease," *Arquivos de Neuro-Psiquiatria*, vol. 72, no. 5, pp. 356–359, 2014.

[15] N. Okubadejo, A. Britton, C. Crews et al., "Analysis of Nigerians with apparently sporadic Parkinson disease for mutations in LRRK2, PRKN and ATXN3," *PLoS ONE*, vol. 3, no. 10, Article ID e3421, 2008.

[16] S. Bardien, A. Marsberg, R. Keyser et al., "LRRK2 G2019S mutation: frequency and haplotype data in South African Parkinson's disease patients," *Journal of Neural Transmission*, vol. 117, no. 7, pp. 847–853, 2010.

[17] N. Change, G. Mercier, and G. Lucotte, "Genetic screening of the G2019S mutation of the LRRK2 gene in southwest European, North African, and sephardic Jewish subjects," *Genetic Testing*, vol. 12, no. 3, pp. 333–339, 2008.

[18] A. Orr-Urtreger, C. Shifrin, U. Rozovski et al., "The LRRK2 G2019S mutation in Ashkenazi Jews with Parkinson disease: is there a gender effect?" *Neurology*, vol. 69, no. 16, pp. 1595–1602, 2007.

[19] L. N. Clark, Y. Wang, E. Karlins et al., "Frequency of LRRK2 mutations in early- and late-onset Parkinson disease," *Neurology*, vol. 67, no. 10, pp. 1786–1791, 2006.

[20] S. Punia, M. Behari, S. T. Govindappa et al., "Absence/rarity of commonly reported LRRK2 mutations in Indian Parkinson's disease patients," *Neuroscience Letters*, vol. 409, no. 2, pp. 83–88, 2006.

[21] J. J. Ferreira, L. C. Guedes, M. M. Rosa et al., "High prevalence of LRRK2 mutations in familial and sporadic Parkinson's disease in Portugal," *Movement Disorders*, vol. 22, no. 8, pp. 1194–1201, 2007.

[22] S. Goldwurm, M. Zini, A. Di Fonzo et al., "LRRK2 G2019S mutation and Parkinson's disease: a clinical, neuropsychological and neuropsychiatric study in a large Italian sample," *Parkinsonism and Related Disorders*, vol. 12, no. 7, pp. 410–419, 2006.

[23] S. Belarbi, N. Hecham, S. Lesage et al., "LRRK2 G2019S mutation in Parkinson's disease: a neuropsychological and neuropsychiatric study in a large Algerian cohort," *Parkinsonism and Related Disorders*, vol. 16, no. 10, pp. 676–679, 2010.

[24] C. Schulte and T. Gasser, "Genetic basis of Parkinson's disease: inheritance, penetrance, and expression," *Application of Clinical Genetics*, vol. 4, pp. 67–80, 2011.

[25] W. C. Nichols, N. Pankratz, D. Hernandez et al., "Genetic screening for a single common LRRK2 mutation in familial Parkinson's disease," *Lancet*, vol. 365, no. 9457, pp. 410–412, 2005.

[26] S. Lesage, P. Ibanez, E. Lohmann et al., "G2019S LRRK2 mutation in French and North African families with Parkinson's disease," *Annals of Neurology*, vol. 58, no. 5, pp. 784–787, 2005.

[27] L. Ishihara, R. A. Gibson, L. Warren et al., "Screening for Lrrk2 G2019S and clinical comparison of Tunisian and North American Caucasian Parkinson's disease families," *Movement Disorders*, vol. 22, no. 1, pp. 55–61, 2007.

[28] L. Warren, R. Gibson, L. Ishihara et al., "A founding LRRK2 haplotype shared by Tunisian, US, European and Middle Eastern families with Parkinson's disease," *Parkinsonism and Related Disorders*, vol. 14, no. 1, pp. 77–80, 2008.

[29] S. Lesage, S. Belarbi, A. Troiano et al., "Is the common LRRK2 G2019S mutation related to dyskinesias in North African Parkinson disease?" *Neurology*, vol. 71, no. 19, pp. 1550–1552, 2008.

[30] M. M. Hulihan, L. Ishihara-Paul, J. Kachergus et al., "LRRK2 Gly2019Ser penetrance in Arab-Berber patients from Tunisia: a case-control genetic study," *The Lancet Neurology*, vol. 7, no. 7, pp. 591–594, 2008.

[31] A. J. Hughes, S. E. Daniel, L. Kilford, and A. J. Lees, "Accuracy of clinical diagnosis of idiopathic Parkinson's disease: a clinicopathological study of 100 cases," *Journal of Neurology Neurosurgery and Psychiatry*, vol. 55, no. 3, pp. 181–184, 1992.

[32] C. L. Tomlinson, R. Stowe, S. Patel, C. Rick, R. Gray, and C. E. Clarke, "Systematic review of levodopa dose equivalency reporting in Parkinson's disease," *Movement Disorders*, vol. 25, no. 15, pp. 2649–2653, 2010.

[33] J.-W. Cho, S.-Y. Kim, S.-S. Park, and B. S. Jeon, "The G2019S LRRK2 mutation is rare in Korean patients with Parkinson's disease and multiple system atrophy," *Journal of Clinical Neurology (Korea)*, vol. 5, no. 1, pp. 29–32, 2009.

[34] R. N. Alcalay, A. Mirelman, R. Saunders-Pullman et al., "Parkinson disease phenotype in Ashkenazi jews with and without LRRK2 G2019S mutations," *Movement Disorders*, vol. 28, no. 14, pp. 1966–1971, 2013.

[35] A. Puschmann, "Monogenic Parkinson's disease and parkinsonism: clinical phenotypes and frequencies of known mutations," *Parkinsonism and Related Disorders*, vol. 19, no. 4, pp. 407–415, 2013.

[36] N. L. Khan, S. Jain, J. M. Lynch et al., "Mutations in the gene LRRK2 encoding dardarin (PARK8) cause familial Parkinson's disease: clinical, pathological, olfactory and functional imaging and genetic data," *Brain*, vol. 128, no. 12, pp. 2786–2796, 2005.

[37] E. M. Gatto, V. Parisi, D. P. Converso et al., "The LRRK2 G2019S mutation in a series of Argentinean patients with Parkinson's disease: clinical and demographic characteristics," *Neuroscience Letters*, vol. 537, pp. 1–5, 2013.

[38] C. Marras, B. Schuele, R. P. Munhoz et al., "Phenotype in parkinsonian and nonparkinsonian *LRRK2* G2019S mutation carriers," *Neurology*, vol. 77, no. 4, pp. 325–333, 2011.

[39] L. L. Kilarski, J. P. Pearson, V. Newsway et al., "Systematic review and UK-based study of PARK2 (parkin), PINK1, PARK7 (DJ-1) and LRRK2 in early-onset Parkinson's disease," *Movement Disorders*, vol. 27, no. 12, pp. 1522–1529, 2012.

[40] W. Regragui, L. Lachhab, R. Razine et al., "Profile of idiopathic Parkinson's disease in Moroccan patients," *International Archives of Medicine*, vol. 7, no. 1, article 10, 2014.

[41] M. Ehrminger, S. Leu-Semenescu, F. Cormier et al., "Sleep aspects on video-polysomnography in LRRK2 mutation carriers," *Movement Disorders*, vol. 30, no. 13, pp. 1839–1843, 2015.

[42] C. Pont-Sunyer, A. Iranzo, C. Gaig et al., "Sleep disorders in parkinsonian and nonparkinsonian LRRK2 mutation carriers," *PLoS ONE*, vol. 10, no. 7, Article ID e0132368, 2015.

[43] D.-W. Li, Z. Gu, C. Wang et al., "Non-motor symptoms in Chinese Parkinson's disease patients with and without LRRK2 G2385R and R1628P variants," *Journal of Neural Transmission*, vol. 122, no. 5, pp. 661–667, 2015.

14

The Outcomes of Total Hip Replacement in Patients with Parkinson's Disease: Comparison of the Elective and Hip Fracture Groups

Pavel Šponer,[1,2] Tomáš Kučera,[1,2] Michal Grinac,[1,2]
Aleš Bezrouk,[3] and Daniel Waciakowski[4]

[1]Department of Orthopaedic Surgery, Charles University in Prague, Faculty of Medicine in Hradec Králové, Šimkova 870,
500 38 Hradec Králové, Czech Republic
[2]Department of Orthopaedic Surgery, University Hospital Hradec Králové, Sokolská 581, 500 05 Hradec Králové, Czech Republic
[3]Department of Medical Biophysics, Charles University in Prague, Faculty of Medicine in Hradec Králové, Šimkova 870,
500 38 Hradec Králové, Czech Republic
[4]Department of Orthopaedics and Traumatology, Kreiskrankenhaus Greiz GmbH, Wichmannstraße 12, 07973 Greiz, Germany

Correspondence should be addressed to Pavel Šponer; sponer.p@seznam.cz

Academic Editor: Mayela Rodríguez-Violante

Introduction. The aim of the study was to compare the clinical outcomes following elective and traumatic total hip arthroplasty in Parkinson's disease patients. *Materials and Methods.* Ten patients with osteoarthritis comprise the elective group (mean age at operation 74 years; mean follow-up 82 months). Thirteen patients with femoral fracture comprise the hip fracture group (mean age 76 years; mean follow-up 54 months). All patients were followed up at 6 and 36 months postoperatively and at the time of the latest follow-up. *Results.* Despite the significant improvement in Merle d'Aubigné-Postel and pain scores, disability related to Parkinson's disease increased during the follow-up. Whereas more than 1/3 of hip fracture patients and all elective patients walked independently at 36 months after total hip arthroplasty, 43% of living patients from both groups were able to walk independently at the time of the latest follow-up. The medical complications were seen mainly in patients with hip fracture. *Conclusions.* Excellent pain relief with preserved walking ability without support of another person and acceptable complication profile was observed in Parkinson's disease patients at 36 months after elective total hip arthroplasty. This procedure may be indicated in Parkinson's disease patients after careful and individualized planning.

1. Introduction

The prevalence of Parkinson's disease and the incidence of hip fractures mirror an ageing population living longer [1, 2]. Parkinson's disease patients with hip fractures stay at higher risk of mortality and surgical and medical complications [3]. Short- and long-term results in patients with Parkinson's disease following hip fracture are generally described to be worse than in patients without this disease [4]. The advancement in pharmacotherapy and surgical treatment has improved the life spans in patients with Parkinson's disease [5]. Nowadays we encounter in our practice Parkinson's disease patients suffering from hip joint osteoarthritis and avascular necrosis

of femoral head, or complications of the hip arthroplasty implanted before the onset of Parkinson's disease such as symptomatic aseptic loosening or periprosthetic fracture of the femur [6]. Contemporary total hip arthroplasty is one of the highly efficient surgical techniques leading to improvement in the patient's quality of life [7]. Nonetheless, reports of the outcomes of elective total hip arthroplasty in patients with Parkinson's disease in the literature are sparse [8, 9]. But it is reasonable to be aware that orthopaedic surgeons will increasingly be required to evaluate the suitability of patients with Parkinson's disease for total hip arthroplasty.

The aim of the study was to compare the short- to mid-term clinical outcomes following elective and traumatic total

TABLE 1: Demographics of patients included in the study.

	Elective group	Hip fracture group
Number of patients	10	13
Number of hips	10	14
Mean age in years (range)	74 (65–82)	76 (67–83)
Gender		
Female	8	7
Male	2	6
Right side	5	5
Left side	5	9
ASA score, average	2.50	2.62
Hoehn-Yahr scale, average	2.30	2.31

TABLE 2: Details of implants used in the study.

	Elective group	Hip fracture group
Acetabular component		
Cemented	8	13
Cementless	2	1
Acetabular liner		
Standard	7	8
With elevated rim/lipped	3	6
Femoral stem		
Cemented	9	12
Cementless	1	2
Head diameter		
28 mm	7	13
32 mm	3	1

hip arthroplasty in patients with Parkinson's disease focusing on the assessment of risks and benefits of surgery.

2. Materials and Methods

2.1. Patients. All patients with a confirmed diagnosis of Parkinson's disease having total hip arthroplasty at our institution between January 2005 and December 2012 were enrolled in a retrospective analysis. In total, 24 total hip arthroplasties were implanted in 23 patients, 8 men (35%) and 15 women (65%). The primary indication for surgery was osteoarthritis for 10 hips; these 10 patients comprise the "elective group" with a mean age at operation 74 years (65 to 82). Thirteen patients underwent total hip arthroplasty for proximal femoral fracture (one patient had hip fracture subsequently on both sides); they comprise the "hip fracture group" with a mean age at operation 76 years (67 to 83) (Table 1). The research was carried out in compliance with the Helsinki Declaration. Written informed consent was obtained from all patients included in the study.

2.2. Surgical Procedure. All the procedures were performed via a standard anterolateral Watson-Jones approach to the hip joint. In order to maximize sample size in the elective and hip fracture groups, implant design was not a controlled variable. The details of components with regard to stability of the implanted nonconstrained total hip arthroplasty are depicted in Table 2. All patients received prophylactic intravenous antibiotics for 24 hours postoperatively. Venous thromboprophylaxis was with low-molecular-weight heparin for 5 weeks. Standard postoperative rehabilitation as for any THA was started on the first postoperative day including mobilization in high vertical walker.

2.3. Outcome Assessments. Outcome measure analysed in the study included Charnley's modified Merle d'Aubigné and Postel scoring system [10]. As a result of Merle d'Aubigné and Postel scoring system is a composite score including objective clinical parameters different from pain, the pain score component of the Charnley's modified Merle d'Aubigné and Postel score was also evaluated separately. The disability caused by the Parkinson's disease was classified according to Hoehn and Yahr [11]. Furthermore, a functional status was based on assessment of independent ability to walk and

was also analysed distinguishing between the following two findings [12]:

(1) Maintained independent ability to walk: being able to walk without support from another person (with aids if necessary).

(2) Not maintained: support from another person or use of a wheelchair required.

Complications were recorded throughout the follow-up period. All patients were followed up prospectively before surgery, at 6 months and 36 months postoperatively, and at the time of the latest follow-up.

In the elective group consisting of 10 hips, the mean follow-up was 82 (33–143) months. One patient in the elective group died at 33 months postoperatively from causes unrelated to the surgery (pulmonary tumor). For 14 hips in the hip fracture group, the mean follow-up was 54 (1–143) months. Five patients in the hip fracture group died during follow-up at 1, 3, 4, 11, and 30 months postoperatively.

2.4. Statistical Analysis. Measurement data were processed and statistically evaluated with the help of MS Excel 2013 (Microsoft Corp, Redmond WA, USA) and NCSS 2007 (Hintze, J. (2007). NCSS 2007. NCSS LLC, Kaysville, Utah, USA. https://www.ncss.com). Since the type of data of all the tested parameters is ordinal, we opted for using the Wilcoxon signed-rank test. A value of $P < 0.05$ was considered to be significant. For the purpose of comparison of the elective with the hip fracture group, only the data of the patients who survived until the last follow-up (median 82 months for the hip fracture and 72 months for the elective group) were used.

3. Results

The statistically significant difference between the medians of Merle d'Aubigné and Postel score in the elective and hip fracture group was recorded preoperatively, at 6 and 36 months after total hip arthroplasty. There was no statistically significant difference between the two groups during the last follow-up (Figure 1). The improvement in Merle d'Aubigné and Postel score preoperatively to 6 months postoperatively

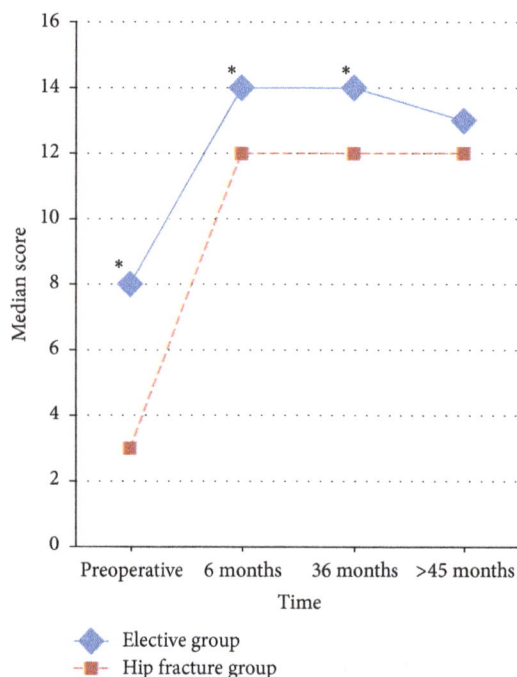

FIGURE 1: Line graph of Merle d'Aubigné and Postel scores by time in the elective and hip fracture group. Comparison of the progress of the medians of Merle d'Aubigné and Postel score during follow-up. The asterisk (*) indicates the statistically significant difference between the compared groups.

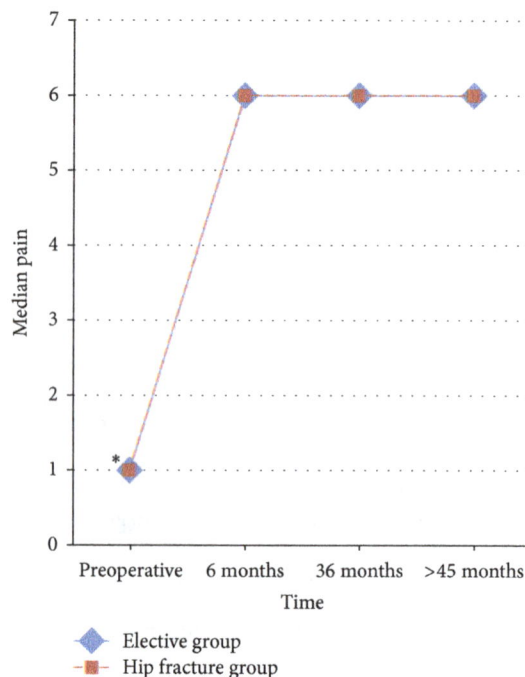

FIGURE 2: Line graph of pain scores by time in the elective and hip fracture group. Comparison of the progress of the medians of pain score during follow-up. The asterisk (*) indicates the statistically significant difference between the compared groups.

was statistically significant ($P < 0.001$) for both groups; there was no difference between the 6 months and 36 months and between the 36 months and latest follow-up Merle d'Aubigné and Postel scores in the elective group and in the hip fracture group too.

The elective group had preoperatively significantly higher pain score when compared with the hip fracture group. There was no statistically significant difference between the two groups during the 6 months, 36 months, and the last follow-up (Figure 2). The improvement in pain score preoperatively to 6 months postoperatively was statistically significant ($P < 0.001$) for both groups with no differences between the 6 months and 36 months pain scores and between the 36 months and latest follow-up scores in the elective group and in the hip fracture group too. Of the 20 patients (21 hips) of both groups followed up at 6 months, 18 hips had no pain and 3 hips had only slight pain. Of the 17 patients (18 hips) of both groups followed up at 36 months, 17 hips had no pain and 1 hip had only slight pain. There was no pain observed in 18 hips of both groups at the time of latest follow-up.

Despite the improvement in Merle d'Aubigné and Postel and pain scores, disability related to Parkinson's disease increased during the follow-up; neurological progression was noted in 83% of all our patients. At the time of latest follow-up 57% of all the patients had progressed to functional stage IV or V (Table 3).

All patients in both groups were able to walk independently before surgery and functional status deteriorated over time as seen in Figure 3. Whereas 7 patients (54%) in

the hip fracture group were able to walk independently, 9 patients (90%) in the elective group walked without support of another person at 6 months after surgery. Whereas 5 patients (38%) in the hip fracture group were able to walk without support of another person at 36 months after total hip arthroplasty, 9 patients (100%) in the elective group walked independently. At the time of the latest follow-up, 10 of living patients from both groups (43%) were still able to walk independently of another person with aid of forearm crutches.

The complications are listed in Table 4. Whereas the surgical complications were observed in both groups, the medical complications were seen mainly in patients undergoing total hip arthroplasty for femoral fracture. Two dislocations occurred within the first 3 months postoperatively, one dislocation in each group. Treatment was closed reduction in one patient of the elective group. One patient of the hip fracture group developed instability after a fatal cerebrovascular accident. Two periprosthetic fractures (one patient of hip fracture group fell 2 months after total hip arthroplasty and one patient of elective group 32 months after initial surgery) were treated operatively by osteosynthesis. One late periprosthetic infection occurred 26 months postoperatively in the hip fracture group and antimicrobial suppression was chosen because comorbidities did not allow additional surgery. Throughout the whole follow-up period, urinary tract infection and pneumonia were the most frequent medical complications in the hip fracture group (coincident respiratory and urinary tract infections were recorded in 4 patients) and were treated with antibiotics.

TABLE 3: Details of patients included in the study.

(a) Elective group

Case	A	B	C	D	E	F	G	H	I	J
1	2	75	2	33	3/4	1/2	1 + 4	70/80	30/20	7 + 4
2	2	71	2	123	2/5	1/2	1 + 5	70/100	0/30	6 + 8
3	1	66	3	143	2/3	1/1	2 + 4	95/90	35/40	10 + 3
4	1	77	3	99	2/2	1/1	1 + 5	90/95	20/20	8 + 6
5	2	70	3	132	2/4	1/2	1 + 5	70/90	30/30	8 + 7
6	2	82	2	60	2/2	1/1	1 + 5	60/90	15/30	6 + 8
7	2	77	3	72	3/3	1/1	2 + 4	120/90	30/40	9 + 4
8	2	82	2	52	2/3	1/1	2 + 3	95/90	30/30	12 + 0
9	2	65	2	53	3/4	1/1	1 + 5	80/90	25/30	7 + 6
10	2	74	3	48	2/3	1/2	2 + 4	85/120	20/30	10 + 4

(b) Hip fracture group

Case	A	B	C	D	E	F	G	H	I	J
1	1	70	3	1	3/5	1/2	1 + *	*/**	*/**	3 + *
2	1	75	3	4	3/5	1/2	1 + *	*/**	*/**	3 + *
3	2	80	3	143	2/3	1/1	1 + 5	*/95	*/30	3 + 12
4	2	73	2	93	2/5	1/2	1 + 5	*/90	*/30	3 + 9
5 left	2	80	3	53	3/3	1/1	1 + 5	*/80	*/20	3 + 9
5 right	2	80	3	53	3/3	1/1	1 + 4	*/70	*/20	3 + 8
6	2	78	2	85	2/4	1/2	1 + 5	*/90	*/30	3 + 10
7	2	67	3	82	2/5	1/2	1 + 5	*/90	*/15	3 + 9
8	1	83	3	87	3/5	1/2	1 + 5	*/90	*/40	3 + 10
9	1	77	3	11	2/5	1/2	1 + 5	*/90	*/15	3 + 9
10	2	75	2	3	2/5	1/2	1 + *	*/**	*/**	3 + *
11	1	75	2	61	2/3	1/1	1 + 5	*/70	*/25	3 + 9
12	2	74	2	45	1/2	1/1	1 + 5	*/60	*/30	3 + 9
13	1	82	3	30	3/4	1/2	1 + 5	*/60	*/25	3 + 9

A: gender: 1: male; 2: female; B: age at total hip arthroplasty (years); C: ASA score; D: follow-up (months); E: Hoehn and Yahr functional stage preoperatively/at the time of latest follow-up; F: functional status preoperatively/at the time of latest follow-up: 1: maintained independent ability to walk; 2: not maintained independent ability to walk; G: preoperative pain score ± the postoperative increase at 6 months postoperatively (points); * the data were not available (short follow-up); H: hip flexion preoperatively/at 6 months postoperatively (degrees); * indicates that the hip joint was not moved in sagittal plane due to fracture; ** indicates that the data were not available (short follow-up); I: hip abduction preoperatively/at 6 months postoperatively (degrees); * indicates that the hip joint was not moved in frontal plane due to fracture; ** indicates that the data were not available (short follow-up); J: preoperative Merle d'Aubigné and Postel score ± the postoperative increase at 6 months postoperatively (points); * indicates that the data were not available (short follow-up).

TABLE 4: Complications.

Complication	Elective group (10 hips; 10 patients)	Hip fracture group (14 hips; 13 patients)
Dislocation	1	1
Periprosthetic fracture	1	1
Periprosthetic infection	0	1
Cerebrovascular accident	0	1
Postoperative confusion	0	2
Urinary tract infection	0	9
Pneumonia	0	4
Vulvovaginitis	1	0
Pressure sores	1	2
Decompensation of diabetes mellitus	1	0
Total	*5*	*21*

Six patients (five in the hip fracture group) had two complications each. Two patients in the hip fracture group had four complications.

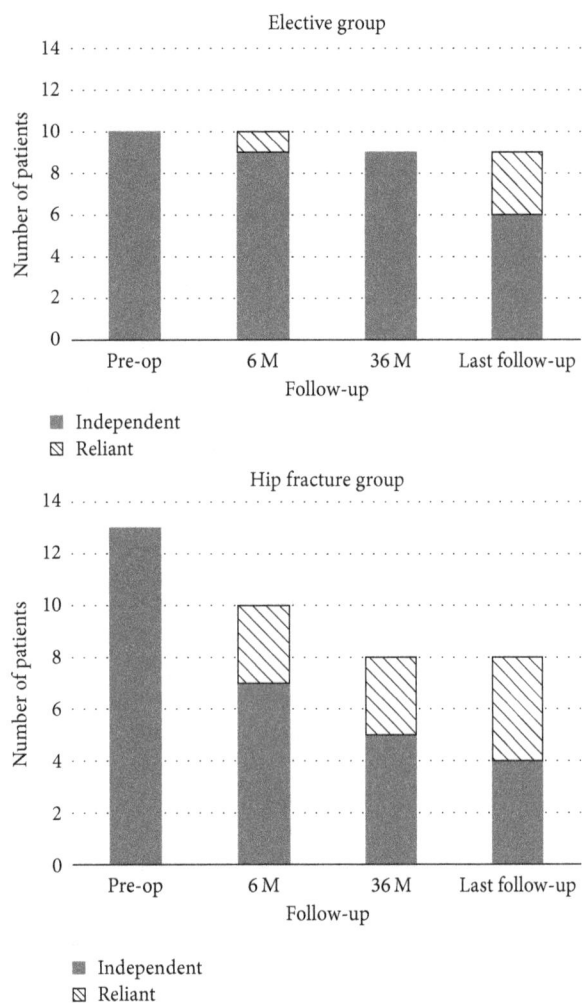

FIGURE 3: Distribution of independent and reliant patients in the elective and hip fracture groups during follow-up.

Four patients in the hip fracture group died during first year after surgery: three of pneumonia and one of cerebrovascular accident. The overall 1-year mortality for the hip fracture group was 28.6%.

4. Discussion

Total hip arthroplasty is one of the major successes of modern medicine [7]. As a result of progress in the implant designs and the precise surgical techniques, the indications for this procedure are continually expanding [13]. Total hip arthroplasty may be now considered also in patients with different neurological dysfunctions which would previously have been managed by salvage procedures. Several studies have evaluated the outcome of hemiarthroplasty in Parkinson's disease patients with hip fractures [14–16]. Unfortunately these surveys are not accurately applicable to an elective total hip arthroplasty. In order to support the current evidence regarding the outcome of total hip arthroplasty in Parkinson's disease patients we carried out a present study.

Our study demonstrates a clear improvement in hip pain following total hip arthroplasty in patients with Parkinson's disease as supported by improved Merle d'Aubigné and Postel and pain scores. This improvement was maintained from 6 months after surgery to the latest follow-up in the elective and hip fracture group. Although the functional status of Parkinson's disease patients deteriorated over time, we observed that patients in the elective group benefited from excellent pain relief and were able to walk without support of another person at 36 months after total hip arthroplasty which was indicated for osteoarthritis with severe hip joint pain preventing activities of daily living. Ten of living patients from both groups (43%) were still able to walk without support of another person at the time of the latest follow-up.

Although variable mortality following hip fracture in Parkinson's disease patients has been reported, we found it comparable with 1-year mortality published in non-Parkinson's disease patients [3, 17]. However, the morbidity with an increased complication rate was observed in our hip fracture group [18]. The most frequently recorded medical complication (64% of patients in the hip fracture group throughout the whole follow-up period) was urinary tract infection. The neurogenic detrusor overactivity is common in Parkinson's disease patients (45–93%) and bladder dysfunction plays important role in development of urinary tract infection [19]. In large retrospective study of neurogenic bladder patients, more than one-third (36%) of patients were diagnosed with a lower urinary tract infection at least one year after neurogenic bladder diagnosis [20].

Obstructive respiratory pattern due to neuromuscular dysfunction predisposes to retained secretion, atelectasis, and pulmonary infection [21]. We found pneumonia in 29% of Parkinson's disease patients with femoral fractures. High pulmonary infection rates (40–43%) were reported also by Eventov et al. and Staeheli et al. [15, 16]. Immobility, constant pressure, friction, reduced muscle mass, and low skin turgor contribute to development of pressure sores. Historically, high rates of pressure sores (25–49%) were published in Parkinson's disease patients after hip fracture [14, 15]. Despite early mobilization, we observed pressure sores in 12.5% of Parkinson's disease patients after total hip arthroplasty.

The musculoskeletal manifestation of Parkinson's disease include tremor, rigidity, contractures, bradykinesia, dystonia, and postural instability which theoretically predispose patients to dislocation of the hip [13]. Historically, high rate of hemiarthroplasty dislocation (37%) was published in Parkinson's disease patients who were not mobilized in the first week after hip fracture surgery [14]. The results in these patients after surgery for hip fractures were poor, mainly because of medical complications with high rates of morbidity and mortality. Later studies described lower rates of hemiarthroplasty dislocation in Parkinson's disease patients (2–11%) suggesting that these better outcomes may have been due to pharmacotherapy aimed at maintaining muscle tone [16, 22].

Recently Parkinson's disease patients had an approximately twofold risk of hip dislocation [23]. Adduction contracture is an important finding in these patients which can be overlooked during the procedure [6]. Due to pain and muscle spasm following hip fracture, it is not possible to assess the hip abduction prior to surgery. For this reason, careful intraoperative hip stability testing consisting of extension with external rotation motions, subsequent flexion with internal rotation motions, and check for telescoping of the components should be emphasized [24]. To prevent instability, adductor or psoas tenotomies for severe flexion contracture were recommended [8]. Based on thorough intraoperative assessment, the stability of all our total hip arthroplasties was adequate and no pelvifemoral muscle contractures were observed. Therefore adductor tenotomies were thought to be not necessary to prevent hip joint instability in our patients.

Despite early mobilization started on the first postoperative day, intensive postoperative rehabilitation, and patient's care, the dislocation rate of nonconstrained total hip arthroplasty in our study (8.3%) is comparable with recently reported rate in nationwide registry-based case-controlled study (6.1%) [23]. Both are significantly greater than has been published in patients without neurological dysfunction [25]. Therefore certain innovative implant designs, such as dual mobility acetabular cup and large-diameter heads, should be considered to reduce the incidence of dislocation in patients with Parkinson's disease [26, 27].

Most Parkinson's disease patients experience falls as a result of disease symptoms and many have recurrent episodes [28]. It was estimated that 60.5% of patients with Parkinson disease experience at least one episode and 39% have recurrent falls [29]. The high frequency of falls consequently contributes to the increased fracture risk. Falls in the period after total hip arthroplasty may result in serious periprosthetic fractures of the femur as is seen in 8.3% of hip joints in our study. Surgical treatment of periprosthetic fractures belongs to the most difficult orthopaedic procedures due to the extensive surgery with increased blood loss, high frequency of other complications, and series of unfavorable outcomes, such as disability and death [30].

With increasing prevalence of Parkinson's disease, falls and fractures are anticipated to have a major impact on health care systems in the coming decades [28]. Severity of disease and functional impairment might be substantial determinants of the risk of falls and fractures. However, neurodegenerative diseases and especially cognitive disorders substantially compromise individuals' physical reserves important for adaptation to changes in health state and acute stress, such as hip fracture [23]. In addition, patients with Parkinson's disease have poorer initial physical condition. In the setting of acute trauma for displaced femoral neck fractures, our study did not entirely support total hip arthroplasty in Parkinson's disease patients. During the period of the study, hemiarthroplasty was routinely used in moderate to low functioning elderly patients with displaced femoral neck fractures. Based on the results of our study, Parkinson's disease patients with hip fractures have poorer prognosis due to the disease progression with inevitable functional disability and therefore hemiarthroplasty remains an appropriate option [31].

This retrospective study is limited by the small patient numbers and short duration of follow-up. Nevertheless the follow-up was sufficient to reveal a clinical outcome following elective and traumatic total hip arthroplasty in patients with Parkinson's disease. Total hip arthroplasty is a viable alternative for these patients if the surgery is individualized and carefully planned. A multidisciplinary team comprised of health professionals, including the neurologist, geriatrician, and physiotherapist, should be involved to maximize patient outcome [32]. Early discussion with the patient and his family regarding the difficulty of prolonged rehabilitation process, as well as the potential need of prolonged stay in nursing home, should be emphasized in effort to optimize surgical outcomes in Parkinson's disease patients [5]. Before an elective procedure, tremor and other symptoms related to Parkinson's disease should be well controlled to minimize postoperative complications and enhance rehabilitation process. To be recognized as a potential key element for arthroplasty success, rehabilitation process should be started preoperatively with subsequent early postoperative mobilization and physical therapy [33]. The patients should be also carefully monitored for common complications, such as urinary tract infection, pulmonary infection, and pressure sores [5]. Finally, improving the patient bone density or preventing bone loss is important before joint arthroplasty is considered in Parkinson's disease patients.

5. Conclusions

In conclusion, total hip arthroplasty in patients with Parkinson's disease is challenging due to higher risk of medical complications which were seen mainly in patients with hip fracture. Excellent pain relief with preserved walking ability without support of another person and acceptable complication profile was observed in Parkinson's disease patients at 36 months after elective total hip arthroplasty. Elective total hip arthroplasty may be indicated in patients with Parkinson's disease after careful and individualized planning.

Acknowledgments

This study was supported by the Program PROGRES Q40/04.

References

[1] T. Pringsheim, N. Jette, A. Frolkis, and T. D. L. Steeves, "The prevalence of Parkinson's disease: a systematic review and meta-analysis," *Movement Disorders*, vol. 29, no. 13, pp. 1583–1590, 2014.

[2] C. A. Brauer, M. Coca-Perraillon, D. M. Cutler, and A. B. Rosen, "Incidence and mortality of hip fractures in the United States," *The Journal of the American Medical Association*, vol. 302, no. 14, pp. 1573–1579, 2009.

[3] R. J. Critchley, S. K. Khan, A. J. Yarnall, M. J. Parker, and D. J. Deehan, "Occurrence, management and outcomes of hip

fractures in patients with Parkinson's disease," *British Medical Bulletin*, vol. 115, no. 1, pp. 135–142, 2015.

[4] R. W. Walker, A. Chaplin, R. L. Hancock, R. Rutherford, and W. K. Gray, "Hip fractures in people with idiopathic Parkinson's disease: incidence and outcomes," *Movement Disorders*, vol. 28, no. 3, pp. 334–340, 2013.

[5] L. M. Zuckerman, "Parkinson's disease and the orthopaedic patient," *Journal of the American Academy of Orthopaedic Surgeons*, vol. 17, no. 1, pp. 48–55, 2009.

[6] P. G. Mathew, P. Sponer, T. Kucera, M. Grinac, and J. Knízek, "Total HIP arthroplasty in patients with Parkinson's disease," *Acta medica (Hradec Králové)/Universitas Carolina, Facultas Medica Hradec Králové*, vol. 56, no. 3, pp. 110–116, 2013.

[7] B. M. Wroblewski, P. D. Siney, and P. A. Fleming, "Charnley low-friction arthroplasty: Survival patterns to 38 years," *Journal of Bone and Joint Surgery - Series B*, vol. 89, no. 8, pp. 1015–1018, 2007.

[8] M. Weber, M. E. Cabanela, F. H. Sim, F. J. Frassica, and W. S. Harmsen, "Total hip replacement in patients with Parkinson's disease," *International Orthopaedics*, vol. 26, no. 2, pp. 66–68, 2002.

[9] R. Mohammed, K. Hayward, S. Mulay, F. Bindi, and M. Wallace, "Outcomes of dual-mobility acetabular cup for instability in primary and revision total hip arthroplasty," *Journal of Orthopaedics and Traumatology*, vol. 16, no. 1, pp. 9–13, 2015.

[10] J. Charnley, "The long-term results of low-friction arthroplasty of the hip performed as a primary intervention," *The Journal of Bone & Joint Surgery—British Volume*, vol. 54, no. 1, pp. 61–76, 1972.

[11] M. M. Hoehn and M. D. Yahr, "Parkinsonism: onset, progression and mortality," *Neurology*, vol. 17, no. 5, pp. 427–442, 1967.

[12] T. J. Pedersen and J. M. Lauritsen, "Routine functional assessment for hip fracture patients: Are there sufficient predictive properties for subgroup identification in treatment and rehabilitation?" *Acta Orthopaedica*, vol. 87, no. 4, pp. 374–379, 2016.

[13] J. M. Queally, A. Abdulkarim, and K. J. Mulhall, "Total hip replacement in patients with neurological conditions," *The Journal of Bone & Joint Surgery—British Volume*, vol. 91, no. 10, pp. 1267–1273, 2009.

[14] L. Coughlin and J. Templeton, "Hip fractures in patients with Parkinson's disease," *Clinical Orthopaedics and Related Research*, vol. 148, pp. 192–195, 1980.

[15] I. Eventov, M. Moreno, E. Geller, R. Tardiman, and R. Salama, "Hip fractures in patients with parkinson's syndrome," *Journal of Trauma - Injury, Infection and Critical Care*, vol. 23, no. 2, pp. 98–101, 1983.

[16] J. W. Staeheli, F. J. Frassica, and F. H. Sim, "Prosthetic replacement of the femoral head for fracture of the femoral neck in patients who have Parkinson disease," *Journal of Bone and Joint Surgery - Series A*, vol. 70, no. 4, pp. 565–568, 1988.

[17] S. Schnell, S. M. Friedman, D. A. Mendelson, K. W. Bingham, and S. L. Kates, "The 1-year mortality of patients treated in a hip fracture program for elders," *Geriatric Orthopaedic Surgery & Rehabilitation*, vol. 1, no. 1, pp. 6–14, 2010.

[18] Y. L. Manach, G. Collins, M. Bhandari et al., "Outcomes after hip fracture surgery compared with elective total hip replacement," *JAMA - Journal of the American Medical Association*, vol. 314, no. 11, pp. 1159–1166, 2015.

[19] L. Yeo, R. Singh, M. Gundeti, J. M. Barua, and J. Masood, "Urinary tract dysfunction in Parkinson's disease: A review," *International Urology and Nephrology*, vol. 44, no. 2, pp. 415–424, 2012.

[20] A. Manack, S. P. Motsko, C. Haag-Molkenteller et al., "Epidemiology and healthcare utilization of neurogenic bladder patients in a US claims database," *Neurourology and Urodynamics*, vol. 30, no. 3, pp. 395–401, 2011.

[21] L. Lethbridge, G. M. Johnston, and G. Turnbull, "Co-morbidities of persons dying of Parkinson's disease," *Progress in Palliative Care*, vol. 21, no. 3, pp. 140–145, 2013.

[22] R. Turcotte, C. Godin, R. Duchesne, and A. Jodoin, "Hip fractures and Parkinson's disease. A clinical review of 94 fractures treated surgically," *Clinical Orthopaedics and Related Research*, no. 256, pp. 132–136, 1990.

[23] E. Jämsen, T. Puolakka, M. Peltola, A. Eskelinen, and M. U. K. Lehto, "Surgical outcomes of primary hip and knee replacements in patients with Parkinson's disease: A nationwide registry-based case-controlled study," *Bone and Joint Journal*, vol. 96, no. 4, pp. 486–491, 2014.

[24] H. Tanino, H. Ito, M. K. Harman, T. Matsuno, W. A. Hodge, and S. A. Banks, "An In Vivo Model for Intraoperative Assessment of Impingement and Dislocation in Total Hip Arthroplasty," *Journal of Arthroplasty*, vol. 23, no. 5, pp. 714–720, 2008.

[25] R. S. Kotwal, M. Ganapathi, A. John, M. Maheson, and S. A. Jones, "Outcome of treatment for dislocation after primary total hip replacement," *Journal of Bone and Joint Surgery - Series B*, vol. 91, no. 3, pp. 321–326, 2009.

[26] K.-S. Park, J.-K. Seon, K.-B. Lee, and T.-R. Yoon, "Total Hip Arthroplasty Using Large-Diameter Metal-On-Metal Articulation in Patients With Neuromuscular Weakness," *Journal of Arthroplasty*, vol. 29, no. 4, pp. 797–801, 2014.

[27] M. Yassin, A. Garti, M. Khatib, M. Weisbrot, and D. Robinson, "Retentive Cup Arthroplasty in Selected Hip Fracture Patients—A Prospective Series With a Minimum 3-Year Follow-Up," *Geriatric Orthopaedic Surgery & Rehabilitation*, vol. 7, no. 4, pp. 178–182, 2016.

[28] L. Kalilani, M. Asgharnejad, T. Palokangas, and T. Durgin, "Comparing the incidence of falls/fractures in Parkinson's disease patients in the US population," *PLoS ONE*, vol. 11, no. 9, Article ID e0161689, 2016.

[29] N. E. Allen, A. K. Schwarzel, and C. G. Canning, "Recurrent falls in Parkinson's disease: a systematic review," *Parkinson's Disease*, vol. 2013, Article ID 906274, 16 pages, 2013.

[30] M. Korbel, P. Sponer, T. Kucera, E. Procházka, and T. Procek, "Results of treatment of periprosthetic femoral fractures after total hip arthroplasty," *Acta medica (Hradec Králové)/Universitas Carolina, Facultas Medica Hradec Králové*, vol. 56, no. 2, pp. 67–72, 2013.

[31] M. J. Grosso, J. R. Danoff, T. S. Murtaugh, D. P. Trofa, A. N. Sawires, and W. B. Macaulay, "Hemiarthroplasty for Displaced Femoral Neck Fractures in the Elderly Has a Low Conversion Rate," *Journal of Arthroplasty*, vol. 32, no. 1, pp. 150–154, 2017.

[32] R. Skelly, F. Lindop, and C. Johnson, "Multidisciplinary care of patients with Parkinson's disease," *Progress in Neurology and Psychiatry*, vol. 16, no. 2, pp. 10–14, 2012.

[33] A. M. Swank, Joseph B. Kachelman, B. Wendy et al., "Prehabilitation before total knee arthroplasty increases strength and function in older adults with severe osteoarthritis," *Journal of Strength and Conditioning Research*, vol. 25, no. 2, pp. 318–325, 2011.

15

Protective Effects of an Ancient Chinese Kidney-Tonifying Formula against H$_2$O$_2$-Induced Oxidative Damage to MES23.5 Cells

Yihui Xu,[1] Wei Lin,[2] Shuifen Ye,[3] Huajin Wang,[4] Tingting Wang,[5] Youyan Su,[5] Liangning Wu,[6] Yuanwang Wang,[7] Qian Xu,[5] Chuanshan Xu,[8] and Jing Cai[5]

[1]*Second People's Hospital, Fujian University of Traditional Chinese Medicine, Fuzhou, Fujian Province 350003, China*
[2]*Academy of Integrative Medicine, Fujian University of Traditional Chinese Medicine, Fuzhou, Fujian Province 350122, China*
[3]*Longyan First Hospital Affiliated to Fujian Medical University, Longyan, Fujian Province 364000, China*
[4]*Tibet Autonomous Region People's Hospital, Lhasa, Tibet Autonomous Region 850000, China*
[5]*College of Integrative Medicine, Fujian University of Traditional Chinese Medicine, Fuzhou, Fujian Province 350122, China*
[6]*Graduate School, Fujian University of Traditional Chinese Medicine, Fuzhou, Fujian Province 350122, China*
[7]*Quanzhou Orthopedic-Traumatological Hospital, Fujian University of Traditional Chinese Medicine,
 Quanzhou, Fujian Province 362000, China*
[8]*School of Chinese Medicine, Faculty of Medicine, The Chinese University of Hong Kong, Shatin, Hong Kong*

Correspondence should be addressed to Jing Cai; caij1@163.com

Academic Editor: Jin-Tai Yu

Oxidative damage plays a critical role in the etiology of neurodegenerative disorders including Parkinson's disease (PD). In our study, an ancient Chinese kidney-tonifying formula, which consists of *Cistanche*, *Epimedii*, and *Polygonatum cirrhifolium*, was investigated to protect MES23.5 dopaminergic neurons against hydrogen peroxide- (H$_2$O$_2$-) induced oxidative damage. The damage effects of H$_2$O$_2$ on MES23.5 cells and the protective effects of KTF against oxidative stress were evaluated using MTT assay, transmission electron microscopy (TEM), immunocytochemistry (ICC), enzyme-linked immunosorbent assay (ELISA), and immunoblotting. The results showed that cell viability was dramatically decreased after a 12 h exposure to 150 μM H$_2$O$_2$. TEM observation found that the H$_2$O$_2$-treated MES23.5 cells presented cellular organelle damage. However, when cells were incubated with KTF (3.125, 6.25, and 12.5 μg/ml) for 24 h after H$_2$O$_2$ exposure, a significant protective effect against H$_2$O$_2$-induced damage was observed in MES23.5 cells. Using ICC, we found that KTF inhibited the reduction of the tyrosine hydroxylase (TH) induced by H$_2$O$_2$, upregulated the mRNA and protein expression of HO-1, CAT, and GPx-1, and downregulated the expression of caspase 3. These results indicated that KTF may provide neuron protection against H$_2$O$_2$-induced cell damage through ameliorating oxidative stress, and our findings provide a new potential strategy for the prevention and treatment of Parkinson's disease.

1. Introduction

Neurodegenerative diseases have recently become an important public health problem. Parkinson's disease (PD) is a neurodegenerative disease characterized by the progressive loss of dopaminergic neurons in the substantia nigra. Even though the cause of PD remains to be clarified, several lines of evidence strongly suggest that oxidative damage and mitochondrial dysfunction play an important role in the pathological mechanisms of PD [1–3]. Increased oxidative stress results from imbalance between oxidative products such as reactive oxygen species (ROS) and antioxidant molecules in the cell [4]. Enhancing antioxidative capacity of brain cells has become an effective strategy in protecting nervous cells against oxidative stress damage.

PD is a difficult-to-treat disease threatening the elderly worldwide. The current therapeutic drugs have limited efficacy with severe side-effects. Traditional Chinese herbs and formula have been widely used in folk medicine to treat neurodegenerative diseases including PD for a long time. According to Chinese medicine theory, the deficiency of kidney is the main pathological mechanism of PD. *Cistanche deserticola* Y. C. Ma, a species of *Cistanche* which belongs to the Orobanchaceae family, is a well-known herb in traditional Chinese medicine with so-called kidney-tonifying efficacy and is used for the treatment of kidney deficiency, female infertility, morbid leucorrhea, neurasthenia, and senile constipation [5]. It has been reported that *Cistanche* total glycosides exerted protective effects on substantia nigra dopaminergic neuron in mice model and cells of PD [6, 7]. Moreover, the active ingredients of *Cistanche* have been documented to possess neuroprotective effect through enhancing antioxidant capacity and inhibiting apoptosis of neurons [8–15]. *Herba Epimedii* is also a traditional kidney-tonifying Chinese herb with significantly antioxidative activity, which is widely utilized in treating osteoporosis and cardiovascular diseases and improving sexual and neurological functions [16]. *Polygonatum sibiricum* is often employed as an assistant to improve the effectiveness of the monarch drug and minister drug in the traditional Chinese formula. Recent report showed that the water extracts of *Polygonatum sibiricum* are natural antioxidants.

Based on these benefits from the ancient Chinese kidney-tonifying formula (KTF) which consists of *Cistanche*, *Epimedii,* and *Polygonatum cirrhifolium*, we hypothesized that KTF might protect MES23.5 dopaminergic neurons against hydrogen peroxide- (H_2O_2-) induced oxidative damage. Herein, as proof-of-concept, we conducted a series of experiments to examine the effects of KTF on cell death and antioxidant enzymes expression in the H_2O_2-treated MES23.5 cells.

2. Materials and Methods

2.1. Chemicals and Reagents. HO-1, CAT, caspase 3, and β-actin antibodies were obtained from Cell Signaling Technology Inc. (Boston, USA). GPx-1 antibody was from Abcam (Cambridge Science Park, UK). Rabbit Anti-Tyrosine Hydroxylase was from Boster (BA1454, China). Goat anti-rabbit IgG1 conjugated to a horseradish peroxidase label was from Santa Cruz Biotechnology Inc. (California, USA). Dulbecco's modified Eagle's medium (DMEM) was purchased from GIBCO BRL Co. Ltd. (Gaithersburg, MD, USA). All the other reagents, unless otherwise stated, were from Sigma Chemical Co. (St. Louis, MO, USA). RevertAid™ First Strand cDNA Synthesis Kit was from Fermentas Inc. (Burlington, USA). DreamTaq Green PCR Master Mix (2x) was from Fermentas Inc. (Burlington, USA). Bio DL100 was from BioFlux (Tokyo, Japan). Polink-2 plus Polymer HRP Detection System for Rabbit Primary Antibody (PV-9001) and DAB (3, 3′-diaminoobenzidine tetrahydrochloride) (ZLI-9032) were from ZSGB-BIO (Beijing, China). ELISA kits for measuring CAT, GPx-1, and GSH were from Hufeng Biotechnology Inc. (Shanghai, China). *Ginkgo biloba* extracts (GE) were from Shanghai Sine Promod Pharmaceutical Co., Ltd. (Shanghai, China).

2.2. Preparation and Standardization of Kidney-Tonifying Formula. The components of kidney-tonifying formula, *Cistanche deserticola*, *Epimedium brevicornum,* and *Polygonatum sibiricum*, were supplied by Second Affiliated People's Hospital, Fujian University of Traditional Chinese Medicine, and carefully authenticated according to the Chinese pharmacopoeia (The Pharmacopoeia Commission of China, 2005). To prepare KTF samples, *Cistanche deserticola*, *Epimedium brevicornum,* and *Polygonatum sibiricum* at the weight ratio of 1:1:1.2 were mixed and ground into the powder and then immersed in a total volume of 10 times (w/v) distilled water for 1 h and boiled for 2 h. After the solution was filtered, the filtrate was collected. The entire residue was collected and further boiled with a total volume of 8 times (w/v) distilled water for 2 h. The solution was filtered and the two filtrates were combined, concentrated, and freeze-dried. The yield of the final dried extract was 25% (w/w) of the starting raw herbal materials and was stored at −20°C until used. The stock solution KTF (10 mg/ml) was prepared by dissolving KTF in phosphate-buffer solution (PBS), followed by sonication, sterilization at 100°C, and filtration.

2.3. Cell Culture and H_2O_2 Treatment. MES23.5 cells were cultured and exposed to H_2O_2 as described by our previous paper [10]. Briefly, MES23.5 cells were grown in DMEM/F12 (GIBCO BRL Co. Ltd., Gaithersburg, MD, USA) medium containing 5% (vol/vol) FBS (GIBCO BRL Co. Ltd., Gaithersburg, MD, USA), 100 U penicillin/streptomycin, 2 mM L-glutamine (Sigma Chemical Co., St. Louis, MO, USA), and Sato's (50 × Sato's: insulin 25 mg; transferring 25 mg; pyruvic acid, 243 mg; putrescine 20 mg; 1 mg/ml sodium selenate, 25 μl; 0.315 mg/ml progesterone) at 37°C with 5% CO_2. Overnight grown MES23.5 cells were further incubated with 150 μM H_2O_2 for 12 h.

2.4. KTF Treatment. MES23.5 cells were randomly divided into control group (fresh culture medium), H_2O_2 group (H_2O_2 culture medium), *Ginkgo biloba* extract (GE) group (H_2O_2 and GE culture medium), and KTF groups including low dose of KTF treatment, middle dose of FTF treatment, and high dose of KTF treatment. MES23.5 cells at logarithmic phase were seeded in culture plate coated by poly-L-lysine (PLL) for 24 h. The cells in the control group were treated with the fresh culture medium, and those in all other groups were treated with the culture medium containing 150 μM H_2O_2 for 12 h. The cells in the GE group were treated with the culture medium containing 12.5 μg/ml GE, and those in the low dose KTF group, middle dose KTF group, and high dose KTF group were treated with KTF at the concentrations of 3.125, 6.25, and 12.5 μg/ml for 24 h, respectively.

2.5. Cell Viability. After KTF treatment for 20 h, the cells were incubated with MTT (0.5 mg/ml) for 4 h at 37°C, and the media were carefully removed and 150 μL of DMSO was added to each well. The formazan crystals were dissolved for 10 min, and absorbance was measured at 490 nm. Optical density (OD) of each well was measured by spectrophotometer (BIO-TEK ELX 800, BioTek Instruments Inc., Vermont,

USA). Freshly cell culture medium was used as a negative control.

2.6. Ultrastructural Morphology Observation. After KTF treatment for 24 h, the cells were collected, suspended, and fixed with 3% glutaraldehyde in 1.5% paraformaldehyde solution (pH 7.3) at 4°C for 24 h. Cell suspensions were then rinsed twice with PBS and postfixed with 1% osmic acid and 1.5% potassium hexacyanoferrate (II) solution (pH 7.3) and incubated at 4°C for 2 h; then cell suspensions were dehydrated in a graded series of alcohol for 5 min each. The dehydrated pellets were embedded three times with propylene oxide for 1 h and infiltrated with a resin/propylene oxide mixture at 1 : 1 ratio for 2 h and then with resin for 12 h at room temperature. The inclusion was made with epoxy resin 618 and Araldite and polymerization was performed at 60°C for 48 h. Finally, ultrathin sections (80 nm) were stained with uranyl acetate and counterstained with lead citrate for 5 min. The stained cells were examined with the H7650 transmission electron microscope (Hitachi, Japan).

2.7. Immunocytochemical Assay of Tyrosine Hydroxylase (TH). After KTF treatment for 24 h, the cells were washed twice for 2 min with PBS and fixed with 4% paraformaldehyde for 15 min. The fixed cells were washed 3 times and then treated with 0.5% Triton X-100 for 20 min. Afterward, the cells were washed 3 times and treated with 3% H_2O_2 for 10 min. The H_2O_2-treated cells were washed 3 times and then blotted with goat serum for 20 min. After being blotted, rabbit anti-TH (1 : 400) was added to each sample at 4°C overnight. The samples were then washed 3 times and treated with Polymer Helper for 20 min. After Polymer treatment the cells were washed 3 times and treated with poly-HRP anti-rabbit IgG for 20 min. The cells were washed 3 times and treated with DAB for 3 min. Finally, the samples were washed with running water and treated with hematoxylin counterstaining for 1 min and then washed with running water and sealed with permount mounting medium.

2.8. Measurement of Antioxidative Enzymes by ELISA. After KTF treatment for 24 h, the activity level of intracellular CAT, GPx-1, and GSH was measured using an ELISA kit (Hufeng Biotechnology Inc., Shanghai, China) according to the manufacturer's instruction. Briefly, $100 \mu L$ homogenate supernatant of the lysate of the treated cells was added to the ELISA wells and then incubated at 37°C for 30 min. After being washed five times and dried, $50 \mu L$ enzyme-labeled antibody working solution was added to each well (expected control tube). The resultant solution was incubated for 30 min at 37°C and washed five times and dried. Substrate working solution $(150 \mu L)$ was added to each well and incubated for 15 min at 37°C. Finally, stop solution $(50 \mu L)$ was added to each well and the absorbance value was determined at 450 nm using an automatic ELISA reader (XL800, BioTex, Incorporated, Houston, TX, USA).

2.9. Western Blot Analysis. After KTF treatment for 24 h, the cells were washed with ice-cold PBS and proteins were extracted in a lysis buffer containing 50 mM Tris-HCl (pH

7.4), 1 mM EDTA, 150 mM NaCl, 1% Nonidet P-40, 1 mM phenylmethylsulfonyl fluoride, and $10 \mu g/mL$ aprotinin. Protein concentration was determined using BCA Protein Assay Kit (Thermo Scientific Pierce, Rockford, Illinois, USA). Protein were separated by SDS-PAGE electrophoresis and transferred to PVDF (Bio-Rad, Hercules, CA, USA). Blocking was performed with 5% nonfat dried milk; the membrane was incubated with the of rabbit anti-rat HO-1, CAT, caspase 3, β-actin antibody (1 : 1000, Cell Signaling), and rabbit anti-rat GPx-1 antibody (1 : 1000, Abcam) overnight at 4°C. The treated membrane was washed and then exposed to goat anti-rabbit IgG1 conjugated to a horseradish peroxidase label (1 : 5000, Santa Cruz, USA) for 2 h at room temperature. After five more washes, cross-reactivity was visualized using Electrochemiluminescence (ECL) Western blotting detection reagents and analyzed using scanning densitometry in an Image System (Bio-Rad, Hercules, CA, USA).

2.10. RT-PCR Analysis. PCR primer of HO-1, CAT, GPx-1, and β-actin were purchased from Sangon Biotech Co. Ltd. (Shanghai, China). After KTF treatment for 24 h, total RNA of cells was isolated using Trizol reagent according to the manufacturer's instruction. Reverse transcription (RT) was performed using the AMV reverse transcription system (Fermentas, Burlington, USA). cDNA fragment and β-actin were amplified using Green PCR master MIX Kit (Fermentas, Burlington, USA). DNA was amplified immediately with a single cycle at 94°C for 5 min and 30 cycles at 94°C for 30 s and 58°C for 30 s and 72°C for 30 s for β-actin, and a final extension step was taken at 72°C for 10 min. Ethidium bromide stained gels were scanned and qualified using Tanon Image Software. The intensity of each band was normalized against the intensity of β-actin.

2.11. Statistical Analysis. Statistical analysis was done with SPSS 18.0 (SPSS Inc., Chicago, IL). All data were shown as mean ± SD (standard deviation), and statistical significance of difference was performed by one-way ANOVA and LSD (linear standard deviation). A difference was considered to be significant at $P < 0.05$.

3. Results

3.1. The Damage Effects of H_2O_2 on MES23.5 Cells and the Protective Effects of KTF against Oxidative Stress. As shown in Figure 1(a), H_2O_2 exhibited a dose- and time-dependent inhibition in the viability of MES23.5 dopaminergic neuronal cells. After 12 h exposure to $50 \mu M$ H_2O_2, a significant loss of cell viability was noted, and the cell viability loss gradually increased with H_2O_2 dose increasing to $150 \mu M$. However, further increasing H_2O_2 dose from 200 to $500 \mu M$ did not result in significant higher loss of cell viability. Extending MES23.5 cells exposure to H_2O_2 from 12 h to 24 h and 48 h increased the loss of cell viability at lower H_2O_2 concentration. A significant loss of MES23.5 cell viability was noted after 24 h exposure to $25 \mu M$ H_2O_2 and 48 h exposure to $12.5 \mu M$ H_2O_2. A time-dependent manner of cell viability loss was observed in all tested concentration of H_2O_2.

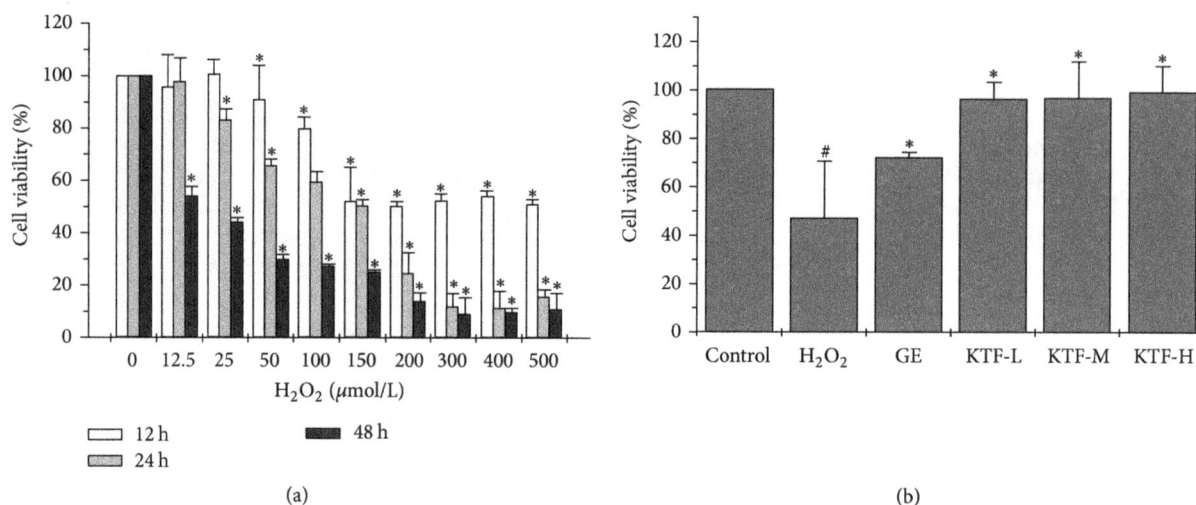

FIGURE 1: The damage effects of H_2O_2 on MES23.5 cells and the protective effects of KTF against oxidative stress were evaluated using MTT assay. (a) Effects of different concentrations of H_2O_2 treatment on cell damage. MES23.5 cells were treated with 12.5, 25, 50, 100, 150, 200, 300, 400, and 500 μMol/L H_2O_2 for 12, 24, and 48 h. (b) Protective effects of different concentrations of KTF treatment on H_2O_2-induced cell damage. Treatment of KTF resulted in increase of MES23.5 cells viability after H_2O_2 addition. MES23.5 cells were incubated with GE (12.5 μg/ml) or KTF (3.125, 6.25, 12.5 μg/ml) for 24 h after the addition of H_2O_2. The cell viability was measured with MTT. Data are expressed as mean $\pm$ SD (standard deviation) in three independent experiments. $^{\#}P < 0.05$ compared to the control group. $^{*}P < 0.05$ compared to the H_2O_2-treat group.

Exposing MES23.5 cells to KTF alone did not have significant cytotoxic effect even when KTF concentration was up to 100 μg/ml. MES23.5 cells cocultured with 150 μM H_2O_2 for 12 h caused cell viability loss of 46.76%. Cytotoxic effect of H_2O_2 on MES23.5 cells was significantly attenuated upon KTF treatment for 24 h (Figure 1(b)). Augmented viability of H_2O_2 treated MES23.5 cells was restored to 95.86% $\pm$ 7.18%, 96.49% $\pm$ 15.07%, and 99.04% $\pm$ 10.57% by a treatment with KTF at concentrations of 3.125, 6.25, and 12.5 μg/ml, respectively.

TEM showed that normal cells in control group exhibited oval shape with intact cell membrane which has many corrugations and microvilli-like structures. Cell nucleus was elliptic in the center with a single nucleolus and had normal euchromatin and scattered heterochromatin. Mitochondria exhibited rod-like or elliptic, scattered, and with normal cristae mitochondriate. Rough endoplasmic reticulum was well developed and had no obvious degranulation (Figure 2(a)). However, the cells treated with H_2O_2 presented typical oxidative damage with smaller, irregular nucleus, and swelled mitochondria. Obvious degranulation was found in rough endoplasmic reticulum (Figure 2(b)). In the cells treated by KTF ameliorated H_2O_2-induced oxidative damage, mitochondria exhibited rod-like or elliptic, scattered, and with more cristae mitochondriate. Rough endoplasmic reticulum had no obvious degranulation (Figures 2(d), 2(e), and 2(f)).

3.2. Increasing Expression of TH in MES23.5 Cells after KTF Treatment. TH is a critical catalyzing enzyme in the conversion of the amino acid L-tyrosine to L-3,4-dihydroxyphenylalanine (L-DOPA) which is the precursor to the neurotransmitters dopamine. The normal expression of TH

is the mark of active neuron. Therefore, we compared the TH expression in the H_2O_2-incubated MES23.5 cells with or without following KTF treatment by immunohistochemistry. The result showed that H_2O_2 decreased TH expression in the MES23.5 cells, and following KTF treatment could improve TH expression significantly (Figure 3). This indicates that KTF treatment was able to restore the function of the H_2O_2-treated MES23.5 cells.

3.3. KTF Suppressed H_2O_2-Induced Caspase 3 Activation in MES23.5 Cells. For further investigating the mechanism of MES23.5 cell damage, we evaluated the expression of proapoptosis factor caspase 3 by immunoblotting. Result showed that H_2O_2 treatment markedly downregulated the expression of procaspase 3 and upregulated the expression of caspase 3. In contrast, KTF treatment restored the procaspase 3 and caspase 3 balance by increasing the expressions of procaspase 3 and decreasing the expression of caspase 3 (Figure 4). These findings demonstrate that KTF treatment effectively inhibited caspase 3 activation.

3.4. Increased Expression of Antioxidative Enzymes in MES23.5 Cells by KTF Treatment. ELISA assay revealed that intracellular CAT, GPx-1, and GSH were downregulated after 150 μM H_2O_2 treatment in MES23.5 cells. Of note, following treatment of KTF restored intracellular CAT, GPx-1, and GSH expression. RT-PCR analysis indicated that H_2O_2 treatment downregulated CAT and GPx-1 mRNA expression; however, KTF treatment restored the expressions of CAT and GPx-1 mRNA in MES23.5 cells. Immunoblot with specific antibodies also confirmed that CAT and GPx-1 protein expression in MES23.5 cells were downregulated by H_2O_2 treatment, and KTF treatment was able to restore CAT and

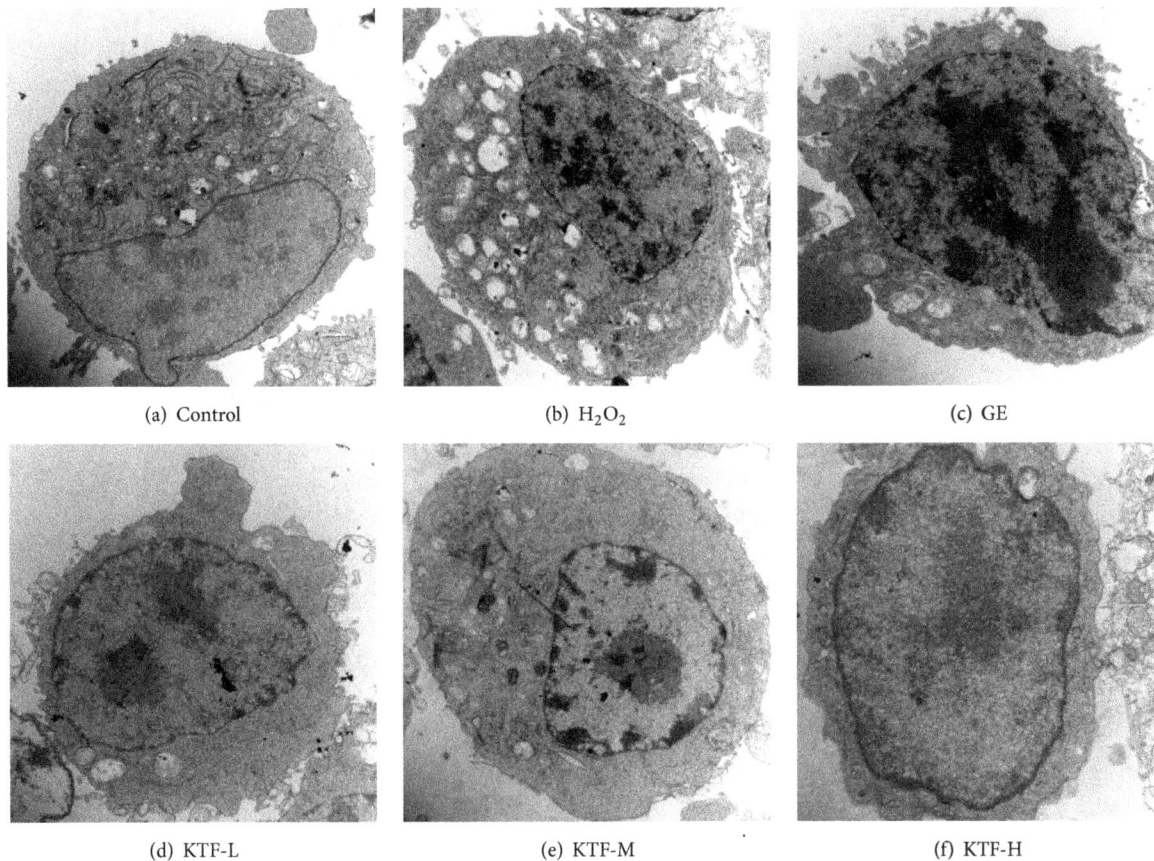

FIGURE 2: Effect of KTF on cellular ultrastructure in H_2O_2-induced MES23.5 cells. Cellular ultrastructure was observed under TEM. Normal morphology of cytoplasm, cell organelles in control group ((a), ×15,000), characteristic ultrastructural morphology of oxidative damage in H_2O_2-treated group ((b), ×15,000), treatment with KTF group (3.125, 6.25, and 12.5 μg/ml, respectively) ((d), (e), (f), ×15,000), or *Ginkgo* extract (12.5 μg/ml) ((c), ×15,000).

GPx-1 protein expression. Moreover, mRNA expression of oxidative stress responding protein HO-1 was also inhibited after H_2O_2 treatment and then was restored by following KTF treatment. Immunoblotting also proved that HO-1 protein expression was markedly downregulated by H_2O_2, but KTF treatment was able to restore HO-1 protein expression. As expected, the highest KTF concentration used in our investigation has the best effect on restoring CAT, GPx-1, GSH, and HO-1 expression (Figures 5 and 6). Taken together, the obtained results demonstrate that KTF treatment significantly upregulated antioxidant substrates in the H_2O_2-treated MES23.3 cells.

4. Discussion

As an important component of redox system, ROS play important roles in regulating cell function. Moderate levels of ROS may function as signals to promote cell proliferation and survival. Under physiologic conditions, the balance between generation and elimination of ROS maintains the proper function of redox-sensitive signaling system. Redox homeostasis can be disrupted by increase of ROS production or decrease of ROS-scavenging capacity, leading to an overall

increase in oxidative stress [17, 18], subsequently causing an irreversible damage of intracellular structure and inducing cell death.

High consumption of O_2 in brain leads to accumulation of ROS; thus, neurons are particularly vulnerable to the attack of oxidative stress. Postmortem investigations have shown lipid peroxidation and oxidative damage to brain cells in PD patients [19]. Growing studies confirm that oxidative damage plays a critical role in the pathogenesis of neuron degenerative diseases, such as AD, PD, HD, and ALS [18, 20]. In the present study, a significant loss of cell viability was observed in MES23.5 dopaminergic neuronal cell after exposure to 50 μM H_2O_2 for 12 h, 25 μM H_2O_2 for 24 h, or 12.5 μM H_2O_2 for 48 h. As shown by morphology observation, the cells exposed 12 h to 150 μM H_2O_2 exhibited a typical oxidative injury including multiple membranous vacuoles in the cytoplasm, disruption of endoplasmic reticulum and mitochondrion, and condensing euchromatin in cell nucleus.

According to Chinese medicine theory, the deficiency of kidney is the main pathological mechanism of PD. Invigorating the kidney is an important strategy in the treatment of PD. In the present study, we found that traditional kidney-tonifying formula KTF, which consists of *Cistanche, Epimedii,*

(a)

(b)

(c)

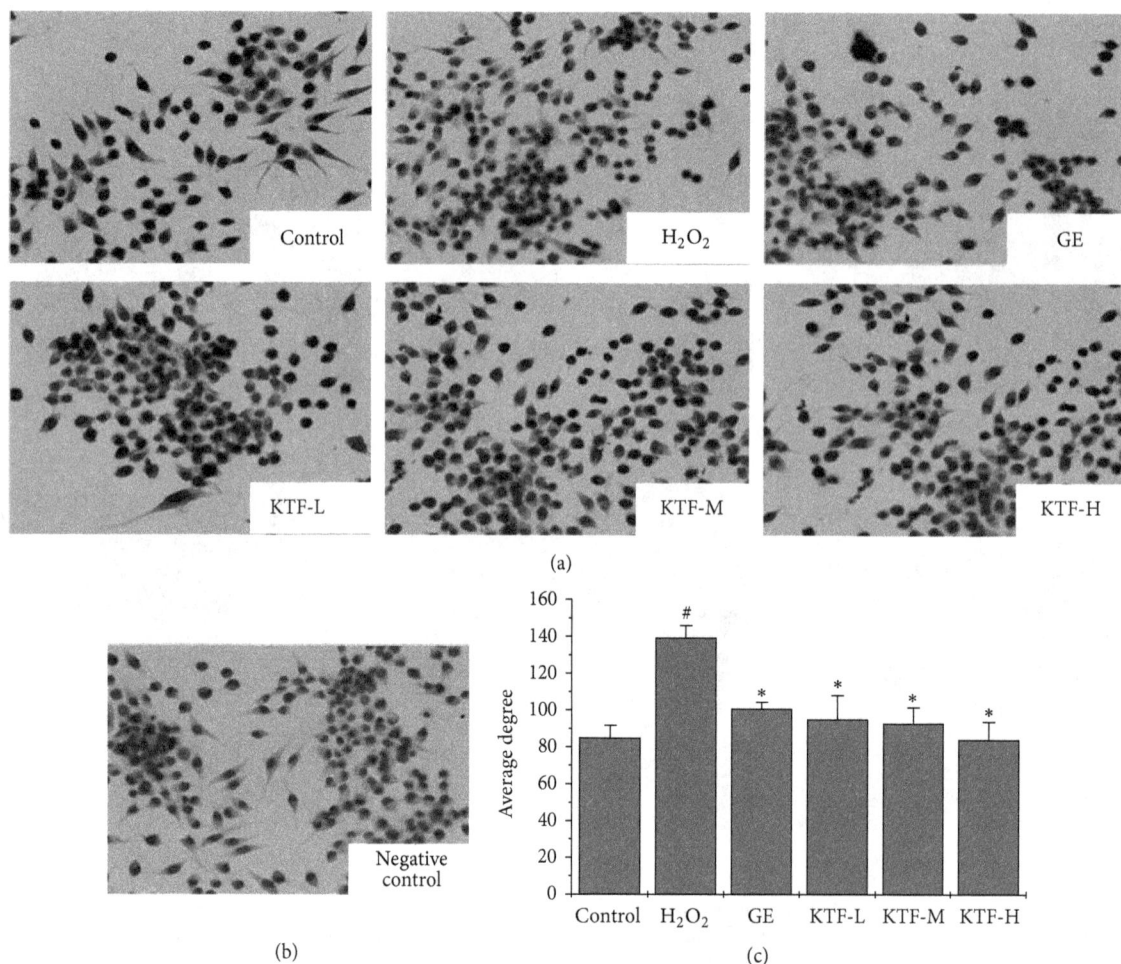

FIGURE 3: KTF ameliorated H_2O_2-induced reduction of TH in MES23.5 cells. Cells were fixed with 4% paraformaldehyde and the expression of TH was detected by immunocytochemistry. (a) Tan represents the TH positive expression (×400). (b) Negative control. (c) Results are expressed as average grey degree. Data are mean ± SD in three independent experiments. $^\#P < 0.05$ compared to the control group. $^*P < 0.05$ compared to the H_2O_2-treat group.

and *Polygonatum sibiricum*, significantly enhanced cell viability and the expression of TH of H_2O_2-treated MES23.5 cells.

Cell apoptosis is a mode of programmed cell death upon various stimuli which activate either extrinsic or intrinsic pathways. Cysteinyl aspartate-specific proteases (caspases) are highly conserved in multicellular organisms and function as central regulators of apoptosis. Activation of caspases is the main axis of all apoptosis events. Among those caspases, caspase 3 has been identified as a key mediator and indicator of cell apoptosis. Like other caspases, caspase 3 usually exists as an inactive proenzyme (precaspase 3). After proteolytic processing, it will produce two subunits which can dimerize to form active caspase 3, subsequently evoking many of the biochemical and biophysical changes to induce cell apoptosis [21]. Our present study revealed that H_2O_2 treatment significantly upregulated caspase 3, but this trend was reversed by KTF treatment in MES23.5 cells, indicating that KTF reduced cell apoptosis of H_2O_2-treated MES23.5 cells.

Antioxidative enzymes, such as superoxide dismutase (SOD), CAT, GPx-1, GSH, and HO-1, are important defense mechanism of cells against the oxidative stress. As an antioxidative enzyme, SOD can transform superoxide radicals to hydrogen peroxide which was subsequently converted to H_2O by CAT and GPx [22]. GSH is also an important antioxidant. Catalytic conversion of reduced glutathione (GSH) to oxidized glutathione (GSSG) by GPx is helpful to convert H_2O_2 to O_2. It has been reported that the activity of the antioxidant was decreased in PD model mice [23–25]. Therefore, drugs that regulate expression of enzymatic antioxidants may serve as potential candidates for the treatment of PD. Our data showed that H_2O_2 treatment suppressed CAT, GPx, GSH, and HO-1 in MES23.5 cells, while KTF treatment at different concentration effectively restored the expression of CAT, GPx, GSH, and HO-1.

In conclusion, our findings demonstrate that traditional Chinese herb kidney-tonifying formulation, which consists of *Cistanche*, *Epimedii*, and *Polygonatum sibiricum*, has strong antioxidative capacity and significant neuroprotective effects. This study provides a clue for developing the kidney-tonifying formulation as a potential therapeutic agent to prevent and treat Parkinson's disease.

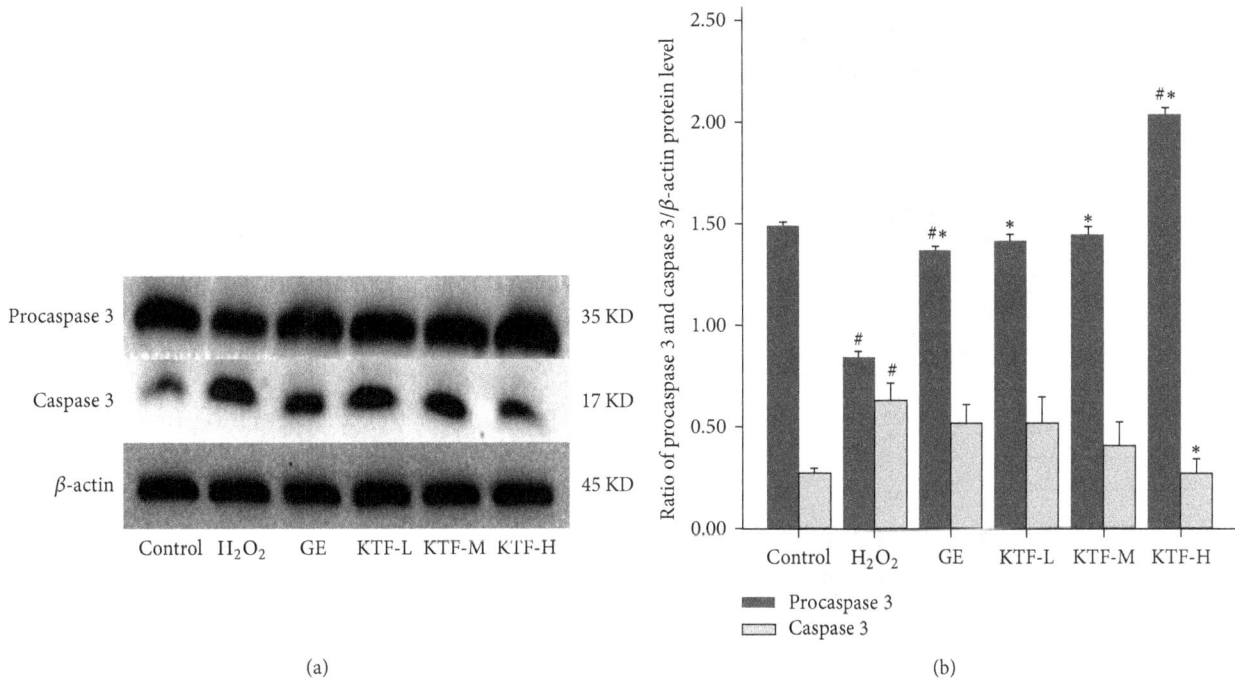

(a)

(b)

FIGURE 4: Effect of KTF on the protein expression of caspase 3 in H_2O_2-induced MES23.5 cells. (a) The protein expression of caspase 3 was determined with western blot and quantified in (b). Data are expressed as mean ± SD in three independent experiments. [#]$P < 0.05$ compared to the control group. [*]$P < 0.05$ compared to the H_2O_2 -treat group.

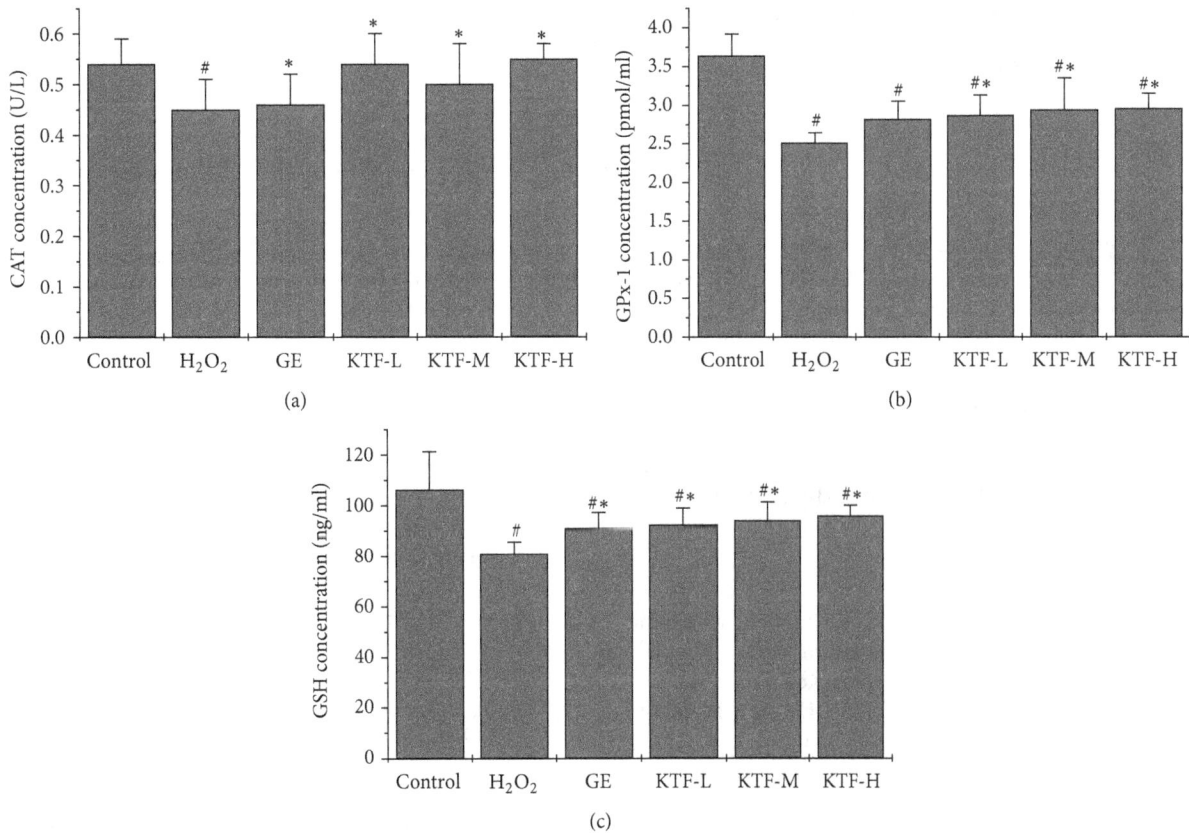

(a)

(b)

(c)

FIGURE 5: Effect of KTF on the level of intracellular CAT, GPx-1, and GSH in H_2O_2-induced MES23.5 cells. The activity level of intracellular CAT, GPx-1, and GSH was measured using an ELISA kit. Data are expressed as mean ± SD in three independent experiments. [#]$P < 0.05$ compared to the control group. [*]$P < 0.05$ compared to the H_2O_2-treat group.

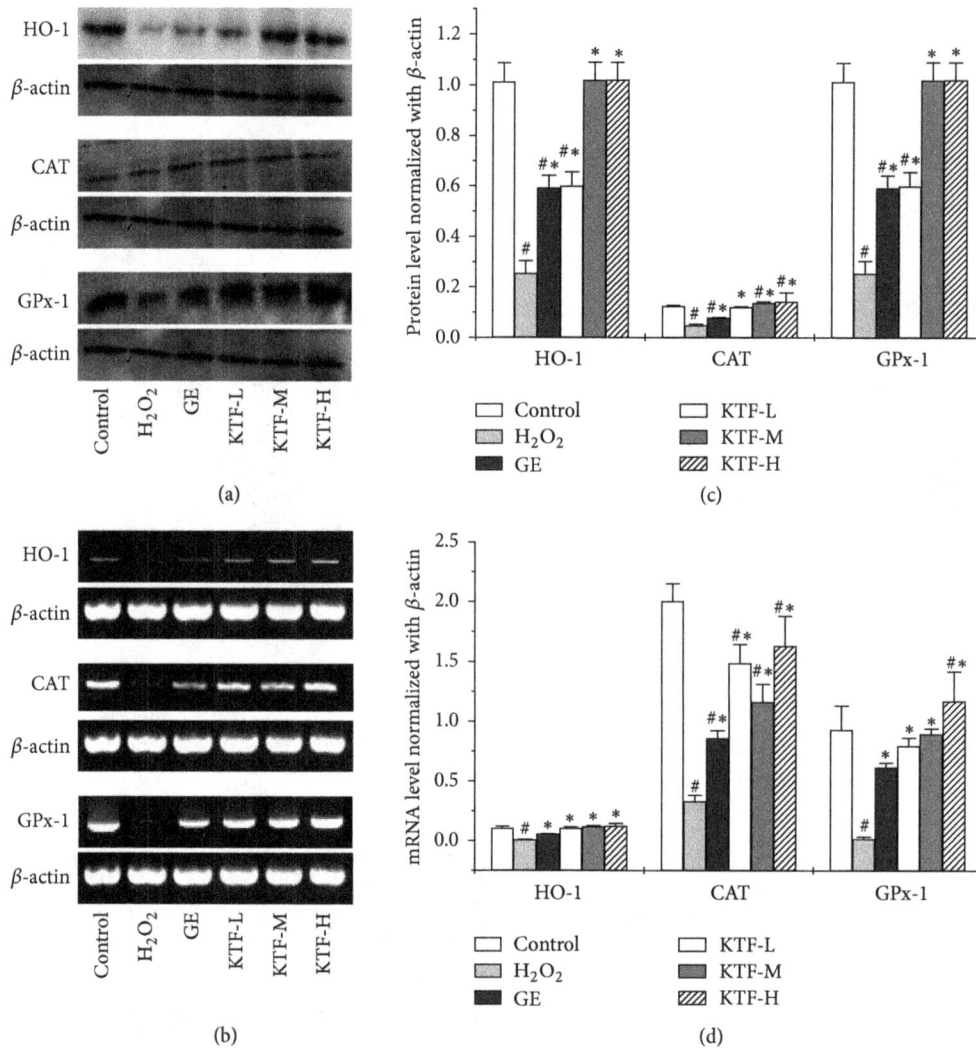

(a)

(b)

(c)

(d)

FIGURE 6: KTF increased the protein and mRNA expression of antioxidant enzymes in H_2O_2-induced MES23.5 cells. (a) The protein expressions of HO-1, CAT, and GPx-1 were determined with Western blot and quantified in (c). (b) The mRNA expressions of HO-1, CAT, and GPx-1 were determined with RT-PCR and quantified in (d). Data are expressed as mean ± SD in three independent experiments. [#]$P < 0.05$ compared to the control group. [*]$P < 0.05$ compared to the H_2O_2 -treat group.

Authors' Contributions

Yihui Xu and Wei Lin share the same contribution to the article. Chuanshan Xu is the cocorresponding author.

Acknowledgments

This work was supported by Scientific Fund of National Health and Family Planning Commission of the People's Republic of China (WKJ-FJ-38), Chen Keji Development Fund Of Integrative Medicine (CKJ2014012), and Fund Of Key Disciplinary (X2014010-xueke). The authors express their sincere thanks to Miss Xin Pan for her helpful assistance.

References

[1] S. Fahn and G. Cohen, "The oxidant stress hypothesis in Parkinson's disease: evidence supporting it," *Annals of Neurology*, vol. 32, no. 6, pp. 804–812, 1992.

[2] P. Jenner and C. W. Olanow, "Oxidative stress and the pathogenesis of Parkinson's disease," *Neurology*, vol. 47, supplement 3, pp. S161–S170, 1996.

[3] Y. Akaneya, M. Takahashi, and H. Hatanaka, "Involvement of free radicals in MPP+ neurotoxicity against rat dopaminergic neurons in culture," *Neuroscience Letters*, vol. 193, no. 1, pp. 53–56, 1995.

[4] J. Emerit, M. Edeas, and F. Bricaire, "Neurodegenerative diseases and oxidative stress," *Biomedicine & Pharmacotherapy*, vol. 58, no. 1, pp. 39–46, 2004.

[5] Chinese Pharmacopoeial Commission, *Pharmacopoeia of the Peoples Republic of China*, vol. 1, People's Medical Publishing House, Beijing, China, 2010.

[6] J. Cai, Y. Tian, R. Lin, X. Chen, Z. Liu, and J. Xie, "Protective effects of kidney-tonifying Chinese herbal preparation on substantia nigra neurons in a mouse model of Parkinson's disease," *Neural Regeneration Research*, vol. 7, no. 6, pp. 413–420, 2012.

[7] W. W. Li, R. Yang, and D. F. Cai, "Protective effects of Cistanche total glycosides on dopaminergic neuron in substantia nigra of

model mice of Parkinson's disease," *Zhongguo Zhong Xi Yi Jie He Za Zhi*, vol. 28, no. 3, pp. 248–251, 2008.

[8] W. Wei and C. Jing, "An analysis of TCM pattern and formula for parkinson's disease," *Journal of Traditional Chinese Medicine*, vol. 54, no. 20, pp. 1778–1782, 2013.

[9] Y. Tian, J. Cai, and X. Chen, "Protection of kidney-tonifying Chinese herb on the nigra striatal neurons mice with Parkinson's disease," *Chinese Journal of Gerontology*, vol. 31, no. 3, pp. 440–443, 2011.

[10] S. G. Lin, S. F. Ye, J. M. Huang et al., "How do Chinese medicines that tonify the kidney inhibit dopaminergic neuron apoptosis?" *Neural Regeneration Research*, vol. 8, no. 30, pp. 2820–2826, 2013.

[11] H. Wang, W.-W. Li, D.-F. Cai, and R. Yang, "Protecting effect of Cistanche extracts on MPP+-induced injury of the Parkinson's disease cell model," *Journal of Chinese Integrative Medicine*, vol. 5, no. 4, pp. 407–411, 2007.

[12] X. Geng, X. Tian, P. Tu, and X. Pu, "Neuroprotective effects of echinacoside in the mouse MPTP model of Parkinson's disease," *European Journal of Pharmacology*, vol. 564, no. 1–3, pp. 66–74, 2007.

[13] X.-F. Tian and X.-P. Pu, "Phenylethanoid glycosides from Cistanches salsa inhibit apoptosis induced by 1-methyl-4-phenylpyridinium ion in neurons," *Journal of Ethnopharmacology*, vol. 97, no. 1, pp. 59–63, 2005.

[14] X. Geng, L. Song, X. Pu, and P. Tu, "Neuroprotective effects of phenylethanoid glycosides from Cistanches salsa against 1-methyl-4-phenyl-1,2,3,6-tetrahydropyridine (MPTP)-induced dopaminergic toxicity in C57 mice," *Biological and Pharmaceutical Bulletin*, vol. 27, no. 6, pp. 797–801, 2004.

[15] H. S. Wong and K. M. Ko, "Herba Cistanches stimulates cellular glutathione redox cycling by reactive oxygen species generated from mitochondrial respiration in H9c2 cardiomyocytes," *Pharmaceutical Biology*, vol. 51, no. 1, pp. 64–73, 2013.

[16] S. C. Wing Sze, Y. Tong, T. B. Ng, C. L. Yin Cheng, and H. P. Cheung, "Herba Epimedii: anti-oxidative properties and its medical implications," *Molecules*, vol. 15, no. 11, pp. 7861–7870, 2010.

[17] D. Trachootham, W. Lu, M. A. Ogasawara, N. R.-D. Valle, and P. Huang, "Redox regulation of cell survival," *Antioxidants and Redox Signaling*, vol. 10, no. 8, pp. 1343–1374, 2008.

[18] D. J. Moore, A. B. West, V. L. Dawson, and T. M. Dawson, "Molecular pathophysiology of Parkinson's disease," *Annual Review of Neuroscience*, vol. 28, pp. 57–87, 2005.

[19] J. Sian, D. T. Dexter, A. J. Lees et al., "Alterations in glutathione levels in Parkinson's disease and other neurodegenerative disorders affecting basal ganglia," *Annals of Neurology*, vol. 36, no. 3, pp. 348–355, 1994.

[20] B. Halliwell and J. M. C. Gutteridge, "Role of free radic in human diseases: an overview," *Methods in Enzymology*, vol. 186, pp. 1–85, 1990.

[21] K. Venderova and D. S. Park, "Programmed cell death in Parkinson's disease," *Cold Spring Harbor Perspectives in Medicine*, vol. 2, no. 8, Article ID a009365, 2012.

[22] I. Fridovich, "Fundamental aspects of reactive oxygen species, or what's the matter with oxygen?" *Annals of the New York Academy of Sciences*, vol. 893, pp. 13–18, 1999.

[23] Q. Xiong, S. Kadota, T. Tani, and T. Namba, "Antioxidative effects of phenylethanoids from Cistanche deserticola," *Biological and Pharmaceutical Bulletin*, vol. 19, no. 12, pp. 1580–1585, 1996.

[24] S. Koppula, H. Kumar, S. V. More, H.-W. Lim, S.-M. Hong, and D.-K. Choi, "Recent updates in redox regulation and free radical scavenging effects by herbal products in experimental models of Parkinson's disease," *Molecules*, vol. 17, no. 10, pp. 11391–11420, 2012.

[25] Z. Fang and Y. Wang, "Effect of isatin on the activities of antioxidase in PD model mice," *China Pharmacy*, vol. 19, no. 22, pp. 1696–1697, 2008.

16

Quantitative Analysis of Parkinsonian Tremor in a Clinical Setting Using Inertial Measurement Units

Donatas Lukšys ⓘ, Gintaras Jonaitis, and Julius Griškevičius

Faculty of Mechanics, Department of Biomechanical Engineering, Vilnius Gediminas Technical University, Basanavičiaus str. 28, LT-03224 Vilnius, Lithuania

Correspondence should be addressed to Donatas Lukšys; donatas.luksys@vgtu.lt

Academic Editor: Cristine Alves da Costa

Background. Parkinson's disease (PD) is a neurodegenerative disorder that affects human voluntary movements. Tremor is one of the most common symptoms of PD and is expressed as involuntary oscillation of the body. Tremors can be analysed in the frequency domain. *Objective.* The aim of the current study was to examine selected tremor parameters (frequency, root mean square, and approximated entropy) in order to quantify the characteristics of patients diagnosed with PD, compared to a healthy control group, and to compare the parameters by dividing the subjects according to UPDRS assessment. *Methods.* The subjects were divided into two groups: a group of people diagnosed with PD ($n = 19$) and a control group consisting of healthy volunteers (CO = 12). Each subject performed motor tasks specific to certain tremors: the finger-to-nose test. Each subject performed a motor task three times. A nine degree of freedom (DOF) wireless inertial measurement unit was used for the measurement of upper limb motor tasks. For the quantitative estimation of kinetic and postural tremors, dominant frequency, root means square, and approximation entropy were selected and calculated from the measured angular velocity and linear acceleration signals. A one-way ANOVA with a significance level of $\alpha = 0.05$ was used to test the null hypothesis that the means of the tremor metrics were the same between the PD and CO groups. *Results.* Statistically significant differences between PD patients and control groups were observed in ApEn acceleration signal of kinetic tremor, ApEn angular velocity signal of kinetic tremor, ApEn angular velocity of postural tremor, frequency acceleration signal of postural tremor, and RMS angular speed kinetic tremor. *Conclusion.* Application of inertial measurement units for clinical research of patients and PD tremor evaluation allows providing quantitative information for diagnostic purposes, during screening in a clinical setting that differentiates between PD patients and controls.

1. Introduction

Parkinson's disease (PD) is a disorder of certain nerve cells in the part of the brain that produces dopamine. PD usually begins in middle or later life (after age 50) [1]. PD is the second most common neurodegenerative movement disorder [2]. Tremor, in addition to rigidity, bradykinesia, and postural instability, is generally considered to be one of the cardinal features of PD [3].

Tremor is defined as rhythmical and involuntary oscillatory movement of a body part; detection of tremors plays a crucial role in the management and treatment of PD patients. There are three types of PD tremor:

(1) rest tremor, which occurs in a body segment while this body segment is relaxed;

(2) action (kinetic) tremor, which is associated with any voluntary movement;

(3) postural tremor, which occurs when a person maintains a position against gravity, such as holding their arms outstretched.

Postural or action tremors can happen together with rest tremors, but with different frequencies. A rest tremor can occur with a postural tremor, but disappears during an action tremor task [4].

The Unified Parkinson's Disease Rating Scale (UPDRS) allows evaluation of motor and nonmotor symptoms in PD. This scale has standardised movements and tasks; thus, doctors do not need to use any special devices to evaluate specific movements. The severity of the disease is evaluated only according to the competence of the doctor. Each

TABLE 1: Demographic and clinical characteristic of subjects.

Group	n	Total UDPRS score (mean ± SD)	UPDRS III score (mean ± SD)	Age (mean ± SD)	Hoehn and Yahr scale score (mean ± SD)
PD	19 (M/F: 8/11)	40.21 ± 15.97	28.42 ± 11.21	61.53 ± 10.81	2.10 ± 0.54
CO	12 (M/F: 6/6)	—	—	57.83 ± 7.58	—

M, male; F, female.

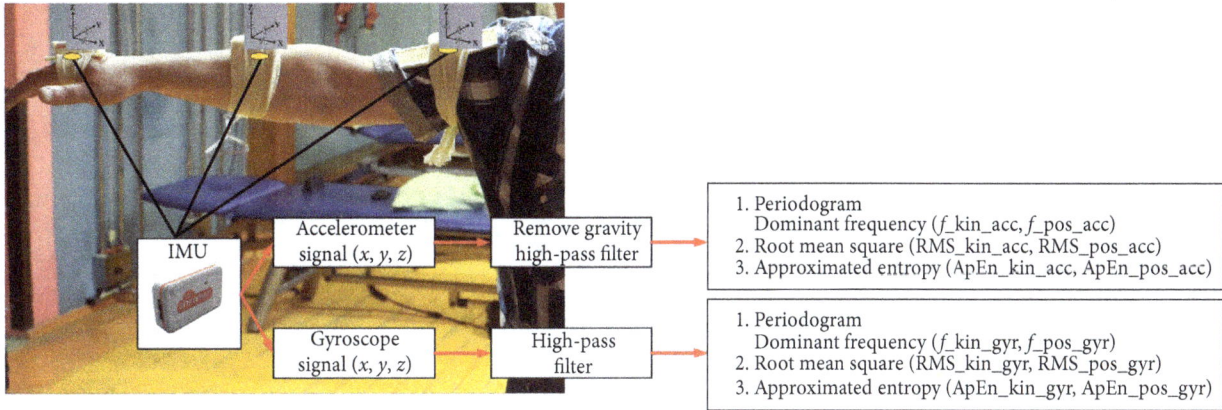

FIGURE 1: Placement of the inertial measurement unit (IMU) sensors on the upper extremity and the calculation algorithm.

motor task is rated from 0 to 4, where 0 is normal and 4 is severe.

Various motion capture equipment can be used to quantify tremors. An accelerometer is one of the most commonly used sensors for tremor detection [5]. Electromyography (EMG) is also used to detect tremors of the limbs [6], and laser displacement sensors can be used to measure and quantify tremors [7]. There are also systems that allow the registration of tremors and the parameters associated with disease rating scales [8]. Inertial measurement units (IMUs) are increasingly used to detect tremors, as they combine several types of sensors: accelerometers, gyroscopes, and magnetometers. In some studies, angular velocity is used to quantify tremors instead of the acceleration signal [9].

PD can be diagnosed incorrectly and can be confused with other diseases such as essential tremor (ET) [10]. Therefore, studies use data classification techniques to discriminate different diseases. A support vector machine has been used successfully to classify PD and ET tremor characteristics [11]. Classical statistical techniques such as binary logistic linear regression and linear discriminant analysis can also be applied [12]. Researchers often use artificial neural network methods which can automatically detect PD resting tremor using EMG and a recurrent neural network classifier [13].

Tremor signal analysis can be divided into several types: time-domain analysis [14], spectral analysis [15], time-frequency analysis [16], and nonlinear analysis [17].

Amplitude and frequency are the main parameters that describe a tremor [18]. These parameters allow researchers to distinguish between different types of tremors and to assess the severity of the disease. Fast Fourier transformation is used to obtain frequency characteristics. This is a mathematical technique for transforming a signal from the time domain to the frequency domain. Most research analyses only a single limb, usually the one that is most affected, or analyses one segment of the upper limb. Further studies often use a combination of parameters in order to separate PD patients from the control group. In addition, quantification of tremors is often performed using a dominant frequency, which is calculated using the power spectral density function or root mean square (RMS). One of the most commonly used nonlinear analysis parameters is the approximated entropy, which allows estimation of the complexity of the signal.

The aim of the current study was to examine selected parameters (dominant frequency (f), root mean square (RMS), and approximated entropy (ApEn)) in order to quantify the characteristics of patients with PD, compared to a control group, and to compare the parameters by dividing the subjects according to UPDRS assessment (kinetic or postural tremor). Finally, this study aimed to compare which side and segment (s) were most affected.

2. Materials and Methods

The data were collected at the Vilnius University Hospital "Santaros Klinikos" Centre of Neurology. Subjects were divided into two groups: a group of subjects diagnosed with PD and healthy subjects. The control subjects did not have any illnesses and injuries that would impair movement or coordination. The inclusion criterions were person older than 18 years of age, able to walk independently without assisting devices, and disease severity, according to the Hoehn and Yahr scale, at 2-3. The exclusion criterions were cardiologic pathologies and other diseases that would impair movement. The experimental protocol was approved by the local ethical committee and all the subjects gave their written

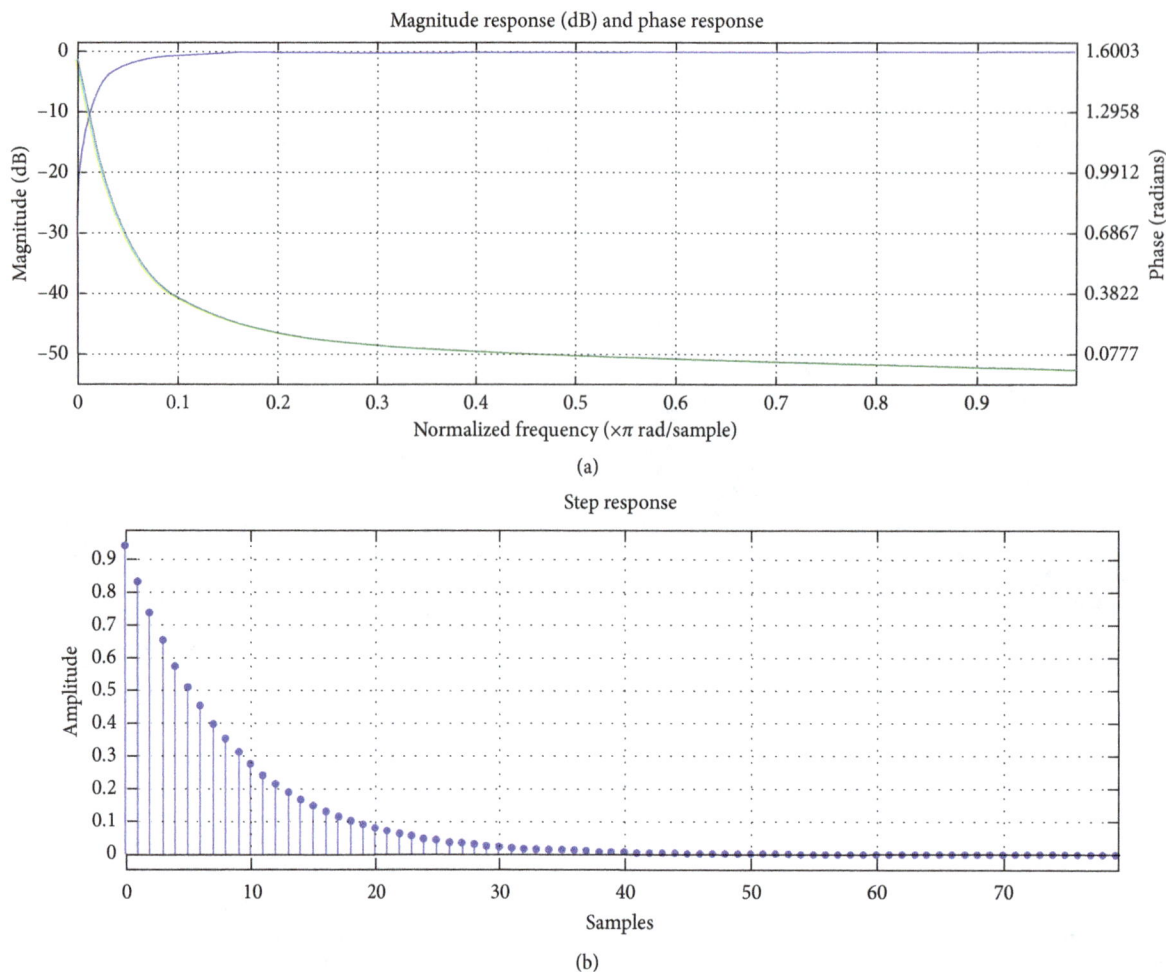

Figure 2: (a) Frequency-domain digital filter; (b) time-domain digital filter.

informed consent before participating. Subject data are presented in Table 1.

A nine degree of freedom (DOF) wireless inertial measurement unit (Shimmer Research, Dublin, Ireland) was used for the measurement of upper limb motor tasks. Six wireless sensors were attached to the subjects' right and left arm, forearm, and hand (Figure 1).

Each sensor measured linear acceleration (three-axis acceleration, FreeScale MM7361, and accelerometer limit ± 6 g), angular velocity (three-axis gyroscope, InvenSense 500 MEMs Gyro, angular velocity limit ± 500°/s, and sensibility 2 mV/°), and magnetic heading (three-axis magnetometer, Honeywell HMX5843, and input field boundaries = −0.7–4.5 Ga). The data from the sensors were received via a Bluetooth wireless connection, at a sampling frequency (F_s) of 51.2 Hz, and were stored on a computer.

Each subject performed motor tasks specific to certain tremors: the finger-to-nose test for examining kinetic tremor features and holding an outstretched arm for examination of postural tremor features. Each subject performed a motor task three times.

Data processing was performed using Matlab (MathWorks, Inc., 2013). Prior to the analysis, all data recordings were high-pass filtered with a cut-off frequency of 1 Hz (1st order Butterworth filter). The cut-off frequency was chosen considering the digital signal processing to the IMU. Further, the gravitational component was removed from the acceleration signal. Figure 2 shows time and frequency response of a digital filter.

For the quantitative estimation of kinetic and postural tremors, several parameters were selected and calculated from the measured angular velocity and linear acceleration signals:

(i) Dominant frequency (frequency kinetic tremor acceleration signal (f_{kin_acc}), frequency postural tremor acceleration signal (f_{pos_acc}), frequency kinetic tremor gyroscope signal (f_{kin_gyr}), and frequency postural tremor gyroscope signal (f_{pos_gyr}))

(ii) Root mean square (RMS kinetic tremor acceleration signal (RMS_{kin_acc}), RMS postural tremor acceleration signal (RMS_{pos_acc}), RMS kinetic tremor gyroscope signal (RMS_{kin_gyr}), and RMS postural tremor gyroscope signal (RMS_{pos_gyr}))

(iii) Approximated entropy (ApEn kinetic tremor acceleration signal ($ApEn_{kin\_acc}$), ApEn postural tremor acceleration signal ($ApEn_{pos\_acc}$), ApEn kinetic tremor gyroscope signal ($ApEn_{kin\_gyr}$), and ApEn postural tremor gyroscope signal ($ApEn_{pos\_gyr}$)).

TABLE 2: Comparison of approximation entropy between PD and CO.

Segment	Group	ApEn_kin_acc (mean ± SD)	ApEn_pos_acc (mean ± SD)	ApEn_kin_gyr (mean ± SD)	ApEn_pos_gyr (mean ± SD)
Right upper arm	CO	0.452 ± 0.139	0.967 ± 0.168	0.394 ± 0.107	0.455 ± 0.188
	PD	0.578 ± 0.208	0.947 ± 0.154	0.416 ± 0.175	0.552 ± 0.135
Left upper arm	CO	**0.368 ± 0.195**	0.991 ± 0.153	**0.329 ± 0.097**	0.541 ± 0.223
	PD	**0.552 ± 0.198**	0.860 ± 0.181	**0.475 ± 0.119**	0.577 ± 0.168
Right forearm	CO	**0.240 ± 0.081**	0.859 ± 0.201	0.383 ± 0.178	**0.429 ± 0.151**
	PD	**0.387 ± 0.194**	0.906 ± 0.217	0.375 ± 0.098	**0.573 ± 0.197**
Left forearm	CO	0.297 ± 0.115	0.891 ± 0.229	**0.279 ± 0.069**	0.516 ± 0.183
	PD	0.491 ± 0.227	0.858 ± 0.281	**0.369 ± 0.104**	0.579 ± 0.200
Right hand	CO	0.343 ± 0.112	0.776 ± 0.156	0.283 ± 0.070	0.402 ± 0.124
	PD	0.400 ± 0.181	0.762 ± 0.210	0.311 ± 0.139	0.494 ± 0.179
Left hand	CO	0.373 ± 0.111	0.804 ± 0.180	0.291 ± 0.095	0.463 ± 0.180
	PD	0.447 ± 0.155	0.754 ± 0.194	0.321 ± 0.103	0.482 ± 0.169

TABLE 3: Comparison of root mean square between PD and CO.

Segment	Group	RMS_kin_acc (mean ± SD)	RMS_pos_acc (mean ± SD)	RMS_kin_gyr (mean ± SD)	RMS_pos_gyr (mean ± SD)
Right upper arm	CO	1.617 ± 0.958	0.275 ± 0.095	34.078 ± 19.754	0.394 ± 0.107
	PD	1.629 ± 1.007	0.267 ± 0.159	36.018 ± 21.575	0.416 ± 0.175
Left upper arm	CO	2.349 ± 1.595	0.256 ± 0.130	43.031 ± 20.821	**0.329 ± 0.097**
	PD	1.576 ± 1.008	0.317 ± 0.289	31.536 ± 16.057	**0.475 ± 0.119**
Right forearm	CO	1.909 ± 1.006	0.344 ± 0.198	45.722 ± 23.602	0.383 ± 0.178
	PD	1.772 ± 0.882	0.281 ± 0.157	42.203 ± 16.655	0.375 ± 0.098
Left forearm	CO	1.834 ± 0.831	0.271 ± 0.215	63.640 ± 25.549	**0.279 ± 0.069**
	PD	1.469 ± 0.794	0.239 ± 0.101	44.170 ± 16.903	**0.369 ± 0.104**
Right hand	CO	2.429 ± 1.350	0.392 ± 0.204	70.972 ± 39.044	0.283 ± 0.070
	PD	2.703 ± 1.587	0.395 ± 0.209	86.217 ± 48.488	0.310 ± 0.139
Left hand	CO	2.446 ± 1.588	0.377 ± 0.283	70.419 ± 35.286	0.290 ± 0.095
	PD	2.462 ± 1.230	0.476 ± 0.406	88.970 ± 44.162	0.321 ± 0.103

As can be seen, selected parameters (ApEn, dominant frequency, and RMS) allowed us to distinguish between PD and CO groups. Therefore, these parameters allow quantification of tremor characteristics.

Spectral analysis was performed to identify dominant frequencies. The signal strength in a specific frequency spectrum is shown using power spectral density (PSD). The dominant frequency of a tremor is evident as a visible peak in the PSD [19]. A periodogram was used for the evaluation of PSD. A periodogram is a nonparametric estimate of power spectral density, which is based on the Fourier transform of the based estimate of the autocorrelation sequence. A rectangular window is used for calculating the PSD. A periodogram is defined as

$$P_{xx}(f) = \frac{1}{LF_S} \left| \sum_{n=0}^{L-1} x_L(n) e^{-i2\pi fn/F_s} \right|^2, \tag{1}$$

where $x_L(n)$ is the signal, L is the length, and F_S is the sampling frequencies.

If the dominant frequency in different axes is not the same, the valid dominant frequency in the axis with the highest peak power is regarded as the dominant frequency of all axes.

Approximate entropy (ApEn) is a technique that quantifies the degree of irregularity and the unpredictability of fluctuations in time series data [20]. This is a popular tool for analysing the complexity of time series data, especially in

clinical research. Low ApEn values indicate predictability and high regularity of time series data, whereas high ApEn values indicate incalculable and random time series data. In this study, we calculated ApEn values for all data sets using $m = 2$ and $r = 0.45$ of SD of the individual subjects' time series. This value is recommended [21], and ApEn is defined as

$$\text{ApEn}(S_n, m, r) = \ln \left[\frac{c_m(r)}{c_{m+1}(r)} \right], \tag{2}$$

where S_n gives a sequence consisting of N instantaneous measurements, m specifies the pattern length, r defines the criterion of similarity, and $C_{im}(r)$ is the fraction of patterns of length m that is similar to the pattern of the same length that starts at interval i.

RMS is used to evaluate intensity of tremors. RMS interprets actual vibration levels, while PSD results indicate the dominant frequency that contributes the most to the tremor. Because tremors are based on a dominant frequency, the advantages of PSD compared to a statistical measure (quadratic mean) are that it isolates the tremor signals from noise and other movements, by analysis of the frequency dimension, and it provides a squared value for the signals.

TABLE 4: Comparison of dominant frequencies between PD and CO.

Segment	Group	f_{kin_acc} (mean ± SD)	f_{pos_acc} (mean ± SD)	f_{kin_gyr} (mean ± SD)	f_{pos_gyr} (mean ± SD)
Right upper arm	CO	3.278 ± 1.565	6.558 ± 3.213	2.175 ± 0.752	4.164 ± 2.162
	PD	3.516 ± 2.094	7.610 ± 2.730	2.519 ± 1.075	5.715 ± 2.836
Left upper arm	CO	3.101 ± 1.374	5.788 ± 2.775	2.007 ± 0.866	**3.195 ± 1.633**
	PD	3.925 ± 1.882	7.588 ± 3.627	2.814 ± 1.377	**5.421 ± 2.081**
Right forearm	CO	1.534 ± 0.396	**3.196 ± 1.949**	1.829 ± 0.623	2.693 ± 1.662
	PD	1.878 ± 0.890	**5.234 ± 2.947**	2.364 ± 1.405	4.248 ± 2.654
Left forearm	CO	1.944 ± 0.827	3.958 ± 3.373	2.079 ± 0.749	**2.639 ± 1.834**
	PD	2.173 ± 1.112	6.617 ± 4.504	2.722 ± 2.155	**5.074 ± 2.841**
Right hand	CO	1.750 ± 0.415	2.287 ± 1.771	1.296 ± 0.649	2.316 ± 2.062
	PD	1.653 ± 0.488	3.857 ± 2.682	1.037 ± 0.347	3.484 ± 2.400
Left hand	CO	1.939 ± 0.656	4.009 ± 3.151	1.548 ± 0.723	2.396 ± 1.211
	PD	1.882 ± 1.014	2.892 ± 1.889	1.662 ± 1.726	3.333 ± 2.479

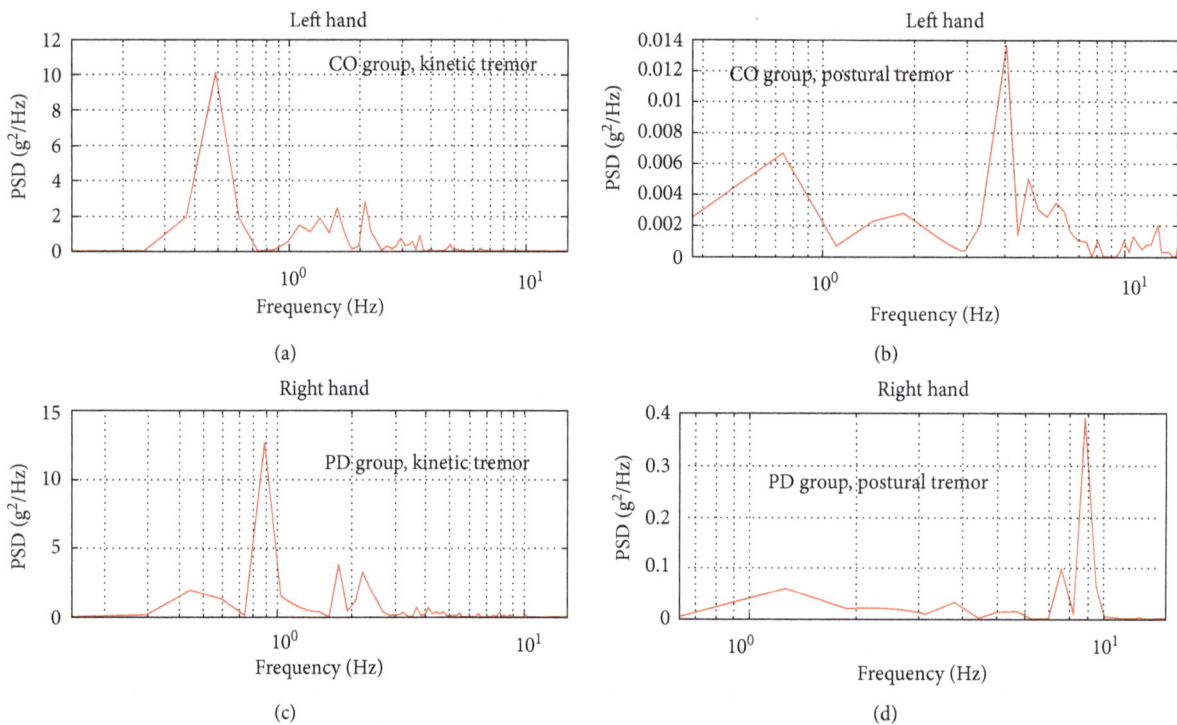

FIGURE 3: The power spectrum based power spectral density (PSD) plot. (a, b) Postural and kinetic tremor in the CO group, (c, d) kinetic and postural tremor in the PD group.

Data from PD patients were divided into groups according to a clinical assessment: Right 0, Right 1, Left 0, and Left 1. Statistical analysis of the metrics was performed using IBM's SPSS v22 software. A one-way ANOVA with a significance level of $\alpha = 0.05$ was used to test the null hypothesis that the means of the tremor metrics were the same between the PD and CO groups.

3. Results

Significant differences ($\alpha < 0.05$) between the PD and CO groups are shown in Tables 2–4 (bold values have statistical significance).

Data from PD patients were further divided into groups according UPDRS clinical assessment (action or postural tremor of hand and UPDRS III motor task 21). This motor task is evaluated in numbers from 0 to 4 (0: no tremor; 4: severe tremor). This motor task is assessed by the right and left side of subjects. This assessment was received from a doctor. Clinical assessment was performed, and the upper limbs from both sides were evaluated; each segment was then scored (upper arm, forearm arm, and hand). Each participant was classified according to the clinical assessment (Right 0 ($n = 14$), Right 1 ($n = 4$), Left 0 ($n = 14$), and Left 1 ($n = 4$)). The data were grouped as follows: Left 0 versus Left 1 and Right 0 versus Right 1. Figure 3 shows the PSD calculation from the acceleration signal.

TABLE 5: Tremor parameters between the PD groups with regard to the UPDRS assessment.

Parameter	Segment	Right 0 (mean ± SD)	Right 1 (mean ± SD)	Segment	Left 0 (mean ± SD)	Left 1 (mean ± SD)
$f_{\_kin\_gyr}$	Right upper arm	2.486 ± 0.891	3.077 ± 1.423	Left upper arm	2.804 ± 1.303	3.335 ± 1.551
	Right forearm	2.082 ± 1.189	2.842 ± 1.915	Left forearm	2.354 ± 1.388	2.756 ± 3.245
	Right hand	1.063 ± 0.378	0.890 ± 0.236	Left hand	1.160 ± 0.363	1.954 ± 2.140
$f_{\_kin\_acc}$	Right upper arm	3.800 ± 2.234	3.177 ± 1.361	Left upper arm	3.512 ± 1.514	4.146 ± 1.568
	Right forearm	1.940 ± 0.982	1.759 ± 0.693	Left forearm	2.561 ± 0.914	1.232 ± 0.994
	Right hand	1.709 ± 0.528	1.585 ± 0.336	Left hand	2.103 ± 1.101	1.277 ± 0.198
$f_{\_post\_gyr}$	Right upper arm	5.730 ± 2.901	6.835 ± 1.654	Left upper arm	5.111 ± 1.802	7.224 ± 2.090
	Right forearm	3.861 ± 2.598	6.342 ± 1.882	Left forearm	5.103 ± 2.724	6.101 ± 2.843
	Right hand	2.927 ± 2.534	5.373 ± 0.708	Left hand	2.692 ± 2.177	5.238 ± 2.99
$f_{\_post\_acc}$	Right upper arm	7.263 ± 3.065	8.476 ± 1.338	Left upper arm	7.210 ± 3.962	9.109 ± 2.638
	Right forearm	4.642 ± 3.149	6.960 ± 1.711	Left forearm	6.883 ± 5.155	5.987 ± 2.281
	Right hand	**2.881 ± 2.2821**	**6.463 ± 1.884**	Left hand	**2.189 ± 1.5860**	**4.716 ± 1.281**
$RMS_{\_kin\_gyr}$	Right upper arm	37.44 ± 21.235	38.85 ± 22.193	Left upper arm	33.69 ± 13.926	29.344 ± 22.912
	Right forearm	**45.37 ± 16.075**	**38.445 ± 13.822**	Left forearm	**48.706 ± 15.478**	**34.746 ± 15.483**
	Right hand	94.38 ± 50.830	75.52 ± 27.201	Left hand	**102.949 ± 41.806**	**53.629 ± 23.809**
$RMS_{\_kin\_acc}$	Right upper arm	1.5377 ± 0.684	2.237 ± 1.755	Left upper arm	1.741 ± 0.981	1.301 ± 1.100
	Right forearm	1.8329 ± 0.628	1.912 ± 1.500	Left forearm	1.641 ± 0.803	1.024 ± 0.677
	Right hand	2.6642 ± 1.335	3.395 ± 2.262	Left hand	2.729 ± 1.107	2.017 ± 1.382
$RMS_{\_post\_gyr}$	Right upper arm	4.8751 ± 3.650	5.218 ± 3.298	Left upper arm	3.974 ± 2.542	4.452 ± 2.172
	Right forearm	5.1201 ± 3.841	5.870 ± 1.942	Left forearm	3.983 ± 2.160	4.518 ± 1.867
	Right hand	8.261 ± 7.465	6.589 ± 1.707	Left hand	8.774 ± 7.580	7.808 ± 6.445
$RMS_{\_post\_acc}$	Right upper arm	0.238 ± 0.087	0.389 ± 0.303	Left upper arm	0.296 ± 0.209	0.411 ± 0.546
	Right forearm	**0.292 ± 0.178**	**0.259 ± 0.073**	Left forearm	**0.249 ± 0.110**	**0.203 ± 0.078**
	Right hand	0.423 ± 0.212	0.351 ± 0.210	Left hand	0.504 ± 0.436	0.438 ± 0.376
$ApEn_{\_kin\_gyr}$	Right upper arm	0.381 ± 0.134	0.514 ± 0.291	Left upper arm	**0.443 ± 0.108**	**0.585 ± 0.116**
	Right forearm	**0.364 ± 0.097**	**0.407 ± 0.123**	Left forearm	**0.351 ± 0.114**	**0.434 ± 0.041**
	Right hand	0.307 ± 0.144	0.283 ± 0.130	Left hand	0.305 ± 0.109	0.375 ± 0.087
$ApEn_{\_kin\_acc}$	Right upper arm	0.556 ± 0.196	0.561 ± 0.210	Left upper arm	0.513 ± 0.167	0.600 ± 0.252
	Right forearm	**0.333 ± 0.152**	**0.462 ± 0.190**	Left forearm	**0.445 ± 0.183**	**0.593 ± 0.352**
	Right hand	0.389 ± 0.181	0.353 ± 0.133	Left hand	0.405 ± 0.116	0.522 ± 0.207
$ApEn_{\_post\_gyr}$	Right upper arm	0.564 ± 0.152	0.542 ± 0.056	Left upper arm	0.579 ± 0.187	0.579 ± 0.138
	Right forearm	**0.570 ± 0.186**	**0.645 ± 0.233**	Left forearm	**0.549 ± 0.201**	**0.678 ± 0.216**
	Right hand	0.476 ± 0.179	0.532 ± 0.210	Left hand	0.445 ± 0.166	0.595 ± 0.162
$ApEn_{\_post\_acc}$	Right upper arm	0.970 ± 0.129	0.845 ± 0.227	Left upper arm	0.879 ± 0.177	0.803 ± 0.232
	Right forearm	**0.898 ± 0.201**	**0.698 ± 0.309**	Left forearm	**0.867 ± 0.273**	**0.678 ± 0.386**
	Right hand	0.738 ± 0.199	0.792 ± 0.273	Left hand	0.750 ± 0.144	0.745 ± 0.364

Statistically significant differences between the PD groups with regard to the UPDRS assessment are shown in Table 5 (bold values have statistical significance).

4. Discussion

Application of inertial measurement units for clinical research of patients and PD tremor evaluation allows providing quantitative information for diagnostic purposes, during screening in a clinical setting that differentiates between PD patients and controls. Three basic parameters (frequency, RMS, and approximation entropy) can be used to separate two different groups and for quantitative tremor assessment according to the UPDRS score.

As can be seen from the results obtained (Tables 2–4) to find statistically significant differences between the calculated parameters between PD and CO groups, ApEn is the best way to separate the groups from each other. The result obtained for ApEn values is higher in the PD group, which indicates that the movement is more unpredictable and more incidental. Higher values of ApEn between the subjects and the different sides indicate which side and segment are more severe in the PD group. RMS values show tremor intensity. The result shows that the intensity of the postural tremor is larger on the left side of the angular velocity signal. The dominant frequency is one of the main characteristics for estimating PD tremor, and the obtained result indicates that postural tremor detection is a more appropriate angular velocity signal than the acceleration signal.

Divided PD patients according UDPRS clinical assessment showed a statistically difference. The higher values of the calculated parameter indicate that the values set by the medical doctor correspond to the difference between the calculated values, and their values are higher among the estimates.

Acknowledgments

Special thanks are due to the Clinics of Neurology and Neurosurgery of Vilnius University Hospital Santaros Klinikos medical doctors Rūta Kaladytė–Lokominienė, Dalius Jatužis, and Ramunė Bunevičiūtė.

References

[1] G. Rigas, A. T. Tzallas, D. G. Tsalikakis, S. Konitsiotis, and D. I. Fotiadis, "Real-time quantification of resting tremor in the Parkinson's disease," *Proceedings of the 31st Annual International Conference of the IEEE Engineering in Medicine and Biology Society. IEEE Engineering in Medicine and Biology Society. Annual Conference*, vol. 2009, pp. 1306–1309, 2009.

[2] M. El-Gohary, J. McNames, K. Chung, M. Aboy, A. Salarian, and F. Horak, "Continuous at-home monitoring of tremor in patients with Parkinson's disease," in *Proceedings of Biosignal 2010: Analysis of Biomedical Signals and Images*, vol. 20, pp. 420–424, 2010.

[3] T. Heida, E. Wentink, and E. Marani, "Power spectral density analysis of physiological, rest and action tremor in Parkinson's disease patients treated with deep brain stimulation," *Journal of NeuroEngineering and Rehabilitation*, vol. 10, no. 1, p. 70, 2013.

[4] H. Dai, P. Zhang, and T. C. Lueth, "Quantitative assessment of Parkinsonian tremor based on an inertial measurement unit," *Sensors*, vol. 15, no. 10, pp. 25055–25071, 2015.

[5] V. Ruonala, A. Meigal, S. M. Rissanen, O. Airaksinen, M. Kankaanp, and P. A. Karjalainen, "EMG signal morphology and kinematic parameters in essential tremor and Parkinson's disease patients," *Journal of Electromyography and Kinesiology*, vol. 24, no. 2, pp. 300–306, 2014.

[6] G. Grimaldi and M. Manto, "Neurological tremor: sensors, signal processing and emerging applications," *Sensors*, vol. 10, no. 2, pp. 1399–1422, 2010.

[7] C. Duval, "Rest and postural tremors in patients with Parkinson's disease," *Brain Research Bulletin*, vol. 70, no. 1, pp. 44–48, 2006.

[8] G. Mostile, J. P. Giuffrida, O. R. Adam, A. Davidson, and J. Jankovic, "Correlation between kinesia system assessments and clinical tremor scores in patients with essential tremor," *Movement Disorders*, vol. 25, no. 12, pp. 1938–1943, 2010.

[9] C. Thanawattano, R. Pongthornseri, C. Anan, S. Dumnin, and R. Bhidayasiri, "Temporal fluctuations of tremor signals from inertial sensor: a preliminary study in differentiating Parkinson's disease from essential tremor," *BioMedical Engineering OnLine*, vol. 14, no. 1, p. 101, 2015.

[10] E. J. Sternberg, R. N. Alcalay, O. A. Levy, and E. D. Louis, "Postural and intention tremors: a detailed clinical study of essential tremor vs. Parkinson's disease," *Frontiers in Neurology*, vol. 4, pp. 1–8, 2013.

[11] D. Surangsrirat, C. Thanawattano, R. Pongthornseri, S. Dumnin, C. Anan, and R. Bhidayasiri, "Support vector machine classification of Parkinson's disease and essential tremor subjects based on temporal fluctuation," *Proceedings of the 38th Annual International Conference of the IEEE Engineering in Medicine and Biology Society. IEEE Engineering in Medicine and Biology Society. Annual Conference*, vol. 2016, pp. 6389–6392, 2016.

[12] R. G. Ramani and G. Sivagami, "Parkinson's Disease classification using data mining algorithms," *Int. J. Comput. Appl*, vol. 32, pp. 17–22, 2011.

[13] R. Arvind, B. Karthik, N. Sriraam, and J. Kamala-Kannan, "Automated detection of PD resting tremor using PSD with recurrent neural network classifier," *Proceedings of the 2nd International Conference in Advances in Recent Technologies in Communication and Computing (ARTCom)*, vol. 2010, pp. 414–417, 2010.

[14] A. Salarian, H. Russmann, C. Wider, P. R. Burkhard, F. J. G. Vingerhoets, and K. Vingerhoets, "Quantification of tremor and bradykinesia in Parkinson's disease using a novel ambulatory monitoring system," *IEEE Transactions on Biomedical Engineering*, vol. 54, no. 2, pp. 313–322, 2007.

[15] J. K. Florian Amtage, "Spectral and higher-order spectral analysis of tremor time series," *Clinical and Experimental Pharmacology and Physiology*, vol. 4, 2014.

[16] D. Surangsrirat, A. Intarapanich, C. Thanawattano, R. Bhidayasiri, S. Petchrutchatachart, and C. Anan, "Tremor assessment using spiral analysis in time-frequency domain," *Proceedings of IEEE Southeastcon*, vol. 1, pp. 1–6, 2013.

[17] L. M. Gil, T. P. Nunes, A. C. D. Faria, and P. L. Melo, "Analysis of human tremor in patients with Parkinson disease using entropy measures of signal complexity," in *Annual International Conference of the IEEE Engineering in Medicine and Biology*, vol. 1, pp. 2786–2789, 2010.

[18] B. Wilk, "Assessment of a hand tremor based on analysis of the accelerometer signal," *Przegląd Elektrotechniczny*, vol. 1, no. 11, pp. 146–149, 2016.

[19] J. Sanchez-Ramos, D. Reimer, T. Zesiewicz, K. Sullivan, and P. A. Nausieda, "Quantitative analysis of tremors in welders," *International Journal of Environmental Research and Public Health*, vol. 8, no. 5, pp. 1478–1490, 2011.

[20] B. Abhinaya and D. Charanya, "Feature extraction and selection of a combination of entropy features for real-time epilepsy detection," *International Journal Of Engineering And Computer Science*, vol. 5, pp. 16073–16078, 2016.

[21] K. Chon, C. Scully, and S. Lu, "Approximate entropy for all signals," *IEEE Engineering in Medicine and Biology Magazine*, vol. 28, pp. 18–23, 2009.

17

Mutation Analysis of *HTRA2* Gene in Chinese Familial Essential Tremor and Familial Parkinson's Disease

Ya-Chao He, Pei Huang, Qiong-Qiong Li, Qian Sun, Dun-Hui Li, Tian Wang, Jun-Yi Shen, Juan-Juan Du, Shi-Shuang Cui, Chao Gao, Rao Fu, and Sheng-Di Chen

Department of Neurology and Collaborative Innovation Center for Brain Science, Ruijin Hospital, Shanghai Jiao Tong University School of Medicine, Shanghai 200025, China

Correspondence should be addressed to Sheng-Di Chen; chen_sd@medmail.com.cn

Academic Editor: Hélio Teive

Background. HTRA2 has already been nominated as PARK13 which may cause Parkinson's disease, though there are still discrepancies among these results. Recently, Gulsuner et al.'s study found that *HTRA2* p.G399S is responsible for hereditary essential tremor and homozygotes of this allele develop Parkinson's disease by examining a six-generation family segregating essential tremor and essential tremor coexisting with Parkinson's disease. We performed this study to validate the condition of *HTRA2* gene in Chinese familial essential tremor and familial Parkinson's disease patients, especially essential tremor. *Methods.* We directly sequenced all eight exons, exon-intron boundaries, and part of the introns in 101 familial essential tremor patients, 105 familial Parkinson's disease patients, and 100 healthy controls. *Results.* No exonic variant was identified, while one exon-intron boundary variant (rs2241028) and one intron variant (rs2241027) were detected, both with no clinical significance and uncertain function. There was no difference in allele, genotype, and haplotype between groups. *Conclusions.* HTRA2 exonic variant might be rare among Chinese Parkinson's disease and essential tremor patients with family history, and HTRA2 may not be the cause of familial Parkinson's disease and essential tremor in China.

1. Introduction

As two of the most prevalent tremor disorders, essential tremor (ET) and Parkinson's disease (PD), which are estimated to constitute 0.9% and 0.3% of worldwide population, respectively, are considered as distinctively different entities formerly [1, 2]. Several lines of evidence showed that there are remarkable overlaps in clinical features, epidemiology, imaging, genetics, and pathology between PD and ET, including a fourfold increase of risk developing Parkinson's disease in essential tremor cases [3, 4].

ET is widely regarded as caused by genetic with no disease-causing gene ever been focused; Contrarily, though PD is mainly sporadic, up to now 22 PARK loci have been identified [5, 6]. To be specific, 50% of ET patients demonstrate familial aggregation, while less than 15% of PD patients have affected first-degree relatives [7–9]. Due to the overlap phenomena between ET and PD, investigations into the relationship between PD risk variants and ET patients have

been done, involving *LINGO1, LINGO2, LRRK2, SLC1A2,* and *HTRA2* genes [3, 10–12].

HTRA2 has already been nominated as PARK13 which may cause Parkinson's disease, though there are still discrepancies among these results. Recently, a research by Gulsuner and colleagues examining a six-generation family segregating ET and ET coexisting with PD revealed that *HTRA2* p.G399S is responsible for hereditary essential tremor and homozygotes for this allele develop Parkinson's disease [13]. Replications conducted in Western Norway and Asian population to address the association between p.G399S and ET, PD, ET/PD, and tremulous cervical dystonia failed to reach a consensus [14, 15]. In addition, report from a small sample (29 FETs) in Germany adopting coding exon Sanger sequencing did not reconfirm it either [16]. To validate the condition in Chinese familial essential tremor (FET) and familial Parkinson's disease (FPD) patients, we performed a Sanger sequencing of eight exons and exon-intron boundaries of *HTRA2* instead of just one variant (p.G399S).

TABLE 1: Demographics of participants.

Details	FET	FPD	ET-PD	Control
Total	101	105	15	100
Age[a] (range, p^b value)	61.24 ± 12.62 (28–90, 0.12)	59.28 ± 11.21 (36–84, 0.86)	67.80 ± 8.65 (56–79, NA)	59.06 ± 6.21 (49–74, NA)
Male/female, p^b value	51/50, 0.52	53/52, 0.52	12/3, N/A	46/54, N/A

N/A: not applicable; [a]data are mean ± SD; [b]data are compared with control; FPD: familial PD; FET: familial ET; ET-PD: ET coexisting with PD.

TABLE 2: Primers of HTRA2.

Name	Forward	Reverse	Products
1	GTC TCA CAA CTC GCG TCC G	GCC TGA AAT GGA GGG AAA GCA	Exon 1 and boundaries
2	TCG AGA TCC TGG ACC GGT AA	GGC CAC ATT TTT GCA GCC TAA	Exons 2, 3 and intron 2; boundaries
3	GCA GCT ATT GAT GTG CGT CC	TGA AGG GAG ACA GCT CTT GTG	Exons 4, 5, 6 and introns 4, 5; boundaries
4	ACT CAG CCA ACC TGA TTT CCT AC	TTC AGA GCC CAG GAG TCA GT	Exons 7, 8 and intron 7; boundaries

2. Methods

2.1. Patients.
This study enrolled 221 unrelated Chinese patients, including 105 PD patients with autosomal dominant inheritance (2 or more affected relatives in 2 consecutive generations), 101 ET patients with family history, and 15 patients of ET coexisting with PD. All patients were from the Movement Disorder Clinic of Department of Neurology at Ruijin Hospital affiliated to Shanghai Jiao Tong University School of Medicine. PD and ET patients were diagnosed by senior movement disorder specialist on the basis of MDS clinical diagnostic criteria for Parkinson's disease and Consensus Statement on Tremor of the Movement Disorders Society, respectively [17, 18]. Patients presenting secondary Parkinsonism, Parkinson-plus syndrome, or hyperthyroidism were excluded from the study. We also included 100 healthy controls without any symptom of movement disorders. The demographic information of patients is shown in Table 1. We received approval from the Ethics Committee of Ruijin Hospital affiliated to Shanghai Jiao Tong University School of Medicine. Written informed consents were obtained from all patients and controls participating in the study as well.

2.2. DNA Sequencing and Mutation Analysis.
Genomic DNA was extracted from venous blood applying standardized phenol/chloroform extraction method from patients and controls. The 8 coding sequences, exon-intron boundaries, and part of introns were sequenced by Sanger sequencing in 4 products of PCR (polymerase chain reaction) amplification using 4 pairs of primers (Table 2). DNASTAR Lasergene MegAlign (v7.1.0) and Chromas (v2.33) were used to conduct sequence alignment, and the chromatograms were double checked to avoid missing any variants. Variants detected were searched in NCBI to get access to their clinical significance and MAF in ExAC and 1000 Genomes Projects database.

2.3. Statistical Analysis.
Statistical analysis was performed with Statistical Analysis System V8 (SAS V8). Difference of age was assessed applying t-test or t'-test. Hardy-Weinberg equilibrium (HWE) was calculated by Chi-square analysis. Chi-square or Fisher's exact test was used to test the differences in genotype and gender between groups. Odds ratios

(ORs) and 95% confidence intervals (95% CI) were evaluated by Mantel-Haenszel Chi-squared test to verify the association between variants and FPD or FET. The evaluation of the association was also conducted using logistic regression under different genetic models adjusted for age and gender. Online SHEsis program was used to conduct haplotype analysis [19]. Two-tailed p value < 0.05 was considered significant. The statistical power was performed using Quanto.

3. Results

The patients and controls in the study are well matched for mean age ($p = 0.12$ for FET and $p = 0.86$ for FPD) and sex distribution ($p = 0.52$ for FET and $p = 0.52$ for FPD) (Table 1). By sequencing all the four products in all 221 patients (FET, FPD, and ET-PD) and 100 controls, no exonic variant was identified, while one exon-intron boundary variant (rs2241028) and one intron variant (rs2241027) were detected. In NCBI SNP database, MAF of rs2241027 and rs2241028 were 0.05/0.10, 0.06/0.07, respectively, from ExAC/1000 Genomes Project, both with no clinical significance. The function of both variants was defined as uncertain by MyGenostics. The variants distribution was within the range of Hardy-Weinberg equilibrium in controls ($p = 0.82$, 0.71 resp., Table 3). Given the present sample sizes, we have 80% power to detect an odds ratio of 1.83 in both PD and ET for rs2241027 adopting an additive model and OR of 1.91 in both PD and ET for rs2241028 adopting an additive model. What is worth noting is that there are big differences in MAFs between our control and database in both two variants, which may be caused by ethnical diversity, so we calculate the power considering MAFs of 0.28 and 0.21, respectively, in our control, which is higher than in database; otherwise, it would require much bigger sample sizes. Additionally, we only have 34% power to detect an OR of 1.44 (the OR in Krüger et al.'s study) for rs2241028.

As for allele and genotype distribution of both variants, we failed to detect any significant differences either in FET versus controls or in FPD versus controls (Tables 3 and 4). No significant difference was observed in the logistic regression either (data not shown). Moreover, haplotypes of two variants showed hardly any association with the risk

TABLE 3: Statistics of minor allele frequency (MAF).

| RS number | Position | Function | MAF | | | | ExAC/1000 Genomes MAF | HWE (p^a) | OR (95% CI), p value | |
			FET	FPD	ET-PD	Control			FET versus control	FPD versus control
rs2241027	Intron	Uncertain	0.33	0.29	0.33	0.28	0.05/0.10	0.82	1.28 (0.83–1.96), 0.26	0.80 (0.47–1.35), 0.40
rs2241028	Exon-intron boundary	Uncertain	0.14	0.16	0.23	0.21	0.06/0.07	0.71	1.08 (0.70–1.66), 0.73	0.70 (0.42–1.16), 0.17

[a]HWE for controls.

TABLE 4: Statistics of genotype.

| Participants | Genotype (rs2241027/rs2241028) | | | p^a value | |
	GG	GA	AA	rs2241027	rs2241028
FET	44/75	48/23	9/3	0.50	0.29
FPD	53/73	43/31	9/1	0.77	0.14
ET-PD	8/9	4/5	3/1	N/A	N/A
Control	51/64	43/30	6/6	N/A	N/A

[a] p value compared with controls.

TABLE 5: Haplotype analysis.

Haplotype	FET (%)	FPD (%)	Control (%)	χ^2 value[a/b]	Fisher's $p^{a/b}$	Pearson's $p^{a/b}$	OR (95% CI)[a/b]
A-A	0	0	0	—	—	—	—
A-G	33	29	28	1.28/0.12	0.26/0.73	0.26/0.73	1.28 (0.83–1.96)/1.08 (0.70–1.66)
G-A	14	16	21	3.05/1.92	0.08/0.17	0.08/0.17	0.63 (0.38–1.06)/0.70 (0.42–1.16)
G-G	53	55	52	0.09/0.58	0.77/0.45	0.77/0.45	1.06 (0.72–1.57)/1.16 (0.79–1.71)

[a/b] value for FET versus controls/FPD versus controls.

of FET or FPD (Table 5). Regarding ET-PD, in which we attempted to investigate the situation of *HTRA2* in case there were some dramatic mutations, owing to the limitation of sample size, we quitted further statistical analysis.

4. Discussion

The high temperature requirement A2 (*HTRA2*), known as a mitochondria protein, plays distinct different roles in mitochondria homeostasis and cellular apoptosis regulation [20]. As one study indicated, deficiency of *HTRA2* can cause damage and mutation of mitochondria DNA [21]. Another study revealed that *HTRA2* was regulated by *PINK1*, which might contribute to early-onset PD, in the proteolytic activity [22].

Many researches concerning the association of PD with *HTRA2* variants have been done. The earliest mutation screening of *HTRA2* in PD patients was done in a German population after the finding that targeted disruption of HTRA2 can cause neurodegeneration and a Parkinsonian phenotype in mice, which resulted in the identification of two mutations (G399S and A141S) related to the risk of PD [23, 24]. Later on, replications with contradictory consequences have been conducted [25–31], and one large scale genetic association study is worth noting, which showed no evidence for an overall association of common variants in *HTRA2* with PD [32], while Gulsuner et al.'s study of a six-generation family provides further evidence for the probability of *HTRA2* acting as a cause for PD and ET, especially those with family history [13]. So the aim of our study is to investigate the situation of *HTRA2* by Sanger sequencing of the whole coding sequence in FET, FPD, and ET-PD in Chinese population, especially FET and ET-PD.

Our study detected two variants (rs2241028, rs2241027). Variant rs2241028 has been reported in several studies with similar negative results except for Krüger et al.'s study, in which rs2241028 was considered as a susceptible factor for PD in the Scandinavian population and their descent from

USA [32], while there is no report of this variant in studies about ET. Since rs2241028 is near the splicing region, it may affect the transcript efficiency of HTRA2 to some extent or influence the expression of HTRA2 in some other way, so it would be promising to do some research into the function of this variant and the relationship with PD. Variant rs2241027 has never been mentioned in the previous study no matter about PD or ET. Our study showed that neither of two variants was related to the risk of developing ET or PD, and two variants were defined as no clinical significance in database. Meanwhile, we have not detected mutations (G399S and A141S) mentioned in other studies. So we provided no evidence of association of *HTRA2* with FET and FPD. As for ET-PD, the result of our study was not so convincing due to the sample size though we found nothing significant as well. Admittedly, there are some limitations in our study. On the one hand, the sample sizes were only able to detect a moderate correlation with enough power and not for a relatively weaker correlation, which may cause false negative error. On the other hand, it would be more persuasive if the promoter of HTRA2 gene has been sequenced as well.

In conclusion, *HTRA2* might not be a cause of familial ET or PD in China. Studies with larger sample size are needed to investigate thoroughly the role of *HTRA2* in ET and ET-PD in China and other places in the world.

Authors' Contributions

Ya-Chao He and Pei Huang contributed equally to this work as first authors.

Acknowledgments

The authors are grateful to all the participants recruited in this study for their donation of blood samples without which the research could not be conducted. The study was supported by National Natural Science Fund (81430022, 91332107, and 81371407). The Sanger sequencing was performed by MyGenostics and Biosune.

References

[1] E. D. Louis and J. J. Ferreira, "How common is the most common adult movement disorder? Update on the worldwide prevalence of essential tremor," *Movement Disorders*, vol. 25, no. 5, pp. 534–541, 2010.

[2] J.-F. Schmouth, P. A. Dion, and G. A. Rouleau, "Genetics of essential tremor: from phenotype to genes, insights from both human and mouse studies," *Progress in Neurobiology*, vol. 119-120, pp. 1–19, 2014.

[3] M. A. Thenganatt and J. Jankovic, "The relationship between essential tremor and Parkinson's disease," *Parkinsonism and Related Disorders*, vol. 22, supplement 1, pp. S162–S165, 2016.

[4] J. Benito-León, E. D. Louis, and F. Bermejo-Pareja, "Risk of incident Parkinson's disease and parkinsonism in essential tremor: A Population Based Study," *Journal of Neurology, Neurosurgery and Psychiatry*, vol. 80, no. 4, pp. 423–425, 2009.

[5] K. Kalinderi, S. Bostantjopoulou, and L. Fidani, "The genetic background of Parkinson's disease: current progress and future prospects," *Acta Neurologica Scandinavica*, vol. 134, no. 5, pp. 314–326, 2016.

[6] M. Funayama, K. Ohe, T. Amo et al., "CHCHD2 mutations in autosomal dominant late-onset Parkinson's disease: a genome-wide linkage and sequencing study," *The Lancet Neurology*, vol. 14, no. 3, pp. 274–282, 2015.

[7] S. K. McDonnell, D. J. Schaid, A. Elbaz et al., "Complex segregation analysis of Parkinson's disease: the Mayo Clinic Family Study," *Annals of Neurology*, vol. 59, no. 5, pp. 788–795, 2006.

[8] N. R. Whaley, J. D. Putzke, Y. Baba, Z. K. Wszolek, and R. J. Uitti, "Essential tremor: phenotypic expression in a clinical cohort," *Parkinsonism and Related Disorders*, vol. 13, no. 6, pp. 333–339, 2007.

[9] C. Wider, O. A. Ross, and Z. K. Wszolek, "Genetics of Parkinson disease and essential tremor," *Current Opinion in Neurology*, vol. 23, no. 4, pp. 388–393, 2010.

[10] Y. X. Chao, E. Y. Ng, L. Tan et al., "Lrrk2 R1628P variant is a risk factor for essential tremor," *Scientific Reports*, vol. 5, article 9029, 2015.

[11] S.-W. Yu, C.-M. Chen, Y.-C. Chen et al., "SLC1A2 variant is associated with essential tremor in taiwanese population," *PLoS ONE*, vol. 8, no. 8, article e71919, 2013.

[12] E. García-Martín, C. Martínez, H. Alonso-Navarro et al., "No association of the SLC1A2 rs3794087 allele with risk for essential tremor in the Spanish population," *Pharmacogenetics and Genomics*, vol. 23, no. 11, pp. 587–590, 2013.

[13] H. U. Gulsuner, S. Gulsuner, F. N. Mercan et al., "Mitochondrial serine protease HTRA2 p.G399S in a kindred with essential tremor and Parkinson disease," *Proceedings of the National Academy of Sciences of the United States of America*, vol. 111, no. 51, pp. 18285–18290, 2014.

[14] C. Tzoulis, T. Zayats, P. M. Knappskog et al., "HTRA2 p.G399S in Parkinson disease, essential tremor, and tremulous cervical dystonia," *Proceedings of the National Academy of Sciences of the United States of America*, vol. 112, no. 18, Article ID E2268, 2015.

[15] Y. X. Chao, E. Y. Ng, J. N. Foo, J. Liu, Y. Zhao, and E.-K. Tan, "Mitochondrial serine protease HTRA2 gene mutation in Asians with coexistent essential tremor and Parkinson disease," *Neurogenetics*, vol. 16, no. 3, pp. 241–242, 2015.

[16] F. Hopfner, S. H. Müller, D. Lorenz et al., "Mutations in HTRA2 are not a common cause of familial classic ET," *Movement Disorders*, vol. 30, no. 8, pp. 1149–1150, 2015.

[17] R. B. Postuma, D. Berg, M. Stern et al., "MDS clinical diagnostic criteria for Parkinson's disease," *Movement Disorders*, vol. 30, no. 12, pp. 1591–1601, 2015.

[18] G. Deuschl, P. Bain, and M. Brin, "Consensus statement of the Movement Disorder Society on Tremor. Ad Hoc Scientific Committee," *Movement Disorders*, vol. 13, supplement 3, pp. 2–23, 1998.

[19] Z. Li, Z. Zhang, Z. He et al., "A partition-ligation-combination-subdivision em algorithm for haplotype inference with multiallelic markers: update of the SHEsis (http://analysis.bio- x.cn)," *Cell Research*, vol. 19, no. 4, pp. 519–523, 2009.

[20] L. Vande Walle, M. Lamkanfi, and P. Vandenabeele, "The mitochondrial serine protease HtrA2/Omi: an overview," *Cell Death and Differentiation*, vol. 15, no. 3, pp. 453–460, 2008.

[21] H.-G. Goo, M. K. Jung, S. S. Han, H. Rhim, and S. Kang, "HtrA2/Omi deficiency causes damage and mutation of mitochondrial DNA," *Biochimica et Biophysica Acta (BBA)—Molecular Cell Research*, vol. 1833, no. 8, pp. 1866–1875, 2013.

[22] H. Plun-Favreau, K. Klupsch, N. Moisoi et al., "The mitochondrial protease HtrA2 is regulated by Parkinson's disease-associated kinase PINK1," *Nature Cell Biology*, vol. 9, no. 11, pp. 1243–1252, 2007.

[23] K. M. Strauss, L. M. Martins, H. Plun-Favreau et al., "Loss of function mutations in the gene encoding Omi/HtrA2 in Parkinson's disease," *Human Molecular Genetics*, vol. 14, no. 15, pp. 2099–2111, 2005.

[24] J. M. Jones, P. Datta, S. M. Srinivasula et al., "Loss of Omi mitochondrial protease activity causes the neuromuscular disorder of mnd2 mutant mice," *Nature*, vol. 425, no. 6959, pp. 721–727, 2003.

[25] V. Bogaerts, K. Nuytemans, J. Reumers et al., "Genetic variability in the mitochondrial serine protease HTRA2 contributes to risk for Parkinson disease," *Human Mutation*, vol. 29, no. 6, pp. 832–840, 2008.

[26] O. A. Ross, A. I. Soto, C. Vilariño-Güell et al., "Genetic variation of Omi/HtrA2 and Parkinson's disease," *Parkinsonism and Related Disorders*, vol. 14, no. 7, pp. 539–543, 2008.

[27] J. Simón-Sánchez and A. B. Singleton, "Sequencing analysis of OMI/HTRA2 shows previously reported pathogenic mutations in neurologically normal controls," *Human Molecular Genetics*, vol. 17, no. 13, pp. 1988–1993, 2008.

[28] C.-H. Lin, M.-L. Chen, G. S. Chen, C.-H. Tai, and R.-M. Wu, "Novel variant Pro143Ala in HTRA2 contributes to Parkinson's disease by inducing hyperphosphorylation of HTRA2 protein in mitochondria," *Human Genetics*, vol. 130, no. 6, pp. 817–827, 2011.

[29] C.-Y. Wang, Q. Xu, L. Weng et al., "Genetic variations of Omi/HTRA2 in Chinese patients with Parkinson's disease," *Brain Research*, vol. 1385, pp. 293–297, 2011.

[30] J.-Y. Tian, J.-F. Guo, L. Wang et al., "Mutation analysis of LRRK2, SCNA, UCHL1, HtrA2 and GIGYF2 genes in Chinese patients with autosomal dorminant Parkinson's disease," *Neuroscience Letters*, vol. 516, no. 2, pp. 207–211, 2012.

18

Cognitive Training in Parkinson's Disease: A Review of Studies from 2000 to 2014

Daniel Glizer[1] and Penny A. MacDonald[1,2]

[1]*MacDonald Lab, Brain and Mind Institute, University of Western Ontario, London, ON, Canada*
[2]*Clinical Neurological Sciences, Schulich School of Medicine and Dentistry, University of Western Ontario, London, ON, Canada*

Correspondence should be addressed to Daniel Glizer; dglizer@uwo.ca

Academic Editor: Yuan-Han Yang

Cognitive deficits are prevalent among patients with Parkinson's disease (PD), in both early and late stages of the disease. These deficits are associated with lower quality of life, loss of independence, and institutionalization. To date, there is no effective pharmacological treatment for the range of cognitive impairments presented in PD. Cognitive training (CT) has been explored as an alternative approach to remediating cognition in PD. In this review we present a detailed summary of 13 studies of CT that have been conducted between 2000 and 2014 and a critical examination of the evidence for the effectiveness and applicability of CT in PD. Although the evidence shows that CT leads to short-term, moderate improvements in some cognitive functions, methodological inconsistencies weaken these results. We discuss several key limitations of the literature to date, propose methods of addressing these questions, and outline the future directions that studies of CT in PD should pursue. Studies need to provide more detail about the cognitive profile of participants, include larger sample sizes, be hypothesis driven, and be clearer about the training interventions and the outcome measures.

1. Introduction

Parkinson's disease (PD) is a disorder characterized by degeneration of dopamine-producing cells in the substantia nigra (SN) and to a much lesser degree in the ventral tegmental area (VTA). This deficiency produces the cardinal motor symptoms of tremor, rigidity, and bradykinesia [1]. Additionally, cognitive symptoms are now also recognized as an undisputable feature of PD [2, 3].

The pathophysiology of cognitive deficits in PD is complex. It seems likely that at least some cognitive deficits result from striatal dopamine deficiency [4–6]. Dopaminergic drugs used to treat motor symptoms in PD have also been implicated in diverse cognitive deficits, proposed to be due to an overdosing of the relatively spared VTA [7–12]. In addition to dopaminergic pathways, dysregulation in cholinergic [13, 14], serotoninergic [15, 16], and noradrenergic [17–19] pathways potentially contributes to cognitive deficits in PD. Alpha-synuclein-containing Lewy bodies deposited in

SN and cortex have also been strongly associated with the development of dementia in PD in early and especially at later stages of the disease [20–22].

Although motor impairments are well addressed by dopaminergic medications and deep brain stimulation [23, 24], cognitive symptoms, perhaps due to their complexity and variability from patient to patient, lack clearly effective therapies. Dopaminergic medications improve some cognitive functions but worsen others [7, 10, 23–26]. Further, the clinical significance of these effects has not been systematically studied in placebo-controlled randomized trials. Finally, cholinesterase inhibitors improve cognition and quality of life (QOL; for review, see [27]) but these therapies are limited to patients who are diagnosed with clinically significant dementia and not lesser cognitive impairment. Additionally, the effects on cognitive dysfunction are minimal, not sustained with advancing disease, or sufficient to produce truly meaningful enhancements of function [28]. In sum, neither dopaminergic treatments nor cholinesterase inhibitors modify disease progression, being merely prescribed for symptomatic relief. Investigating effective nonpharmacological treatment options for cognitive decline in lieu of or to enhance available pharmacological treatment in PD is therefore an important area of research.

To better understand what treatments might be useful for cognitive decline in PD, there is a need to better characterize the cognitive impairments associated with this disease. Cognitive decline in PD includes impairments in diverse functions and skills. To date, there is considerable evidence of impairments in executive functions such as working memory (WM), attention, reasoning, and planning even in early, nondemented PD patients [29–32]. Additionally, more basic perceptual visuospatial and verbal processes have been shown consistently to be impaired in PD [32–35]. Impairments in memory have also been documented [36].

Cognitive deficits are very prevalent in PD patients. Even at the time of PD diagnosis, approximately 30–50% of patients already exhibit symptoms consistent with mild cognitive impairment (MCI) or dementia [37] and from 60 to 80% of cases develop into full dementia within 10 years [38, 39]. Cognitive impairments are strongly related to lower QOL ratings and challenges in activities of daily living in patients [40–43]. These deficits present challenges to everyday functioning [41, 44] and are a major cause of loss of independence and institutionalization in PD [45]. Consequently, effective therapies for cognitive impairment in PD are an important but unmet need [23, 45]. Exploration and empirical testing of interventions to address cognitive decline in PD are imperative.

Over the last decade, nonpharmacological treatments that aim to improve cognition have increasingly been a focus in healthy aging as well as in various clinical populations other than PD. Cognitive training (CT), a nonpharmacological intervention, has generated significant interest and engendered a wealth of research. CT is an approach that broadly encompasses the idea that repeated performance of cognitive tasks leads to strategy development or brain changes that improve cognitive functions either within a specific domain or in general.

In healthy populations, evidence suggests that CT can benefit older adults through either restorative or protective factors [46–51], although other studies appear to find modest or no effects following CT [52, 53]. Thus, it remains to be seen whether a CT intervention can be developed that leads to meaningful effects in a healthy population. A thorough review of this controversy, however, is beyond the scope of the current review, which will focus more on CT in PD.

CT in Clinical Populations. In contrast to studies in healthy controls, in clinical populations, CT has shown much more promising and consistent results. CT and attention training have been found to improve visuospatial and language abilities in patients with aphasia and neglect syndromes following traumatic brain injury (TBI; [54, 55]). Several reviews and meta-analyses of TBI treatments concluded that CT approaches have potential as remediation strategies after stroke but noted that further research is warranted [56, 57]. In conjunction with other approaches, CT has been successfully

employed in the treatment of disorders such as schizophrenia [58–60], Attention Deficit Hyperactivity Disorder (ADHD), and various addictions and mood disorders [61–64]. Finally, in at-risk populations, such as older adults susceptible to Alzheimer's disease and dementia, various forms of CT show protective effects and even improvements in select cognitive functions [49, 51, 65–67].

There have now been a number of studies investigating the effect of CT on cognitive dysfunction in PD. In this review, we present and summarize each study individually, discuss the potential of CT as a therapy for cognitive impairment in PD, highlight knowledge gaps, and make recommendations for future studies. We will critically evaluate the design and methods of studies of CT in PD. The ultimate goal of this review is to focus the research on CT in PD, to suggest guidelines for future studies, and to highlight common issues that are noted in the literature.

Literature Search. To identify all studies that investigated CT to treat cognitive symptoms of PD, we conducted a search in PubMed and PsycINFO using the following key terms and combinations: cognit* train* AND Parkinson*; memory train* AND Parkinson*; attention train* AND Parkinson*; cognit* rehabilitation AND Parkinson*; memory rehabilitation AND Parkinson*; attention rehabilitation AND Parkinson*; cognit* remediation AND Parkinson*; memory remediation AND Parkinson*; attention remediation AND Parkinson*. We selected for further inspection studies that included information on (1) the training group(s), (2) the training intervention, (3) the outcome measures, and (4) specifically used CT interventions, alone or in combination with (an)other nonpharmacological therapy in PD. We found only 13 studies that met all of these criteria. In each study, we examined whether (1) there was a control group or comparison intervention, (2) training was multimodal, computerized, or pen and paper, (3) CT was combined with another intervention, (4) CT was standardized or individually tailored, and (5) QOL changes were assessed. Table 1 lists the identified studies and categorizes them according to design.

2. Results

2.1. Single Group, Uncontrolled Studies. In a small preliminary study of CT with inpatients, Sinforiani et al. [68] examined the effects of a rehabilitation program consisting of motor and cognitive training in patients with early stages of PD and mild cognitive decline but not dementia. They used Training Neuropsicologico (TNP; [82])—a computerized CT program aimed at improving attention, abstract reasoning, and visuospatial abilities. The PD patients ($N = 20$) who enrolled in the program for 12 sessions showed significant improvement on measures of verbal processing and verbal memory as well as on one measure of abstract reasoning. These improvements remained when examined at a six-month follow-up. However, without a control group, it is impossible to attribute improvement to CT specifically. Alternatively, change in function could have owed to nonspecific effects of being enrolled and followed in a study, to the

TABLE 1: Classification of studies of CT in PD according to design.

Single group, uncontrolled studies	Waitlist-controlled studies	Studies comparing CT to standard treatments	Comparing different CT interventions
		Sammer et al., [74]	
Sinforiani et al., [68]	Nombela et al., [71]	París et al., [75]	Reuter et al., [79]
Mohlman et al., [69]	Naismith et al., [72]	Pompeu et al., [76]	Petrelli et al., [80]
Disbrow et al., [70]	Edwards et al., [73]	Peña et al., [77]	Zimmermann et al., [81]
		Cerasa et al., [78]	

passage of time, to fluctuations in clinical disease with regression to mean behaviour, or to decreased anxiety or stress of performing with repeated exposure to the setting. Additionally, participants were an inpatient group at a rehabilitation centre, making them a special subset of the PD population. This scenario enhances the possibility that improvement represented regression to mean performance, with the passage of time of the inciting event or circumstance leading to admission to a rehab setting and later testing. Other confounds exist due to the rehabilitation setting. The group received motor rehabilitation in addition to the CT program so the influence of the two cannot be teased apart. Additionally, it is important to note that *a majority of the measures of cognition yielded no significant improvement, including measures of overall cognition (Mini-Mental State Examination score, MMSE), WM (digit span, Corsi block), and measures of cognitive flexibility (Wisconsin Card Sorting Test, WCST)*, and the authors did not indicate if corrections for multiple comparisons were applied.

In another study, Mohlman et al. [69] examined the acceptability and feasibility of administering CT to patients with PD. Participants ($N = 16$) completed neuropsychological tests and psychometric questionnaires before and after training to assess changes in cognition and mood. The neuropsychological battery consisted of the digit span forward and backward tasks, the Stroop Color Word Test, the Trail Making Test (TMT), and the Controlled Oral Word Association Test (COWAT). The psychometric tests included the Penn State Worry Questionnaire, the Beck Anxiety Inventory (BAI), the trait scale of the State-Trait Anxiety Inventory (STAI), and the Beck Depression Inventory (BDI). During the training period, which lasted one month, with 90 minutes of training per week, participants came to the lab on university campus and performed the Attention Process Training (APT-II) Intervention, a computerized CT program. The modules included in the APT-II focused on training sustained attention, selective attention, alternating attention, and divided attention. Participants also received daily homework assignments throughout the month. The main focus of the study was to determine the acceptability and feasibility of the CT across 4 dimensions: fatigue, effort, progress, and enjoyment. Findings indicated that participants showed good acceptance and completion of the training program. In addition, *all participants' scores on the 4 neuropsychological tasks improved from pre- to postintervention (though no statistics were provided)*. As the main focus was on acceptability of the CT, the article did not include information about the cognitive performance of the group before or after training.

A study by Disbrow and colleagues [70] investigated the effects of executive function and motor focused CT on performance of a similar motor sequence learning task, as well as measures of cognitive flexibility, verbal fluency, and timed instrumental activities of daily living (TIADL). They enrolled 30 PD patients and 21 age matched controls. During pre-training, participants performed a motor sequence learning task (which also served as the training task), the TMT, the Delis-Kaplan Executive Function Scale (D-KEFS), and the Timed-Up-and-Go Test (TUG). In the motor sequence task, participants had to press on a keypad the sequence of numbers corresponding to the sequence that was displayed on the screen (e.g., 1-3-4). Sequence length varied between 1 and 4 digits and included two conditions, the Externally Cued (EC) condition, where feedback was displayed on the screen every trial, and an Internally Represented (IR) condition, where feedback was not displayed on the screen every trial. Based on performance on the motor sequence task, PD patients were split into two groups for further analyses, an impaired performance group ($N = 14$) and an unimpaired performance group ($N = 16$). Outcome measures for the motor sequence learning task were time to initiate motor response, time to end sequence, and number of errors. During the training period, participants performed the motor sequence task for 10 sessions each taking 40 minutes, over the course of about two weeks.

Results showed that training benefitted both the EC and the IR conditions in all groups. Although after training the impaired PD patients still had slower initiation and completion times in the EC condition than the unimpaired PD patients and controls, their performance in the IR condition improved after training and was not significantly different from the other two groups. This indicates that the training improved motor performance dependent on executive function, as required when participants internally represent and plan a sequence but not a simpler version of motor performance when feedback and digit sequence are shown. The previously impaired PD patients also made fewer errors after completing training, similar to the unimpaired PD group and the control group. Training did not have an effect on the D-KEFS, the TIADL, or the TUG. There was a main effect on training on the TMT B minus A scores; however, the impaired PD patients still showed impaired performance after the training compared to the other two groups.

Overall, the results of this study suggest that patients with specific impairments can particularly benefit from specialized, focused training. It is important to note that the training and outcome tasks were nearly identical; thus, it is unclear whether the effects of this type of training transfer to other functions.

Improvement on the TMT suggests that there may be some degree of transfer although no effects were found on measures of QOL and other motor tasks. Moreover, there was no waitlist PD group so it is impossible to attribute improvement solely to the training rather than repeated testing or the passage of time.

2.2. Waitlist-Controlled Studies. In a study employing neuroimaging to investigate CT, Nombela et al. [71] scanned participants using fMRI before and after training. Ten participants with PD and ten healthy age-matched controls completed a variation of the Stroop task at baseline and after training. Half of the PD patients were enrolled in a training intervention ($N = 5$), and half served as the untrained waitlist control group ($N = 5$). Training consisted of a series of Sudoku puzzles completed at home every day for the duration of six months, with weekly meetings with the researchers to go over the puzzles. During baseline assessment, participants completed an easy Sudoku puzzle, the modified Stroop task, and several questionnaires evaluating cognition and PD symptoms (MMSE, Unified Parkinson's Disease Rating Scale (UPDRS), Montgomery-Asberg Rating Scale). PD patients had slower response times (RTs) on the Stroop task, more missed trials, and poorer performance overall. They also took longer to complete the easy Sudoku puzzle compared to controls. Functional neuroimaging revealed more extensive brain activation in patients than in controls and less activation in the left precentral gyrus, left medial frontal gyrus, right precuneus, and the left inferior parietal gyrus. After the six-month training period, the trained PD group had faster RTs on the Stroop task, more correct answers, and fewer missed trials than the untrained patients. Their RTs and correct and missed trials were also better than during their baseline assessment. Further, they completed the Sudoku puzzles more quickly than the untrained PD group. The brain activation of the trained PD group during the Stroop task was more similar to that of the healthy control group. The results of this study suggest that daily performance of cognitive exercises can improve performance on these exercises as well as other related cognitive tasks, but the study is limited by a small sample size and a very unusual and time consuming intervention. Additionally, the assignment to the training group was not random but voluntary, leading possibly to fundamental differences between the training and untrained groups, with the former being more engaged and enthusiastic participants.

A study by Naismith et al. [72] combined psychoeducation and CT and found that, compared to a waitlist control group ($N = 15$), the treatment group ($N = 35$) improved on measures of learning and memory retention. The CT intervention was based on the Neuropsychological Educational Approach to Remediation (NEAR), was individualized to each participant, and comprised a wide array of commercially available computer-based programs depending on the individual's strengths and weaknesses. Participants completed 14 training sessions over two weeks in a lab group-setting. The primary outcome variable was episodic memory measured through the Logical Memory subtest of the

Wechsler Memory Scale III (LOGMEM). Secondary measures consisted of psychomotor speed and mental flexibility (TMT), verbal fluency (COWAT), general cognition (MMSE, National Adult Reading Test), and knowledge about PD assessed using a multiple choice questionnaire. Results revealed that the CT group improved more than the waitlist group on LOGMEM (learning and memory retention). There was no improvement on measures of psychomotor speed, mental flexibility, verbal fluency, or depressive symptoms. The results lend support to CT as a viable intervention to possibly slow down memory decline in PD patients and improve performance on some memory and learning tasks. Due to the difficulty of administering such a comprehensive and individually tailored intervention as well as the high degree of variability in terms of the intervention between patients, it is difficult to assert whether these effects might generalize to PD patients broadly.

A randomized, waitlist-controlled study by Edwards and colleagues [73] investigated the effect of a processing speed training intervention on useful field of view (UFOV), self-rated cognition, and depressive symptoms. One group of PD patients received Speed of Processing Training (SOPT; $N = 44$), and a second group of PD patients served as a waitlist control ($N = 43$). The groups did not differ on any motor, cognitive, or demographic measures at pretraining. The training intervention consisted of a SOPT program (InSight, Posit Science, Inc., San Francisco, CA) which included five exercises focusing on rapid processing of visual stimuli, selective attention, and visual working memory. Training was self-administered, computerized, and completed at home. The intervention lasted for three months, with a recommended schedule of three sessions per week, each session taking an hour. Outcome measures were UFOV, the Cognitive Self-Report Questionnaire, and the Centre for Epidemiological Studies Depressive Symptoms Scale (CES-D). *Analyses revealed that although both the SOPT and the waitlist group showed significantly improved performance on the UFOV task, the SOPT group improved significantly more from pre- to posttraining than the waitlist group. The other two measures, self-reported cognition and depressive symptoms, did not show any changes.* The results of this study provide evidence that SOPT, even when self-administered and completed at home, can lead to improvement in similar tasks, more than can be accounted for by test-retest effects. An important caveat the authors mention is that the effects were most strongly associated with factors accounting for less severe PD stage (e.g., age at onset, disease duration, and L-dopa equivalent dosage). Additionally, none of the patients had symptoms consistent with MCI; thus it will be helpful to conduct a similar study with MCI patients to evaluate whether the SOPT program can benefit more severe stages of PD or cognitive decline.

2.3. Studies Comparing CT to Standard Treatments. Sammer et al. [74] investigated the effectiveness of CT with inpatients at a rehabilitation centre. Participants were divided into two groups: one group ($N = 12$) received a treatment focusing on executive functions; the other group ($N = 14$) completed a standard treatment comprised of occupational therapy, physiotherapy, and physical treatment sessions. The executive function intervention consisted of a range of both standardized and novel tasks training WM, abstract reasoning, problem solving, visuospatial processing, and verbal processing. After 10 training sessions over the course of a 3-4-week hospital stay, only the executive function treatment group improved on some measures of executive function and WM (Behavioural Assessment of the Dysexecutive Syndrome-rule shift and 6-element subtests). However, there were other measures of WM and executive function (TMT and a face-name learning task) and a measure of attention, on which neither group improved. There was also no change in ratings of well-being or depression between the two groups. The results of this study provide some limited evidence that CT can lead to enhancements of executive function. However, it is necessary to identify why some tasks of executive function showed improvement whereas other tasks of executive function did not. With no corrections for multiple comparisons, it is possible to find statistically significant differences in a subset of many tasks due to chance alone, which cannot be ruled out in this case.

In a randomized, controlled, experimenter-blinded study of CT in patients with PD, París and colleagues [75] compared the effects of an intensive individualized CT program (N = 12) to a speech therapy intervention (N = 12). Each participant in the CT group received individual training using a platform of 28 tasks (i.e., SmartBrain computerized program) focusing on specific cognitive domains known to be impaired in PD patients such as memory, attention, WM, executive functions, visuospatial abilities, and psychomotor speed. They also trained on nonspecific tasks that tapped overall cognition including language, simple calculations, and culture. Additionally, participants received homework exercises to be completed outside the sessions. The speech therapy participants received group-sessions focusing on communication difficulties as a result of PD. The intervention program for both CT and speech therapy groups consisted of 12 sessions over four weeks, each session lasting 45 minutes. The CT group also received 20 weekly homework exercises to stimulate cognition. At a baseline assessment, participants completed a comprehensive battery of tasks measuring overall cognition (e.g., MMSE), attention and WM (e.g., digit span), information processing speed (e.g., TMT), verbal and visual processing, learning, and executive functions (e.g., Tower of London (TOL), Stroop test), as well as questionnaires assessing QOL and mood. *Following the training period, the CT group showed significantly more improvement than the speech therapy group on measures of attention, processing speed, memory, visuospatial abilities, executive function, and semantic and verbal fluency. There was no difference between the groups on measures of QOL or mood.* More importantly, although many outcome measures were included, not all measures showed improvement, and there was no indication that analyses were corrected for multiple comparisons. Despite describing aspects of cognition that the training program focused on, the specifics of each training task were not included in the manuscript, thwarting widespread implementation. These details are also needed to

determine how well the trained skills transferred to the outcome measures, and whether the training effect generalized to similar or diverse tasks.

In a study examining the effects of a CT-like intervention on symptoms of PD and independent activities of daily living measured by the UPDRS-II, Pompeu and colleagues [76] divided 32 PD patients into two groups. Both groups received an intervention consisting of 14 sessions of 30 minutes of global physical exercises. The control group (N = 16) received additional 30 minutes of balance exercises, whereas the training group (N = 16) received 30 minutes of training using WiiFit games. WiiFit games focus on motor performance (e.g., Torso twist, soccer heading, basic step, and speed run), though cognitive processes such as planning, decision making, and divided attention are invoked to perform the tasks. The main outcome measure, *performance of activities of daily living as assessed by the self-report on the UPDRS-II,* revealed *no difference between the two groups before training, after training, or at 60-day follow-up* evaluations. Both groups indicated improvement on the UPDRS-II, leading the authors to conclude that training using the WiiFit games does not lead to any improvement over performance of general balance exercises. However, the WiiFit games are designed primarily to focus on motor performance rather than cognitive processes. It is likely that the chosen WiiFit games did not have a clear focus on any aspect of cognition *per se* and instead the cognitive training occurred as a by-product of performing the motor task. Although the authors claim that the WiiFit games trained cognition, the CT tasks and the cognitive evaluations were a secondary measure and were not clearly defined.

Another study conducted by Peña et al. [77] compared a structured, pen and paper CT program to occupational activities. Outcome measures were processing speed (TMT-A, Salthouse Letter Comparison Test), verbal learning and memory (Hopkins Verbal Learning Test), visual learning and memory (Brief Visual Memory Test), executive function (Stroop), and Theory of Mind (Happé test). The CT group (N = 22) received a standardized intervention (REHACOP, a Spanish cognitive rehabilitation program for psychosis) focused on improving attention, memory, language, verbal processing, executive function, and theory of mind, as well as general cognition and functional disability ratings. The occupational therapy group (N = 22) performed activities such as drawing, reading the newspaper, and arts and crafts. Both groups completed 39 sessions over 13 weeks, three per week, with each session taking an hour. They found that, following training, the *CT group showed more improvement than the occupational therapy group on measures of processing speed, visual memory, theory of mind, and functional disability.* This provides further evidence that structured CT is more beneficial than interventions not explicitly focused on cognitive improvement. Also, the improvement on the functional disability scale suggests that CT might lead to benefits that generalize to functional activities. However, the training program is quite a bit longer than those usually studied in CT so results are difficult to compare to other studies.

A study by Cerasa and colleagues [78] compared a computerized CT program designed to rehabilitate attention in patients with multiple sclerosis (REHACOM) to a group performing a simple visuomotor coordination tapping task. Participants were also scanned using fMRI at resting state before and after training. Both the CT group ($N = 8$) and the PD control group ($N = 7$) completed 12, one-hour training sessions over six weeks. On the outcome measures, which included a range of tasks assessing verbal memory, spatial memory, verbal fluency, information processing speed, visuospatial processing, mood, cognition, and QOL, the CT group improved more than the control group on two tests. In some cases improvement was found in only some tests but not others from the same cognitive domain, or even tests that are similar to each other (e.g., digit span forward improved whereas digit span backward did not). There was also a difference in resting state brain activity in the left dorsolateral prefrontal cortex within the left central executive network between the CT and the PD control group. Overall, results from the study provide weak evidence that CT can lead to improvements in cognition and some changes in brain activation. However, no differences between the groups were found on most cognitive measures, and also on measures of QOL and mood, so these effects do not seem to benefit daily functioning.

2.4. Studies Comparing Different Forms of CT. Reuter et al. [79] conducted a large scale study of CT with inpatients and their caregivers, examining the effects of three intervention programs on tests of memory, language, reasoning, attention, executive function, and visuospatial processing, measured with the Alzheimer Disease Assessment Scale-Cognition (ADAS-Cog) and the Scale for Outcomes in Parkinson's Disease-Cognition (SCOPA-Cog) testing batteries. Measures of general cognitive function (Parkinson Neuropsychometric Dementia Assessment (PANDA) and MMSE), QOL, and activities of daily living (Parkinson's disease questionnaire (PDQ-39)) were also taken to assess the overall impact of the training programs on cognition. Patients completed the training while staying at a hospital for four weeks, for a total of at least 14 training sessions, and were assessed before, after, and at six-month follow-up.

Group "A" ($N = 71$) completed an array of individually tailored tasks focused generally on executive functions, memory, reasoning, WM, attention and concentration, and planning (for a list of tasks please see Table 2). Group "B" ($N = 75$) received the same program as well as transfer training that aimed to improve management of activities of daily living and increase self-confidence through the use of strategies such as mnemonics, decision making, handling of money, reading comprehension, and other tasks that patients identified as challenging. Group "C" ($N = 76$) received the CT, the transfer training, and motor training, which consisted of games and tasks that focus on inhibitory control, coordination, speed, perception, orientation, WM, attention, and visuospatial abilities. The caregivers of participants from each group also received educational sessions pertaining to the skills practiced with the patients.

All groups showed improvement on the outcome measures; however, Group C, the group receiving all interventions, showed significantly more improvement than Group A or B across all measures. Participants in each group also showed *increases in rated QOL*, with Group C reporting the most improvement. At the six-month follow-up, a larger proportion of participants in Group C had retained their skills and improved performance compared to Groups A and B. The results strongly suggest that multimodal rehabilitation programs can lead to significant improvements across a variety of cognitive functions, and that carefully designed, individualized CT programs can generalize to improvement on untrained but similar cognitive tasks. However, there are limitations to such an approach. First, it is difficult to understand and clearly attribute benefits to individual components of the intervention given that all groups received multiple components of active treatment. Such an intervention is very time and resource consuming, because training programs have to be tailored to each participant and therefore widespread application seems unfeasible. Additionally, it requires a significant time commitment from the patients who complete the training program, ranging from four hours per week with a trained professional for Group A, and upward of six hours per week for participants in Groups B and C, which showed the most change.

In a randomized controlled study Petrelli and colleagues [80] examined the effects of a structured and an unstructured CT intervention relative to a waitlist control group on measures of memory, attention, and executive functions, as well as QOL and mood. One group received a structured CT program ($N = 22$) administered using the NeuroVitalis software. A second group received an unstructured CT program ($N = 22$) administered using the MentallyFit program. Finally, a third group was a waitlist control ($N = 21$). Training sessions were completed in a group setting led by a supervisor, and training lasted 12 sessions which took 90 minutes each. At pre- and posttraining evaluations, participants completed a comprehensive battery of cognitive tests and neurological assessments. Primary outcome measures were performance on the Brief Test of Attention (BTA), DemTect, a cognitive screening tool, and Memo, a verbal processing test. Secondary measures included visuoconstruction (Complex Figure Test), depression scores (BDI), and QOL (PDQ-39).

When compared to the waitlist control, the group receiving the structured CT program showed improvement in measures of WM and short term memory, whereas the unstructured CT group showed trends in improvement on verbal memory and fluency. The *unstructured CT group also showed a decrease in depression scores.* The structured CT group showed significantly more improvement than either group on WM measures, as well as a trend in verbal short term memory. This study supports CT as an intervention that can improve performance on untrained measures of cognition and suggests that a structured program leads to more benefits than an unstructured one. The use of many outcome measures that overlap in domains and the fact that some WM tasks showed improvement whereas others did not, weakens the conclusions drawn somewhat. Additionally, the training interventions included various tasks completed in group sessions which reduces the specificity of the intervention and

TABLE 2: Summary of studies of CT in PD.

Article by	Participants	Description of training intervention	Outcome measures	Results on outcome measures (# significant differences/total # of measures)	Description of setting # weeks|# sessions|session length (minutes)|total intervention length (hours)	Combined intervention or only CT	Standardized intervention	Assessed QOL
Sinforiani et al., 2004 [68]	20 PD-MCI MMSE~25 No dementia H&Y 1.5	TNP software, focus on attention, abstract reasoning, visuospatial abilities, different level of complexity.	MMSE Digit span Corsi's test COWAT FAS Babcock's story Raven's matrices WCST Stroop test	Pre-post improvement: 3/8 Babcock's story;* COWAT FAS;** Raven's matrices *	Computerized, hospital program 6|12|60|12	CT and motor rehabilitation	Yes, TNP software.	No
Sammer et al., 2006 [74]	12 PD CT 14 PD standard treatment MMSE~27 No dementia H&Y 2-3	CT - BADS (unused subtests); Raven's matrices; picture arrangement tasks, picture completion tasks, block design, object assembly (from WISC); short stories & discussions; pictures prompting stories. Standard treatment, occupational therapy, physiotherapy, and physical treatment.	BADS, rule shifting BADS, six elements CET, German version TMT, German version Face name learning test Attention Wellbeing scale Verbal intelligence scale Hamilton Rating Scale for Depression	Pre-post improvement: 2/5 CT more than standard treatment, improved on BADS rule shifting* CT and standard treatment groups, improved on BADS six elements***	Noncomputerized, hospital program 3-4|10|30|5	Only CT in hospital versus standard treatment	Not standardized intervention. Additionally, task difficulty was adjusted according to each participant's performance level.	Yes. No change (mood questionnaire)
Nombela et al., 2011 [71]	5 PD CT 5 PD untrained 10 healthy controls MMSE 25-26 H&Y 2.5	PD untrained & healthy controls, waitlist CT, one easy level Sudoku puzzle (4 × 4 grid, 2 × 2 blocks) daily for six months. Weekly meetings.	UPDRS MMSE Stroop accuracy Stroop RT Sudoku RT Brain activation	Posttraining PD CT versus PD untrained: Sudoku, faster solving time* Stroop, more correct answers*, fewer missing answers**, lower RT** PD CT group showed brain activation pattern more similar to controls.	Noncomputerized, at home with weekly meetings to discuss progress, Sudoku table 1/day, for 6 months Impossible to calculate total training time	Only CT	No, Sudoku plus weekly meetings, much longer duration than traditional CT.	No
Mohlman et al., 2011 [69]	16 PD MMSE 28 No dementia	Attention Process Training II (APT-II), audio CDs, pen and paper worksheets, response clickers. Training sustained attention, divided attention, alternating attention, and selective attention.	Acceptability Feasibility COWAT Stroop Digit span f & b TMT B	Pre-post improvement. No statistics	Computerized + daily practice, in lab, assisted 4|4|90|6	Only CT but not assessing effectiveness	Yes, APT-II.	Not reported

TABLE 2: Continued.

Article by	Participants	Description of training intervention	Outcome measures	Results on outcome measures (# significant differences/total # of measures)	Description of setting # weeks|# sessions|session length (minutes)|total intervention length (hours)	Combined intervention or only CT	Standardized intervention	Assessed QOL
Paris et al., 2011 [75]	16 PD CT 12 PD control Excluded MMSE <23, some MCI in both groups H&Y 2.37, 2.25	*PD CT:* SmartBrain intervention as well as pen and paper homework. Individualized from a platform of 28 tasks focusing on attention, WM, executive function, memory, visuospatial abilities, psychomotor speed. Also training in language, calculations, and culture. *PD control:* speech therapy, focus on speech and communication difficulties.	MMSE ACE *Attention and WM:* (i) WAIS III Digit Span f & b (ii) CVLT II-List AI *Information processing speed:* (i) SDMT (ii) TMT A (iii) Stroop, word subtest *Verbal memory:* (i) CVLT-II-Short-Delay Free Recall (ii) CVLT-II-Long-Delay Free Recall (iii) Logical Memory subtest I (iv) Logical Memory subtest II *Learning:* (i) CVLT-II-List A Total *Visual memory:* (i) ROCFT-Immediate Recall (ii) ROCFT-Delayed Recall *Visuoconstructive abilities:* (i) ROCFT-Copy *Visuospatial Abilities:* (i) RBANS-Line Orientation *Verbal fluency:* (i) Phonemic-COWAT FAS (ii) Semantic-COWAT Animals *Executive functions:* (i) TMT-B (ii) TOL-Total Moves (iii) TOL-Total Correct (iv) TOL-Rules Violations (v) Stroop Test-Interference PDQ-39 Mood, geriatric depression scale Cognitive difficulties in activities of daily living, Cognitive Deficits Scale	SmartBrain group improved on 10/23 measures compared to PD control group. *Attention and WM 1/4:* digit span forward* *Information processing speed 1/3:* Stroop word*** *Visual memory 2/4:* ROCFT, immediate** and delayed* *Verbal 1/2:* Semantic-Animals** but not Phonemic-FAS *Executive functions 3/5:* TMT-B*, TOL Total Moves **, and Total Correct**	Computerized and noncomputerized plus homework tasks, in lab and at home 4|12|45|9 Plus homework for unspecified amount of time	Only CT versus speech therapy	No, selection of tasks plus SmartBrain, individualized for each participant.	Yes. No change on PDQ39, on measure of mood, or of activities of daily living

TABLE 2: Continued.

Article by	Participants	Description of training intervention	Outcome measures	Results on outcome measures (# significant differences/total # of measures)	Description of setting # weeks|# sessions|session length (minutes)|total intervention length (hours)	Combined intervention or only CT	Standardized intervention	Assessed QOL.
Pompeu et al., 2012 [76]	16 PD General balance 16 PD WiiFit H&Y 1-2 MOCA 22-impaired	*WiiFit and cognition* (cognition as part of the game's requirements, not specifically trained). Games used: Single Leg Extension, Torso Twist, Table Tilt, Tilt City, Soccer Heading, Penguin Slide, Rhythm Parade, Obstacle Course, Basic Step, Basic Run. *General Balance:* Similar motor requirements as the Wii games.	UPDRS-II (activities of independent living) MOCA Static and dynamic balance measures	WiiFit and general balance exercise groups both showed improvement in UPDRS II* (independent activities of daily living scale) and MOCA scores*. No difference between groups before, after, or at 60-day follow-up.	Computerized-sessions led by an instructor 7|14|60|14	Combined with global exercises. Computerized but not cognitive focused.	Yes, WiiFit games.	Yes. Both groups improved on UPDRS II-activities of independent living
Reuter et al., 2012 [79]	71 PD CT (group A) 75 PD CT + transfer (group B) 76 CT + transfer + motor (group C) MCI in all groups	*CT* - BADS (unused subtests); Raven's matrices; picture arrangement tasks, picture completion tasks, block design, object assembly (from WISC); short stories & discussions; pictures prompting stories. *CT + transfer:* same as above + daily tasks such as grocery shopping, tending to a vegetable patch, and so forth. *CT + transfer + motor:* same as above + games and tasks to enhance inhibitory control, WM, coordination, and so forth.	ADAS- Cog SCOPA – Cog BADS- six element BADS – zoo map BADS – instruction PASAT Goal Attainment Scale PDQ – 39 UPDRS	No detailed statistics, all groups improved. The more involved groups (groups B and C) improved more. There was a significant group × time interaction, suggesting group C improved more than other groups on ADAS-Cog *** and SCOPA-Cog***	Computerized and noncomputerized, hospital and at home, at least 14 sessions, 4/week, 60 minutes, then at home, 3/week, 45 minutes each. Minimum: 4|16|60|16	Only CT versus CT + transfer training versus CT + transfer training + psychomotor training	No Individualized	Yes. Improvement in order of magnitude C > B > A
Disbrow et al., 2012 [70]	14 PD CT impaired 16 PD CT unimpaired 21 Controls	*Two-phase button press task,* a motor sequence learning task, participants had to press numbered keys corresponding to the number sequence shown on screen. Sequence length varied between 1 and 4 digits.	Motor sequence learning task TIADL TMT D-KEFS TUG	Posttraining, the impaired PD group showed significant improvement in time for sequence initiation, time for sequence completion, and number of errors in the internally represented condition of the task.	Computerized, adaptive difficulty, completed at home 2|10|40| ~6.5	Only CT	Yes, but adaptive difficulty.	Yes. No changes in time to complete instrumental activities of daily living

TABLE 2: Continued.

Article by	Participants	Description of training intervention	Outcome measures	Results on outcome measures (# significant differences/total # of measures)	Description of setting # weeks|sessions|session length (minutes)|total intervention length (hours)	Combined intervention or only CT	Standardized intervention	Assessed QOL
Naismith et al., 2013 [72]	35 PD CT + psychoeducation 15 PD waitlist MMSE 27	*Neuropsychological Educational Approach to Remediation (NEAR)*, individualized, computer based training program devised according to their test results, using a mix of commercially available CT interventions and software programs.	Wechsler Memory Scale III: LOGMEM I - Immediate LOGMEM II - Delayed TMT A TMT B COWAT FAS BDI	CT > waitlist improvement on 2/7 measures: LOGMEM I – Immediate* LOGMEM II – Delayed*	Computerized, in lab group sessions 7|14|120|28	CT combined with psychoeducation	No Individualized	Yes No effects on depression BDI.
Edwards et al., 2013 [73]	44 PD Speed of Processing Training (SOPT) 43 PD waitlist H&Y 1-3 MMSE 28	SOPT, self-administered, computer based training program that includes 5 exercises aimed at training speed of information processing. The exercises adapt in difficulty according to performance.	UFOV Cognitive Self-Report Questionnaire Depressive symptoms (CES-D)	SOPT > waitlist improvement on 1/3 measures: UFOV**	Computerized, self-administered, at home 12|36|60| ≥20	Only CT	Standardized program (InSight), individually adaptive difficulty levels.	Yes No effects on depression CES-D
Petrelli et al., 2014 [80]	22 PD NeuroVitalis (NV) 22 PD mentally fit (MF) 21 PD waitlist H&Y 1-3 No dementia MMSE 28	*Structured:* Psychoeducation, group games, individual and group tasks, focusing on attention, memory, and executive functions. *Unstructured:* Group conversation, group games, individual and group tasks, focusing on attention, memory, executive functions, language, and creative thinking. Tasks for each session chosen at random.	DemTect MMSE Brief Test of Attention Memo Complex figure-ROCFT and Taylor COWAT FAS BDI PDQ-39	NV > waitlist improved on 2/12: Memo-Verbal short term attention score *** and DemTect, digit span reverse*. MF > waitlist improved on BDI*. NV > MF improved on DemTect, digit span reverse**.	Computerized, pen and paper and activities, in lab group sessions 6|12|90|18	Only CT	NV group standardized intervention. MF unstandardized, unstructured.	Yes. MF improved on BDI scores. No changes in PDQ-39
Zimmermann et al. 2014 [81]	19 PD CogniPlus 20 PD WiiFit MMSE 29 H&Y 1-2	CogniPlus-focused attention; N-Back; planning and action; response inhibition. WiiFit-tennis, swordplay, archery, air sports.	Tests of Attentional Performance-Alertness Tests of Attentional Performance-WM TMT Block design test CVLT	No overall test of improvement for each group separately. WiiFit group improved over CogniPlus group on 1/5 measures: Tests of Attentional Performance-Alertness*.	Computerized, in lab supervised by assistant 4|12|40|8	Only CT versus pure Wii sports	Yes, both interventions.	No

TABLE 2: Continued.

Article by	Participants	Description of training intervention	Outcome measures	Results on outcome measures (# significant differences/total # of measures)	Description of setting # weeks|sessions|session length (minutes)|total intervention length (hours)	Combined intervention or only CT	Standardized intervention	Assessed QOL
Peña et al., 2014 [77]	22 PD REHACOP 22 PD occupational therapy MMSE 27	REHACOP, group sessions including focus on attention, memory (visual and verbal, recall and recognition), language and verbal processing, executive functions (planning and logical reasoning), social cognition and Theory of Mind.	*Processing speed:* TMT A Salthouse letter comparison test *Verbal memory:* Hopkins verbal learning test, learning and long term recall *Visual memory:* Brief visual memory test, learning and long term recall *Executive function:* Stroop word color, interference scores Theory of Mind: Happé test	REHACOP > occupational therapy improved on 4/9 measures. Processing speed* Visual memory* Theory of Mind* Functional disability*	Noncomputerized, psychologist led group sessions 13|39|60|39	Only CT	Yes, REHACOP modules.	Yes. Functional disability scores improved in REHACOP group more than occupational therapy group
Cerasa et al., 2014 [78]	8 PD RehaCom 7 PD coordinated tapping task	RehaCom, computer assisted training of attention and information processing. Tapping task, also computerized, using in-house software.	ROCFT Selective Reminding Test Judgement Line Orientation COWAT SDMT PASAT Digit span f & b Stroop TMT A & B	RehaCom > control tapping group improved on 2/20 measures. Digit span forward* SDMT**	Computerized, group sessions with weekly meetings 6|12|60|12	Only CT	Yes, RehaCom training.	Yes. No changes in PDQ-39 scores or measures of mood

P value indicators:
*: <0.05.
**: <0.01.
***: <0.001.

limits the accessibility and independent performance of the CT regimen.

In a controlled, randomized, participant-blinded study, Zimmermann and colleagues [81] compared the effects of a structured CT program and an alternative, nonspecific treatment intervention, on measures of attention, executive function, visuoconstruction, and episodic memory. The CT group (N = 19) performed a series of training tasks on the computer using the CogniPlus software. The alternative treatment group (N = 20) played an interactive videogame which involved physical activity (WiiSports). Both training interventions ran for 12 sessions over the course of four weeks, each session taking 40 minutes and supervised by a psychologist or trained student, who were not blinded to group allocation. Neuropsychological assessment included parts of the Tests of Attentional Performance battery (alertness, working memory), the TMT, the Block Design Test from the Wechsler Intelligence Scale for Adults, and the California Verbal Learning Test. The alternative treatment group that completed training using the WiiSports games showed significant improvement on the alertness portion of the Tests of Attention relative to the CT group and a trend level improvement on tests of visuoconstruction and episodic memory. These results suggest that a *nonspecific training intervention might be as effective as a CT intervention in improving attention*. However, it is likely that the WiiSports tasks were more novel and engaging than the standardized CT program delivered using CogniPlus, which could explain the improvement in attention. Finally, as the authors note, there is increasing evidence that physical activity promotes cognition [83, 84], potentially accounting for these findings because performance of WiiSports games involves physical activity.

A summary of the studies discussed above is presented in Table 2. Due to largely varied methodologies and relatively small sample sizes it remains unclear whether CT is effective as a wide-spread, cognitive intervention in PD. Reviews of earlier CT studies noted similar limitations [85, 86]. Based on the research published to date, there is insufficient information to determine which training program or schedule is most likely to promote improvements, what outcome measures best estimate the impact of CT, and which cognitive functions benefit most from training.

Due to lack of standardized training programs in this field, there was little consistency or convergence between training tasks or outcome measures, making cross-experimental comparisons difficult and eliminating the opportunity for true replication. Moreover, some studies found improvement across a wide array of tasks and cognitive skills, whereas others found more modest and domain-specific effects. Even when there was improvement on outcome measures, it was seldom explained from a theoretical perspective by the cognitive elements that were targeted by the training regimen. Further, training did not often generalize to other untrained aspects of cognition.

More recent studies of CT in PD used active control groups and compared different CT interventions to one another, as well as to alternative interventions such as psychoeducation, physiotherapy, skill transfer training, and video-

games [72, 76–81]. However, there is still crucial information lacking that would enable predictions to the larger PD population or permit widespread and faithful application beyond the study. Studies need to (1) be clear about exact details of the intervention applied to the training group, (2) include larger sample sizes, (3) describe more fully the patient population characteristics in case only subgroups are expected to benefit, and (4) examine effects on QOL and long term outcomes. Providing detailed information about the methodology and task administration will enable comparisons of results across studies.

It is clear that there is burgeoning interest in CT as an intervention in PD, yet due to lack of methodological consistency even the positive results are difficult to evaluate across studies. This problem appears to permeate all areas of research of CT, in healthy younger and older populations, as well as in studies with clinical patients [57, 87]. Several reviews still note that methodological limitations are holding the field back [66, 87, 88], and these need to be addressed so that CT can be examined with the scientific rigor and standardized protocol that many pharmaceutical and behavioural interventions currently undergo. In effect, there are no clear replications and consequently the legitimacy of CT as a therapy for cognitive impairment in PD has not been conclusively determined. This is in line with a recent meta-analysis suggesting that the evidence for CT in PD is not robust and more research is needed [88]. In the discussion that follows we examine several of these issues in more depth and provide suggestions for unifying the research in this field.

3. Discussion

3.1. Cognitive and Demographic Profile of Participants and Implications for CT Effects. If investigations of CT in PD hope to address the ambiguity regarding training effects and the extent to which training can benefit individuals, there is a need to consider the cognitive and demographic profile of the studied sample. Demographic and clinical characterization of participants in future studies should more clearly describe the groups under study as these patient features might interact with CT effects. This will also define the groups to which findings might be applicable because PD patients can vary vastly in their cognitive aptitudes depending upon stage of disease, and some interventions might be more suitable to relatively unimpaired patients, whereas others could be particularly beneficial for patients showing more severe decline. Therefore, studies need to clearly describe the severity of disease and provide measures indicating the extent of cognitive decline, both as an overall score and ideally as a composite of different cognitive domains as recommended by the MDS Task Force [89]. It is also necessary to consider the effect different disease severity (as measured by the Hoehn and Yahr scale or the UPDRS) can have on the ability to complete the training intervention either autonomously or with assistance, and how this might impact performance on outcome measures.

Many studies of CT in PD exclude patients with dementia or MCI, enrolling only PD patients who are clinically cognitively intact. Considering that baseline cognitive function is a variable that will likely strongly impact CT effects, full characterization of PD patients included in studies needs to be disclosed. Finally, studies that explicitly contrast PD groups, formed on the basis of cognitive abilities, are needed to directly investigate this issue though only one has been conducted to date [70]. Of the studies reviewed, some included participants with MCI and others included only cognitively healthy patients (see Table 2). Since the effects of CT are likely different for cognitively healthy versus cognitively impaired participants, it is impossible to make conclusions about the effectiveness of CT when one study employs a cognitively healthy population and another employs patients with MCI. The interpretation of the results is limited further when the participants are not thoroughly defined in terms of their cognitive abilities or disease severity.

3.2. Mechanisms Underlying CT.

Over the last decade several studies found that CT can lead to functional and structural brain changes. Most commonly and reliably, fMRI studies have shown improvement-correlated changes in activation in frontostriatal networks, the dorsolateral prefrontal cortex (dlPFC), medial PFC (mPFC), and the parietal cortex (PC) following CT [61, 71, 90–94]. Functional connectivity (FC) analyses have revealed increased connectivity following CT in areas of the PFC, PC, and the basal ganglia [95, 96]. Studies have also observed functional changes using measures of cerebral blood flow (CBF) in the Default Mode Network (DMN) and the External Attention System, as well as globally [96, 97].

Recently, Chapman and colleagues [97] observed both functional and structural changes in healthy seniors following CT. The authors found increased global and regional CBF in the DMN and the central executive network as well as greater connectivity in these regions, compared to a waitlist group. They also found differences suggesting changes in white matter integrity, which could be due to increased axonal myelination. More support for structural changes comes from McNab and colleagues [98], who used Positron Emission Tomography (PET) and found changes in dopamine D1 receptor density and binding potentials in the PFC and PC after 14 hours (across five weeks) of training. These changes were correlated with behavioural improvement in WM tasks. Finally, in nonhuman primates, WM training has been shown to lead to changes in neuronal firing patterns, leading to the recruitment of more neurons but a less variable and correlated firing rate (for review, please see [99]).

These findings that CT leads to brain changes and potentially normalization of activation and connectivity patterns are intriguing and increasing the plausibility of CT as an effective therapy (see review in [91]). However, more research is needed to understand the nature of these changes. There is as of yet no consensus that these changes reflect actual restorative processes of impaired brain function/structure integrity in clinical populations. An alternative explnatio is that brain changes could reflect protection from cognitive decline given that these alterations occur in healthy older adults

performing CT who show less decline than a waitlist comparison group [97, 100]. The changes in brain activation and structure notwithstanding, at a behavioural level, CT likely imparts consciously and/or unconsciously developing cognitive strategies that permit more effective task performance. One such example could be the use of mnemonics or other memory aids, as well as chunking of items to reduce memory load (e.g., as in [93]). Ultimately, whatever the mechanism, whether due to neural alterations or acquisition of new, more effective cognitive strategies, it remains unclear whether these alterations are long lasting or temporary, and whether they correlate with improvement in daily tasks.

3.3. Selecting and Characterizing Outcome Measures of CT.

Before CT can be established as a therapeutic or preventative measure of cognitive dysfunction in PD, it is necessary to demonstrate that completion of a CT program translates into improvements in untrained contexts and activities. To evaluate the effectiveness of CT, there needs to be some indication that general skills or functions improve *and* that this improvement transfers to other untrained activities. Discussing CT-mediated changes with reference to learning and transfer of learning literatures (e.g., [91, 101, 102]), training on one task should, at a minimum, lead to improvements in similar tasks that invoke the same cognitive processes or strategies. This is termed *near transfer*. An example of near transfer would be improvement on an N-back task, requiring WM maintenance and updating, following training on a digit span task, also requiring WM maintenance. Though these are different tasks on the surface, both engage and depend on WM processes. In this way, improvements in one task following training of the other presumably result from general enhancement of WM processes. An ideal CT regimen, however, would not only produce near transfer effects but in fact optimize performance of very different tasks or skills, relying on quite disparate cognitive processes from those that were trained. This is referred to as *far transfer*. An example of far transfer would include practice on a digit span task augmenting efficiency of designing a multistep plan to achieve a goal in the Tower of Hanoi task. Far transfer effects potentially arise due to shared cognitive processes or strengthening of more general cognitive processing. CT-related improvements only on trained tasks that do not translate to benefits outside the specific experimental context, termed *direct transfer* or simply *training effects*, would be trivial, having little importance given the aim of addressing cognitive impairment in PD in the real world. That is, though training effects can have value in some scenarios where skill learning is the focus, for example, in learning to fly a plane, these would be insufficient to merit investment of time or resources for the stated purpose of preventing or remedying cognitive dysfunction in PD. Studies investigating CT effects need to state clearly the degree of transfer effects that they have achieved so their value can be understood.

Although there is some evidence of what might constitute far transfer of skills in PD in some of the studies that were reviewed, these effects are difficult to ascertain because often multiple tasks are included in training interventions without explicit design to test far transfer. In part this relates to the fact that most studies use training paradigms that are unfocussed, incorporating tasks that train many cognitive domains within a single regimen to increase the probability of a successful outcome. While pragmatic, this approach unfortunately makes it very difficult to identify the specific component(s) of the training intervention that promotes improvement. Future studies should employ the concepts of direct, near, and far transfer explicitly in their hypotheses, choice of interventions, and corresponding outcome measures to investigate these issues more clearly and provide a context for the results.

Ultimately, it is important to test whether CT leads to any QOL changes. Studies that have found improvement on these measures delivered CT either in a social group setting or in one-on-one sessions with an instructor (e.g., [69, 76, 77, 79]). In this way, the improvement was potentially confounded by increased social contacts and a greater sense of involvement in a community rather than the specific CT regimen. Although from a practical perspective these improvements are desirable regardless of the underlying cause, from the perspective of gaining theoretical understanding and for evolving recommendations regarding the most effective approaches, the specific effect of a CT regimen on QOL and mood needs to be isolated from other nonspecific effects. To tease apart these influences, it would be necessary to compare the same CT when self-administered versus when it was delivered in a group, attending to QOL changes related to each intervention. Future studies must establish whether CT specifically enhances QOL and performance of daily activities, as these are ultimately the changes that are most important to patients with cognitive impairments. Subjective benefit in real life function is an important endpoint. Many studies to date did not examine the effect of CT-derived improvements in PD on everyday QOL.

3.4. Description of Interventions. There is a significant lack of clarity, detail, and consistency regarding CT interventions in PD. No gold-standard CT program has been developed to date; consequently many different CT interventions have been investigated. A variety of tasks tend to be used as part of any given CT regimen. In some studies, the intervention comprised a developed standalone CT program, whereas in others, the intervention consisted of a multitude of training tasks with no overarching theoretical basis for inclusion. Additionally, when including a task as an outcome measure, it should be noted why this task is chosen and what is the expected outcome (e.g., decrease in reaction time, higher accuracy, and fewer steps taken). Interventions and outcome measures tend to be chosen due to convenience and availability, and no true replications have been achieved. There is a dire need for consistency in the literature so that results of different studies can be synthesized and compared in a more meaningful way. The design of future CT studies should be more programmatic and theoretically motivated. Ideally, the training regimen should consider known cognitive impairments in PD. The specificity of the target training regimen should be determined by comparing to a task or set of tasks that train cognitive skills that are not known to be impaired in PD. Finally, outcome measures should be selected to represent broad cognitive function to evaluate near and far transfer effects. Following this more reasoned approach, the probability of deriving CT programs that are effective and impactful seems increased.

A related issue is that some studies individually tailored CT to each participant, whereas others used the same tasks and levels of difficulty for all participants. Although tailored training in theory might be expected to lead to better outcomes, this has not been proven and therefore the time-consuming and costly nature of this approach is not empirically justified yet. To fully explore this, a study would need to directly compare a group receiving a tailored intervention (based on deficits in baseline performance) taken from a battery of standardized tasks, with another equivalent group receiving a random selection from the same battery of tasks. If the patients that received the individualized training benefit more from the intervention than the random training group, there will be merit in adjusting a training program for each participant on an individual basis. We offer that until such a study has been conducted, a middle ground would be selection of tasks and CT programs that take into account the cognitive profile of PD patients. That is, CT would be tailored not to each individual, but to the PD population as a whole. It appears that recent studies do indeed employ such an approach; however, there needs to be stronger theoretical backing for training task and outcome measure selection as described in the preceding paragraph. Finally, studies should attempt to select tasks and programs that have parallel versions to control for test-retest effects between baseline and posttraining. Again, direct transfer or practice effects are of little value given the aim of rehabilitating cognition in PD outside of the experimental context.

One of the challenges of CT programs is that they tend to be time-consuming and generally require the presence of an administrator to lead the session, especially during group sessions. This might limit the accessibility and availability of the CT program for patients who live remotely, mobilize with difficulty, or for other reasons are unable to attend the sessions. Some might simply prefer the convenience of in-home regimens. Computerized CT programs have been developed with these notions in mind and allow participants to complete the program on a variety of electronic devices, including home computers, laptops, and even tablets or phones. Computerized CT is potentially more convenient for some patients, allowing for more accessibility and conferring a feeling of autonomy. On the other hand, some patients might feel daunted by the technology which could be a disadvantage. Studies of computerized CT programs in healthy older adults and individuals with TBI, schizophrenia, and PD show that these computerized programs can be as effective as or even more effective than traditional pen and paper programs [48, 50, 56, 67, 94, 103]. It remains undetermined which approach is more effective in PD, however, without head-to-head comparisons. This is an important empirical question that needs to be resolved given the expense of one-on-one administration of some programs. Once again, a direct comparison of the same CT delivered by an administrator or in a pencil and paper version versus a computerized format is necessary to address this question. Until then, this remains a confounding factor with some studies administering computerized CT whereas others spend face-to-face time with patients to provide training.

Finally, there has been no investigation of the appropriate length of an individual training session or the number of sessions that are needed to produce positive effects. Further, the question of whether promoted changes are enduring remains unanswered. The duration of training courses seems chosen for practical reasons (e.g., the duration of admission to a rehabilitation center) or at random with virtually no justification for the parameters that were chosen. Going forward, investigating dose effects, by varying and comparing effects of more or less intense and prolonged CT regimens, will be needed.

3.5. Replication and Multiple Comparisons. Despite the many comparisons conducted in each CT study, there is seldom a statistical adjustment for multiple comparisons. This greatly weakens our confidence in the results, as performing a large number of comparisons will inflate the chance of finding differences in pre-post intervention measures or across comparison groups due to chance alone. This confidence would be increased if on an *a priori* basis a chosen regimen was predicted to improve some skills relative to others. Further, greater confidence would be inspired by similar effects of CT on outcome measures that gage the same cognitive domain. In our review, we often found inconsistent effects of CT on measures tapping into a common cognitive domain, though more often studies were simply not designed to allow for this conceptual replication. Most studies of CT train participants on a variety of popular and widely used tasks divided broadly into the areas of WM, attention, reasoning, planning, visuospatial processing, and verbal processing. Some studies find improvement across a wide array of tasks and cognitive skills, whereas others find more modest effects in only a subset of the outcome measures. In some studies, out of the many comparisons, only a few actually reveal any change or benefit, raising concern for the possibility of a Type 1 error.

4. Conclusion

Patients with PD are at an increased risk of cognitive decline. MCI and dementia are significantly more prevalent in PD relative to age-matched controls, and pharmacological treatments for these symptoms are modest at best. Consequently, developing alternative or adjunctive therapies is vital. To date, the small literature investigating CT in patients with PD suggests that these interventions are promising, at least in the immediate or short term for some cognitive domains. However, there remain many unanswered questions. Owing to a lack of consistency across studies in terms of participants included, outcome measures and training interventions selected, and modes of administration with few direct comparisons across alternative groups, regimens, or methods of administration, the efficacy of CT and the expected impact in PD remains largely unknown.

Indeed, it remains unclear if any element(s) in a CT regimen render it effective. The literature is mostly silent on the dosage of intervention required to produce changes and whether any improvements are enduring. There is also a vital need to address the generalizability of CT effects within the framework of transfer of learning. We highly recommend examining transfer of trained skills to practical and functional outcomes that are more similar to daily activities. Examination of QOL changes is also of utmost importance because ultimately the goal is for cognitive improvements to lead to an increased functionality and QOL. Lastly, and most importantly, to advance CT in PD literature, future studies need to provide clear and detailed justification and operationalization of outcome measures and training tasks. Significant changes in outcome measures achieved by training regimens that are rational, theoretically motivated, and hypothesis driven will inspire greatest confidence. Based on the current literature, it is premature to make recommendations for immediate and practical clinical application of CT in PD. This area of research remains in its initial stage but it is crucial that future investigations incorporate clear and appropriate controls, well-described and justified training and outcome tasks, and replications within and between studies.

Abbreviations

ACE:	Addenbrooke Cognitive Examination
ADAS-Cog:	Alzheimer's assessment scale
BADS:	Behavioral assessment of the dysexecutive syndrome
BDI:	Beck Depression Inventory
CES-D:	Centre for Epidemiological Studies-Depression Scale
CET:	Cognitive estimation test
COWAT:	Controlled Oral Word Association Test
CT:	Cognitive training
CVLT:	California Verbal Learning Test
D-KEFS:	Denis-Kaplan Executive Function Scale
f & b:	Forward and backward
H&Y:	Hoehn and Yahr Scale
MCI:	Mild cognitive impairment
MF:	Mentally fit
MMSE:	Mini-Mental State Examination
MOCA:	Montreal cognitive assessment
NV:	NeuroVitalis
PASAT:	Paced auditory serial attention test
PD:	Parkinson's disease
PDQ-39:	Parkinson's disease questionnaire
RBANS:	Repeatable battery for the assessment of neuropsychological status
ROCFT:	Rey Osterrieth complex figure test
RT:	Reaction time
SCOPA-Cog:	Scales for outcome of Parkinson's disease
SDMT:	Symbol digit modality test

SOPT: Speed of Processing Training
TIADL: Timed instrumental activities of daily
         living
TMT: Trail Making Test
TNP: Training
TOL: Tower of London
TUG: Timed-Up-and-Go Test
UFOV: Useful field of view
UPDRS: Unified Parkinson's disease rating
         scale
WAIS: Weschler adult intelligence scale
WCST: Wisconsin card sorting task
WISC: Wechsler intelligence scale-children's
         version
WM: Working memory.

Acknowledgments

This work was supported by a Canada Graduate Scholarship from the Canadian Institutes of Health Research awarded to Daniel Glizer and a CRC Tier 2 in Cognitive Neurosciences and Neuroimaging CRC Grant no. 950-230372 awarded to Penny A. MacDonald.

References

[1] J. Jankovic, "Parkinson's disease: clinical features and diagnosis," *Journal of Neurology, Neurosurgery and Psychiatry*, vol. 79, no. 4, pp. 368–376, 2008.

[2] D. Aarsland and M. W. Kurz, "The epidemiology of dementia associated with Parkinson's disease," *Brain Pathology*, vol. 20, no. 3, pp. 633–639, 2010.

[3] D. Aarsland, K. Andersen, J. P. Larsen, A. Lolk, H. Nielsen, and P. Kragh-Sørensen, "Risk of dementia in Parkinson's disease: a community-based, prospective study," *Neurology*, vol. 56, no. 6, pp. 730–736, 2001.

[4] P. Barone, D. Aarsland, D. Burn, M. Emre, J. Kulisevsky, and D. Weintraub, "Cognitive impairment in nondemented Parkinson's disease," *Movement Disorders*, vol. 26, no. 14, pp. 2483–2495, 2011.

[5] J. L. W. Bosboom, D. Stoffers, and E. C. Wolters, "Cognitive dysfunction and dementia in Parkinson's disease," *Journal of Neural Transmission*, vol. 111, no. 10-11, pp. 1303–1315, 2004.

[6] N. Caballol, M. J. Martí, and E. Tolosa, "Cognitive dysfunction and dementia in Parkinson disease," *Movement Disorders*, vol. 22, no. 17, pp. S358–S366, 2007.

[7] R. Cools, "Dopaminergic modulation of cognitive function-implications for L-DOPA treatment in Parkinson's disease," *Neuroscience and Biobehavioral Reviews*, vol. 30, no. 1, pp. 1–23, 2006.

[8] A. Costa, A. Peppe, G. Dell'Agnello et al., "Dopaminergic modulation of visual-spatial working memory in Parkinson's disease," *Dementia and Geriatric Cognitive Disorders*, vol. 15, no. 2, pp. 55–66, 2003.

[9] P. A. MacDonald, A. A. MacDonald, K. N. Seergobin et al., "The effect of dopamine therapy on ventral and dorsal striatum-mediated cognition in Parkinson's disease: support from functional MRI," *Brain*, vol. 134, no. 5, pp. 1447–1463, 2011.

[10] P. A. MacDonald and O. Monchi, "Differential effects of dopaminergic therapies on dorsal and ventral striatum in Parkinson's disease: implications for cognitive function," *Parkinson's Disease*, vol. 2011, Article ID 572743, 18 pages, 2011.

[11] A. A. MacDonald, O. Monchi, K. N. Seergobin, H. Ganjavi, R. Tamjeedi, and P. A. MacDonald, "Parkinson's disease duration determines effect of dopaminergic therapy on ventral striatum function," *Movement Disorders*, vol. 28, no. 2, pp. 153–160, 2013.

[12] J. B. Rowe, L. Hughes, B. C. P. Ghosh et al., "Parkinson's disease and dopaminergic therapy—differential effects on movement, reward and cognition," *Brain*, vol. 131, no. 8, pp. 2094–2105, 2008.

[13] N. I. Bohnen, D. I. Kaufer, R. Hendrickson et al., "Cognitive correlates of cortical cholinergic denervation in Parkinson's disease and parkinsonian dementia," *Journal of Neurology*, vol. 253, no. 2, pp. 242–247, 2006.

[14] S. Gilman, R. A. Koeppe, B. Nan ct al., "Cerebral cortical and subcortical cholinergic deficits in parkinsonian syndromes," *Neurology*, vol. 74, no. 18, pp. 1416–1423, 2010.

[15] P. Huot, S. H. Fox, and J. M. Brotchie, "The serotonergic system in Parkinson's disease," *Progress in Neurobiology*, vol. 95, no. 2, pp. 163–212, 2011.

[16] Z. Ye, E. Altena, C. Nombela et al., "Selective serotonin reuptake inhibition modulates response inhibition in Parkinson's disease," *Brain*, vol. 137, no. 4, pp. 1145–1155, 2014.

[17] K. Del Tredici and H. Braak, "Dysfunction of the locus coeruleus-norepinephrine system and related circuitry in Parkinson's disease-related dementia," *Journal of Neurology, Neurosurgery and Psychiatry*, vol. 84, no. 7, pp. 774–783, 2013.

[18] E. M. Vazey and G. Aston-Jones, "The emerging role of norepinephrine in cognitive dysfunctions of Parkinson's disease," *Frontiers in Behavioral Neuroscience*, vol. 6, article 48, 2012.

[19] D. Weintraub, S. Mavandadi, E. Mamikonyan et al., "Atomoxetine for depression and other neuropsychiatric symptoms in Parkinson disease," *Neurology*, vol. 75, no. 5, pp. 448–455, 2010.

[20] H. Apaydin, J. E. Ahlskog, J. E. Parisi, B. F. Boeve, and D. W. Dickson, "Parkinson disease neuropathology: later-developing dementia and loss of the levodopa response," *Archives of Neurology*, vol. 59, no. 1, pp. 102–112, 2002.

[21] W. J. Schulz-Schaeffer, "The synaptic pathology of α-synuclein aggregation in dementia with Lewy bodies, Parkinson's disease and Parkinson's disease dementia," *Acta Neuropathologica*, vol. 120, no. 2, pp. 131–143, 2010.

[22] J. J. Zarranz, J. Alegre, J. C. Gómez-Esteban et al., "The new mutation, E46K, of α-synuclein causes parkinson and Lewy body dementia," *Annals of Neurology*, vol. 55, no. 2, pp. 164–173, 2004.

[23] K. Seppi, D. Weintraub, M. Coelho et al., "The movement disorder society evidence-based medicine review update: treatments for the non-motor symptoms of Parkinson's disease," *Movement Disorders*, vol. 26, no. 3, pp. S42–S80, 2011.

[24] S. Vale, "Current management of the cognitive dysfunction in Parkinson's disease: how far have we come?" *Experimental Biology and Medicine*, vol. 233, no. 8, pp. 941–951, 2008.

[25] T. W. Robbins and R. Cools, "Cognitive deficits in Parkinson's disease: a cognitive neuroscience perspective," *Movement Disorders*, vol. 29, no. 5, pp. 597–607, 2014.

[26] D. M. E. Torta, L. Castelli, M. Zibetti, L. Lopiano, and G. Geminiani, "On the role of dopamine replacement therapy in decision-making, working memory, and reward in Parkinson's disease: does the therapy-dose matter?" *Brain and Cognition*, vol. 71, no. 2, pp. 84–91, 2009.

[27] D. Aarsland, U. P. Mosimann, and I. G. McKeith, "Role of cholinesterase inhibitors in Parkinson's disease and dementia with Lewy bodies," *Journal of Geriatric Psychiatry and Neurology*, vol. 17, no. 3, pp. 164–171, 2004.

[28] H. O. Tayeb, H. D. Yang, B. H. Price, and F. I. Tarazi, "Pharmacotherapies for Alzheimer's disease: beyond cholinesterase inhibitors," *Pharmacology and Therapeutics*, vol. 134, no. 1, pp. 8–25, 2012.

[29] J. Green, W. M. McDonald, J. L. Vitek et al., "Cognitive impairments in advanced PD without dementia," *Neurology*, vol. 59, no. 9, pp. 1320–1324, 2002.

[30] A. Kudlicka, L. Clare, and J. V. Hindle, "Executive functions in Parkinson's disease: systematic review and meta-analysis," *Movement Disorders*, vol. 26, no. 13, pp. 2305–2315, 2011.

[31] K. Pigott, J. Rick, S. X. Xie et al., "Longitudinal study of normal cognition in Parkinson disease," *Neurology*, vol. 85, no. 15, pp. 1276–1282, 2015.

[32] D. J. Zgaljardic, J. C. Borod, N. S. Foldi, and P. Mattis, "A review of the cognitive and behavioral sequelae of Parkinson's disease: relationship to frontostriatal circuitry," *Cognitive and Behavioral Neurology*, vol. 16, no. 4, pp. 193–210, 2003.

[33] D. Aarsland, K. Brønnick, and T. Fladby, "Mild cognitive impairment in Parkinson's disease," *Current Neurology and Neuroscience Reports*, vol. 11, no. 4, pp. 371–378, 2011.

[34] A. McKinlay, R. C. Grace, J. C. Dalrymple-Alford, and D. Roger, "Characteristics of executive function impairment in Parkinson's disease patients without dementia," *Journal of the International Neuropsychological Society*, vol. 16, no. 2, pp. 268–277, 2010.

[35] D. Muslimović, B. Post, J. D. Speelman, and B. Schmand, "Cognitive profile of patients with newly diagnosed Parkinson disease," *Neurology*, vol. 65, no. 8, pp. 1239–1245, 2005.

[36] A. A. MacDonald, K. N. Seergobin, A. M. Owen et al., "Differential effects of Parkinson's disease and dopamine replacement on memory encoding and retrieval," *PLoS ONE*, vol. 8, no. 9, Article ID e74044, 2013.

[37] D. Aarsland, J. T. Kvaløy, K. Andersen et al., "The effect of age of onset of PD on risk of dementia," *Journal of Neurology*, vol. 254, no. 1, pp. 38–45, 2007.

[38] D. Aarsland, K. Andersen, J. P. Larsen, A. Lolk, and P. Kragh-Sørensen, "Prevalence and characteristics of dementia in Parkinson disease: an 8-year prospective study," *Archives of Neurology*, vol. 60, no. 3, pp. 387–392, 2003.

[39] T. C. Buter, A. Van Den Hout, F. E. Matthews, J. P. Larsen, C. Brayne, and D. Aarsland, "Dementia and survival in Parkinson disease: A 12-Year Population Study," *Neurology*, vol. 70, no. 13, pp. 1017–1022, 2008.

[40] J. B. Leverenz, J. F. Quinn, C. Zabetian, J. Zhang, K. S. Montine, and T. J. Montine, "Cognitive impairment and dementia in patients with Parkinson disease," *Current Topics in Medicinal Chemistry*, vol. 9, no. 10, pp. 903–912, 2009.

[41] A. Schrag, M. Jahanshahi, and N. Quinn, "How does Parkinson's disease affect quality of life? A comparison with quality of life in the general population," *Movement Disorders*, vol. 15, no. 6, pp. 1112–1118, 2000.

[42] N. Klepac, V. Trkulja, M. Relja, and T. Babić, "Is quality of life in non-demented Parkinson's disease patients related to cognitive performance? A clinic-based cross-sectional study," *European Journal of Neurology*, vol. 15, no. 2, pp. 128–133, 2008.

[43] W. Reginold, S. Duff-Canning, C. Meaney et al., "Impact of mild cognitive impairment on health-related quality of life in Parkinson's disease," *Dementia and Geriatric Cognitive Disorders*, vol. 36, no. 1-2, pp. 67–75, 2013.

[44] K. Bronnick, U. Ehrt, M. Emre et al., "Attentional deficits affect activities of daily living in dementia-associated with Parkinson's disease," *Journal of Neurology, Neurosurgery & Psychiatry*, vol. 77, no. 10, pp. 1136–1142, 2006.

[45] D. Aarsland, J. P. Larsen, E. Tandberg, and K. Laake, "Predictors of nursing home placement in Parkinson's disease: A Population-Based, Prospective Study," *Journal of the American Geriatrics Society*, vol. 48, no. 8, pp. 938–942, 2000.

[46] K. Ball, D. B. Berch, K. F. Helmers et al., "Effects of cognitive training interventions with older adults: a randomized controlled trial," *The Journal of the American Medical Association*, vol. 288, no. 18, pp. 2271–2281, 2002.

[47] R. Nouchi, Y. Taki, H. Takeuchi et al., "Brain training game improves executive functions and processing speed in the elderly: a randomized controlled trial," *PLoS ONE*, vol. 7, no. 1, Article ID e29676, 2012.

[48] G. E. Smith, P. Housen, K. Yaffe et al., "A cognitive training program based on principles of brain plasticity: results from the improvement in memory with plasticity-based adaptive cognitive training (IMPACT) study," *Journal of the American Geriatrics Society*, vol. 57, no. 4, pp. 594–603, 2009.

[49] S. L. Willis, S. L. Tennstedt, M. Marsiske et al., "Long-term effects of cognitive training on everyday functional outcomes in older adults," *The Journal of the American Medical Association*, vol. 296, no. 23, pp. 2805–2814, 2006.

[50] A. M. Kueider, J. M. Parisi, A. L. Gross, and G. W. Rebok, "Computerized cognitive training with older adults: a systematic review," *PLoS ONE*, vol. 7, no. 7, article e40588, 2012.

[51] L. Mowszowski, J. Batchelor, and S. L. Naismith, "Early intervention for cognitive decline: can cognitive training be used as a selective prevention technique?" *International Psychogeriatrics*, vol. 22, no. 4, pp. 537–548, 2010.

[52] A. M. Owen, A. Hampshire, J. A. Grahn et al., "Putting brain training to the test," *Nature*, vol. 465, no. 7299, pp. 775–778, 2010.

[53] T. W. Thompson, M. L. Waskom, K.-L. A. Garel et al., "Failure of working memory training to enhance cognition or intelligence," *PLoS ONE*, vol. 8, no. 5, article e63614, 2013.

[54] C. A. Coelho, "Direct attention training as a treatment for reading impairment in mild aphasia," *Aphasiology*, vol. 19, no. 3–5, pp. 275–283, 2005.

[55] M. P. Sinotte and C. A. Coelho, "Attention training for reading impairment in mild aphasia: a follow-up study," *NeuroRehabilitation*, vol. 22, no. 4, pp. 303–310, 2007.

[56] K. D. Cicerone, D. M. Langenbahn, C. Braden et al., "Evidence-based cognitive rehabilitation: updated review of the literature from 2003 through 2008," *Archives of Physical Medicine and Rehabilitation*, vol. 92, no. 4, pp. 519–530, 2011.

[57] M. L. Rohling, M. E. Faust, B. Beverly, and G. Demakis, "Effectiveness of cognitive rehabilitation following acquired brain injury: a meta-analytic re-examination of Cicerone et al.'s (2000, 2005) systematic reviews," *Neuropsychology*, vol. 23, no. 1, pp. 20–39, 2009.

[58] O. Grynszpan, S. Perbal, A. Pelissolo et al., "Efficacy and specificity of computer-assisted cognitive remediation in schizophrenia: a meta-analytical study," *Psychological Medicine*, vol. 41, no. 1, pp. 163–173, 2011.

[59] M. M. Kurtz, "Cognitive remediation for schizophrenia: current status, biological correlates and predictors of response," *Expert Review of Neurotherapeutics*, vol. 12, no. 7, pp. 813–821, 2012.

[60] J. Dang, J. Zhang, Z. Guo et al., "A pilot study of iPad-assisted cognitive training for schizophrenia," *Archives of Psychiatric Nursing*, vol. 28, no. 3, pp. 197–199, 2014.

[61] E. Hoekzema, S. Carmona, V. Tremols et al., "Enhanced neural activity in frontal and cerebellar circuits after cognitive training in children with attention-deficit/hyperactivity disorder," *Human Brain Mapping*, vol. 31, no. 12, pp. 1942–1950, 2010.

[62] T. Klingberg, H. Forssberg, and H. Westerberg, "Training of working memory in children with ADHD," *Journal of Clinical and Experimental Neuropsychology*, vol. 24, no. 6, pp. 781–791, 2002.

[63] E. Hoekzema, S. Carmona, J. A. Ramos-Quiroga et al., "Training-induced neuroanatomical plasticity in ADHD: a tensor-based morphometric study," *Human Brain Mapping*, vol. 32, no. 10, pp. 1741–1749, 2011.

[64] M. S. Keshavan, S. Vinogradov, J. Rumsey, J. Sherrill, and A. Wagner, "Cognitive training in mental disorders: update and future directions," *American Journal of Psychiatry*, vol. 171, no. 5, pp. 510–522, 2014.

[65] S. L. Naismith, K. Diamond, P. E. Carter et al., "Enhancing memory in late-life depression: the effects of a combined psychoeducation and cognitive training program," *American Journal of Geriatric Psychiatry*, vol. 19, no. 3, pp. 240–248, 2011.

[66] M. Valenzuela and P. Sachdev, "Can cognitive exercise prevent the onset of dementia? Systematic review of randomized clinical trials with longitudinal follow-up," *The American Journal of Geriatric Psychiatry*, vol. 17, no. 3, pp. 179–187, 2009.

[67] F. D. Wolinsky, M. W. Vander Weg, M. B. Howren, M. P. Jones, and M. M. Dotson, "A randomized controlled trial of cognitive training using a visual speed of processing intervention in middle aged and older adults," *PLoS ONE*, vol. 8, no. 5, Article ID e61624, 2013.

[68] E. Sinforiani, L. Banchieri, C. Zucchella, C. Pacchetti, and G. Sandrini, "Cognitive rehabilitation in Parkinson's disease," *Archives of Gerontology and Geriatrics. Supplement*, vol. 9, no. 9, pp. 387–391, 2004.

[69] J. Mohlman, D. Chazin, and B. Georgescu, "Feasibility and acceptance of a nonpharmacological cognitive remediation intervention for patients with Parkinson disease," *Journal of Geriatric Psychiatry and Neurology*, vol. 24, no. 2, pp. 91–97, 2011.

[70] E. A. Disbrow, K. A. Russo, C. I. Higginson et al., "Efficacy of tailored computer-based neurorehabilitation for improvement of movement initiation in Parkinson's disease," *Brain Research*, vol. 1452, pp. 151–164, 2012.

[71] C. Nombela, P. J. Bustillo, P. F. Castell, L. Sanchez, V. Medina, and M. T. Herrero, "Cognitive rehabilitation in Parkinson's disease: evidence from neuroimaging," *Frontiers in Neurology*, vol. 2, article 82, 2011.

[72] S. L. Naismith, L. Mowszowski, K. Diamond, and S. J. G. Lewis, "Improving memory in Parkinson's disease: a healthy brain ageing cognitive training program," *Movement Disorders*, vol. 28, no. 8, pp. 1097–1103, 2013.

[73] J. D. Edwards, R. A. Hauser, M. L. O'Connor, E. G. Valdés, T. A. Zesiewicz, and E. Y. Uc, "Randomized trial of cognitive speed of processing training in Parkinson disease," *Neurology*, vol. 81, no. 15, pp. 1284–1290, 2013.

[74] G. Sammer, I. Reuter, K. Hullmann, M. Kaps, and D. Vaitl, "Training of executive functions in Parkinson's disease," *Journal of the Neurological Sciences*, vol. 248, no. 1-2, pp. 115–119, 2006.

[75] A. P. París, H. G. Saleta, M. de la Cruz Crespo Maraver et al., "Blind randomized controlled study of the efficacy of cognitive training in Parkinson's disease," *Movement Disorders*, vol. 26, no. 7, pp. 1251–1258, 2011.

[76] J. E. Pompeu, F. A. D. S. Mendes, K. G. D. Silva et al., "Effect of Nintendo Wii™-based motor and cognitive training on activities of daily living in patients with Parkinson's disease: a randomised clinical trial," *Physiotherapy*, vol. 98, no. 3, pp. 196–204, 2012.

[77] J. Peña, N. Ibarretxe-Bilbao, I. García-Gorostiaga, M. A. Gomez-Beldarrain, M. Díez-Cirarda, and N. Ojeda, "Improving functional disability and cognition in parkinson disease randomized controlled trial," *Neurology*, vol. 83, no. 23, pp. 2167–2174, 2014.

[78] A. Cerasa, M. C. Gioia, M. Salsone et al., "Neurofunctional correlates of attention rehabilitation in Parkinson's disease: an explorative study," *Neurological Sciences*, vol. 35, no. 8, pp. 1173–1180, 2014.

[79] I. Reuter, S. Mehnert, G. Sammer, M. Oechsner, and M. Engelhardt, "Efficacy of a multimodal cognitive rehabilitation including psychomotor and endurance training in Parkinson's disease," *Journal of Aging Research*, vol. 2012, Article ID 235765, 15 pages, 2012.

[80] A. Petrelli, S. Kaesberg, M. T. Barbe et al., "Effects of cognitive training in Parkinson's disease: a randomized controlled trial," *Parkinsonism and Related Disorders*, vol. 20, no. 11, pp. 1196–1202, 2014.

[81] R. Zimmermann, U. Gschwandtner, N. Benz et al., "Cognitive training in Parkinson disease: cognition-specific vs nonspecific computer training," *Neurology*, vol. 82, no. 14, pp. 1219–1226, 2014.

[82] M. Tonetta, *Il TNP: Un Software che opera in ambiente Windows. Atti del 4 Congresso Nazionale Informatica Didatticae Disabilita*, New Magazine Edizioni, Naples, Italy, 1995 (Italian).

[83] K. E. Cruise, R. S. Bucks, A. M. Loftus, R. U. Newton, R. Pegoraro, and M. G. Thomas, "Exercise and Parkinson's: benefits for cognition and quality of life," *Acta Neurologica Scandinavica*, vol. 123, no. 1, pp. 13–19, 2011.

[84] J. R. Nocera, L. J. P. Altmann, C. Sapienza, M. S. Okun, and C. J. Hass, "Can exercise improve language and cognition in Parkinson's disease? A case report," *Neurocase*, vol. 16, no. 4, pp. 301–306, 2010.

[85] J. Calleo, C. Burrows, H. Levin, L. Marsh, E. Lai, and M. K. York, "Cognitive rehabilitation for executive dysfunction in Parkinson's disease: application and current directions," *Parkinson's Disease*, vol. 2012, Article ID 512892, 6 pages, 2012.

[86] J. V. Hindle, A. Petrelli, L. Clare, and E. Kalbe, "Nonpharmacological enhancement of cognitive function in Parkinson's disease: a systematic review," *Movement Disorders*, vol. 28, no. 8, pp. 1034–1049, 2013.

[87] C. C. Walton, L. Mowszowski, S. J. G. Lewis, and S. L. Naismith, "Stuck in the mud: time for change in the implementation of cognitive training research in ageing?" *Frontiers in Aging Neuroscience*, vol. 6, article 43, 2014.

[88] I. H. K. Leung, C. C. Walton, H. Hallock, S. J. G. Lewis, M. Valenzuela, and A. Lampit, "Cognitive training in Parkinson

disease: a systematic review and meta-analysis," *Neurology*, vol. 85, no. 21, pp. 1843–1851, 2015.

[89] I. Litvan, J. G. Goldman, A. I. Tröster et al., "Diagnostic criteria for mild cognitive impairment in Parkinson's disease: movement Disorder Society Task Force guidelines," *Movement Disorders*, vol. 27, no. 3, pp. 349–356, 2012.

[90] E. Dahlin, A. S. Neely, A. Larsson, L. Bäckman, and L. Nyberg, "Transfer of learning after updating training mediated by the striatum," *Science*, vol. 320, no. 5882, pp. 1510–1512, 2008.

[91] T. Klingberg, "Training and plasticity of working memory," *Trends in Cognitive Sciences*, vol. 14, no. 7, pp. 317–324, 2010.

[92] Z.-C. Lin, J. Tao, Y.-L. Gao, D.-Z. Yin, A.-Z. Chen, and L.-D. Chen, "Analysis of central mechanism of cognitive training on cognitive impairment after stroke: resting-state functional magnetic resonance imaging study," *Journal of International Medical Research*, vol. 42, no. 3, pp. 659–668, 2014.

[93] P. J. Olesen, H. Westerberg, and T. Klingberg, "Increased prefrontal and parietal activity after training of working memory," *Nature Neuroscience*, vol. 7, no. 1, pp. 75–79, 2004.

[94] K. Subramaniam, T. L. Luks, C. Garrett et al., "Intensive cognitive training in schizophrenia enhances working memory and associated prefrontal cortical efficiency in a manner that drives long-term functional gains," *NeuroImage*, vol. 99, pp. 281–292, 2014.

[95] Y. Sun, F. Taya, Y. Chen, I. Delgado Martinez, N. Thakor, and A. Bezerianos, "Topological changes of the effective connectivity during the working memory training," in *Proceedings of the 36th Annual International Conference of the IEEE Engineering in Medicine and Biology Society (EMBC '14)*, pp. 6242–6245, Chicago, Ill, USA, August 2014.

[96] H. Takeuchi, Y. Taki, R. Nouchi et al., "Effects of working memory training on functional connectivity and cerebral blood flow during rest," *Cortex*, vol. 49, no. 8, pp. 2106–2125, 2013.

[97] S. B. Chapman, S. Aslan, J. S. Spence et al., "Neural mechanisms of brain plasticity with complex cognitive training in healthy seniors," *Cerebral Cortex*, vol. 25, no. 2, pp. 396–405, 2015.

[98] F. McNab, A. Varrone, L. Farde et al., "Changes in cortical dopamine D1 receptor binding associated with cognitive training," *Science*, vol. 323, no. 5915, pp. 800–802, 2009.

[99] X.-L. Qi and C. Constantinidis, "Neural changes after training to perform cognitive tasks," *Behavioural Brain Research*, vol. 241, no. 1, pp. 235–243, 2013.

[100] D. C. Park and G. N. Bischof, "The aging mind: neuroplasticity in response to cognitive training," *Dialogues in Clinical Neuroscience*, vol. 15, no. 1, pp. 109–119, 2013.

[101] S. M. Barnett and S. J. Ceci, "When and where do we apply what we learn? A taxonomy for far transfer," *Psychological Bulletin*, vol. 128, no. 4, pp. 612–637, 2002.

[102] A. B. Morrison and J. M. Chein, "Does working memory training work? The promise and challenges of enhancing cognition by training working memory," *Psychonomic Bulletin and Review*, vol. 18, no. 1, pp. 46–60, 2011.

[103] V. K. Günther, P. Schäfer, B. J. Holzner, and G. W. Kemmler, "Long-term improvements in cognitive performance through computer-assisted cognitive training: a pilot study in a residential home for older people," *Aging and Mental Health*, vol. 7, no. 3, pp. 200–206, 2003.

19

Determinants of Dyadic Relationship and Its Psychosocial Impact in Patients with Parkinson's Disease and Their Spouses

Michaela Karlstedt,[1] Seyed-Mohammad Fereshtehnejad,[1,2] Dag Aarsland,[3] and Johan Lökk[1]

[1] Karolinska Institutet, Department of Neurobiology, Care Sciences and Society, Division of Clinical Geriatrics, Novum Pl 5, Blickagången 6/Hälsovägen 7, 14157 Huddinge, Sweden
[2] Department of Neurology and Neurosurgery, McGill University, Montreal, QC, Canada
[3] Karolinska Institutet, Department of Neurobiology, Care Sciences and Society, Division of Neurogeriatrics, Novum Pl 5, Blickagången 6/Hälsovägen 7, 14157 Huddinge, Sweden

Correspondence should be addressed to Michaela Karlstedt; michaela.karlstedt@ki.se

Academic Editor: Hélio Teive

The caregiver-care receiver relationship (mutuality) in Parkinson's disease (PD) and its association with motor and non-motors symptoms, health-related quality of life (HRQoL), and caregiver burden have not fully been investigated. The aim of our study was to explore if (1) the level of mutuality perceived by PD-patients and PD-partners differs, (2) different factors are associated with perceived mutuality by PD-patients and PD-partners, and (3) mutuality is associated with PD-patients health-related quality of life (HRQoL) and caregiver burden. We collected data on motor signs (UPDRS III), non-motor manifestations (NMSQuest), PD-patients' cognition (IQCODE), mutuality scale (MS), PD-patients' HRQoL (PDQ8), and caregiver burden (CB) from 51 PD dyads. Predictors were identified using multivariate regression analyses. Overall, the dyads rated their own mutuality as high with no significant difference between the dyads except for the dimension of reciprocity. PD-patients' MS score ($p = .001$) and NMSQuest ($p \leq .001$) were significant predictors of PDQ8. Strongest predictor of CB was PD-partners' MS score (<.001) and IQCODE ($p = .050$). In general, it seems that non-motor symptoms contribute to a larger extent to the mutual relationship in PD-affected dyads than motor disabilities.

1. Introduction

Parkinson's disease (PD) is a complex neurodegenerative disorder resulting in a combination of motor impairment and a wide range of non-motor manifestations. Non-motor symptoms (NMS) can emerge from nearly all organ systems, such as neuropsychiatric, gastrointestinal, urogenital, and other autonomic presentations partly due to extrastriatal brain changes [1].

A body of evidence suggests that PD as a progressive disabling condition may lead to not only lack of autonomy due to increasing dependency but also placing an increased burden on caregivers and consequently has an impact on the care dyads' health-related quality of life (HRQoL) [1–5]. The construct of HRQoL is complex but can be defined as the "perception and self-evaluation regarding the impact of the disease and its consequences on his/her life in the terms of physical, psychological and social aspects" [4, 6].

Not all family members may regard themselves as caregivers, especially when symptoms are less severe in the early stage of PD. However, the inevitable course of the disease may result in functional dependency and need of help in order to perform daily activities. This can transform the quotidian caregiving activities and lead to emotional, social, and economic strain [7, 8].

An important aspect of caregiving situation is the relationship between the caregiver and care receiver. Research has demonstrated that the quality of relationship can affect caregiver outcomes [9, 10]. Mutuality, defined by Archbold and colleges as the positive quality of relationship, is now widely used to signify relationship quality [10–12]. Mutuality has four dimensions: love and affection, shared pleasurable activities, shared values, and reciprocity [11, 12]. A review suggests that high mutuality can be an important protective factor against caregiver burden in progressive conditions such as PD [10]. Conversely, low mutuality can be a risk factor for increased caregiving burden and depression for the caregivers. So far, the effect of mutuality has mainly been explored in PD caregiver samples [9, 13, 14]. Very few studies have explored mutuality from the perspective of the PD-patients and their partners and these studies have mainly been based on small sample sizes. Nonetheless, their result has suggested that perceived dyadic benefits of living with PD are associated with greater marital quality and that mutuality may act as mediator of PD-patients HRQoL [15, 16]. In contrast to studies with frail elderly and stroke patients [17, 18] Ricciardi et al. found PD-patients to be less satisfied with relationship than their partner. Furthermore, they did not find any association between mutuality and PD motor impairment or disease duration [19]. More research is needed particularly on the relationship of mutuality and motor and NMS.

Therefore, the aim of this study was to identify factors associated with mutuality, HRQoL, and caregiver burden. We used the modified stress-appraisal model proposed by Greenwell et al. (2015) to guide us in our analytic plan [9, 20]. The model suggests that primary stressors (e.g., disease-related factors) and the individuals' appraisal of the situation (e.g., carer involvement, coping strategies) have direct and indirect effects via protective factors such as mutuality on caregiver burden and HRQoL. Mutuality is also proposed to have a direct effect on caregiver burden and HRQoL. In the present study we only explored primary stressors association with mutuality and outcomes such as PD-patients HRQoL and caregiver burden. We hypothesized that there are (1) differences of perceived level of mutuality by PD-patients and PD-partners, (2) differences in factors associated with the mutuality of PD-patients and PD-partners, and (3) a relationship between mutuality perceived by PD-patients and PD-partners as well as PD-patients' HRQoL and caregiver burden.

2. Materials and Method

2.1. Participants. In the present study, we report results from baseline data of a longitudinal study. Fifty-one PD dyads were recruited during 2014-2015, from the movement disorders clinics at Karolinska University Hospital (n = 42), Sweden, and through advertisement in the journal of the Swedish Parkinson's Disease Association (n = 9). The study was approved by the local research ethics committee (registration number: 2013/1812-31/3) and was conducted in accordance with the declaration of Helsinki.

2.2. Eligibility Criteria. To be included in the study, a specialist in movement disorders should have diagnosed the PD-patient. They should be living together as partners (≥3 years), aged ≥55, but should not be in the phase of parenting small children. Furthermore, none of the PD-partners should be employed as a caregiver. Other eligibility criteria consisted of acceptable cognition based on Montreal Cognitive

Assessment (MoCA, [score ≥ 23]) and no severe medical conditions other than PD affecting daily life, which was judged by MK.

2.3. Procedure. The clinical examinations were performed by MK. The care dyads filled out the questionnaires' separately and individually, in the presence of the first author, at the outpatient clinic or during a home visit whichever was most convenient for the dyads. The questionnaires were filled out after having obtained, read, and signed a written consent. Descriptive and sociodemographic data was also collected.

2.4. Measurements

2.4.1. Dependent Variables. PD-specific HRQoL was measured with the Parkinson's Disease Questionnaire-Short Form (PDQ8). The scale comprises 8 items, using 5-point Likert scale, and covers domains as mobility, activities of daily life, emotional wellbeing, stigma, social support, cognition, communication, and bodily discomfort. A summary index (PDQ8SI) was calculated as the sum of items divided by maximum per item times number of items and then multiplied by 100. Higher scores, ranging from 0 to 100% indicate worse quality of life [21].

The caregiver's burden scale (CBS) was used to measure the PD-partners' reaction to caregiving. The scale contains 22 items and is answered using a 4-point Likert scale (1 = not at all to 4 = often). It covers domains such as general strain, isolation, disappointment, and emotional involvement. The total scale score ranges from 22 to 88. Higher score indicates more feelings of stress and burden in the caregiving situation [22]. The CBS has been used in samples of patients with Parkinson's disease and other neurological disorders [22–24].

2.4.2. Dependent and Predictor Variable. The quality of the caregiver-care receiver relationship was measured through the mutuality scale (MS) [11, 12]. The scale contains 15 items, where each item is answered using a 5-point Likert scale (0 = not at all to 4 = a great deal). It covers domains such as love and affection (3 items), shared pleasurable activates (4 items), shared values (2 items), and reciprocity (6 items) [12, 18]. The summary score is calculated as the mean value of all the individual items' scores for the whole scale and the above-mentioned domains. The total scale score ranges from 0 to 4. Higher scores indicate better quality of mutual relationship between the care dyads [11, 12]. We have recently reported the psychometric properties of the Swedish version of MS [25].

2.4.3. Predictor Variables. We used the Hoehn and Yahr (H/Y) scale to determine stage of PD. It contains 6 stages where 0 indicates no visible symptoms and 5 represents a PD-patient who is unable to walk unless assisted [26].

The Unified Parkinson's Disease Rating Scale-Part III (UPDRS III) was used to evaluate severity of PD-specific motor signs. The scale contains 14 items and is answered using a 5-point Likert scale. Higher scores indicate more severe motor signs [27].

The Non-motor Symptom Questionnaire (NMSQuest) was used to detect PD-specific non-motor manifestations in domains such as gastrointestinal, urinary, sexual function, cardiovascular, attention/memory, hallucination, depression/ anxiety, sleep/fatigue, and miscellaneous. The scale contains 30 items scored "yes" or "no." Higher score indicates higher frequency of non-motor manifestations [28].

Informant Questionnaire on Cognitive Decline in the Elderly (IQCODE) uses information from the caregiver to assess functional changes associated with cognitive functioning in the patients under care. The scale contains 26 items and is answered using a 5-point Likert scale. The individual score is calculated by the mean across all item scores, ranging between 1 and 5. Higher score (>3) indicates decline in cognitive functioning [29].

The PD-patients' physical functioning and level of dependency were assessed by the PD-partner using the modified form of the extended Katz index [30]. The scale comprises items assessing grooming/dressing, bathing, food intake, toileting, walking/transferring, housekeeping, and shopping. The scale is answered using a 4-point Likert scale (0 = no help to 3 = need all help). A dichotomous variable (0 = independent and 1 = dependent) was created aiming to assess dependency.

We also created a pooled dichotomous variable of the level of education of the PD-patient and the PD-partner (0 = either elementary, secondary, or only one with university education, 1 = both with university education).

2.4.4. Montreal Cognitive Assessment (MoCA).
To assess cognitive functioning, the MoCA screening instrument was used. Scores above 26 are considered to be normal [31].

2.5. Statistical Analysis.
Continuous and discrete numerical variables are described using mean and standard deviation (SD), whereas stages of PD assessed by H/Y are presented as the median and interquartile range (IQR). Nominal and categorical data are reported as relative frequency and percentages. Prior to the main analyses, we explored the normality of the distribution of all the dependent variables (DVs). Most of the dependent variables' total score were normally distributed with no excessive skewness or kurtosis. Spearman correlation coefficient was calculated to assess direction and magnitude of the correlation between potential predictors and the DVs. Correlation coefficients between 0.1 and 0.29 were considered as weak, 0.3 and 0.49 as medium, and >0.5 as strong [32]. Predictors with correlation coefficients > 0.1 were entered into the multivariate regression models. Our a priori hypotheses on the relationship between the included variables were guided by the aim of the study and the stress-appraisal model [20]. This means that disease-related factors, PD-patients, and PD-partners mutuality may be potential predictors of PD-patients' HRQoL and caregiver burden. Furthermore, disease-related factors may also predict mutuality.

Separate regression analyses were performed for each group and for each dependent variable; that is, we performed one regression analysis including predictors of PD-patients' MS and one including predictors of PD-patients' HRQoL. Furthermore, one regression analysis was performed with predictors of PD-partners' MS and one including predictors of caregiver burden. PD-partners' gender, age, and education

were used for statistical adjustments. Assumptions of linearity, normality, and homoscedasticity were examined through histogram and scatterplots of residuals (Table 5). No influential multivariate outliers were detected using Mahalanobis and Cook's distance (<1) [33]. The Mann–Whitney U test was used to test the differences of MS total scores and the dimension scores between PD-patients and PD-partners. Prior to data collection, sample size was calculated based on available data from previous studies reporting differences in MS scores between caregivers and care receivers [13, 17]. To detect a standardized difference of 0.63 between PD-patients and PD-partners, with a power of 80% and a two-sided significance level of 0.05, a total of 40 subjects in each group is required. To take into account possible drop-outs due to the longitudinal design of the project, 51 dyads were recruited. All data analyses were conducted using IBM SPSS Statistics for Windows, version 23 (IBM Corp., Armonk, NY, USA).

3. Results

3.1. Missing Data.
Two single missing items by two subjects within the NMSQuest scale were identified. These study subjects had individual scores larger than the samples median. To avoid case-wise deletion and loss of power, these missing values were imputed with a zero score.

3.2. Baseline Characteristics.
Mean age for the PD-patients was 70.9 (SD = 8.5) and 70.7 (SD = 9.3) years for the partners. Mean length of cohabitation was 38.4 (SD = 14.5) years. Other sociodemographic and clinical features are presented in Table 1. The most frequent reported NMS was nocturia (78.4%) and urgency (74.5%) (Table 2). Of the PD-patients 35/51 (68.6%) needed some form of supervision or help in daily activities. When help was needed the PD-partner was the main provider of that help. Instrumental activities such as shopping (32/51) or cooking/cleaning (28/51) were the most frequent tasks requiring help from the PD-partners (Table 3). Two PD-patients out of 51 (4%) were unable to be left alone in the home and 33% (17/51) could be alone between 2 and 12 hours. The remaining 63% (32/51) were able to be alone unlimited time.

3.3. Dyadic Differences in Total MS Score and Dimension Score.
There was no significant difference between the total scores of the MS in PD-patients (median = 3.4) and PD-partners (median = 3.1). Regarding dimensions of the MS, only reciprocity (median = 3.3 versus median = 2.8, $p = .014$) was significantly higher rated by PD-patients (Table 1).

3.4. Bivariate Correlations.
Table 4 summaries bivariate correlation coefficients between predictors and dependent variables. There was a significant correlation between PD-partners MS score and PD-patients MS score (rho = .524, $p \leq .001$). PD-patients' MS score had a significantly inverse correlation with PDQ8S (rho = −.516, $p \leq .001$) and UPDRS III (rho = −.311, $p = .026$) but not with caregiver burden and NMSQuest. PD-partners' MS score showed a significant inverse correlation with caregiver burden (rho = −.631, $p \leq .001$), PDQ8SI (rho = −.409, $p = .003$), and IQCODE

TABLE 1: Demographics and clinical features. n = 51 dyads.

		PD-patient	PD-partner
Female	n (%)	22 (43.1)	29 (56.9)
Level of education			
Elementary	n (%)	8 (15.7)	6 (11.8)
Secondary	n (%)	11 (21.6)	16 (31.4)
University	n (%)	32 (62.7)	29 (56.9)
Level of income (SEK)			
0–199,000	n (%)	13 (25.5)	13 (25.5)
200,000–450,000	n (%)	27 (52.9)	30 (58.8)
>450,000	n (%)	11 (21.6)	8 (15.7)
Retired*	n (%)	45 (88.2)	39 (76.5)
Working	n (%)	10 (19.6)	16 (31.4)
Total MS	m (SD)	3.2 (0.65)	2.9 (0.77)
Dimension of MS			
Love	md (IQR)	3.6 (0.67)	3.6 (1.0)
Shared pleasurable activities	md (IQR)	3.2 (1.25)	3.0 (1.25)
Shared values	md (IQR)	3.0 (1.0)	3.0 (1.5)
Reciprocity	md (IQR)	3.3 (1.0)	2.8 (1.67)
Total CBS	m (SD)		42.5 (15.8)
PD-duration	m (SD)	8.4 (6.4)	
PDQ8SI	m (SD)	27.4 (14.6)	
IQCODE	M (SD)	3.2 (.53)	
Hohen & Yahr	md (IQR)	2.0 (1)	
NMSQuest	m (SD)	12.1 (4.6)	
UPDRS III	m (SD)	18.1 (5.8)	
PD-patients self-rating of motor signs			
Tremor	n (%)	28 (54.9)	
Bradykinesia	n (%)	43 (84.3)	
Rigidity	n (%)	38 (74.5)	
Gait	n (%)	35 (68.6)	

Notes: PD: Parkinson's disease, MS: mutuality scale, CBS: caregiver burden scale, PDQ8SI: the Parkinson's Disease Questionnaire Summery Index, IQCODE: Informant Questionnaire on Cognitive Decline in the Elderly, NMSQuest: Non-motor Symptoms Questionnaire, and UPDRS III: the Unified Parkinson's Disease Rating Scale-Part III.
*Some of the study subjects were still working.

(rho = −.529, $p \leq$ .001) but not with NMSQuest and UPDRS III. Hoehn and Yahr stages had a significant correlation with mutuality, PD-patients' HRQoL, and caregiver burden.

3.5. Multivariate Linear Regression Analysis. Suspect multicollinearity (tolerance = ≤ .5, rho = ≥ .5) was detected between some of the included predictors. They were removed one by one and the variable that remained was the one with tolerance >.5, highest adjusted R^2 value, and the best fit regarding the assumptions of regression analysis. Contribution of each predictor to explain variance in the final multivariate regression models is presented in Table 5.

3.5.1. PD-Patients' Mutuality. In the final model with PD-patients' MS as the DV, the included predictors explained 31.6% of the variance. Of them, PD-partners' MS score (beta = .419, p = .002) and gender of the PD-partners (beta = .332, p = .017) contributed most of the explained variance.

Consequently, PD-patients' mutuality score was higher in those with a male partner and partners with high level of mutuality.

3.5.2. PD-Patients' HRQoL. With PDQ8SI as the DV, the included predictors explained 49.7% of the variance. PD-patients' MS score (beta = −.433, p = .001) and NMSQuest score (beta = .498, $p \leq$ .001) contributed significantly to the explained variance of PDQ8SI scores. In other words, patients with high level of mutuality had significantly better HRQoL (lower PDQ8SI), while an increasing frequency of NMS decreases the HRQoL.

3.5.3. PD-Partners' Mutuality. The included predictors explained 28.9% of the variability in PD-partners' MS scores. PD-patients' MS score (beta = .461, p = .002) and increased impairment of cognition (beta = −.314, p = 0.016) contributed significantly to PD-partners' mutuality.

TABLE 2: PD-patients* self-rated frequency of non-motor symptoms. $n = 51$.

	Yes n (%)
Dribbling	22 (43.1)
Taste/smelling	*28 (54.9)*
Swallowing	19 (37.3)
Vomiting	7 (13.7)
Constipation	25 (49.0)
Bowel incontinence	8 (15.7)
Bowel emptying incomplete	*26 (51.0)*
Urgency	*38 (74.5)*
Nocturia	*40 (78.4)*
Pain	17 (33.3)
Weight	12 (23.5)
Remembering	25 (49.0)
Loss of interest	12 (23.5)
Hallucinations	15 (29.4)
Concentrating	*28 (54.9)*
Sad, blues	24 (47.1)
Anxiety	20 (39.2)
Sex drive	16 (31.4)
Sex difficulty	*27 (52.9)*
Dizzy	*33 (64.7)*
Falling	25 (49.0)
Day time sleepiness	11 (21.6)
Insomnia	*28 (54.9)*
Intense vivid dreams	16 (31.4)
Acting out during dreams	18 (35.3)
Restless legs	*27 (52.9)*
Swelling	12 (23.5)
Sweating	14 (27.5)
Diplopia	20 (39.2)
Delusions	6 (11.8)

*PD: Parkinson's disease.
Italics: frequency > 50%.

3.5.4. Caregiver Burden. The explained variance of the included predictors in the model with CBS as the DV was calculated as 52.7%. PD-partners with high MS score (beta = $-.559$, $p \leq .001$) experienced less caregiver burden. A worsening of PD-patients' cognition increased the CBS score although it did not reach statistical significance (beta = .219, $p = .050$).

4. Discussion

4.1. Major Findings. Consistent with the result of other dyadic research with stroke patients and frail elderly, the average MS score was quite high and the patients tend to rate their mutuality higher than their caregivers [17, 18, 34]. However, in the present study the difference was not significant except for the dimension of reciprocity. This is

the first study, to the best of our knowledge, to explore mutuality from the PD-patient's perspective. We found that PD-patients with high level of mutuality also experienced high HRQoL. Similar result has been shown in a study of patients with dementia [35]. Furthermore, having a male partner was associated with higher rated level of mutuality, but not with better HRQoL. Research so far is inconsistent regarding gender and HRQoL even if Martinez-Martin et al. (2008) observed more anxiety and worse HRQoL in female caregivers [4, 36]. Mutuality has also been reported as a protective factor of caregiver burden, which is in line with our result showing that PD-partners who perceived high mutuality also experience lower caregiver burden [9, 11, 37, 38].

Both motor and NMS were correlated with the MS, PDQ8SI, and CBS scores even though neither H/Y nor UPDRS III significantly contributed to the explained variances in the subsequent regression analysis. According to prior research, it seems that NMS such as depression, impaired cognition, sleep disorders, and fatigue have a larger impact on PD-patients' HRQoL than motor symptoms [3, 5, 39–41]. Similar result has also been reported regarding caregivers' mutuality showing gait impairment correlating with mutuality but not as a significant predictor [14]. The negative impact of NMS on PD-patients' HRQoL and impaired cognition on caregiver burden was expected and has also been reported in an extensive literature review by Chaudhuri [1].

Another interesting finding which has not been reported, as far as we know, was that mutuality scored by one member of the dyad was the strongest contributor of the level of mutuality experienced by the other member of the dyad. Using the modified stress-appraisal model but with a dyadic perspective [9, 20], some of our results could hypothetically be explained by the relatively high reported frequencies of NMS such as sleeping difficulties (55%), nocturia (78%), and restless legs (53%). These NMS, if protracted and severe enough, may not only disturb the PD-patients but also negatively affect their partners in various aspects such as sleep quality. Furthermore, impaired concentration (55%) and dizziness (65%), which were commonly reported in this study, may also affect the partners' wellbeing through worries of fall and need of adaptation or adjustment of daily activities. On the other hand, it may also affect the patients' wellbeing due to an increased experience of dependency and loss of the role as a partner. Altogether, the balance of responsibilities, interdependency, and roles may alter and put a strain on the relationship. This is reflected in our results by the significant difference in the MS dimension of reciprocity. However, if the dyads succeed to find gratification, meaning, and support, high mutuality may ameliorate negative outcomes such as burden and improve HRQoL even though the disease severity worsens by time. Overall, our results encourage a dyadic perspective due to the potential impact perceived mutuality has on HRQoL and caregiving burden when evaluating PD-symptoms and tailoring interventions. Paying attention to the experience of mutuality by both members of the dyad will allow clinicians to detect high risk dyads and look for interventions that address the patient's and their partner's

TABLE 3: Frequency of PD-patients* who need help in different daily activities. $n = 51$.

	No help		Supervision		Some help		All help	
	n	(%)	n	(%)	n	(%)	n	(%)
Grooming/dressing	40	78.4	6	11.8	4	7.8	1	2.0
Bath/shower	38	74.5	6	11.8	5	9.8	2	3.9
Food intake	44	86.3	2	3.9	5	9.8	0	
Toileting	42	82.4	3	5.9	5	9.8	1	2.0
Walking/transferring	28	54.9	6	11.8	15	29.4	2	3.9
Cooking/cleaning	23	45.1	2	3.9	16	31.4	10	19.6
Shopping	19	37.3	1	2.0	21	41.2	10	19.6

*PD: Parkinson's disease.

TABLE 4: Spearman rank correlation coefficients between independent variables and dependent variables. $n = 51$ dyads.

	PD-patient MS		PDQ8SI		PD-partner MS		CBS	
	Rho	p value	Rho	p value	Rho	p value	Rho	p value
PD-patient MS	1.00							
PDQ8SI	−.516	<.001	1.00					
PD-partner MS	.524	<.001	−.409	.003	1.00			
CBS	−.262	.063	.292	.038	−.631	<.001	1.00	
UPDRS III	−.311	.026	.322	.021	−.255	.071	.286	.042
H/Y	−.290	.039	.413	.003	−.309	.027	.336	.016
NMSQuest	−.178	.212	.631	<.001	−.252	.074	.258	.067
IQCODE	−.229	.107	.285	.042	−.529	<.001	.618	<.001
Cohabitation	.056	.695	−.013	.925	.072	.614	−.296	.035
PD-duration	−.199	.171	.085	.563	−.100	.495	.053	.715

Notes: PD: Parkinson's disease, PDQ8SI: the Parkinson's Disease Questionnaire Summery Index, MS: mutuality scale, CBS: caregiver burden scale, NMSQuest: the Non-motor Symptom Questionnaire, UPDRS III: the Unified Parkinson's Disease Rating Scale-Part III, H/Y: Hohen & Yahr, and IQCODE: Informant Questionnaire on Cognitive Decline in the Elderly.

wellbeing. Interventions such as social support, respite care, couple therapy, or counseling may help the couple to adapt and adjust to the ever changing care situation and find inner strength to cope. This will allow the medical system to provide a quality collaborative care that can improve patient outcomes and ameliorate caregiver burden.

4.2. Limitations. The present study has some limitations. First, we have only explored disease-related factors and mutuality association with the dependent variables of interest in our study. This is shown by the relatively low explained variance in the regression models. Future research would benefit from exploring models with measurement of both PD-related and general factors affecting the caregiving situation. However, our results provide a starting point for future studies with a dyadic perspective in PD. Secondly, the cross-sectional design and the rather small sample size with predominance of patients with mild to moderate PD limit the generalizability and possibility of causal inferences. Nevertheless, this was the initial analysis of baseline data within an ongoing longitudinal study, and we are anticipating data that will enable assessment of changes during the follow-up. Thirdly, the use of PDQ8 as measurement of

HRQoL may not assess all suggested domains of the concept HRQoL. However, PDQ8 is a validated and a commonly used questionnaire in PD research and enabled us to compare our research with others.

5. Conclusion

The main findings of our study suggest that high level of mutuality experienced by the PD-patient was associated with their HRQoL. This was also shown in the PD-partner sample with an association between mutuality and burden. Furthermore, level of mutuality scored by one member of the dyad was shown to be a dominant contributor to the other member's mutuality. We do acknowledge that more research is needed including both PD-related and general factors in different PD settings. In general, it seems that NMS contribute to a larger extent to the mutual relationship in PD-affected dyads than motor disabilities.

TABLE 5: Multiple linear regression analysis to find predictors of the Parkinson's Disease Summary Index (PDQ8SI), caregiver burden scale, PD-patient mutuality, and PD-partner mutuality. n = 51 dyads.

	Unstandardized coefficients	Standardized coefficients	p value	95% CI	Tolerance/VIF
Dependent variable = PD-patient MS Adj R^2 = .316					
Predictors					
PD-partner MS	.356	.419	*.002*	.143–.569	.882/1.134
UPDRS III	−.023	−.205	.113	−.052–.006	.852/1.174
NMS	−.025	−.176	.169	−.061–.011	.866/1.155
*PD-partner gender**	.434	.332	*.017*	.080–.788	.759/1.318
Education**	.144	.110	.366	−.173–.461	.938/1.066
PD-partner age	−.001	−.016	.902	−.020–.018	.768/1.302
Dependent variable = PDQ8SI Adj R^2 = .497					
Predictors					
PD-patient MS	−9.655	−.433	*.001*	−14.862−−4.449	.752/1.330
UPDRS III	.090	.036	.749	−.475–.655	.814/1.228
NMS	1.592	.498	*<.001*	.871–2.313	.803/1.245
IQCODE	.034	.032	.762	−.190–.257	.911/1.097
PD-partner gender*	−4.329	−.148	.234	−11.565–2.907	.666/1.500
Education**	−3.353	−.115	.275	−9.471–2.766	.924/1.083
PD-partner age	−.190	−.121	.293	−.551–.171	.778/1.285
Dependent variable = PD-partner MS Adj R^2 = .289					
Predictors					
PD-patient MS	.542	.461	*.002*	.216–.869	.752/1.330
UPDRS III	−.013	−.101	.450	−.049–.022	.814/1.228
NMS	.011	.066	.621	−.034–.056	.803/1.245
IQCODE	−.017	−.314	*.016*	−.031−−.003	.911/1.097
PD-partner gender*	.039	.025	.865	−.415–.492	.666/1.500
Education**	−.117	−.076	.543	−.500–.267	.924/1.083
PD-partner age	−.009	−.104	.446	−.031–.014	.778/1.285
Dependent variable = CBS Adj R^2 = .527					
Predictors					
PD-partner MS	−11.541	−.559	*<.001*	−16.149−−6.933	.771/1.296
UPDRS III	.447	.163	.129	−.136–1.030	.852/1.174
NMS	.282	.081	.449	−.462–1.026	.839/1.191
IQCODE	.251	.219	.050	.000–.503	.802/1.247
PD-partner gender*	3.023	.095	.400	−4.143–10.188	.756/1.322
Education**	1.178	.037	.713	−5.250–7.607	.931/1.074
PD-partner age	−.253	−.148	.191	−.636–.131	.768/1.302

Notes: PD: Parkinson's disease, PDQ8SI: the Parkinson's Disease Questionnaire Summery Index, MS: mutuality scale, CBS: caregiver burden scale, NMSQuest: the Non-motor Symptom Questionnaire, UPDRS III: the Unified Parkinson's Disease Rating Scale-Part III, and IQCODE: Informant Questionnaire on Cognitive Decline in the Elderly. Italics: significant predictors.
* PD-partner gender = 0 = female, 1 = male.
** Education = 0 = either elementary, secondary, or only one with university education and 1 = both with university education.

Acknowledgments

The authors would like to thank all the participants. The study was supported by The Parkinson Foundation in Sweden with Grant no. 663/14.

References

[1] K. R. Chaudhuri, *Handbook of Non-Motor Symptoms in Parkinson's Disease*, Springer, Dordrecht, The Netherlands, 2012.

[2] J. Lökk, "Caregiver strain in Parkinson's disease and the impact of disease duration," *European Journal of Physical and Rehabilitation Medicine*, vol. 44, no. 1, pp. 39–45, 2008.

[3] D. Aarsland, J. P. Larsen, K. Karlsen, N. G. Lim, and E. Tandberg, "Mental symptoms in Parkinson's disease are important contributors to caregiver distress," *International Journal of Geriatric Psychiatry*, vol. 14, no. 10, pp. 866–874, 1999.

[4] P. Martinez-Martin, C. Rodriguez-Blazquez, and M. J. Forjaz, "Quality of life and burden in caregivers for patients with Parkinson's disease: concepts, assessment and related factors,"

Expert Review of Pharmacoeconomics & Outcomes Research, vol. 12, no. 2, pp. 221–230, 2012.

[5] B. Müller, J. Assmus, K. Herlofson, J. P. Larsen, and O.-B. Tysnes, "Importance of motor vs. non-motor symptoms for health-related quality of life in early Parkinson's disease," *Parkinsonism and Related Disorders*, vol. 19, no. 11, pp. 1027–1032, 2013.

[6] P. Martinez-Martin, "An introduction to the concept of 'quality of life in Parkinson's disease'," *Journal of Neurology*, vol. 245, supplement 1, pp. S2–S6, 1998.

[7] S. Carretero, J. Garcés, F. Ródenas, and V. Sanjosé, "The informal caregiver's burden of dependent people: theory and empirical review," *Archives of Gerontology and Geriatrics*, vol. 49, no. 1, pp. 74–79, 2009.

[8] L. K. George and L. P. Gwyther, "Caregiver well-being: a multidimensional examination of family caregivers of demented adults," *The Gerontologist*, vol. 26, no. 3, pp. 253–259, 1986.

[9] B. Goldsworthy and S. Knowles, "Caregiving for Parkinson's disease patients: an exploration of a stress-appraisal model for quality of life and burden," *Journals of Gerontology—Series B Psychological Sciences and Social Sciences*, vol. 63, no. 6, pp. P372–P376, 2008.

[10] E. O. Park and K. L. Schumacher, "The state of the science of family caregiver-care receiver mutuality: a systematic review," *Nursing Inquiry*, vol. 21, no. 2, pp. 140–152, 2014.

[11] P. G. Archbold, B. J. Stewart, M. R. Greenlick, and T. Harvath, "Mutuality and preparedness as predictors of caregiver role strain," *Research in Nursing & Health*, vol. 13, no. 6, pp. 375–384, 1990.

[12] P. Archbold, B. J. Stewart, M. R. Greenlick, and T. A. Harvath, "The clinical assessment of mutuality and prepardness in family caregivers to frail older people," in *Key Aspects of Elder Care: Managing Falls, Incontinence, and Cognitive Impairment*, Funk SG, E. M. Tornquist, M. T. Champagne, and R. A. Wise, Eds., pp. 328–339, Springer, New York, NY, USA, 1992.

[13] J. H. Carter, B. J. Stewart, P. G. Archbold et al., "Living with a person who has Parkinson's disease: the spouse's perspective by stage of disease," *Movement Disorders*, vol. 13, no. 1, pp. 20–28, 1998.

[14] H. Tanji, K. E. Anderson, A. L. Gruber-Baldini et al., "Mutuality of the marital relationship in Parkinson's disease," *Movement Disorders*, vol. 23, no. 13, pp. 1843–1849, 2008.

[15] S. Mavandadi, R. Dobkin, E. Mamikonyan, S. Sayers, T. Ten Have, and D. Weintraub, "Benefit finding and relationship quality in Parkinson's disease: a pilot dyadic analysis of husbands and wives," *Journal of Family Psychology*, vol. 28, no. 5, pp. 728–734, 2014.

[16] C. D. Morrow, K. Smentkowski, S. Schwartz et al., "Does spouse participation influence quality of life reporting in patients with Parkinson's disease?" *Quality of Life Research*, vol. 24, no. 1, pp. 245–249, 2015.

[17] K. S. Lyons, A. G. Sayer, P. G. Archbold, M. C. Hornbrook, and B. J. Stewart, "The enduring and contextual effects of physical health and depression on care-dyad mutuality," *Research in Nursing and Health*, vol. 30, no. 1, pp. 84–98, 2007.

[18] G. Pucciarelli, H. G. Buck, C. Barbaranelli et al., "Psychometric characteristics of the mutuality scale in stroke patients and caregivers," *The Gerontologist*, vol. 56, no. 5, pp. e89–e98, 2016.

[19] L. Ricciardi, M. Pomponi, B. Demartini et al., "Emotional awareness, relationship quality, and satisfaction in patients with parkinson's disease and their spousal caregivers," *Journal of Nervous and Mental Disease*, vol. 203, no. 8, pp. 646–649, 2015.

[20] K. Greenwell, W. K. Gray, A. van Wersch, P. van Schaik, and R. Walker, "Predictors of the psychosocial impact of being a carer of people living with Parkinson's disease: a systematic review," *Parkinsonism and Related Disorders*, vol. 21, no. 1, pp. 1–11, 2015.

[21] C. Jenkinson, R. Fitzpatrick, V. Peto, R. Greenhall, and N. Hyman, "The PDQ-8: development and validation of a short-form parkinson's disease questionnaire," *Psychology and Health*, vol. 12, no. 6, pp. 805–814, 1997.

[22] S. Elmståhl, B. Malmberg, and L. Annerstedt, "Caregiver's burden of patients 3 years after stroke assessed by a novel caregiver burden scale," *Archives of Physical Medicine and Rehabilitation*, vol. 77, no. 2, pp. 177–182, 1996.

[23] M. Caap-Ahlgren and O. Dehlin, "Factors of importance to the caregiver burden experienced by family caregivers of Parkinson's disease patients," *Aging Clinical and Experimental Research*, vol. 14, no. 5, pp. 371–377, 2002.

[24] U. S. Manskow, S. Sigurdardottir, C. Røe et al., "Factors affecting caregiver burden 1 year after severe traumatic brain injury: A Prospective Nationwide Multicenter Study," *Journal of Head Trauma Rehabilitation*, vol. 30, no. 6, pp. 411–423, 2015.

[25] M. Karlstedt, S. M. Fereshtehnejad, E. Winnberg, D. Aarsland, and J. Lökk, "Psychometric properties of the mutuality scale in Swedish dyads with Parkinson's disease," *Acta Neurologica Scandinavica*, 2016.

[26] M. M. Hoehn and M. D. Yahr, "Parkinsonism: onset, progression, and mortality," *Neurology*, vol. 17, no. 5, pp. 427–442, 1967.

[27] "Recent developments in Parkinson's disease. Edited by S. Fahn, C. D. Mardsen, P. Jenner, and P. Teychenne New York, Raven Press, 1986 375 pp, illustarted," *Edited*, vol. 22, no. 5, p. 672, 1987.

[28] K. R. Chaudhuri, P. Martinez-Martin, A. H. V. Schapira et al., "International multicenter pilot study of the first comprehensive self-completed nonmotor symptoms questionnaire for Parkinson's disease: The NMSQuest Study," *Movement Disorders*, vol. 21, no. 7, pp. 916–923, 2006.

[29] A. F. Jorm, "The informant questionnaire on cognitive decline in the elderly (IQCODE): a review," *International Psychogeriatrics*, vol. 16, no. 3, pp. 275–293, 2004.

[30] K. H. Asberg and U. Sonn, "The cumulative structure of personal and instrumental ADL. A study of elderly people in a health service district," *Scandinavian Journal of Rehabilitation Medicine*, vol. 21, no. 4, pp. 171–177, 1988.

[31] Z. S. Nasreddine, N. A. Phillips, V. Bédirian et al., "The montreal cognitive assessment, MoCA: a brief screening tool for mild cognitive impairment," *Journal of the American Geriatrics Society*, vol. 53, no. 4, pp. 695–699, 2005.

[32] J. Cohen, *Statistical Power Analysis for the Behavioral Sciences*, L. Erlbaum Associates, Hillsdale, NJ, USA, 1988.

[33] B. G. Tabachnick, *Using Multivariate Statistics*, Pearson Education, Boston, Mass, USA, 2012.

[34] S. K. Ostwald, M. P. Bernal, S. G. Cron, and K. M. Godwin, "Stress experienced by stroke survivors and spousal caregivers during the first year after discharge from inpatient rehabilitation," *Topics in Stroke Rehabilitation*, vol. 16, no. 2, pp. 93–104, 2009.

[35] H.-L. Huang, L.-C. Weng, Y.-H. Tsai et al., "Predictors of self- and caregiver-rated quality of life for people with dementia living in the community and in nursing homes in northern Taiwan," *International Psychogeriatrics*, vol. 27, no. 5, pp. 825–836, 2015.

[36] P. Martinez-Martin, S. Arroyo, J. M. Rojo-Abuin et al., "Burden, perceived health status, and mood among caregivers of Parkinson's disease patients," *Movement Disorders*, vol. 23, no. 12, pp. 1673–1680, 2008.

[37] Y.-I. L. Shyu, C.-T. Yang, C.-C. Huang, H.-C. Kuo, S.-T. Chen, and W.-C. Hsu, "Influences of mutuality, preparedness, and balance on caregivers of patients with dementia," *The journal of nursing research : JNR*, vol. 18, no. 3, pp. 155–163, 2010.

[38] C.-Y. Hsiao and Y.-F. Tsai, "Caregiver burden and satisfaction in families of individuals with schizophrenia," *Nursing Research*, vol. 63, no. 4, pp. 260–269, 2014.

[39] Z. Qin, L. Zhang, F. Sun et al., "Health related quality of life in early Parkinson's disease: impact of motor and non-motor symptoms, results from Chinese levodopa exposed cohort," *Parkinsonism and Related Disorders*, vol. 15, no. 10, pp. 767–771, 2009.

[40] G. W. Duncan, T. K. Khoo, A. J. Yarnall et al., "Health-related quality of life in early Parkinson's disease: the impact of nonmotor symptoms," *Movement Disorders*, vol. 29, no. 2, pp. 195–202, 2014.

[41] S.-M. Fereshtehnejad, M. Shafieesabet, F. Farhadi et al., "Heterogeneous determinants of quality of life in different phenotypes of Parkinson's disease," *PLoS ONE*, vol. 10, no. 9, Article ID e0137081, 2015.

20

Health-Related Quality of Life Subdomains in Patients with Parkinson's Disease: The Role of Gender

Anja Ophey ⓘ,[1] Carsten Eggers,[2,3] Richard Dano,[1] Lars Timmermann,[2,3] and Elke Kalbe ⓘ[1]

[1]Department of Medical Psychology | Neuropsychology and Gender Studies and Center for Neuropsychological Diagnostics and Intervention (CeNDI), University Hospital Cologne, Kerpener Str. 68, 50937 Cologne, Germany
[2]Department of Neurology, University Hospital Cologne, Kerpener Str. 62, 50937 Cologne, Germany
[3]Department of Neurology, University Hospital Gießen Marburg, Baldingerstraße, 35043 Marburg, Germany

Correspondence should be addressed to Elke Kalbe; Elke.Kalbe@uk-koeln.de

Academic Editor: Seyed-Mohammad Fereshtehnejad

The most frequently used instrument to assess health-related quality of life (HrQoL) in Parkinson's disease (PD) is the Parkinson's Disease Questionnaire 39 (PDQ-39). However, both the dimensionality of the eight PDQ-39 subscales and their summary score recently faced criticism. Furthermore, data on disease-related and neuropsychological determinants and the role of gender on HrQoL in PD are inconclusive yet. Therefore, our aim was to reevaluate the PDQ-39 structure and to further explore determinants of HrQoL in PD. 245 PD patients (age: $M = 69.64$, SD = 8.43; 62.9% male; H&Y: Md = 3.00; cognitive assessment with PANDA: $M = 24.82$, SD = 3.57) from the baseline database of the Cologne Parkinson Network were used to reevaluate the dimensionality of the PDQ-39 with a principal component analysis (PCA). Multiple regression analyses were conducted to clarify general and domain-specific relationships between clinical, (neuro)psychological, and sociodemographic variables, gender in particular, and HrQoL. The PCA identified three HrQoL domains: physical-functioning, cognition, and socioemotional HrQoL. Depressive symptoms were identified as the most important determinant of HrQoL across all models. Disease-related HrQoL determinants (UPDRS-III, H&Y stage, and LEDD) were less strong and consistent HrQoL determinants than nonmotor symptoms. Analyses did not reveal a global gender effect; however, female gender was a negative predictor for physical-functioning and socioemotional HrQoL, whereas male gender was a negative predictor for cognition HrQoL. Our analyses suggest the consideration of a reevaluation of the PDQ-39. Only the full understanding of HrQoL, its determinants, and their interrelationships will allow the development of PD intervention strategies focusing on what matters the most for patients' HrQoL. Gender is one relevant variable that should be considered in this context.

1. Introduction

Still considered as a paradigmatic movement disorder, Parkinson's disease (PD) is associated with cognitive dysfunctions, depressive symptoms, and a broad spectrum of other nonmotor symptoms (NMS; [1]), as well. Focusing on quality of life in relation to the impact of disease on patients' physical, mental (i.e., emotional and cognitive), and social well-being after diagnosis and treatment, health-related quality of life (HrQoL) has become the preferred concept, when assessing the impact of disease and treatment on the lives of patients [2–4].

To assess HrQoL as a health outcome in PD patients, the Parkinson's Disease Questionnaire 39 (PDQ-39; [5, 6]) was

identified as the most appropriate, thoroughly tested, and used questionnaire [7]. The PDQ-39 comprises eight HrQoL subscales [5], commonly summarized by a PDQ-39 summary score [6]. However, recent evidence challenges the validity and interpretability of this summary index. Hagell and Nilsson [8] found that neither Rasch analysis nor confirmatory factor analysis supports for the unidimensionality of the PDQ-39, thus questioning the PDQ-39 summary index. Similarly, the eight-dimensional structure of the PDQ-39 faces criticism to be over-complex and the integration of HrQoL dimensions to a more theoretical framework is demanded [9]. Therefore, one goal of this study was to summarize the eight predefined HrQoL domains to a more meaningful and less complex domain structure based on statistical procedures to reduce data dimensionality. The recent review of Martinez-Martin [2] emphasized the general importance of a critical evaluation of (Hr)QoL instruments in terms of appropriateness, validity, and psychometric properties.

In a systematic review on HrQoL determinants in PD patients, the influence of NMS to HrQoL, especially depressive symptoms, was highlighted [10]. The negative influence of depression on HrQoL does act not only directly but also indirectly by increasing disability and cognitive dysfunction, which are themselves considered to be negative HrQoL determinants [11–13]. Disease-related HrQoL determinants such as the severity of motor impairment, the overall disease severity, and the levodopa equivalent daily dose (LEDD) were typically less strong and consistent HrQoL determinants than the NMS including depression [10, 14–16]. Concerning demographic variables, heterogeneous results occur, and more studies are necessary to evaluate the influence of age and gender, for example.

Especially for NMS, the existence of gender differences is commonly assumed [17, 18]. However, only a minority of studies was able to identify gender as an independent HrQoL determinant, as the special association of female gender with NMS frequently accounted for observed gender differences in HrQoL [19]. Those findings get even more complex, when gender differences in specific HrQoL domains are taken into account [20, 21]. Emerging evidence for general versus domain-specific relationships in HrQoL determinants is another reason, why an assessment of domain-specific HrQoL determinants might be of special scientific interest: whereas mental health variables were found to be independent HrQoL determinants across all HrQoL dimensions, more domain-specific effects were found in motor-related HrQoL domains [14, 15].

Taken together, the potential of scientific access into the relationships of clinical and sociodemographic HrQoL determinants is far from fully utilized. Thus, the aims of this study were (i) to reevaluate the structure of the PDQ-39 by reducing the number of HrQoL subscales on the basis of the already existing eight-dimensional structure, to further clarify (ii) general and (iii) domain-specific relationships between clinical and sociodemographic variables, gender in particular, and HrQoL of PD patients, and (iv) to explore gender-specific manifestations and moderating effects of depressive symptoms and cognitive impairment onto those relationships. For this purpose, analyses were conducted in use of a large clinical database of the Cologne Parkinson Network (CPN, http://www.koelner-parkinson-netzwerk. uk-koeln.de; [22]).

2. Materials and Methods

2.1. Participants. For this study, baseline data from the CPN were used. Participants were recruited between January 2012 and July 2015 at the University Hospital of Cologne, Germany, in cooperation with community-based neurologists in greater Cologne. After signing the informed consent form, participants were assessed clinically and neuropsychologically by movement disorder-specialized neurologists or a PD nurse.

To be eligible for enrolment in the CPN study, participants had to be aged 25–85 years, be diagnosed with idiopathic PD according to UK Parkinson's Disease Society Brain Bank diagnostic criteria [23], and have sufficient language ability in German. Exclusion criteria were psychiatric or neurological disorders, severe depressive symptoms operationalized by the Beck's Depression Inventory II [24] (BDI-II; cutoff ≥29), and severe cognitive impairment operationalized by the Parkinson Neuropsychometric Dementia Assessment (PANDA; cutoff ≤14; [25]).

2.2. Clinical and Neuropsychological Assessment

2.2.1. Health-Related Quality of Life Assessment. The PDQ-39 [5, 6], a disease-specific, self-evaluative HrQoL instrument, was used to assess HrQoL, with each of the 39 items to be scored on a 5-level scale from 0 (never) to 4 (always). Eight subscale scores and a global HrQoL summary score can be calculated, with all answers being transformed to a 0–100 scale and higher scores representing worse HrQoL. The eight PDQ-39 subscales are mobility, activities of daily living, emotional well-being, stigma, social support, cognitive impairment, communication, and bodily discomfort.

2.2.2. Assessment of Cognition and Nonmotor Symptoms. Global cognitive functioning was assessed with the PANDA (maximum score = 30; [25]), a PD specific cognitive screening tool to assess typical cognitive dysfunctions resulting in mild cognitive impairment in PD (PD-MCI, score 15–17) and dementia (cutoff ≤14). To assess depressive symptoms, the BDI-II (maximum score = 63; [24]), a 21-item self-evaluation questionnaire, was used. A BDI-II score of 9 to 13 reflects minimal depressive symptoms, a score of 14 to 19 mild depressive symptoms, a score of 20 to 28 moderate depressive symptoms, and a score of ≥29 accounts for a severe depressive symptomology. The presence and severity of other NMS was evaluated with the Nonmotor Symptom Scale (NMSS; maximum score = 360; [26]), a 30-item self-evaluation questionnaire.

2.2.3. Clinical Assessment. Disease duration as the time since diagnosis and medication was recorded, as well as the LEDD summarizing the patient's total dopaminergic treatment [27]. Motor impairment was assessed with the motor examination of the Unified Parkinson's Disease Rating Scale Part III (UPDRS-III; [28]) and the Hoehn and Yahr (H&Y; [29]) scale.

2.3. Ethical Approval. The study was conducted in compliance with the World Medical Association Declaration of Helsinki (1975). The study protocol was approved by the Ethics Committee of the Medical Faculty of the University of Cologne (Number 11-233) and registered in the German Clinical Trials Register (DRKS00003452).

TABLE 1: Summary of study sample characteristics and gender comparisons ($n = 245$).

	Max. score	M (SD) range			p
		Total ($n = 245$)	Women ($n = 91$)	Men ($n = 154$)	
Age	—	69.64 (8.43) 41–86	70.16 (7.42) 47–86	69.34 (8.99) 41–83	0.955[b]
PDQ-39	100	26.23 (15.08) 0–79.95	26.97 (14.32) 0–79.95	25.79 (15.54) 1.67–67.61	0.341[b]
PDQ-39 physical-functioning[a]	100	31.80 (20.17) 0–86.94	33.61 (19.34) 0–79.17	30.73 (20.63) 0–86.94	0.154[b]
PDQ-39 cognition[a]	100	26.62 (17.66) 0–83.34	22.77 (15.70) 0–66.66	28.90 (18.40) 0–83.34	**0.017**[b]
PDQ-39 socioemotional[a]	100	20.36 (15.40) 0–89.58	23.02 (16.01) 0–89.58	18.79 (14.85) 0–56.25	**0.032**[b]
PANDA	30	24.82 (3.57) 14–30	25.60 (3.09) 17–30	24.36 (3.76) 14–30	**0.020**[b]
BDI-II	63	12.10 (7.80) 0–38	13.03 (7.67) 0–37	11.55 (7.84) 0–38	0.090[b]
NMSS	360	57.31 (31.76) 6–198	55.62 (26.15) 8–122	58.32 (34.69) 6–198	0.987[b]
UPDRS-III	108	28.09 (8.94) 9–65	26.87 (8.36) 11–51	28.81 (9.21) 9–65	0.087[b]
Disease duration	—	5.88 (5.73)	6.20 (5.76)	5.69 (5.72)	0.426[b]
H&Y	5	0: 25 1: 29 2: 87 3: 106 4: 23	0: 23 1: 11 2: 34 3: 35 4: 11	0: 25 1: 18 2: 53 3: 71 4: 12	0.563[c]
LEDD	—	610.07 (408.29) 0–2065	580.94 (433.05) 0–2065	627.28 (393.36) 0–1780	0.204[b]

Note. Significant gender comparisons appear in bold. BDI-II = Beck's Depression Inventory II; H&Y = Hoehn and Yahr stage; LEDD = levodopa equivalent daily dose; NMSS = Nonmotor Symptom Scale; PANDA = Parkinson Neuropsychometric Dementia Assessment; PDQ-39 = Parkinson's Disease Questionnaire 39; UPDRS-III = Unified Parkinson's Disease Rating Scale Part III. [a]For a detailed description of PDQ-39 physical-functioning, cognition, and socioemotional component scores, see principal component analysis; [b]comparison between women and men with the Mann–Whitney U test; [c]comparison between women and men with the chi-square test.

2.4. Statistical Analyses. Statistical analyses were conducted using R (http://www.r-project.org). Normal distributions were tested using the Shapiro–Wilk test. Sample characteristics were calculated and compared between genders with Mann–Whitney U tests and chi-square tests, each with a significance level of $\alpha = 0.05$. Correlation coefficient r was reported as effect size for Mann–Whitney U tests.

A higher-order principal component analysis (PCA) was conducted on the eight PDQ-39 subscales, as for example used to develop and validate the PDQ-39 summary score [6, 30]. However, we used Jolliffe's instead of Kaiser's criterion to extract the underlying number of components. Furthermore, to ensure interpretability of the extracted components, and as we assume substantial interrelations between the HrQoL dimensions, we conducted oblique promax rotation on the identified components. Multiple regressions were then used to analyze HrQoL determinants. Baseline HrQoL operationalized by the PDQ-39 total score and the HrQoL domains identified by the PCA, with component scores calculated as mean score of the contributing PDQ-39 subscales, were used as dependent variables in distinct models. Based on the current literature, gender, age, PANDA score, BDI-II score, NMSS score, UPDRS-III score, disease duration, H&Y stage, and LEDD were integrated in the regression models. To further explore

relationships between HrQoL determinants, moderated domain-specific HrQoL models extending the domain-specific basic models by gender-specific effects were explored. Significance level for multiple regression analyses was set at $\alpha = 0.05$. Unstandardized (B) and standardized (β) regression coefficients, t-tests for regression coefficients, relative importance of each determinant (R^2), multiple R^2, and adjusted R^2 were reported for each model. Global model fit was tested via F-tests. Assumptions for multiple regressions were checked.

3. Results

3.1. Study Sample Characteristics. Our sample from the baseline data set of the CPN study included 245 patients (37.1% women). Sociodemographic and clinical data of the study sample and gender comparisons are displayed in Table 1. As indicated by Shapiro–Wilk-tests, sample characteristics were not assumed to be normally distributed ($ps < 0.001$). Corresponding q-q plots for all variables are displayed in Figure S1 (Supplementary Materials). Patients were aged 41 to 86 years ($M = 69.64$, SD = 8.43) with disease duration ranging from just recently to 25 years ($M = 5.88$, SD = 5.73). More than 90% of the patients' PANDA scores fell in the range of normal cognitive functioning ($M = 24.82$,

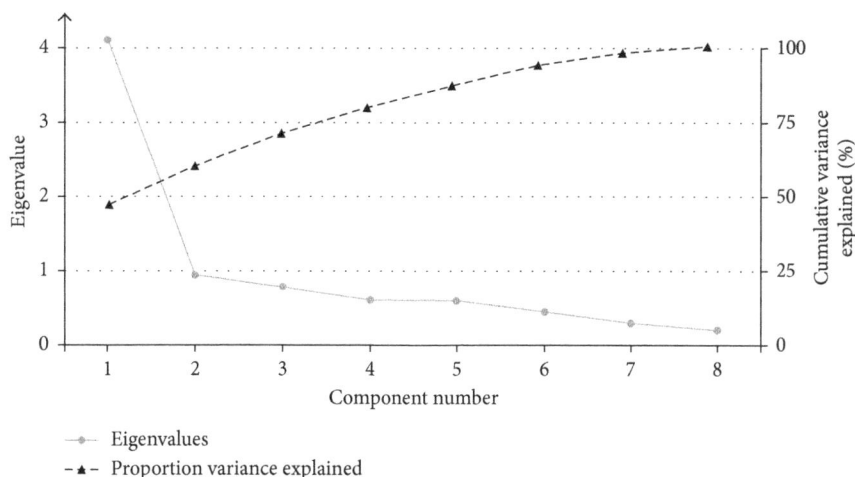

FIGURE 1: Screeplot of the eigenvalues obtained in the principal component analysis on the eight subscales of the Parkinson's Disease Questionnaire and cumulative variance explained across the eight components.

SD = 3.57) and on average, depressive symptoms rated with the BDI-II were minimal to mild ($M = 12.10$, SD = 7.80).

Men and women did not significantly differ in terms of age, reported global HrQoL, severity of NMS, disease duration, and LEDD. The distribution of disease severity according to H&Y stages was comparable between genders. However, PANDA scores were significantly higher for women than for men ($W = 8248$, $p = 0.020$, $r = 0.15$). Additionally, results revealed a nonsignificant tendency for women reporting more severe depressive symptoms than men (BDI-II, $W = 7915$, $p = 0.090$, $r = 0.11$) and men showing more severe motor impairment than women (UPDRS-III, $W = 6090$, $p = 0.087$, $r = 0.11$).

3.2. Principal Component Analysis. A PCA was conducted on the eight subscales of the PDQ-39. During an initial analysis without rotation and the maximum number of eight components, only one component had an eigenvalue over Kaiser's criterion of 1 and explained 51% of the variance, which converges well with evidence from earlier studies evaluating the dimensionality of the PDQ-39 [6, 31, 32]. However, three components had eigenvalues over Jolliffe's criterion of 0.70 and in combination explained 73% of the variance, exceeding the 60% criterion [33]. The eigenvalues of each component are displayed in the screeplot of Figure 1, as well as the cumulative variance explained by each of the initial eight components.

As a three-component structure is also compatible with emerging criticism concerning the PDQ-39 structure [8, 9], three components were retained in the subsequent PCA with oblique promax rotation. The PDQ-39 subscales that cluster on the same components suggest that component 1 featuring the PDQ-39 subscales bodily discomfort, mobility, and activities of daily living represents physical-functioning HrQoL (eigenvalue = 2.27, Cronbach's $\alpha = .81$), component 2 featuring the PDQ-39 subscales communication and cognitive impairment represents cognition HrQoL (eigenvalue = 1.91, Cronbach's $\alpha = 0.76$), and component 3 featuring the PDQ-39 subscales emotional well-being,

stigma, and social support represents socioemotional HrQoL (eigenvalue = 1.67, Cronbach's $\alpha = 0.72$). Tables S2 and S3 (Supplementary Materials) display the factor loadings of the pattern and structure matrix after oblique promax rotation.

3.3. Basic Health-Related Quality of Life Models. Four basic HrQoL models with PDQ-39 summary score, physical-functioning, cognition, and socioemotional scores as dependent variables were calculated. The multiple regression models for global (g), physical-functioning (p), cognition (c), and socioemotional (s) HrQoL explained 65.1%, 59.6%, 54.7%, and 46.8% of the total variance (adjusted $R^2 g$: 63.72%, p: 58.0%, c: 52.8%, and s: 44.7%). Increasing depressive symptoms as indicated by BDI-II scores were a significant negative HrQoL determinant in all four models ($\beta_g = 0.49$, $\beta_p = 0.32$, $\beta_c = 0.51$, and $\beta_s = 0.59$). More severe NMS as indicated by NMSS scores were a significant negative HrQoL determinant in three models ($\beta_g = 0.21$, $\beta_p = 0.22$, and $\beta_c = 0.17$). Motor impairment as assessed by the UPDRS-III score occurred as a negative HrQoL determinant in only two models (UPDRS-III: $\beta_g = 0.13$ and $\beta_p = 0.25$), as well as a higher LEDD ($\beta_g = 0.15$ and $\beta_p = 0.18$). Female gender was a negative predictor for physical-functioning and socioemotional HrQoL ($\beta_p = -0.11$ and $\beta_s = -0.11$), whereas male gender was a negative predictor for cognition HrQoL ($\beta_c = 0.19$). Less consistent significant HrQoL determinants across all models included a lower cognitive state as indicated by the PANDA total score for cognition HrQoL ($\beta_c = -0.11$) and, only marginally significant, younger age for socioemotional HrQoL ($\beta_s = -0.09$). Disease duration and H&Y stage were not identified as a significant independent HrQoL determinant in any of the multiple regression models. The number of significant predictors per model varied between two and five. A detailed summary of the multiple regression models is displayed in Table 2.

With regard to the dimension specificity of HrQoL determinants, distributions of relative importance values varied

TABLE 2: Results of the multiple regression analyses: basic models.

	Predictor	B	SE	t	p	R^2
Global health-related quality of life (n = 242)	Intercept	10.99	3.35	3.28	<0.001***	
	Gender: male[b]	−1.10	1.20	−0.92	0.361	0.00
	Age[a]	−0.00	0.07	−0.00	0.995	0.00
	Disease duration	0.05	0.14	0.35	0.726	0.02
	PANDA[a]	−0.26	0.17	−1.58	0.116	0.01
	BDI-II	0.93	0.09	10.44	<0.001***	0.28
	NMSS[a]	0.09	0.02	4.04	<0.001***	0.16
	UPDRS-III[a]	0.22	0.09	2.29	0.023*	0.05
	H&Y	1.72	1.24	1.39	0.167	0.07
	LEDD[a]	0.01	0.00	2.81	0.005**	0.05
	$F(9,232) = 48.02$, $p < 0.001$				Multiple R^2	0.65
					Adjusted R^2	0.64
Physical-functioning health-related quality of life (n = 241)	Intercept	16.99	4.95	3.43	<0.001***	0.01
	Gender: male[b]	−4.67	1.79	−2.61	0.010**	0.01
	Age[a]	0.03	0.10	0.26	0.798	0.01
	Disease duration	−0.04	0.22	−0.17	0.868	0.03
	PANDA[a]	−0.09	0.25	−0.38	0.706	0.01
	BDI-II	0.81	0.13	6.23	<0.001***	0.15
	NMSS[a]	0.13	0.03	3.90	<0.001***	0.13
	UPDRS-III[a]	0.56	0.14	3.98	<0.001***	0.10
	H&Y	3.02	1.84	1.64	0.101	0.10
	LEDD[a]	0.01	0.00	3.19	0.002**	0.06
	$F(9,231) = 37.80$, $p < 0.001$				Multiple R^2	0.60
					Adjusted R^2	0.58
Cognition health-related quality of life (n = 240)	Intercept	0.99	4.63	0.21	0.831	
	Gender: Male[b]	6.97	1.66	4.21	<0.001***	0.03
	Age[a]	0.14	0.09	1.52	0.131	0.01
	Disease duration	0.16	0.20	0.82	0.416	0.01
	PANDA[a]	−0.55	0.23	−2.40	0.017*	0.02
	BDI-II	1.16	0.13	9.07	<0.001***	0.26
	NMSS[a]	0.09	0.03	2.86	0.005**	0.13
	UPDRS-III[a]	−0.13	0.13	−1.00	0.318	0.02
	H&Y	2.80	1.70	1.65	0.100	0.04
	LEDD[a]	0.00	0.00	0.75	0.453	0.02
	$F(9,230) = 53.68$, $p < 0.001$				Multiple R^2	0.55
					Adjusted R^2	0.53
Socioemotional health-related quality of life (n = 241)	Intercept	9.56	4.18	2.29	0.023*	
	Gender: Male[b]	−3.36	1.51	−2.23	0.027*	0.01
	Age[a]	−0.17	0.09	−1.94	0.053	0.01
	Disease duration	0.12	0.17	0.66	0.510	0.01
	PANDA[a]	−0.25	0.21	−1.23	0.220	0.01
	BDI-II	1.13	0.11	10.14	<0.001***	0.32
	NMSS[a]	0.02	0.03	0.72	0.471	0.07
	UPDRS-III[a]	0.20	0.12	1.73	0.085	0.02
	H&Y	−0.43	1.53	−0.28	0.779	0.02
	LEDD[a]	0.00	0.00	0.83	0.407	0.01
	$F(9,231) = 22.58$, $p < 0.001$				Multiple R^2	0.47
					Adjusted R^2	0.45

Note. Parkinson's Disease Questionnaire 39 (PDQ-39) total score and the PDQ-39 component scores physical-functioning, cognition, and socioemotional HrQoL (as revealed by the principal component analysis) were used as dependent variables. BDI-II = Beck's Depression Inventory II; H&Y = Hoehn and Yahr stage; LEDD = levodopa equivalent daily dose; NMSS = Nonmotor Symptom Scale; PANDA = Parkinson Neuropsychometric Dementia Assessment; UPDRS-III = Unified Parkinson's Disease Rating Scale Part III. [a]Variable was mean-centered; [b]gender was dummy coded with female gender as the baseline group; * $p \leq 0.05$; ** $p \leq 0.01$; *** $p \leq 0.001$.

across HrQoL dimensions. On average, depressive symptoms accounted for 46.0% of the total variance explained in HrQoL (g: 43.0%, p: 25.1%, c: 47.5%, and s: 68.4%). NMS accounted for around 21.3% of the total variance explained in HrQoL (g: 24.6%, p: 21.8%, c: 23.8%, and s: 15.0%). On average, disease-related variables (UPDRS-III, H&Y stage, and LEDD)

accounted for 23.8% of the total variance explained in HrQoL (g: 26.1%, p: 43.6%, c: 14.6%, and s: 10.7%).

3.4. *Moderated Domain-Specific Health-Related Quality of Life Models.* Multiple regression analyses and model comparisons between hierarchical nested models revealed moderating effects of gender on physical-functioning HrQoL determinants, whereas no evidence for moderating effects was observed in cognition and socioemotional HrQoL. Neither the gender-moderated cognition HrQoL model (adjusted $R^2 = 0.53$), $F(12,222) = 16.86$, $p < 0.001$, nor the gender-moderated socioemotional HrQoL model (adjusted $R^2 = 0.44$), $F(17,223) = 11.97$, $p < 0.001$, was significantly better than the corresponding basic model (cognition HrQoL $\Delta R^2 = 0.02$, $F(8,222) = 1.09$, $p = 0.372$; socioemotional HrQoL $\Delta R^2 = 0.01$, $F(8,223) = 0.48$, $p = 0.869$).

Originating the basic physical-functioning HrQoL model, the regression model allowing for gender moderations in all potential HrQoL determinants (adjusted $R^2 = 0.60$), $F(17,223) = 22.42$, $p < 0.001$, was significantly better than its corresponding basic model, $\Delta R^2 = 0.03$, $F(8,223) = 2.67$, $p = 0.008$. Increasing depressive symptoms ($\beta = 0.31$) and a higher LEDD ($\beta = 0.31$) were identified as significant independent negative determinants of physical-functioning HrQoL. Additionally, for both men and women, more severe motor impairment was a significant determinant of physical-functioning HrQoL; however, the relationship was more pronounced for women ($\beta = 0.43$) than for men ($\beta = 0.20$). More severe NMS was a significant negative determinant of physical-functioning HrQoL for men only ($\beta = 0.04$). Note that compared to the basic physical-functioning HrQoL model, gender was not a significant independent determinant of HrQoL anymore. The tendency of women being more affected in the physical-functioning HrQoL domain than men seems to be moderated by the differential influence of the severity of motor symptoms on physical-functioning HrQoL across genders. A detailed summary of the moderated regression model is displayed in Table 3.

4. Discussion

The main findings of this study examining the dimensional structure of the PDQ-39 as well as general and domain-specific relationships between clinical and sociodemographic variables, gender in particular, and HrQoL in a cohort of 245 PD patients were as follows: (i) PCA leads to a well interpretable three-component structure of the PDQ-39 with the domains physical-functioning, cognition, and socioemotional HrQoL; (ii) depression and NMS were the strongest and most consistent determinants of global HrQoL and its subdomains; (iii) for disease-related variables and cognition, domain-specific relationships were obtained; and (iv) despite the lack of a gender effect for global HrQoL, domain-specific gender differences and gender-specific manifestations of HrQoL determinants were found.

Further research is needed to evaluate the validity of the proposed three-dimensional HrQoL structure of the PDQ-39 in comparison with the unidimensional and eight-dimensional structure of the PDQ-39, for example, using confirmatory factor analyses and Rasch analyses. The proposed three-dimensional structure already seems more relatable to the domains of the International Classification of Functioning, Disability and Health [34, 35], where the domain of impairment of body functions and structures is relatable to our physical-functioning HrQoL domain and

TABLE 3: Results of the gender-moderated multiple regression analysis on physical-functioning health-related quality of life ($n = 241$).

	B	SE	t	p
Intercept	15.38	8.38	1.84	0.068
Gender: male[b]	0.01	10.04	<0.01	0.999
Age[a]	0.01	0.18	0.03	0.974
Age gender	0.09	0.22	0.42	0.678
Disease duration	−0.27	0.39	−0.70	0.483
Disease duration gender	0.17	0.47	0.36	0.719
PANDA[a]	0.18	0.47	0.39	0.696
PANDA gender	−0.36	0.55	−0.66	0.511
BDI-II	0.78	0.20	3.87	<0.001***
BDI-II gender	0.01	0.26	0.03	0.978
NMSS[a]	0.01	0.06	0.10	0.920
NMSS gender	0.20	0.07	2.75	0.006**
UPDRS-III[a]	0.95	0.26	3.69	<0.001***
UPDRS-III gender	−0.59	0.31	−1.92	0.046*
H&Y	3.98	3.09	1.29	0.200
H&Y gender	−2.06	3.81	−0.54	0.589
LEDD[a]	0.01	0.01	3.23	0.001**
LEDD gender	−0.01	0.01	−1.55	0.122
Multiple R^2				0.63
Adjusted R^2				0.60

Note. BDI-II = Beck's Depression Inventory II; LEDD = levodopa equivalent daily dose; NMSS = Nonmotor Symptom Scale; UPDRS-III = Unified Parkinson's Disease Rating Scale Part III. [a]Gender was dummy coded with female gender as the baseline group; [b]variable was mean-centered; * $p \leq 0.05$; ** $p \leq 0.01$; *** $p \leq 0.001$.

the domain of activity and participation limitations encompasses the cognition and socioemotional HrQoL domain. The proposed three-dimensional structure also mirrors the HrQoL dimensions proposed by Wood-Dauphinee [3] more generally and by Den Oudsten et al. [4] and Martinez-Martin [2] for PD. However, a limitation of this analysis is its dependency on the eight-dimensional PDQ-39 structure, which is criticized itself [9]. Therefore, we recommend validating the proposed three-dimensional structure from a data-driven point of view that is based on the individual item level.

Depressive symptoms as the most important, independent HrQoL determinant across all regression models support the hypothesis of general relationships between mental health variables and HrQoL [10, 14, 15]. Corroborating results from earlier studies [10, 15], NMS was the second most important determinant of both general HrQoL and its subdomains. However, it must be noted that the NMSS includes a broad range of symptoms, and the total score does not provide information about their nature. Furthermore, the NMSS includes a short assessment of mood and depressive symptoms; thus, a clear distinction of depression and NMS cannot be made with our data.

Other findings of our study point to more specific relationships. Not surprisingly, in line with previous work [14, 15], PD-related HrQoL determinants were strong and consistent HrQoL determinants only in the physical-functioning HrQoL domain. Likewise, global cognitive state was identified as a significant determinant only of cognition HrQoL. However, cognitive impairment in PD is typically associated with poorer HrQoL [12], and the lack of evidence for cognitive state as a determinant of global HrQoL might be due to the skewed range of cognitive abilities of patients in our study.

Our findings revealed a tendency of younger age being a negative determinant of socioemotional HrQoL, which converges well with the hypothesis of younger PD patients having higher HrQoL expectations, facing more difficulties adjusting to disease-related constraints and experiencing more severe psychosocial consequences than older PD patients [36, 37]. Especially the stigma dimension may play a crucial role for reduced socioemotional HrQoL of younger PD patients, whereas opposing effects (i.e., greater disease burden, mobility constraints, and more cognitive impairment for older PD patients) eliminate a global age effect in the other HrQoL domains.

In line with previous literature on domain-specific relationships based on the eight PDQ-39 subscales [20, 21], female gender was a significant negative determinant of physical-functioning and socioemotional HrQoL, whereas male gender was a significant negative determinant of cognition HrQoL, and analyses on global HrQoL revealed no gender effect at all. The moderated regression model of physical-functioning HrQoL further emphasizes the special vulnerability of women concerning their experienced HrQoL through an accentuated negative relationships between motor impairment and physical-functioning HrQoL, possibly due to differential symptom perception and reporting between men and women and the social construction of gender [38].

To the authors' best knowledge, this is the first study evaluating gender-specific manifestations of HrQoL determinants in PD. Although the full spectrum of symptoms should be considered in any patient, knowledge about gender-specific relationships of specific symptoms to HrQoL might sensitize clinicians for symptoms typically reducing HrQoL in men and women and thus to optimize treatment concepts with regard to improving HrQoL. Following the results, the management of depressive symptoms is of outstanding importance in PD interventions for both sexes. Although relevant for all PD patients, the consideration of NMS in the HrQoL context seems especially important for men. Finally, the special vulnerability of men in the cognition HrQoL domain might be due to a close interaction between cognition and communication with job performance and the social construction of male gender [38]. Improving cognitive and communicative abilities, however, might result in an improvement of HrQoL in general and across sexes [39, 40].

Some possible limitations have to be taken into account when interpreting the findings of this study. Even though multiple regression analyses have been the method of choice when evaluating HrQoL determinants [10], they do not take into account the complex interrelationships between HrQoL determinants, as alternative statistical methods such as path analysis and structural modeling could do [41, 42]. Second, despite assessing a wide range of potential variables, some potential HrQoL determinants were not assessed: for example, sociodemographic data on participants' housing situation, marital status, education, and employment status, their quality of sleep, and the nature of NMS and a more detailed assessment of motor complications (e.g., freezing of gate, dyskinesias, and motor fluctuations). Furthermore, assessing symptoms that have to be differentiated from depression, such as apathy and demoralization, could improve the predictive accuracy of HrQoL models [43, 44]. Recently, positive psychological functioning and resilience-related factors have gained attention of HrQoL researchers regarding its protective influence on HrQoL against less modifiable PD symptoms, especially motor ones [14, 45, 46], so that those variables might have accounted for additional variance, most notably in the socioemotional HrQoL domain. Additionally, greater predictive accuracy regarding the relationship of cognition and HrQoL may result from the use of more specific cognitive assessments [47]. Above all, further research is needed to clarify the findings of contributors to HrQoL in a broader sample of PD patients, including individuals with advanced disease (H&Y stage 5) and progressing cognitive impairment (PD-MCI and dementia).

5. Conclusions

This study supports and extends previous findings on HrQoL and its determinants in PD patients. A new PDQ-39 component structure dividing HrQoL into a physical-functioning, cognition, and socioemotional domain was proposed. Multiple regression analyses supported evidence for general and domain-specific relationships, emphasize the outstanding importance of depressive symptoms in the management of PD, and highlight scarcely investigated gender-specific manifestations of HrQoL determinants. Only the full understanding of HrQoL determinants and their interrelationships in such an encompassing way will allow the development of new PD intervention strategies that focus on what matters the most for the patients' HrQoL.

Disclosure

Funding was transferred to the University Hospital Cologne, so that no direct sponsoring of any of the participating team members occurred. The sponsors had no role in study design, data collection, data analysis, data interpretation, or writing the reports.

Authors' Contributions

Anja Ophey and Carsten Eggers contributed equally.

Acknowledgments

The authors in behalf of the CPN study group thank all patients participating in the study and all staff members who contributed to the study. This study was supported by Abbott Pharma GmbH, Archimedes GmbH, Bayer Vital GmbH, Medtronic GmbH, Teva Pharma GmbH, UCB Pharma GmbH, and Zur Rose Pharma GmbH.

References

[1] W. Poewe, "Non-motor symptoms in Parkinson's disease," *European Journal of Neurology*, vol. 15, no. S1, pp. 14–20, 2008.

[2] P. Martinez-Martin, "What is quality of life and how do we measure it? Relevance to Parkinson's disease and movement disorders," *Movement Disorders*, vol. 32, no. 3, pp. 382–392, 2017.

[3] S. Wood-Dauphinee, "Assessing quality of life in clinical research: from where have we come and where are we going?," *Journal of Clinical Epidemiology*, vol. 52, no. 4, pp. 355–363, 1999.

[4] B. L. Den Oudsten, G. L. Van Heck, and J. De Vries, "Quality of life and related concepts in Parkinson's disease: a systematic review," *Movement Disorders*, vol. 22, no. 11, pp. 1528–1537, 2007.

[5] V. Peto, C. Jenkinson, R. Fitzpatrick, and R. Greenhall, "The development and validation of a short measure of functioning and well being for individuals with Parkinson's disease," *Quality of Life Research*, vol. 4, no. 3, pp. 241–248, 1995.

[6] C. Jenkinson, R. Fitzpatrick, V. Peto, R. Greenhall, and N. Hyman, "The Parkinson's disease questionnaire (PDQ-39): development and validation of a Parkinson's disease summary index score," *Age and Ageing*, vol. 26, no. 5, pp. 353–357, 1997.

[7] P. Martinez-Martin, M. Jeukens-Visser, K. E. Lyons et al., "Health-related quality-of-life scales in Parkinson's disease: critique and recommendations," *Movement Disorders*, vol. 26, no. 13, pp. 2371–2380, 2011.

[8] P. Hagell and M. H. Nilsson, "The 39-item Parkinson's disease questionnaire (PDQ-39): is it a unidimensional construct?," *Therapeutic Advances in Neurological Disorders*, vol. 2, no. 4, pp. 205–214, 2009.

[9] P. Hagell and C. Nygren, "The 39 item Parkinson's disease questionnaire (PDQ-39) revisited: implications for evidence based medicine," *Journal of Neurology, Neurosurgery and Psychiatry*, vol. 78, no. 11, pp. 1191–1198, 2007.

[10] S.-E. Soh, M. E. Morris, and J. L. McGinley, "Determinants of health-related quality of life in Parkinson's disease: a systematic review," *Parkinsonism and Related Disorders*, vol. 17, no. 1, pp. 1–9, 2011.

[11] G. M. Pontone, C. C. Bakker, S. Chen et al., "The longitudinal impact of depression on disability in Parkinson disease," *International Journal of Geriatric Psychiatry*, vol. 31, no. 5, pp. 458–465, 2015.

[12] I. Leroi, K. McDonald, H. Pantula, and V. Harbishettar, "Cognitive impairment in Parkinson disease: impact on quality of life, disability, and caregiver burden," *Journal of Geriatric Psychiatry and Neurology*, vol. 25, no. 4, pp. 208–214, 2012.

[13] R. Balestrino and P. Martinez-Martin, "Neuropsychiatric symptoms, behavioural disorders, and quality of life in Parkinson's disease," *Journal of the Neurological Sciences*, vol. 373, pp. 173–178, 2016.

[14] J. Simpson, G. Lekwuwa, and T. Crawford, "Predictors of quality of life in people with Parkinson's disease: evidence for both domain specific and general relationships," *Disability and Rehabilitation*, vol. 36, no. 23, pp. 1964–1970, 2014.

[15] Y. Wu, X. Y. Guo, Q. Q. Wei et al., "Determinants of the quality of life in Parkinson's disease: results of a cohort study from Southwest China," *Journal of the Neurological Sciences*, vol. 340, no. 1-2, pp. 144–149, 2014.

[16] L. Kadastik-Eerme, M. Rosenthal, T. Paju, M. Muldmaa, and P. Taba, "Health-related quality of life in Parkinson's disease: a cross-sectional study focusing on non-motor symptoms," *Health and Quality of Life Outcomes*, vol. 13, no. 1, pp. 83–91, 2015.

[17] M. Picillo, A. Nicoletti, V. Fetoni, B. Garavaglia, P. Barone, and M. T. Pellecchia, "The relevance of gender in Parkinson's disease: a review," *Journal of Neurology*, vol. 264, no. 8, pp. 1583–1607, 2017.

[18] D. Georgiev, K. Hamberg, M. Hariz, L. Forsgren, and G. M. Hariz, "Gender differences in Parkinson's disease: a clinical perspective," *Acta Neurologica Scandinavica* vol. 136, no. 6, pp. 570–584, 2017.

[19] M. Kovács, A. Makkos, Z. Aschermann et al., "Impact of sex on the nonmotor symptoms and the health-related quality of life in parkinson's disease," *Parkinson's Disease*, vol. 2016 Article ID 7951840, 12 pages, 2016.

[20] D. R. Hristova, J. I. Hristov, N. G. Mateva, and J. V. Papathanasiou, "Quality of life in patients with Parkinson's disease," *Folia Medica*, vol. 51, pp. 58–64, 2009.

[21] M. Lubomski, R. L. Rushworth, W. Lee, K. L. Bertram, and D. R. Williams, "Sex differences in Parkinson's disease," *Journal of Clinical Neuroscience*, vol. 21, no. 9, pp. 1503–1506, 2014.

[22] C. Eggers, R. Dano, J. Schill et al., "Patient-centered integrated healthcare improves quality of life in Parkinson's disease patients: a randomized controlled trial," *Journal of Neurology*, vol. 265, no. 4, pp. 764–773, 2018.

[23] A. J. Hughes, S. E. Daniel, L. Kilford, and A. J. Lees, "Accuracy of clinical diagnosis of idiopathic Parkinson's disease: a clinico-pathological study of 100 cases," *Journal of Neurology, Neurosurgery and Psychiatry*, vol. 55, no. 3, pp. 181–184, 1992.

[24] A. T. Beck, R. A. Steer, and G. K. Brown, *Beck Depression Inventory-II*, Vol. 78, Psychological Corporation, San Antonio, TX, USA, 1996.

[25] E. Kalbe, P. Calabrese, N. Kohn et al., "Screening for cognitive deficits in Parkinson's disease with the Parkinson neuropsychometric dementia assessment (PANDA) instrument," *Parkinsonism and Related Disorders*, vol. 14, no. 2, pp. 93–101, 2008.

[26] K. R. Chaudhuri, P. Martinez-Martin, R. G. Brown et al., "The metric properties of a novel non-motor symptoms scale for Parkinson's disease: results from an international pilot study," *Movement Disorders*, vol. 22, no. 13, pp. 1901–1911, 2007.

[27] C. L. Tomlinson, R. Stowe, S. Patel, C. Rick, R. Gray, and C. E. Clarke, "Systematic review of levodopa dose equivalency reporting in Parkinson's disease," *Movement Disorders*, vol. 25, no. 15, pp. 2649–2653, 2010.

[28] S. Fahn, "Unified Parkinson's disease rating scale," in *Recent Developments in Parkinson's Disease*, S. Fahn, C. D. Marsden, M. Goldstein, and D. B. Calne, Eds., pp. 153–163, Macmillan Healthcare Information, Florham Park, NJ, USA, 1987.

[29] M. M. Hoehn and M. D. Yahr, "Parkinsonism: onset, progression, and mortality," *Neurology*, vol. 17, no. 5, pp. 427–442, 1967.

[30] J. E. Ware, M. Kosinski, M. S. Bayliss, C. A. McHorney, W. H. Rogers, and A. Raczek, "Comparison of methods for the scoring and statistical analysis of SF-36 health profile and summary measures: summary of results from the medical outcomes study," *Medical Care*, vol. 33, no. 4, pp. AS264–AS279, 1995.

[31] L. C. Tan, N. Luo, M. Nazri, S. C. Li, and J. Thumboo, "Validity and reliability of the PDQ-39 and the PDQ-8 in English-speaking Parkinson's disease patients in Singapore," *Parkinsonism and Related Disorders*, vol. 10, no. 8, pp. 493–499, 2004.

[32] N. Luo, L. Tan, S. Li, L. Soh, and J. Thumboo, "Validity and reliability of the Chinese (Singapore) version of the Parkinson's disease questionnaire (PDQ-39)," *Quality of Life Research*, vol. 14, no. 1, pp. 273–279, 2005.

[33] J. F. Hair, B. Black, B. Babin, R. E. Anderson, and R. L. Tatham, *Multivariate Data Analysis*, Prentice Hall, Upper Saddle River, NJ, USA, 2009.

[34] WHO, *International Classification of Functioning, Disability and Health: ICF*, World Health Organization, Geneva, Switzerland, 2001.

[35] J. M. Van Uem, J. Marinus, C. Canning et al., "Health-related quality of life in patients with Parkinson's disease—a systematic review based on the ICF model," *Neuroscience and Biobehavioral Reviews*, vol. 61, pp. 26–34, 2016.

[36] R. A. Lawson, A. J. Yarnall, G. W. Duncan et al., "Severity of mild cognitive impairment in early Parkinson's disease contributes to poorer quality of life," *Parkinsonism and Related Disorders*, vol. 20, no. 10, pp. 1071–1075, 2014.

[37] A. Schrag, A. Hovris, D. Morley, N. Quinn, and M. Jahanshahi, "Young-versus older-onset Parkinson's disease: impact of disease and psychosocial consequences," *Movement Disorders*, vol. 18, no. 11, pp. 1250–1256, 2003.

[38] L. M. Verbrugge, "The twain meet: empirical explanations of sex differences in health and mortality," *Journal of Health and Social Behavior*, vol. 30, no. 3, pp. 282–304, 1989.

[39] E. Kalbe and A.-K. Folkerts, "Kognitives Training bei Parkinson-Patienten–eine neue Therapieoption?," *Fortschritte der Neurologie Psychiatrie*, vol. 84, pp. S24–S35, 2016.

[40] I. Reuter, S. Mehnert, G. Sammer, M. Oechsner, and M. Engelhardt, "Efficacy of a multimodal cognitive rehabilitation including psychomotor and endurance training in Parkinson's disease," *Journal of Aging Research*, vol. 2012, Article ID 235765, 15 pages, 2012.

[41] S.-E. Soh, J. L. McGinley, J. J. Watts et al., "Determinants of health-related quality of life in people with Parkinson's disease: a path analysis," *Quality of Life Research*, vol. 22, no. 7, pp. 1543–1553, 2013.

[42] J. Lee, M. Choi, D. Jung, Y. H. Sohn, and J. Hong, "A structural model of health-related quality of life in Parkinson's disease patients," *Western Journal of Nursing Research*, vol. 37, no. 8, pp. 1062–1080, 2015.

[43] B. B. Koo, C. A. Chow, D. R. Shah et al., "Demoralization in Parkinson disease," *Neurology*, vol. 90, no. 18, pp. e1613–e1617, 2018.

[44] S. Robinson, D. W. Kissane, J. Brooker, C. Hempton, and S. Burney, "The relationship between poor quality of life and desire to hasten death: a multiple mediation model examining the contributions of depression, demoralization, loss of control, and low self-worth," *Journal of Pain and Symptom Management*, vol. 53, no. 2, pp. 243–249, 2017.

[45] Y. Barak and A. Achiron, "Happiness and neurological diseases," *Expert Review of Neurotherapeutics*, vol. 9, no. 4, pp. 445–459, 2009.

[46] B. Robottom, A. Gruber-Baldini, K. Anderson et al., "What determines resilience in patients with Parkinson's disease?," *Parkinsonism and Related disorders*, vol. 18, no. 2, pp. 174–177, 2012.

[47] R. A. Lawson, A. J. Yarnall, G. W. Duncan et al., "Cognitive decline and quality of life in incident Parkinson's disease: the role of attention," *Parkinsonism and Related Disorders*, vol. 27, pp. 47–53, 2016.

21

Sleep Quality and Levodopa Intestinal Gel Infusion in Parkinson's Disease: A Pilot Study

Oriol De Fabregues [iD],[1] Alex Ferré,[2] Odile Romero,[2] Manuel Quintana,[1] and José Álvarez-Sabin[1]

[1]*Movement Disorders Unit, Department of Neurology, Hospital Universitari Vall D'Hebron,*
Neurodegenerative Diseases Research Group-Vall D'Hebron Research Institute, Universitat Autònoma de Barcelona,
Barcelona, Spain
[2]*Sleep Unit, Department of Neurophysiology, Hospital Universitari Vall D'Hebron, Barcelona, Spain*

Correspondence should be addressed to Oriol De Fabregues; odefabregues@gmail.com

Academic Editor: Cristine Alves da Costa

Background. Sleep problems in patients with advanced Parkinson's disease (PD) have a deleterious impact on quality of life. *Objective.* To assess the effect of levodopa-carbidopa intestinal gel (LCIG) infusion on sleep quality in advanced PD patients. *Methods.* Seven patients participated in a prospective pilot study. Before and after 6 months of LCIG infusion, an overnight polysomnography was performed and the Epworth Sleepiness Scale, fatigue scale, Pittsburgh Sleep Quality Index, Beck Depression Inventory, and the Hamilton Anxiety Rating Scale were administered. *Results.* PSG showed low sleep efficiency. REM sleep without atony was found in 5 patients. After 6 months of LCIG infusion, the percentage of REM sleep decreased as well as the number of arousals especially due to reduction of spontaneous arousals and periodic leg movements during REM sleep, but differences were not statistically significant. Also, scores of all study questionnaires showed a tendency to improve. *Conclusion.* The results show a trend toward an improvement of sleep quality after 6 months of LCIG infusion, although differences as compared to pretreatment values were not statistically significant. The sleep architecture was not modified by LCIG. Further studies with larger study samples are needed to confirm these preliminary findings.

1. Introduction

Sleep problems are important nonmotor manifestations in patients with Parkinson's disease (PD) at different stages during the course of the disease. Numerous forms of alterations of physiologic sleep patterns have been reported, ranging from increased daytime sleepiness after introduction of a dopamine agonist to the therapeutic regimen to specific sleep-related diagnoses (e.g., restless legs syndrome, rapid eye movement sleep behavior disorder, and periodic limb movements in sleep) or sleep-related breathing disorders (e.g., obstructive sleep apnea) [1–3]. The origin of these sleep disorders is multifactorial including degeneration of the brain areas that modulate sleep, the symptoms of the disease, and the effect of medications [2].

These disturbances can primarily affect the patient's quality of life and may worsen the symptoms of PD [4, 5]. In studies that examine the impact of PD on quality of life, sleep difficulties are independent an important predictor of poor quality of life [6]. In fact, sleep disturbance, depression, and lack of independence are the primary determinants of poor quality of life [5]. Also, sleep disturbances contribute to excessive daytime sleepiness and poor daytime functioning as well as patients' reduced enthusiasm for daily events. Adverse effects have also been observed in the sleep habits and the quality of life of their caregivers [7].

There is little evidence of the impact of treatment modalities for advanced PD on sleep [8]. In relation to deep brain stimulation (DBS), a positive effect of subthalamic DBS on sleep-wake disturbances was found in a systematic review of 38 studies involving 1443 subjects [9]. However, only seven studies used polysomnography (PSG) to objectively assess sleep parameters. In a small pilot study, pallidal DBS showed improving trends in several PSG measures including sleep efficiency and latency to sleep onset [10]. Continuous levodopa-carbidopa intestinal gel (LCIG) infusion is a therapeutic option for advanced PD patients complicated with motor fluctuations refractory to conventional treatment. It has been shown that LCIG infusion improves nonmotor symptoms and quality of life [11]. The specific effects of LCIG infusion on sleep disturbances have been poorly studied. In a small clinical series of 12 PD patients, subjective measures of sleep quality and daytime sleepiness improved with LCIG infusion, although PSG was not performed [12]. There is only one open-label pilot study with a sample size limited to 11 patients that examined PSG characteristics in PD patients on a stable LCIG dose [13]. Main findings included improvement of subjective sleep quality, motor complications, and activities of daily living. PSG showed a reduction of the number of awakenings in sleep, a trend towards a lower apnea-hypopnea index, and no change in sleep latency, total sleep time and sleep efficiency [13].

The present clinical study was conducted to add evidence of sleep disturbances in advanced PD patients treated with LCIG infusion. The objective was to determine whether treatment with LCIG infusion had a beneficial effect on the quality of sleep in patients with advanced PD. In these patients, an overnight PSG was performed before and after 6 months of LCIG infusion therapy. The quality of sleep is a complex phenomenon, the assessment of which should integrate subjective and quantitative objective measures. For this reason, besides overnight PSG, we also evaluated subjective parameters using a series of validated questionnaires.

2. Patients and Methods

2.1. Study Population. Seven consecutive patients with advanced PD were included in a single-center, open-label prospectively pilot study, and were evaluated at baseline and after 6 months of LCIG infusion. The study was conducted in compliance with the ethical standards and was approved by the Ethics Committee for Clinical Research of Hospital Universitari Vall d'Hebron, Barcelona (Spain) and followed the Spanish Law 15/1999 on Personal Character Data Protection concerning confidentiality of Patient's data. The Institutional Review Board Clinical Study registration number was PR(AG)129/2008, and the Clinical Study registration number is NCT03602924. Written informed consent was obtained from all patients.

Patients started LCIG infusion after receiving an implant of percutaneous endoscopic gastrostomy with jejunal extension (PEG-J) following a previously described procedure used in our center [14]. The initial LCIG maintenance dose was calculated according to the levodopa equivalent daily dose; the optimal dose was titrated individually until reaching the best motor performance, controlling motor fluctuations without causing annoying dyskinesia, and getting a stable infusion for less than 16 hours a day, stopped

at night, when patients received an oral nocturnal dose of levodopa.

2.2. Study Procedures. All participants underwent a full overnight PSG at the Sleep Unit of our institution. The recorded parameters included electroencephalography (EEG), electro-occulography (EOG), electromyography (EMG), electrocardiography (ECG), respiratory effort, oronasal airflow, oxygen saturation, snoring sounds, and body position. Sleep scoring was performed by a trained technician according to the American Academy of Sleep Medicine (AASM) scoring criteria 2012 [15]. The reported parameters included sleep efficiency, wake after sleep onset (WASO), sleep latency, REM latency, rapid-eye movement (REM) sleep, nonREM (NREM) sleep (stages 1–3), snoring sounds, apnea-hypopnea index (AHI), arousal index, spontaneous arousals, respiratory effort-related arousals (RERA), leg movement arousals, periodic leg movements in sleep (PLMS), PLMS in REM and NREM, oxygen saturation (SpO_2), and CT90.

2.3. Assessments. Evaluation included the Epworth Sleepiness Scale (ESS) [16], the Fatigue Severity Scale (FSS) [17], the Pittsburgh Sleep Quality Index (PSQI) [18], sleep efficiency, the Beck Depression Inventory (BDI) [19], and the Hamilton Anxiety Rating Scale (HARS) [20]. Also, complete pharmacological data, including antiparkinsonian drugs and treatments potentially influencing sleep and daytime sleepiness (i.e., clonazepam, quetiapine, and serotonin selective reuptake inhibitors) were collected at baseline and at follow-up.

The ESS measures the general level of daytime sleepiness (the sum of 8 item scores, 0–3) with a total score ranging from 0 to 24. The higher the ESS score, the higher the person's average sleep propensity in daily life. The FSS is a 9-item questionnaire with questions related to how fatigue interferes with certain activities and rates its severity. Items are scored on a 7 point scale, with 1 = strongly disagree and 7 = strongly agree, with a total score ranging between 9 and 63. The higher the score, the greater fatigue severity. The PSQI consists of 19 individual items creating 7 component scores and one composite score. Each item is weighted on a 0–3 interval scale. The global PSQI score is then calculated by totaling the 7 component scores, providing an overall score ranging from 0 to 21, where lower scores denote a healthier sleep quality. Subjective sleep efficiency (component #4 of the PSQI) was calculated as number of hours slept/number of hours spent in bed × 100 and expressed as a percentage. The BDI consists of 21 questions about how the subject has been feeling during the last week, and a value of 0 to 3 is assigned for each answer, with total score ranging from 0 to 63 (0–13 minimal, 14–19 mild, 20–28 moderate, 29–63 severe). The HARS consists of 14 items, each of which contains a number of symptoms, which are rated scale of 0 to 4, with 4 being the most severe. The total score ranges from 0 to 56.

Moreover, motor fluctuations, dyskinesia, and other motor and nonmotor clinical aspects were evaluated before starting LCIG infusion (baseline) after 6 months of treatment. Motor fluctuations were assessed by "off" time, in hours, recorded in Parkinson's Disease Diary©. Dyskinesia and other motor symptoms were evaluated using the Unified Parkinson's Disease Rating Scale (UPDRS) [21] part IV–Complications of Therapy, UPDRS part II–Activities of Daily Living in On and Off, UPDRS part III–Motor Examination in On and Off; Hoehn and Yahr stage in On and Off [22]; and the Schwab and England Activities of Daily Living (ADL) scale in On [23]. Nonmotor clinical aspects evaluated were cognitive function using the Mini Mental State Examination (MMSE) test [24] and UPDRS part I–Mental, Behavior, and Mood.

Complete pharmacological data, including antiparkinsonian drugs and treatments potentially influencing sleep and daytime sleepiness (i.e., benzodiazepines (clonazepam, lorazepam), neuroleptic (quetiapine), and serotonin selective reuptake inhibitors) were, recorded at baseline and follow-up.

2.4. Statistical Analysis. Data are expressed as mean and standard deviation (±SD). The Wilcoxon signed-rank test was used for the comparison of paired samples before and after 6 months of LCIG infusion. Statistical analysis was performed with the SPSS version 17.0 (Statistical Package for Social Sciences, SPSS, Inc., Chicago, IL, USA). Statistical significance was set at $P < 0.05$.

3. Results

We studied 6 women and 1 man diagnosed with advanced PD, with a mean age of 69.6 years (range 60–78) and a mean body mass index (BMI) of $24.5\,\text{kg/m}^2$ (range 20–32).

Results of clinical variables are shown in Table 1. A significant improvement in motor fluctuations was observed (daily mean "off" time decreased from 6.3 ± 1.4 h at baseline to 1.1 ± 0.7 h after 6 months, $P < 0.001$). Motor symptoms evaluated with UPDRS part III remained stable and the mean score in "off" stage did not change in any of the patients. Dyskinesia assessed with UPDRS part IV decreased significantly from 5.4 ± 2.4 at baseline to 2.9 ± 1.1 after 6 months of LCIG treatment ($P = 0.028$). None of the patients presented a worsening in the percentage of the waking time with dyskinesia, which was reduced in 2 patients (28.6%) and remained stable in the remaining 5 patients (71.4%). The severity of dyskinesias improved in 3 (42.9%) patients, remained stable in 3 (42.9%), and worsened in 1 (14.3%). Nonmotor cognitive function (UPDRS part I) tended to improve.

As shown in Table 2, at 6 months after LCIG infusion, there was a decrease in scores of the ESS, FSS, and PSQI as compared with baseline, indicating an improvement in daytime sleepiness, fatigue, and sleep quality. Severe score of the PSQI at baseline was recorded in 4 patients (57.1%), 3 of which changed to a moderate score at follow-up. One patient with moderate score at baseline had a normal score at follow-up, and of 2 patients with normal score at baseline, 1 had a mild score at follow-up. Sleep efficiency also improved. Differences, however, were not statistically significant. Changes in the scores of BDI and HARS were not significant either.

TABLE 1: Changes in "off" time hours, UPDRS values, cognitive function, body mass index, and pharmacological therapy at baseline and after 6 months of LCIG infusion.

Variables	Baseline	Follow-up	P value
Off time hours recorded in Parkinson's disease diary© (daily mean "off" time)	6.3 ± 1.4	1.1 ± 0.7	<0.001
UPDRS part IV (dyskinesia)	5.4 ± 2.4	2.9 ± 1.1	0.028
UPDRS part II (activities of daily living)			
On	11.4 ± 5.9	10.9 ± 5.6	0.742
Off	22.9 ± 8.3	22.3 ± 7.5	0.231
UPDRS part III (motor examination)			
On	18 ± 3.7	16.6 ± 4.9	0.245
Off	34.1 ± 11.1	34.1 ± 11.1	—
UPDRS part I (mentation, behavior, and mood)	3.6 ± 3.7	2.4 ± 2.1	0.156
MMSE (cognitive function)	29 (27–30)	29 (27–30)	0.317
Body mass index (BMI)	24.5 ± 4.0	23.8 ± 3.3	0.424
Bedtime drugs, no. patients			
Benzodiazepine drugs	6/7	6/7	1.000
Serotonin selective reuptake inhibitor	4/7	4/7	1.000
Neuroleptic drugs	1/7	2/7	1.000

Data as mean ± standard deviation unless otherwise stated.

TABLE 2: Changes of subjective parameters before and after 6 months of LCIG infusion therapy in 7 patients with advanced PD.

Questionnaires	LCIG infusion therapy		P value
	Before	At 6 months	
ESS	6.4 ± 3.6	4.7 ± 4.1	0.340
PSQI	11.9 ± 6.4	8.9 ± 5.0	0.137
Subjective sleep efficiency	61.9 ± 21.5	57.8 ± 16.0	0.612
BDI	11.7 ± 8.7	14.3 ± 9.4	0.497
HARS	21.6 ± 10.8	22.1 ± 12.4	0.917

Data as mean ± standard deviation. ESS: Epworth Sleepiness Scale; PSQI: Pittsburgh Sleep Quality Index; BDI: Beck Depression Inventory; HARS: Hamilton Anxiety Rating Scale.

Results of PSG showed low generalized sleep efficiency. No significant differences were observed in sleep macrostructure parameters, respiratory events, or periodic leg movements. There was a decrease in the percentage of REM sleep ($16.2 \pm 9.9\%$ vs. $10.4 \pm 6.8\%$, $P = 0.080$) and arousal index (15.0 ± 7.0 vs. 12.9 ± 5.6, $P = 0.115$) especially due to reduction of spontaneous arousals (7.5 ± 3.1 vs. 5.2 ± 5.0, $P = 0.075$) and PLMS during REM sleep (20.7 ± 31.6 vs. 2.9 ± 3.7, $P = 0.285$), but differences were not statistically significant. The percentage of NREM sleep increased from a mean of $83.6 \pm 10.1\%$ at baseline to $89.6 \pm 6.8\%$ after 6 months of LCIG infusion therapy, although differences did not reach statistical significance ($P = 0.080$) (Table 3).

TABLE 3: Comparison of polysomnographic results before and after 6 months of LCIG infusion therapy in 7 patients with advanced PD.

Variables	LCIG infusion therapy		P value
	Before	At 6 months	
Sleep efficiency (%)	66.7 ± 8.4	57.8 ± 16.0	0.173
Wake after sleep onset (WASO) (min)	119.9 ± 74.2	113.0 ± 54.1	0.345
Sleep latency (min)	29.7 ± 40.5	71.2 ± 97.2	0.345
REM latency (min)	147.3 ± 72.4	139.8 ± 63.1	0.893
REM sleep (%)	16.2 ± 9.9	10.4 ± 6.8	0.080
NREM sleep (%)	83.6 ± 10.2	89.6 ± 6.8	0.080
Stage 1	16.8 ± 10.0	23.8 ± 13.7	0.463
Stage 2	52.9 ± 8.4	52.4 ± 12.0	0.345
Stage 3	13.9 ± 7.5	13.0 ± 11.9	0.752
Snoring sounds (number/hour)	323.2 ± 279.3	228.6 ± 226.0	0.715
Apnea-hypopnea index (AHI)	11.8 ± 18.0	12.7 ± 14.0	0.686
Arousal index	15.0 ± 7.0	12.9 ± 5.6	0.115
Spontaneous arousals	7.5 ± 3.1	5.2 ± 5.0	0.075
Respiratory effort-related arousals (RERA)	4.9 ± 7.2	4.8 ± 4.1	0.893
Leg movement arousals	3.1 ± 2.3	2.9 ± 2.5	0.462
Periodic leg movement in sleep (PLMS)	12.5 ± 11.6	7.7 ± 11.1	0.345
PLMS in REM sleep	20.7 ± 31.6	2.9 ± 3.7	0.285
PLMS in NREM sleep	10.3 ± 9.5	8.3 ± 12.4	0.893
Oxygen saturation (SpO$_2$) (%)			
Baseline	95.1 ± 2.3	95.8 ± 2.1	0.339
Mean	93.8 ± 2.0	94.3 ± 2.2	0.461
Minimum	87.0 ± 8.9	86.4 ± 6.6	0.672
Oxygen saturation <90%, CT90 (%)	2.7 ± 4.2	1.7 ± 2.0	0.416

Data as mean ± standard deviation. 6–10: higher normal daytime sleepiness. 11–12: mild excessive daytime sleepiness. 13–15: moderate excessive daytime sleepiness. 16–24: severe excessive daytime sleepiness.

The patients had no previous treatment at the beginning of the infusion with dopamine agonists. Also, monoamine oxidase (Mao) and catechol-O-methyl transferase (COMT) inhibitors were withdrawn in all patients, whereas the use of other drugs potentially influencing the quality of sleep and daytime sleepiness were allowed. The number of patients taken drugs with hypnotic effect before and after treatment with LCIG infusion remained unchanged (Table 1).

4. Discussion

This prospective pilot study in a reduced number of patients with advanced PD treated with LCIG infusion shows that their quality of sleep is poor. Treatment with LCIG infusion did not aggravate the quality of sleep in these patients. We found a decreased time in REM sleep and a tendency of improvement in the number of arousals especially in relation to a reduction of spontaneous arousals and PLMS during REM sleep. Despite a reduction in the percentage of REM sleep, the quality of sleep seems to be better as shown by a decrease of spontaneous arousals and PLMS. These changes in objective parameters may explain the trend towards improvement of subjective measures. Although statistically significant differences in clinical or polysomnographic parameters were not found due to the limited population of 7 patients with advanced PD, the present results regarding maintenance of sleep architecture and a trend toward an improvement of sleep quality after 6 months of LCIG infusion, are similar to results reported by Zibetti et al. [13]. In this respect, two pilot studies with a small sample size (11

patients in the study of Zibetti et al. [13] and 7 in our study) point toward similar findings of amelioration of sleep parameters in advanced PD patients treated with LCIG infusion. In our study, however, differences of objective and subjective variables were not statistically significant. The most likely explanation is that the number of subjects (7 patients) is insufficient to reach statistical significance in any of the PSG measures presented.

Various studies have demonstrated an improvement in nonmotor symptoms, including the sleep/fatigue domain of the Non-Motor Symptoms Scale (NMSS) and quality of life in advanced PD patients treated with LCIG infusion [11, 25–28]. However, based on a recent systematic review of randomized controlled trials (RCTs) and observational studies collected from PubMed and EMBASE until March 2016, the quality of evidence regarding effectiveness of LCIG infusion in improving quality of life is moderate and for reducing nonmotor symptoms is low [29]. Also, there is no evidence of the effectiveness of LCIG infusion in the treatment of subjective fatigue [30].

There is little information on the specific effect of LCIG infusion on the quality of sleep in patients with advanced PD. In a study by Zibetti et al. [12] carried out in a sample of 12 patients, sleep and nocturnal symptoms were evaluated with the modified version of Parkinson's Disease Sleep Scale (PDSS-2) Daytime sleepiness was also assessed with the ESS. A significant improvement in all study variables (PDSS-2 total score, disturbed sleep, motor symptoms at night, PD symptoms at night, and ESS score) was found at 2–4 months of follow-up after starting LCIG infusion therapy. Honig et al. [11] evaluated 24 patients with advanced PD who switched from oral medications to LCIG and were followed for 6 months. Treatment with LCIG reduced motor fluctuations and dyskinesias with statistically significant decreases of the nonmotor symptoms scale (NMSS) and improvement in quality of life (PDQ-8 questionnaire). These results are consistent with the present findings. Although our data should be interpreted considering the reduced number of patients included in the study, it was shown that treatment with LCIG infusion was not associated with a significant amelioration of sleep quality. Overall, the quality of sleep in our patients was poor, but it was not found to be worsened by LCIG infusion therapy.

5. Conclusions

The main finding of this preliminary study of 7 advanced PD patients treated with LCGI is a trend toward an improvement of sleep quality after 6 months of LCIG infusion, although differences as compared to pretreatment values were not statistically significant. The sleep architecture was not modified by LCIG. Further prospective masked studies with larger series of patients on LCIG infusion therapy, not stopped at night, are necessary to clarify the positive influence of LCIG on sleep quality in patients with advanced PD.

Additional Points

Additional supporting information may be obtained under request to the correspondence author, Oriol De Fabregues.

Authors' Contributions

ODF designed the study and performed organization and execution; data acquisition; analysis and interpretation of data; manuscript drafting; and manuscript revision. AF and OR performed execution and data acquisition. MQ performed analysis and interpretation of data. JAS revised the manuscript.

Acknowledgments

The authors thank Marta Pulido, MD, PhD, for editing the manuscript and editorial assistance.

References

[1] M. Menza, R. D. Dobkin, H. Marin, and K. Bienfait, "Sleep disturbances in Parkinson's disease," *Movement Disorders*, vol. 25, no. 1, pp. S117–S122, 2010.

[2] A. Iranzo, "Sleep in neurodegenerative diseases," *Sleep Medicine Clinics*, vol. 11, no. 1, pp. 1–18, 2016.

[3] C. L. Comella, "Sleep disturbances and excessive daytime sleepiness in Parkinson's disease: an overview," *Journal of Neural Transmission. Supplementary*, vol. 70, pp. 349–355, 2006.

[4] M. R. Najafi, A. Chitsaz, Z. Askarian, and M. A. Najafi, "Quality of sleep in patients with Parkinson's disease," *International Journal of Preventive Medicine*, vol. 4, no. 2, pp. 229–233, 2013.

[5] T. Scaravilli, E. Gasparoli, F. Rinaldi, G. Polesello, and F. Bracco, "Health-related quality of life and sleep disorders in Parkinson's disease," *Neurological Sciences*, vol. 24, no. 3, pp. 209-210, 2003.

[6] K. H. Karlsen, E. Tandberg, D. Arsland, and J. P. Larsen, "Health related quality of life in Parkinson's disease: a prospective longitudinal study," *Journal of Neurology, Neurosurgery and Psychiatry*, vol. 69, no. 5, pp. 584–589, 2000.

[7] P. K. Pal, K. Thennarasu, J. Fleming, M. Schulzer, T. Brown, and S. M. Calne, "Nocturnal sleep disturbances and daytime dysfunction in patients with Parkinson's disease and in their caregivers," *Parkinsonism and Related Disorders*, vol. 10, no. 3, pp. 157–168, 2004.

[8] A. W. Amara, R. L. Watts, and H. C. Walker, "The effects of deep brain stimulation on sleep in Parkinson's disease," *Therapeutic Advances in Neurological Disorders*, vol. 4, no. 1, pp. 15–24, 2011.

[9] L. Eugster, P. Bargiotas, C. L. Bassetti, and W. M. M. Schuepbach, "Deep brain stimulation and sleep-wake functions in Parkinson's disease: a systematic review," *Parkinsonism and Related Disorders*, vol. 32, pp. 12–19, 2016.

[10] C. M. Tolleson, K. Bagai, A. S. Walters, and T. L. Davis, "A pilot study assessing the effects of pallidal deep brain stimulation on sleep quality and polysomnography in Parkinson's patients," *Neuromodulation: Technology at the Neural Interface*, vol. 19, no. 7, pp. 724–730, 2016.

[11] H. Honig, A. Antonini, P. Martinez-Martin et al., "Intrajejunal levodopa infusion in Parkinson's disease: a pilot multicenter study of effects of nonmotor symptoms and quality of life," *Movement Disorders*, vol. 24, no. 10, pp. 1468–1474, 2009.

[12] M. Zibetti, M. Rizzone, A. Merola et al., "Sleep improvement with levodopa/carbidopa intestinal gel infusion," *Acta Neurol Scand*, vol. 127, no. 5, pp. e28–e32, 2013.

[13] M. Zibetti, A. Romagnolo, A. Merola et al., "A polysomnographic study in parkinsonian patients treated with intestinal levodopa infusion," *Journal of Neurology*, vol. 264, no. 6, pp. 1085–1090, 2017.

[14] O. De Fabregues, J. Dot, M. Abu-Suboh et al., "Long-term safety and effectiveness of levodopa-carbidopa intestinal gel infusion," *Brain and Behavior*, vol. 7, no. 8, article e00758, 2017.

[15] E. Chiner, J. M. Arriero, J. Signes-Costa, J. Marco, and I. Fuentes, "Validación de la versión española del test de somnolencia epworth en pacientes con síndrome de apnea del sueño," *Archivos de Bronconeumología*, vol. 35, no. 9, pp. 422–427, 1999.

[16] P. O. Valko, C. L. Bassetti, K. E. Bloch, U. Held, and C. R. Baumann, "Validation of the fatigue severity scale in a swiss cohort," *Sleep*, vol. 31, no. 11, pp. 1601–1607, 2008.

[17] F. Hita-Contreras, E. Martínez-López, P. A. Latorre-Román, F. Garrido, M. A. Santos, and A. Martínez-Amat, "Reliability and validity of the Spanish version of the Pittsburgh sleep quality index (PSQI) in patients with fibromyalgia," *Rheumatology International*, vol. 34, no. 7, pp. 929–936, 2014.

[18] J. S. Wiebe and J. A. Penley, "A psychometric comparison of the Beck depression inventory-II in English and Spanish," *Psychological Assessment*, vol. 17, no. 4, pp. 481–485, 2005.

[19] J. C. Ramon-Brieve, "Validación de la versión castellana de Hamilton para la depresión," *Actas Luso Esp Neurol Psiquiatr Cienc Afines*, vol. 14, pp. 324–334, 1989.

[20] R. B. Berry, R. Budhiraja, D. J. Gottlieb et al., "Rules for scoring respiratory events in sleep: update of the 2007 AASM manual for the scoring of sleep and associated events. Deliberations of the sleep apnea definitions task force of the American academy of sleep medicine," *Journal of Clinical Sleep Medicine*, vol. 8, no. 5, pp. 597–619, 2012.

[21] S. Fahn, R. L. Elton, and Members of the UPDRS Development Committee, "Unified Parkinson's disease rating scale," in *Recent Developments in Parkinson's Disease*, S. Fahn, C. D. Marsden, M. Goldstein et al., Eds., pp. 153–163, Macmillan Healthcare Information, Florham Park, NJ, USA, 1987.

[22] M. M. Hoehn and M. D. Yahr, "Parkinsonism: onset, progression and mortality," *Neurology*, vol. 17, no. 5, pp. 427–442, 1967.

[23] R. S. Schwab and A. C. England Jr., "Projection technique for evaluating surgery in Parkinson's disease," in *Third Symposium on Parkinson's Disease*, F. J. Gilingham and I. M. L. Donaldson, Eds., pp. 152–157, E & S Livingstone, Edinburgh, UK, 1969.

[24] M. F. Folstein, S. E. Folstein, and P. R. McHugh, ""Mini-mental state": a practical method for grading the cognitive state of patients for the clinician," *Journal of Psychiatric Research*, vol. 12, no. 3, pp. 189–198, 1975.

[25] M. T. Cáceres-Redondo, F. Carrillo, M. J. Lama et al., "Long-term levodopa/carbidopa intestinal gel in advanced Parkinson's disease," *Journal of Neurology*, vol. 261, no. 3, pp. 561–569, 2014.

[26] O. Băjenaru, A. Ene, B. O. Popescu et al., "The effect of levodopa-carbidopa intestinal gel infusion long-term therapy on motor complications in advanced Parkinson's disease: a multicenter Romanian experience," *Journal of Neural Transmission*, vol. 123, no. 4, pp. 407–414, 2016.

[27] A. Antonini, A. Yegin, C. Preda, L. Bergmann, and W. Poewe, "GLORIA study investigators and coordinators. Global long-term study on motor and non-motor symptoms and safety of levodopa-carbidopa intestinal gel in routine care of advanced Parkinson's disease patients; 12-month interim outcomes," *Parkinsonism and Related Disorders*, vol. 21, no. 3, pp. 231–235, 2015.

[28] S. E. Palhagen, N. Dizdar, T. Hauge et al., "Interim analysis of long-term intraduodenal levodopa infusion in advanced Parkinson disease," *Acta Neurologica Scandinavica*, vol. 126, no. 6, pp. 29–33, 2012.

[29] K. Wirdefeldt, P. Odin, and D. Nyholm, "Levodopa-carbidopa intestinal gel in patients with Parkinson's disease: a systematic review," *CNS Drugs*, vol. 30, no. 5, pp. 381–404, 2016.

[30] R. G. Elbers, J. Verhoef, E. E. van Wegen, H. W. Berendse, and G. Kwakkel, "Interventions for fatigue in Parkinson's disease," *Cochrane Database of Systematic Reviews*, vol. 10, article CD010925, 2015.

22

Potential Therapeutic Drugs for Parkinson's Disease Based on Data Mining and Bioinformatics Analysis

Chuan Xu,[1] **Jiajun Chen,**[1] **Xia Xu,**[2] **Yingyu Zhang,**[1] **and Jia Li**(iD)[1]

[1]*Department of Neurology (III), China-Japan Union Hospital of Jilin University, Changchun 130033, Jilin, China*
[2]*Yiwu Maternal and Child Health Hospital, Yiwu 322000, Zhejiang, China*

Correspondence should be addressed to Jia Li; lijia33233@jlu.edu.cn

Academic Editor: Jan Aasly

The objective is to search potential therapeutic drugs for Parkinson's disease based on data mining and bioinformatics analysis and providing new ideas for research studies on "new application of conventional drugs." Method differential gene candidates were obtained based on data mining of genes of PD brain tissue, original gene data analysis, differential gene crossover, pathway enrichment analysis, and protein interaction, and potential therapeutic drugs for Parkinson's disease were obtained through drug-gene relationship. *Result.* 250 common differential genes were obtained from 3 research studies, and 31 differential gene candidates were obtained through gene enrichment analysis and protein interaction. 10 drugs such as metformin hydrochloride were directly or indirectly correlated to differential gene candidates. *Conclusion.* Potential therapeutic drugs that may be used for prevention and treatment of Parkinson's disease were discovered through data mining and bioinformatics analysis, which provided new ideas for research and development of drugs. Results showed that metformin hydrochloride and other drugs had certain therapeutical effect on Parkinson's disease, and melbine (DMBG) can be used for treatment of Parkinson's disease and type 2 diabetes patients.

1. Introduction

With a high morbidity and a high disability rate, Parkinson's disease is the second degenerative disease of nervous system. Presently, treatment Parkinson's disease focuses on symptomatic treatment, which can just relief the symptoms and can neither effectively inhibit the progression of the disease nor cure it [1, 2]. Research studies on "new application of conventional drugs" based on differential genes of the brain tissue may enable to cure Parkinson's disease (PD). Aspirin is a famous drug with "new application of conventional drugs." Aspirin was first applied to antipyretic-analgesic and anti-inflammatory treatment as a nonsteroidal anti-inflammatory drug. Then, it was found to be able to inhibit antiplatelet aggregation of TXA2, and thus it has been extensively applied to treatment of cardiovascular and cerebrovascular diseases [3, 4]. However, the mining model of indications for drug therapy was different from traditional drug R&D modes. The latter depended on physical tests,

such as cell test, animal test, and clinical test, which were made to determine chemical components of relevant substances, and synthesis of drug compounds and featured high investment, high risk, and long R&D cycle [5, 6]. It was an alternative solution for drug R&D to readjust existing drugs for treatment of other diseases, guarantee of drug safety, lower cost, and higher R&D efficiency [7].

This paper was aimed at providing new drug candidates for PD treatment and providing new methods and ideas for drug screening through data mining and bioinformatics analysis of PD brain tissue.

2. Method

(i) As shown in Figure 1, "PD (Parkinson's disease)" and "gene expression profiling" were retrieved in GEO dataset (gene expression omnibus dataset), and references were screened. Selection criteria for retrieved references: the approval of Ethics Committee was

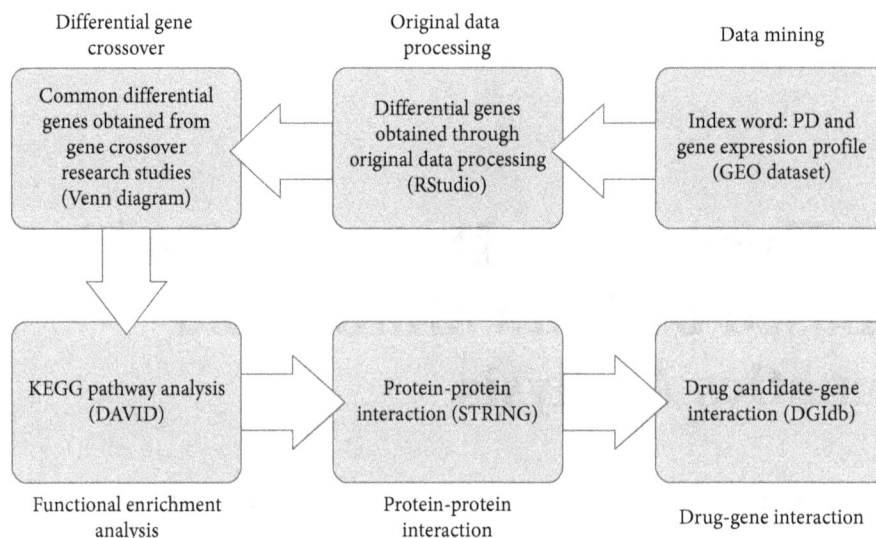

FIGURE 1: Technical route of data mining.

indicated in the research; diagnosis of PD was demonstrated by clinic and neuropathology; the brain tissue of normal people and PD patients was the research object; original gene data can be obtained; original gene chip had high quality. Exclusion criteria: the approval of Ethics Committee was not indicated in the research; diagnosis of PD was not demonstrated by clinic and neuropathology; the research object was not the brain tissue of normal people and PD patients; original gene data cannot be obtained; original gene chip had poor quality. Screened original gene data was obtained and downloaded.

(ii) The quality of original gene data was evaluated using R language and RStudio software, and logFC > 1 or logFC < (−1) was set to obtain differential genes.

(iii) Venn diagram of differential genes obtained in the research studies using bioinformatics and evolutionary genomics (http://bioinformatics.psb.ugent.be/webtools/venn/), and common differential genes were obtained.

(iv) KEGG pathway analysis of common differential genes was made using DAVID (https://david.ncifcrf.gov/) and differential genes closely related to PD were screened [8].

(v) Protein-protein interaction of genes closely related to PD was figured out using STRING (https://string-db.org/), so as to make the protein-protein interaction closer and reduce the range of differential gene candidates. Confidence level ≥ 0.90 was set using STRING and protein-protein interactions, and differential gene candidates were obtained [9].

(vi) Differential gene candidates were inputted into DGIdb dataset (http://dgidb.genome.wustl.edu/) so as to obtain the interrelation between drug and gene and drug candidates for treatment of PD. Relevant information of drug was obtained using PubChem dataset, the approval for clinic or clinical test was searched in ClinicalTrials dataset, and drug candidates were analyzed [10, 11].

3. Result

One hundred sixty-three retrieved results were obtained from the retrieval of "PD (Parkinson's disease)" and "gene expression profiling" in GEO dataset, and based on strict screening, 3 of them conformed the screening requirements and can be applied to our research studies (Moran et al. [12] (chip number: GSE8397); Lewandowski et al. [13] (chip number: GSE19587); Edna et al. [14] (chip number: GSE20333)). 3 searches were analyzed using RStudio software, and 1191, 4484, and 2173 differential genes were obtained, respectively. The Venn diagram of 3 groups of differential genes was drawn using "bioinformatics and evolutionary genomics," as shown in Figure 2, and 250 common differential genes were obtained.

KEGG pathway analysis was made for 250 differential genes using DAVID, and pathways whose P value was less than 0.05 were screened. Figure 3 showed KEGG pathway analysis of 250 differential genes whose P value was less than 0.05. Metabolic pathways, carbon metabolisms, cysteine and methionine metabolism, and Parkinson's disease were 4 KEGG pathways with a smaller P value, and they contained 51, 12, 7, and 12 differential genes, respectively, as shown in Table 1. 82 differential genes of the aforesaid 4 pathways were further analyzed.

Protein-protein interaction of 82 differential genes of the aforesaid 4 pathways was obtained using STRING, and confidence level ≥ 0.90 was set in STRING so as to ensure proteins were closely related. As shown in Figure 4, 31 proteins were closely connected. It indicated that the drug had direct or indirect effect on 31 proteins when it acted on one or more proteins.

31 differential gene candidates were inputted into DGIdb dataset so as to obtain the drug interacting with the aforesaid genes, and 10 drug candidates were obtained through

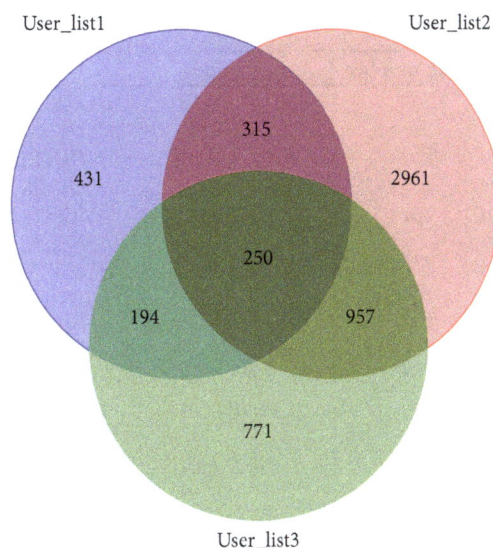

FIGURE 2: Venn diagram of 3 groups of differential genes. List 1, list 2, and list 3 were differential genes of chips GSE8397, GSE19587 and GSE8397, and GSE20333 respectively. 431, 2961, and 771 genes of 3 groups were identified by bioinformatics and evolutionary genomics, respectively, and 3 groups had 250 common differential genes.

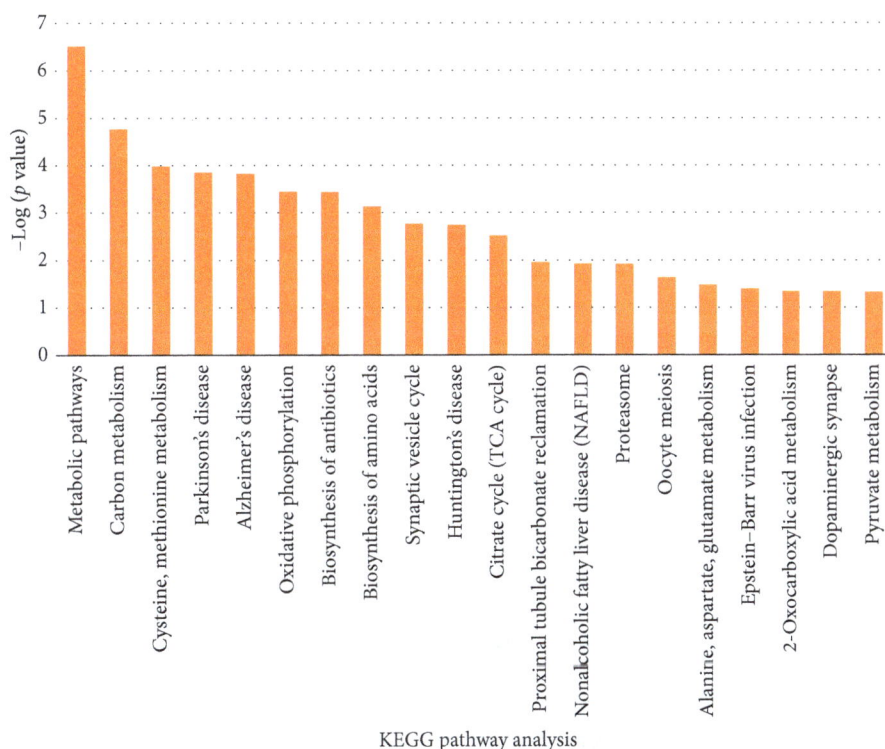

FIGURE 3: KEGG pathway analysis of 250 differential genes whose P value was less than 0.05.

screening their biological characteristics and clinical application. As shown in Table 2, 10 drugs, such as metformin hydrochloride, were directly or indirectly correlated to differential gene candidates.

4. Conclusions

Drugs that may be used for prevention and treatment of PD were discovered through data mining and pathway analysis, which provided new ideas for drug R&D.

Based on the research result and information retrieval relating to drug candidates, 10 drugs such as metformin hydrochloride had certain therapeutical effect on PD, and melbine (DMBG) can be used for treatment of PD and type 2 diabetes patients.

5. Discussion

PD had a high morbidity, and drug therapy represented by dopaminergic drugs was a main treatment method for PD

TABLE 1: Differential genes of 4 DAVID KEGG pathways with a smaller P value.

KEGG pathway	Gene number	P value	Genes
Metabolic pathways	51	$3.08E-07$	UQCRC2, SGSH, LDHA, IMPA1, HMGCR, ATP5B, CYC1, GSS, ALAS1, IDH3G, GOT1, PIGB, PTDSS1, NDUFS1, DHCR24, PLD3, CMAS, PFKP, PFKM, DGUOK, CDO1, NDUFA10, SDS, OAT, MDH2, MDH1, ME3, NDUFB5, SORD, GLUD1, UROS, ASNS, ATP6V1B2, ALDH1A1, ENO2, PAFAH1B1, PTS, PDHX, MTMR4, POLR3F, MSMO1, MOCS2, NDUFA9, NDUFA7, IDH3B, ACLY, ATP6V1E1, NDUFV2, MTR, QPRT, HIBCH
Carbon metabolism	12	$1.70E-0.5$	ME3, GOT1, IDH3G, SDS, GLUD1, ENO2, PFKP, IDH3B, HIBCH, PFKM, MDH2, MDH1
Cysteine and methionine metabolism	7	$1.05E-0.4$	LDHA, GOT1, SDS, MTR, CDO1, MDH2, MDH1
Parkinson's disease	12	$1.40E-0.4$	UQCRC2, NDUFB5, NDUFA9, ATP5B, CYC1, NDUFA7, NDUFV2, UCHL1, SLC18A2, NDUFA10, VDAC3, NDUFS1

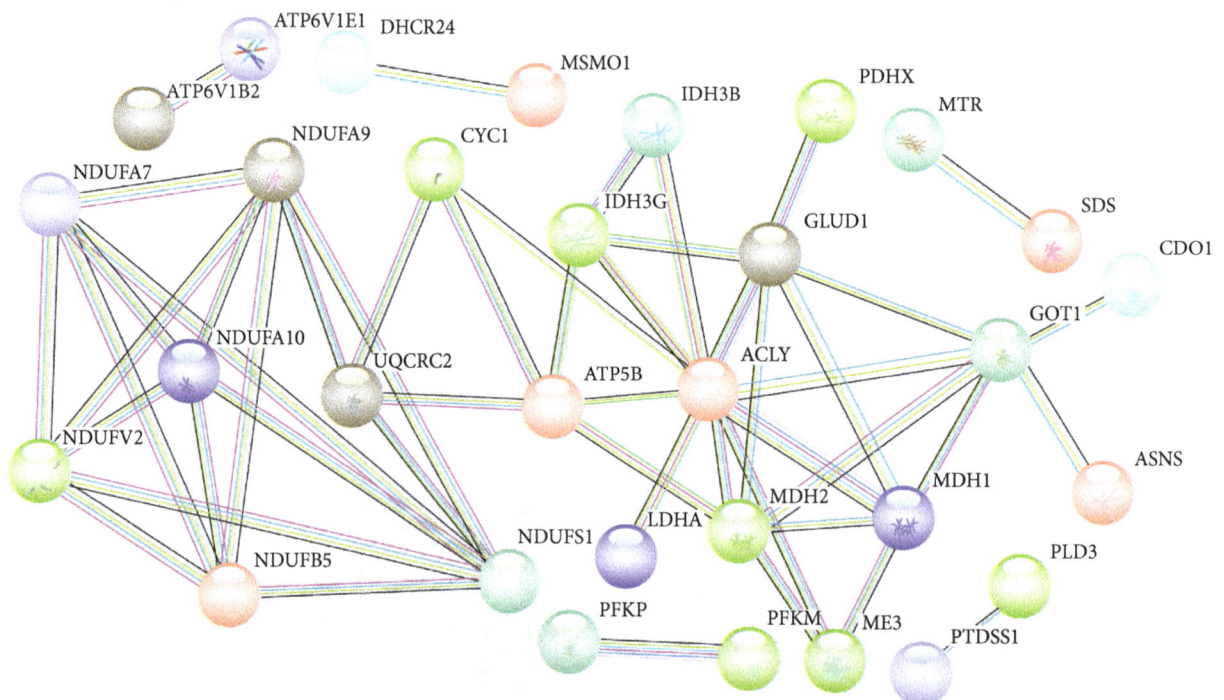

FIGURE 4: Thirty-one protein-protein correlations.

[15]. Nevertheless, anti-Parkinson's disease drugs mainly acted on dopamine metabolism and cholinergic metabolic pathways instead of the apoptosis mechanism of dopaminergic neuron, so it can neither inhibit the progress of the disease effectively nor cure the disease. Whereas traditional drugs synthesized based on physical tests and drug compounds featured long R&D cycle, high investment, high risk, and poor curative effect of clinical test, anti-Parkinson's disease drugs fell behind in drug R&D and could not accommodate to the rapid growth of PDs [16].

Data mining was an emerging research area in recent years that aimed to excavate potential and possible data pattern, internal relation, rule and development trend, etc.

from unorganized data information, extract effective, novel, useful, understandable, and scattered valuable knowledge from text files and to make use of such knowledge for better information organization. Data mining of biomedical literature was construed as effective formation of research hypothesis, since it can reveal a new relationship between gene and pathogenesis. New evidences of adjustment of existing indications for drug therapy can be obtained through data mining combined with other bioinformatics tools [17–19] and reliable conclusions were drawn from drug R&D based on data mining.

In this research, macromining and microanalysis were combined innovatively, the direction of drug screening was

TABLE 2: Thirty-one drug candidates for differential gene prediction (drug-gene connection table).

Drug	Gene	Interaction types	Approved?	Administration	Approved use	PubMed ID
Citric acid	MDH2	N/A	Yes	Oral administration	Anticoagulation	10592235
Folic acid	MTR	N/A	yes	Oral administration	Trophic nerve	
Hydroxocobalamin	MTR	Cofactor	Yes	Oral administration/intravenous drip	Neuroprotection	18565, 1744096, 7599160, 3812589, 9587031
L-glutamate	ASNS, GLUD1, GOT1	N/A	Phase 3	Oral administration	Neuroprotection	17139284, 17016423, 8288265, 17139284, 17016423, 17444813
Metformin hydrochloride	NDUFA10, NDUFA7, NDUFA9, NDUFB5, NDUFS1, NDUFV2	Inhibitor	Yes	Oral administration	Hypoglycemic effect	
Methionine	MTR	Product	Yes	Oral administration	Liver protection	17222188, 16618098, 17615995, 16788729, 17052662
Niacinamide	LDHA	N/A	Yes	Oral administration	Cardiac disease, cognitive disorder	10592235, 17139284, 17016423
Pyridoxal phosphate	GOT1, SDS	Activator	Phase 2	Oral administration	Dyskinesia	11340119, 16925884, 12167474, 11888303, 11752352, 14596599, 15155761, 14646100, 16580895, 15689518
Quercetin	ATP5B	N/A	Phase 1	Oral administration	Pain	10592235
Serine	SDS	N/A	Phase 2	Oral administration	Cognitive improvement	4377655, 14688104, 17139284, 17016423, 500557

determined, and targeting and high efficiency of drug mining were guaranteed based on big data analysis, bioinformatics analysis, and molecular pathology. 3 research studies were included in this research based on data mining of PD in GEO dataset. 250 differential genes were obtained from 3 groups of differential genes after gene crossover based on data mining of original gene and underwent KEGG analysis. KEGG pathway included Parkinson's disease and other pathways. 82 differential genes selected from 4 KEGG pathways with a smaller P value were further analyzed in order to ensure the reliability of differential gene candidates, drug-gene correlation of 31 differential gene candidates was analyzed, and finally 10 drug candidates were screened out.

Some potential therapeutic drugs for PD were discovered in our research studies, among which melbine (DMBG) was worth noting. Current research studies showed that mitochondrial function disorder, abnormal protein aggregation, neuroinflammation increase, and impaired cerebral glucose metabolism were common processes of insulin resistance,

diabetes, and nervous system degeneration and have been identified as the key mechanism for the progress of PD and cognitive disorder [20]. Besides, it has been considered that melbine (DMBG) cannot be applied to treatment of type 2 diabetes through adjustment of glucose metabolism disorder, but it had obvious protective effect on the nerve cells of PD and other nervous system degenerations [21]. This research showed that metformin hydrochloride can be combined with NDUFA10, NDUFA7, NDUFA9, NDUFB5, NDUFS1, NDUFV2, and other acceptors and thus affect the mitochondrial respiratory chain. Information retrieval indicated that melbine (DMBG) had therapeutic effect on the animal model of PD, and epidemiological survey also indicated that it had effect on prevention and treatment of PD. Mark et al. carried out epidemiological survey on type 2 diabetes patients with PD and found that the probability of type 2 diabetes patients suffering PD was 2.2 times higher than normal people. However, melbine (DMBG) could control blood glucose so as to reduce the probability of type 2 diabetes patients suffering PD [22, 23]. Kang et al. discovered that melbine (DMBG) could mediate ATF2/CREB-PGC-1α pathway, induce proteomic change of metabolisms and mitochondria pathways in the substantia nigra, increase mitochondrial protein in the substantia nigra and the corpus striatum, protect dopaminergic neuron in the substantia nigra and the corpus striatum, and improve dyskinesia of PD [24]. Julia et al. discovered that TRAP1 could adjust the mitochondrial function of downstream PINK1 and HTRA2, malfunction of TRAP1 increased free NADH, mitochondria was produced, unfolded protein reaction and membrane potential of mitochondria were triggered, the sensitivity of mitochondria elimination and apoptosis decreased, and PD patients suffered TRAP1 malfunction, while metformin hydrochloride could adjust energy metabolism, produce mitochondria, recover the mitochondrial membrane potential, reverse mitochondrial mitochondrial function arising from TRAP1 mutation of PD, and provide new ideas for mitochondrial pathological change and treatment of PD [22, 25, 26]. Nevertheless, metformin hydrochloride had many untoward effects. Gastrointestinal reaction was the most common untoward effect, and other uncommon untoward effects included lactic acidosis, cutaneous anaphylaxis, hepatorenal damage, hypoglycemia, hematological damage, acute pancreatitis, neural abnormity, etc. [27, 28]. Therefore, metformin hydrochloride may have great clinical effect on treatment of PD, but we suggested using melbine (DMBG) for treatment of PD with type 2 diabetes and paying attention to the side effects.

Other than melbine (DMBG), other potential therapeutic drugs for PD were also discovered in this research. Research studies showed that PD patients lacked V12 but had higher HCY (homocysteine), so V12 could improve cognitive disorder and other symptoms of PD [29]. Clinical tests on vitamin B12 for treating cognitive disorder and other nonmotor symptoms of PD have been terminated [30]. In this research, hydroxocobalamin (namely vitamin B12) had mutual effect with MTR and affected transmethylation of methyl cobalamin to HCY (homocysteine) and consequently it gave play to neuroprotection. Folic acid was similar to hydroxocobalamin, both were the substrates of nerve regression and showed the potential to improve nonmotion functional disorder of PD. Methionine took part in many important physiological processes of human body, it has been rarely reported on PD and may have the potential to treat PD. Citric acid was an anticoagulant drug that took part in tricarboxylic acid cycle, affected the production of mitochondrial energy, and had a certain potential to treat PD [31]. L-glutamate interacted with ASNS, GLUD1, and GOT1. The interaction between dopamine and glutamic acid in the basal ganglion played an important part in the adjustment of motion and cognitive behavior, and functional disorder of dopaminergic-glutamic acid pathway was discovered in PD pathology [32–34]. Serine was an amino acid and research studies indicated that amino acid of D-serine could improve behavior and motor symptoms of PD [35, 36]. Moreover, niacinamide interacted with LDHA. Research studies showed that niacinamide protected dopaminergic neuron from neural degeneration induced by

MPTP in the PD rat model, and it had protective effect on dopaminergic neuron [37, 38]. Niacinamide was a constituent part of coenzyme I and coenzyme II and became a coenzyme of many dehydrogenase. It has been approved to be used for prevention of endemic erythema and aniacinosis. Meanwhile, niacinamide could improve cognitive disorder of Alzheimer disease and has entered the second clinical test stage [39]. Pyridoxal phosphate, namely, vitamin B6, was a coenzyme of aminopherase and decarboxylase in the amino acid metabolism that could promote decarboxylation of glutamic acid. It has been discovered that oral administration of a moderate amount of vitamin B6 had preventive effect on PD [40, 41]. Furthermore, pyridoxal phosphate could relieve tardive dyskinesia of schizophrenia and schizoaffective disorder patients and has entered the second test stage [42]. Quercetin was an active component of many traditional Chinese medicines. It has been approved to be used for reducing the friability of blood corpuscle and had neuroprotective effect on dopaminergic neuron due to antioxygenation [43, 44].

This research still has some disadvantages. It is currently believed that Parkinson's disease is a neurodegenerative disease, caused by a combination of genetic factors, environmental factors, and nervous system aging, through oxidative stress, proteasome dysfunction, inflammation/immune response, mitochondrial dysfunction, calcium homeostasis, excitatory toxins, apoptosis, etc., leading to the degeneration and loss of substantia nigra dopaminergic neurons [45]. The susceptibility gene of Parkinson's disease is part of the pathogenic factor, so the efficacy of Parkinson's disease-based therapeutic drugs based on the Parkinson's disease susceptibility gene needs to be further evaluated. 3 research studies failed to identify the drugs for PD during the lifetime, so differential genes between PD group and the control group may be caused by other pathogenic factors. The drug candidates failed to further verify the potential therapeutical effect on PD. However, this research provided new ideas for R&D of PD drugs and potentially safe drugs for treatment of PD.

In short, drugs that may be used for prevention and treatment of PD can be obtained from data mining and bioinformatics analysis, which provided new ideas for drug R&D and research studies on "new application of conventional drugs." Metformin hydrochloride and other drugs had great clinical effect on treatment of PD, so melbine (DMBG) can be used for treatment of PD and type 2 diabetes patients, which can be proved by more clinical tests.

References

[1] T. Capriotti and K. Terzakis, "Parkinson disease," *Home Healthcare Now*, vol. 34, no. 6, pp. 300–307, 2016.

[2] J. M. Ellis and M. J. Fell, "Current approaches to the treatment of Parkinson's disease," *Bioorganic & Medicinal Chemistry Letters*, vol. 27, no. 18, pp. 4247–4255, 2017.

[3] J. Y. Wick, "Aspirin: a history, a love story," *Consultant Pharmacist*, vol. 27, no. 5, pp. 322–329, 2012.

[4] M. J. R. Desborough and D. M. Keeling, "The aspirin story-from willow to wonder drug," *British Journal of Haematology*, vol. 177, no. 5, pp. 674–683, 2017.

[5] A. Ranga, N. Gjorevski, and M. P. Lutolf, "Drug discovery through stem cell-based organoid models," *Advanced Drug Delivery Reviews*, vol. 69-70, pp. 19–28, 2014.

[6] A. Astashkina and D. W. Grainger, "Critical analysis of 3-D organoid in vitro cell culture models for high-throughput drug candidate toxicity assessments," *Advanced Drug Delivery Reviews*, vol. 69-70, pp. 1–18, 2014.

[7] J. Kirk, N. Shah, B. Noll et al., "Text mining-based in silico drug discovery in oral mucositis caused by high-dose cancer therapy," *Supportive Care in Cancer*, vol. 26, no. 8, pp. 2695–2705, 2018.

[8] D. W. Huang, B. T. Sherman, Q. Tan et al., "DAVID bioinformatics resources: expanded annotation database and novel algorithms to better extract biology from large gene lists," *Nucleic Acids Research*, vol. 35, no. 2, pp. W169–W175, 2007.

[9] D. Szklarczyk, A. Franceschini, S. Wyder et al., "STRING v10: protein-protein interaction networks, integrated over the tree of life," *Nucleic Acids Research*, vol. 43, pp. D447–D452, 2015.

[10] K. C. Cotto, A. H. Wagner, Y.-Y. Feng et al., "DGIdb 3.0: a redesign and expansion of the drug-gene interaction database," *Nucleic Acids Research*, vol. 46, no. D1, pp. D1068–D1073, 2017.

[11] G. Fu, C. Batchelor, M. Dumontier, J. Hastings, E. Willighagena, and E. Bolton, "PubChemRDF: towards the semantic annotation of PubChem compound and substance databases," *Journal of Cheminformatics*, vol. 7, no. 1, p. 34, 2015.

[12] L. B. Moran, D. C. Duke, M. Deprez, D. T. Dexter, R. K. Pearce, and M. B. Graeber, "Whole genome expression profiling of the medial and lateral substantia nigra in Parkinson's disease," *Neurogenetics*, vol. 7, no. 1, pp. 1–11, 2006.

[13] N. M. Lewandowski, S. Ju, M. Verbitsky et al., "Polyamine pathway contributes to the pathogenesis of Parkinson disease," *Proceedings of the National Academy of Sciences*, vol. 107, no. 39, pp. 16970–16975, 2010.

[14] G. Edna, M. Silvia, J. Jasmine et al., "Gene expression profiling of parkinsonian substantia nigra," *GEO*, 2010.

[15] A. Affini, S. Hagenow, A. Zivkovic, J. Marco-Contelles, and H. Stark, "Novel indanone derivatives as MAO B/H3R dual-targeting ligands for treatment of Parkinson's disease," *European Journal of Medicinal Chemistry*, vol. 148, pp. 487–497, 2018.

[16] B. Thrash, K. Thiruchelvan, M. Ahuja, V. Suppiramaniam, and M. Dhanasekaran, "Methamphetamine-induced neurotoxicity: the road to Parkinson's disease," *Pharmacological Reports*, vol. 61, no. 6, pp. 966–977, 2009.

[17] E. L. Berg, "Systems biology in drug discovery and development," *Drug Discovery Today*, vol. 19, no. 2, pp. 113–125, 2014.

[18] E. Mosca, G. Bertoli, E. Piscitelli et al., "Identification of functionally related genes using data mining and data integration: a breast cancer case study," *BMC Bioinformatics*, vol. 10, no. 12, p. S8, 2009.

[19] S. Yu, L.-C. Tranchevent, B. De Moor, and Y. Moreau, "Gene prioritization and clustering by multi-view text mining," *BMC Bioinformatics*, vol. 11, no. 1, p. 28, 2010.

[20] M. R. Ashraghi, G. Pagano, S. Polychronis, F. Niccolini, and M. Politis, "Parkinson's disease, diabetes and cognitive impairment," *Recent Patents on Endocrine, Metabolic & Immune Drug Discovery*, vol. 10, no. 1, pp. 11–21, 2016.

[21] B. Viollet, B. Guigas, N. S. Garcia, J. Leclerc, M. Foretz, and F. Andreelli, "Cellular and molecular mechanisms of metformin: an overview," *Clinical Science*, vol. 122, no. 6, pp. 253–270, 2012.

[22] M. L. Wahlqvist, M.-S. Lee, C.-C. Hsu, S.-Y. Chuang, J.-T. Lee, and H.-N. Tsai, "Metformin-inclusive sulfonylurea therapy reduces the risk of Parkinson's disease occurring with type 2 diabetes in a Taiwanese population cohort," *Parkinsonism & Related Disorders*, vol. 18, no. 6, pp. 753–758, 2012.

[23] M. L. Wahlqvist, M.-S. Lee, S.-Y. Chuang et al., "Increased risk of affective disorders in type 2 diabetes is minimized by sulfonylurea and metformin combination: a population-based cohort study," *BMC Medicine*, vol. 10, no. 1, p. 150, 2012.

[24] H. Kang, R. Khang, S. Ham et al., "Activation of the ATF2/CREB-PGC-1alpha pathway by metformin leads to dopaminergic neuroprotection," *Oncotarget*, vol. 8, no. 30, pp. 48603–48618, 2017.

[25] J. C. Fitzgerald, A. Zimprich, D. A. C. Berrio et al., "Metformin reverses TRAP1 mutation-associated alterations in mitochondrial function in Parkinson's disease," *Brain*, vol. 140, no. 9, pp. 2444–2459, 2017.

[26] H. Kim, J. Yang, M. J. Kim et al., "Tumor necrosis factor receptor-associated protein 1 (TRAP1) mutation and TRAP1 inhibitor gamitrinib-triphenylphosphonium (G-TPP) induce a forkhead box o (FOXO)-dependent cell protective signal from mitochondria," *Journal of Biological Chemistry*, vol. 291, no. 4, pp. 1841–1853, 2016.

[27] S. Alusik and Z. Paluch, "Metformin: the past, presence, and future," *Minerva Medica*, vol. 106, no. 4, pp. 233–238, 2015.

[28] The American College of Physicians, "Summaries for patients: oral drug treatment of type 2 diabetes mellitus: a clinical practice guideline from the American College of Physicians," *Annals of Internal Medicine*, vol. 156, no. 3, p. I36, 2012.

[29] Y. Xie, H. Feng, S. Peng, J. Xiao, and J. Zhang, "Association of plasma homocysteine, vitamin B12 and folate levels with cognitive function in Parkinson's disease: a meta-analysis," *Neuroscience Letters*, vol. 636, pp. 190–195, 2017.

[30] F. Cardoso, "Vitamin B12 and Parkinson's disease: what is the relationship?," *Movement Disorders*, vol. 33, no. 5, pp. 702–703, 2018.

[31] L. P. Leow, L. Beckert, T. Anderson, and M.-L. Huckabee, "Changes in chemosensitivity and mechanosensitivity in aging and Parkinson's disease," *Dysphagia*, vol. 27, no. 1, pp. 106–114, 2012.

[32] M. Amalric, "Targeting metabotropic glutamate receptors (mGluRs) in Parkinson's disease," *Current Opinion in Pharmacology*, vol. 20, pp. 29–34, 2015.

[33] I. Obal et al., "Mental disturbances in Parkinson's disease and related disorders: the role of excitotoxins," *Journal of Parkinson's Disease*, vol. 4, no. 2, pp. 139–150, 2014.

[34] S. D. Pizzi, R. G. Bellomo, S. M. Carmignano et al., "Rehabilitation program based on sensorimotor recovery improves the static and dynamic balance and modifies the basal ganglia neurochemistry: a pilot 1H-MRS study on Parkinson's disease patients," *Medicine*, vol. 96, no. 50, article e8732, 2017.

[35] E. Gelfin, Y. Kaufman, I. Korn-Lubetzki et al., "D-serine adjuvant treatment alleviates behavioural and motor symptoms in Parkinson's disease," *International Journal of Neuropsychopharmacology*, vol. 15, no. 4, pp. 543–549, 2012.

[36] T. Clairembault, W. Kamphuis, L. Leclair-Visonneau et al., "Enteric GFAP expression and phosphorylation in Parkinson's disease," *Journal of Neurochemistry*, vol. 130, no. 6, pp. 805–815, 2014.

[37] J. Xu, SQ. Xu, J. Liang, Y. Lu, J. H. Luo, and J. H. Jin, "Protective effect of nicotinamide in a mouse Parkinson's disease model," *Journal of Zhejiang University*, vol. 41, no. 2, pp. 146–152, 2012.

[38] S. Lehmann, A. C. Costa, I. Celardo, S. H. Y. Loh, and L. M. Martins, "Parp mutations protect against mitochondrial dysfunction and neurodegeneration in a PARKIN model of Parkinson's disease," *Cell Death & Disease*, vol. 7, no. 3, article e2166, 2016.

[39] C. Allone, V. Lo Buono, F. Corallo et al., "Cognitive impairment in Parkinson's disease, Alzheimer's dementia, and vascular dementia: the role of the clock-drawing test," *Psychogeriatrics*, vol. 18, no. 2, pp. 123–131, 2018.

[40] L. Shen, "Associations between B vitamins and Parkinson's disease," *Nutrients*, vol. 7, no. 9, pp. 7197–7208, 2015.

[41] Y. Sato, C. Yasumiishi, T. Chiba, and K. Umegaki, "A systematic review to identify unacceptable intake levels of vitamin B6 among patients taking levodopa," *Food Hygiene and Safety Science*, vol. 58, no. 6, pp. 268–274, 2017.

[42] A. O. Adelufosi, O. Abayomi, and T. M. Ojo, "Pyridoxal 5 phosphate for neuroleptic-induced tardive dyskinesia," *Cochrane Database of Systematic Reviews*, vol. 4, article CD010501, 2015.

[43] K. M. D. Joseph and Muralidhara, "Combined oral supplementation of fish oil and quercetin enhances neuroprotection in a chronic rotenone rat model: relevance to Parkinson's disease," *Neurochemical Research*, vol. 40, no. 5, pp. 894–905, 2015.

[44] M. Ay, J. Luo, M. Langley et al., "Molecular mechanisms underlying protective effects of quercetin against mitochondrial dysfunction and progressive dopaminergic neurodegeneration in cell culture and MitoPark transgenic mouse models of Parkinson's Disease," *Journal of Neurochemistry* vol. 141, no. 5, pp. 766–782, 2017.

[45] A. J. Lees, J. Hardy, and T. Revesz, "Parkinson's disease," *The Lancet*, vol. 373, no. 9680, pp. 2055–2066, 2009.

23

The rs13388259 Intergenic Polymorphism in the Genomic Context of the *BCYRN1* Gene Is Associated with Parkinson's Disease in the Hungarian Population

Sándor Márki (ID),[1] **Anikó Göblös** (ID),[2,3] **Eszter Szlávicz**,[2] **Nóra Török** (ID),[4] **Péter Balicza**,[5] **Benjamin Bereznai**,[5] **Annamária Takáts**,[6] **József Engelhardt**,[4] **Péter Klivényi** (ID),[4] **László Vécsei** (ID),[4,7] **Mária Judit Molnár**,[5] **Nikoletta Nagy** (ID),[1] and **Márta Széll**[1,3]

[1]*Department of Medical Genetics, University of Szeged, Somogyi u. 4, 6720 Szeged, Hungary*
[2]*Department of Dermatology and Allergology, University of Szeged, Korányi fasor 6, 6720 Szeged, Hungary*
[3]*MTA-SZTE Dermatological Research Group, University of Szeged, Korányi fasor 6, 6720 Szeged, Hungary*
[4]*Department of Neurology, University of Szeged, Semmelweis u. 6, 6725 Szeged, Hungary*
[5]*Institute of Genomic Medicine and Rare Disorders, Semmelweis University, Tömő u. 25-29, 1083 Budapest, Hungary*
[6]*Department of Neurology, Semmelweis University, VIII. Balassa J. u. 6, 1083 Budapest, Hungary*
[7]*MTA-SZTE Neuroscience Research Group, University of Szeged, Semmelweis u. 6, 6725 Szeged, Hungary*

Correspondence should be addressed to Anikó Göblös; goblos.aniko@med.u-szeged.hu

Academic Editor: Ivan Bodis-Wollner

Parkinson's disease (PD) is a common neurodegenerative disorder characterized by bradykinesia, resting tremor, and muscle rigidity. To date, approximately 50 genes have been implicated in PD pathogenesis, including both Mendelian genes with rare mutations and low-penetrance genes with common polymorphisms. Previous studies of low-penetrance genes focused on protein-coding genes, and less attention was given to long noncoding RNAs (lncRNAs). In this study, we aimed to investigate the susceptibility roles of lncRNA gene polymorphisms in the development of PD. Therefore, polymorphisms ($n = 15$) of the *PINK1-AS, UCHL1-AS, BCYRN1, SOX2-OT, ANRIL* and *HAR1A* lncRNAs genes were genotyped in Hungarian PD patients ($n = 160$) and age- and sex-matched controls ($n = 167$). The rare allele of the rs13388259 intergenic polymorphism, located downstream of the *BCYRN1* gene, was significantly more frequent among PD patients than control individuals (OR = 2.31; $p = 0.0015$). In silico prediction suggested that this polymorphism is located in a noncoding region close to the binding site of the transcription factor HNF4A, which is a central regulatory hub gene that has been shown to be upregulated in the peripheral blood of PD patients. The rs13388259 polymorphism may interfere with the binding affinity of transcription factor HNF4A, potentially resulting in abnormal expression of target genes, such as *BCYRN1*.

1. Introduction

Parkinson's disease (PD) is the second most common neurodegenerative disease, which belongs to the group of motor system disorders. The key pathological hallmark of PD is the progressive loss of dopamine-producing cells in the substantia nigra pars compacta (located in the midbrain), which results in a dopamine depletion in the striatum. This biochemical imbalance manifests with cardinal motor symptoms including resting tremor, muscle rigidity, bradykinesia, and postural instability [1]. PD affects all populations worldwide with the prevalence of 1-2% among individuals over 65 years of age [2, 3]. Despite the numerous attempts of the last decades, there is still no known cure for the disease [4].

PD is a genetically heterozygous disease. A small portion of PD cases is familial, which can be caused by highly penetrant mutations in Mendelian genes, both with autosomal dominant (*SNCA, LRRK2, VPS35, EIF4G1*, and *CHCHD2*) and with autosomal recessive (*parkin, PINK1, DJ1, ATP13A2, FBXO7, PLA2G6*, and *DNAJC*) modes of inheritance [5, 6]. Mutations in some of these genes may also play a role in cases that appear to be sporadic. However, all known monogenic forms of PD explain only about 30% of familial and 3–5% of sporadic cases [7].

The sporadic forms of PD are linked to polymorphisms of low-penetrance genes [6] identified by case-control studies and lately in genome-wide association studies (GWAS). The single-nucleotide polymorphisms (SNPs) of these susceptibility loci contribute to the development of polygenic PD forms and are referred as risk variants for the disease. The polymorphisms located within common susceptibility variants—the *SNCA*, *MAPT*, *LRRK2*, *GBA*, *PARK16*, *BST1*, *DGKQ*, and *STK39* genes—exhibit the strongest association with sporadic PD [8–11]. These previous studies focused on polymorphisms of protein-coding genes, and little attention was given to polymorphisms of noncoding genes.

Long noncoding RNAs (lncRNAs), defined as nonprotein-coding RNA transcripts longer than 200 nucleotides, are emerging as key regulators of diverse cellular processes [12]. Certain lncRNAs are abundantly expressed in the cells of the central nervous system, providing an additional regulatory layer for fine tuning the cellular outcomes necessary for proper neuronal development and function [13]. Evidence is accumulating that lncRNAs have a pivotal role in PD development [14].

The antisense lncRNA of *PINK1* (*PINK1-AS*) is able to stabilize the expression of a *PINK1* splice variant in neurons and is involved in mitochondrial biogenesis [15]. The antisense lncRNA of the *UCHL* gene (*UCHL1-AS*) is under the regulation of Nurr1, which is a major transcription factor involved in dopaminergic cell differentiation and maintenance [16]. The *brain cytoplasmic RNA 1* lncRNA (*BCYRN1*, also referred to as *BC200*) gene is predominantly expressed in neural tissues and shows an elevated level in variety of tumor types [17] and in Alzheimer's disease (AD) brain samples [18]. BC200 lncRNA functions as translation repressor [19]. Another lncRNA implicated in PD is the overlapping transcript (*SOX2-OT*) of the *SRY-related HMG-box-2* gene (*SOX2*) which regulates the cotranscribed *SOX2* gene expression in neurogenesis and serves as a biomarker for neurodegeneration [14, 20]. The *highly accelerated region 1a* (*HAR1A*) gene marks the evolutionary divergence of humans and chimpanzees and plays a pivotal role in cortical-neuron specification and migration [21]. *ANRIL*, the antisense lncRNA of the *cyclin-dependent kinase inhibitor 2b* (*CDKN2B*) gene, is involved in the development of the melanoma and neural system tumor syndrome, familial melanoma syndrome, and various tumor types; however, its association with PD has not yet been investigated [22].

Although reported data suggest that lncRNAs regulate gene expression in the central nervous system, little is known about the role of their common gene variants in the pathogenesis of PD. Therefore, we aimed to investigate whether polymorphisms located in or close to the *PINK1-AS*, *UCHL1-AS*, *BCYRN1*, *SOX2-OT*, *ANRIL*, and *HAR1A* lncRNA genes are associated with PD.

2. Patients and Methods

2.1. Investigated Individuals. The patients (*n* = 160) participating in this study were recruited from the Department of Neurology, University of Szeged, Szeged, Hungary, and from NEPSY Biobank of the Institute of Genomic Medicine and Rare Disorders at Semmelweis University, Budapest, Hungary. All patients fulfilled the diagnostic criteria for PD. Patients and age- and sex-matched healthy controls (*n* = 167) were of Hungarian ancestry. The average age was 66.4 ± 9.31 years for PD patients and 64.9 ± 8.46 years for healthy controls. The percentage of males was 32.53% for PD patients and 45.50% for controls. The investigation was approved by the Internal Ethical Review Board of the University of Szeged and the Ethical Committee of Semmelweis University. Written informed consent was obtained from patients and healthy controls, and the study was conducted according to the Principles of the Declaration of Helsinki.

2.2. Genotyping. Four lncRNA genes previously implicated in PD (*PINK1-AS* (NR_046507), *UCHL1-AS* (KR709885), *BCYRN1* (NR_001568), and *SOX2-OT* (NR_075091)) and two lncRNA genes linked with neuron differentiation and migration (*ANRIL* (AB548314) and *HAR1A* (NR_003244)) were chosen for genotyping. Polymorphisms selected for genotypic analysis had not been previously studied in any neurodegenerative disorders and were present at a high frequency (global minor allele frequency >0.1) in European populations. The following 15 lncRNA variations were selected for analysis: *PINK1-AS* polymorphisms rs542589, rs1043424, and rs540038; *HAR1A* SNPs rs6089838, rs750697, and rs750696; *ANRIL* polymorphisms rs10738605 and rs564398; *BCYRN1* SNPs rs10865224 and rs13388259; *SOX2-OT* polymorphisms rs6765739 and rs13096623; and *UCHL1* SNPs rs12649180, rs17443616, and rs2342526.

Genomic DNA was isolated from peripheral blood samples using the DNeasy Blood and Tissue Kit (QIAGEN; Hilden, Germany). Genotyping of the lncRNA polymorphisms was based on allelic discrimination assays using the TaqMan SNP Genotyping Assay following the manufacturer's instructions (Thermo Fisher Scientific; Rockford, USA). Each genotyping plate contained samples genotyped in duplicate across all plates. Except *HAR1A* rs750696, all SNPs passed quality control criteria (sample call rate 80%, SNP efficiency > 95%, SNP genotyping accuracy > 99.5%).

2.3. Statistical Analysis. Statistical analysis of PD patients and controls was carried out according to the guidelines of case-control allelic association study design. The statistical significance of the association between the examined SNPs of the investigated lncRNA genes and PD was determined with the Fisher exact probability test. The Bonferroni correction for the multiple hypothesis of the analyzed SNPs (*n* = 14) was also defined. For all SNPs, odds ratios (OR) with 95% confidence intervals (CI) were also determined. All statistical analyses were performed with VassarStats (http://www.faculty.vassar.edu/lowry/vassarstats.html).

3. Results

The 14 polymorphisms passing the quality control criteria were initially assessed in 101 PD patients and 83 controls enrolled at the Department of Neurology and Department of Dermatology and Allergology, University of Szeged, Szeged, Hungary. Three polymorphisms showed promising results with respect to allele distribution among PD patients and controls (Supplementary Table 1). The strongest association with PD was observed for the *BCYRN1* rs13388259 polymorphism (OR = 4.43, CI = 2.0–9.8, Fisher exact probability test $p = 0.00004$), and notable results were observed for the *SOX2-OT* rs6765739 SNP (OR = 1.38, CI = 0.9–2.1, Fisher exact probability test $p = 0.0791$) and the *UCHL1* rs12649180 SNP (OR = 1.63, CI = 0.9–3.0, Fisher exact probability test $p = 0.0907$). No other investigated SNPs exhibited association with PD with respect to allele distribution in the two groups.

Due to these encouraging initial results, further PD patients and control individuals were enrolled into the study at the Department of Neurology, University of Szeged, as well as at the Institute of Genomic Medicine and Rare Disorders, Semmelweis University, Budapest, Hungary. The *BCYRN1* rs13388259 SNP, the *SOX2-OT* rs6765739 SNP, and the *UCHL1* rs12649180 SNP were assessed. For this extended study group ($n = 327$; 160 PD patients and 167 healthy controls), the *BCYRN1* rs13388259 SNP again showed strong association with PD, and its rare allele was significantly more common among PD patients than control individuals (OR = 2.31, CI = 1.3–4.0, Fisher exact probability test $p = 0.0015$, Bonferroni correction $p = 0.021$) (Figure 1). The *SOX2-OT* rs6765739 SNP also showed notable, but not significant differences in allele distribution between PD patients and controls (OR = 1.28, CI = 0.9–1.8, Fisher exact probability test $p = 0.0666$). The alleles of the *UCHL1* rs12649180 SNP did not exhibit notable differences in the distribution in PD patients and controls (Table 1).

The majority of SNPs are located in noncoding regions including introns or intergenic regions [23]. The disease association of SNPs located in noncoding regions sometimes is difficult to interpret. Using different sources, multiple in silico analyses were performed to gain information about the putative functional consequences of the SNP.

According to the Ensembl (http://www.ensembl.org/index.html), UCSC Genome Browser/SNP 147 (http://www.genome.ucsc.edu/), VarSome (https://www.varsome.com), and NCBI/refSNP (https://www.ncbi.nlm.nih.gov/SNP/) databases, rs13388259 has been assigned the functional class of intron variant within *BCYRN1* (ENSG00000236824.1), whereas ALFRED (https://www.alfred.med.yale.edu/alfred/index.asp) and F-SNP (http://www.compbio.cs.queensu.ca/F-SNP) database refer to rs13388259 as an intergenic SNP between the *BCYRN1* and *EPCAM* genes on Chromosome 2. According to the NCBI/SNP Database, the rs13388259 polymorphism is located on chr2:47,343,700 (GRCh38). The difference between the predicted functions of the rs13388259 polymorphism is probably the consequence of the miss-annotation of the *BCYRN1* gene and transcript in various databases. By comparing the data in several databases, we found that two overlapping genes and their corresponding transcripts have been given the name BCYRN1 (BC200): a gene 13,458 nt in length (chr2:47,331,060-47,344,517, GRCh38, Gencode Transcript ENST00000418539.1, and Gencode Gene ENSG00000236824.1) and a gene 200 nt in length (chr2:47,335,315-47,335,514,

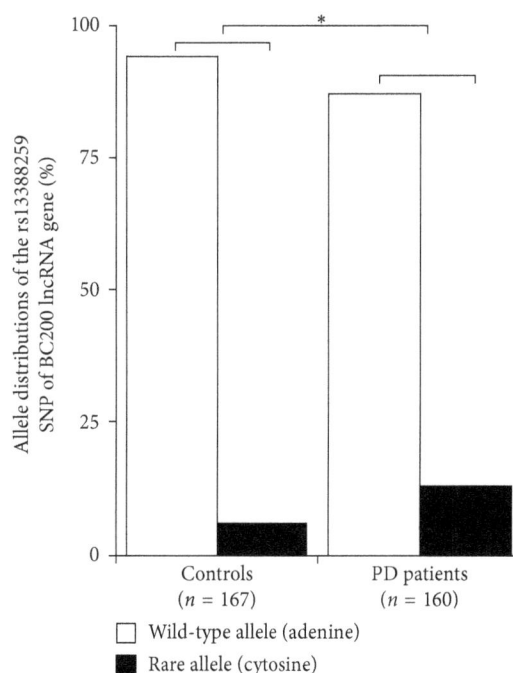

FIGURE 1: Allele distribution of the of the rs13388259 SNP of the *BC200* lncRNA gene among PD patients ($n = 160$) and controls ($n = 167$).

GRCh38, Gencode Transcript ENST00000418539.2, and Gencode Gene ENSG00000236824); the two genes are in the same orientation.

To evaluate if the region containing the rs13388259 polymorphism is transcribed, we designed a primer pair for real-time PCR of that region. Using total RNA isolated from the peripheral blood of healthy individuals ($n = 3$) and chronic lymphoid leukemia (CLL) patients ($n = 3$), cDNA reverse transcription was performed followed by a real-time PCR using the designed primers: no PCR product was detected for the region containing the SNP, although a control using primers for the GAPDH gene was successful (data not shown). Using a primer pair designed for the 200 nt transcript, a PCR product was obtained in samples derived from CLL patients but not in samples from healthy controls (data not shown). This result is in agreement with previous findings that, although BC200 is expressed in normal neural tissue, it is expressed at higher levels in various tumor types. Based on this RT-PCR result, we suppose that rs13388259 is located in an intergenic region.

Results from analysis with the F-SNP software indicated that the rs13388259 SNP is associated with transcriptional regulation. TFBIND software (http://www.tfbind.hgc.jp/) was applied to predict transcription factor binding sites [24], and the analysis revealed that the single-nucleotide alteration in the rs13388259 region (A/C) possibly modifies the binding affinity of a putative transcription factor binding site. To determine the relationships between the identified SNP and regulatory sequences, annotations of regulatory elements containing binding sites were downloaded from the UCSC genome browser [25]. The rs13388259 SNP is located 236 bp downstream of a binding site for the hepatocyte nuclear factor

TABLE 1: Genotype and allele distributions of the rs13388259 SNP of the *BC200* lncRNA gene, the rs6765739 SNP of the *SOX2-OT* lncRNA gene, and the rs12649180 SNP of the *UCHL1* lncRNA gene in PD patients ($n = 160$) and controls ($n = 167$).

	Genotypes (n)			Alleles (n)		Statistical analysis		
	Homozygous wild type	Heterozygous	Homozygous rare	Wild type	Rare	Odds ratio	95% confidence interval	Fisher exact probability test
rs13388259 SNP of the *BC200* lncRNA gene								
PD patients ($n = 160$)	117	43	0	277	43	**2.31**	1.3–4.0	**$p = 0.0015$**
Controls ($n = 167$)	147	19	1	313	21			
rs6765739 SNP of the *SOX2-OT* lncRNA gene								
PD patients ($n = 160$)	17	139	4	173	147	1.28	0.9–1.8	$p = 0.0666$
Controls ($n = 167$)	35	131	1	201	133			
rs12649180 SNP of the *UCHL1* lncRNA gene								
PD patients ($n = 160$)	126	34	0	287	34	1.21	0.8–2.0	$p = 0.2516$
Controls ($n = 167$)	125	42	0	292	42			

4 alpha (HNF4A) transcription factor. According to the ORegAnno DNA regulatory region database, this binding site might be functionally related to the *BCYRN1* gene (OREG1716976 and OREG1741230) (Figure 2). Furthermore, an enhancer region (ID GH02H047342, localization chr2:47,342,469-47,347,454) described in the GeneCard Human Gene Database (http://www.genecards.org) that regulates both the *BCYRN1* and the *EPCAM* genes is located near the rs13388259 SNP. This enhancer region contains binding sites for transcription factors, including HNF4A. The HNF4A transcription factor is associated with gluconeogenesis and diabetes and has been identified as a central regulatory hub gene upregulated in the peripheral blood of PD patients [26].

4. Discussion

As human life spans are prolonged, the incidence of neurodegenerative diseases is increasing. PD is the second most common neurodegenerative diseases worldwide (after Alzheimer's disease) and is currently the most important known risk factor of the elderly with only symptomatic treatment [2, 3]. Therefore, insight into the mechanism of PD is essential. In this study, we contribute to the understanding of the putative roles of lncRNAs, which provide an additional level of gene expression regulation in the development of sporadic, polygenic PD.

We compared the distribution of the rare and wild-type alleles of 15 polymorphisms of the *PINK1-AS*, *UCHL1-AS*, *BCYRN1*, *SOX2-OT*, *ANRIL*, and *HAR1A* lncRNA genes in Hungarian PD patients and ethnicity-, age-, and sex-matched controls. Our results demonstrated strong association between the presences of the rs13388259 intergenic polymorphism and PD. This intergenic SNP is located between the *BCYRN1* and *EPCAM* genes on Chromosome 2, and a functional link to *BCYRN1* has been annotated for the region (http://www.varsome.com, http://www.noncode.org).

The *BCYRN1* lncRNA gene arose after the separation of monkeys and humans in the mammalian linage as

a consequence of the recruitment of the monomeric *Alu* element, which was subjected to retro transposition from an active master gene 35–55 million years ago [27, 28]. BC200 is primate tissue-specific RNA polymerase III transcript [29] exhibiting brain-specific expression in transgenic mice [30]. The BC200 lncRNA is involved in local translational control [31, 32]. Dysfunction of the BC200 lncRNA in neurons—due to either altered expression or mislocalization—results in the deregulation of dendritic mRNA expression, failure of long-term synaptic plasticity, and thus, neurodegeneration [14, 18, 33].

The BCYRN1 lncRNA listed as a 200 nt transcript in the Ensemble Genome Browser (ID: ENST00000418539.2, http://www.ensemble.org) [34]. The rs13388259 SNP is located within an untranscribed region downstream of the BC200 lncRNA and replaces adenine with cytosine (NG_012352.2: g.3538A>C). A binding site for the HNF4A transcription factor is located 236 nt upstream of the SNP, and a short interspersed nuclear element (AluSx) is located 73 nt downstream.

The minor allele frequency (MAF) for the cytosine variant is 0.0865 in the European and in the American population and 0.1807 in Africans. No known clinical significance of this polymorphism has previously been identified by GWAS studies of PD or any other disease.

Previous studies have confirmed that genetic variants in the primary sequence of the lncRNA genes (noncoding RNA transcripts) are highly correlated with human diseases [35, 36]. However, it is difficult to determine the contribution of intronic and intergenic SNPs to the development of disease since these are located outside of the primary RNA sequences. The expression pattern of many lncRNAs shows spatial and temporal specificity, pointing to the strong regulation of lncRNAs expression [37]. Abnormal expression of several lncRNAs is linked to human diseases, for example, elevated level of particular lncRNAs expression closely correlates with several types of cancer formation and/or metastatic activity [38, 39]. SNPs of noncoding genomic regions—either intronic or intergenic—are often located in or closely linked to regulatory regions [23]. They may interfere with host regulatory elements [40, 41] and may affect the expression

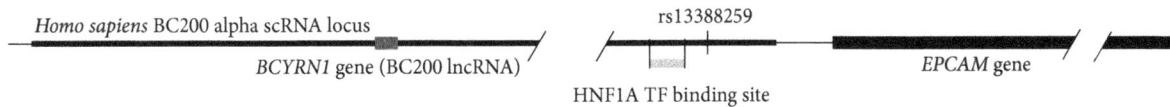

FIGURE 2: The genomic region on Chromosome 2 in which rs13388259 occurs. The rs13388259 SNP is an intergenic polymorphism located on the short arm of Chromosome 2 (Ch2:47,343,700) between the *BCYRN1* and *EPCAM* genes. The 200 nt *BCYRN1* lncRNA gene is located at positions 47,335,315-47,335,514 (ENSG00000236824) and overlaps with the *Homo sapiens* BC200 alpha scRNA locus (accession number AF020057.2; 13,472 bp length; position 47,331,060-47,344,531). The *EPCAM* gene (Chr2:47,345,158-47,387,601; ENSG00000119888) is located 1458 bp downstream of the SNP. The HNF4A transcription factor binding site is located approximately 236 bases upstream of the rs13388259 SNP (Ch2:47,343,088-47,343,464). Genomic positions are relative to GRCh38.

level of lncRNAs implicated in the pathogenesis of certain diseases. The results of our in silico analysis demonstrated that the *BCYRN1* rs13388259 polymorphism lies close to the binding site of the transcription factor HNF4A. HNF4A was identified as a central regulator hub gene upregulated in peripheral blood of PD patient [42]; moreover, the relative abundance of the HNF4A mRNA correlates with the severity of the disease: upon 3-year follow-up constantly increasing HNF4A expression was observed [26]. The *BCYRN1* was predicted as a target gene of HNF4A transcription factor binding site. These data together suggest that the rs13388259 polymorphism may modify the expression level of BC200 lncRNA due to the modification of HNF4A transcription factor binding affinity.

Previous studies linked BC200 lncRNA with neuro-degeneration [18, 36]. This is the first study, however, which confirms the genetic association between the genomic context of the *BCYRN1* lncRNA gene and PD. Our study further emphasizes the increasing awareness of the significance of lncRNAs in the development of human diseases. Further studies are needed to confirm the functional relevance of the identified genetic variants in the expression and/or activity of the BC200 lncRNA and its functions in dopaminergic neurons.

Abbreviations

ANRIL:	Antisense lncRNA of the CDKN2B
BC200/BCYRN1:	Brain cytoplasmic RNA 1 lncRNA
CDKN2B:	Cyclin-dependent kinase inhibitor 2b
HAR1A:	Highly accelerated region 1a
lncRNAs:	Long noncoding RNAs
PD:	Parkinson's disease
PINK1:	Phosphatase- and tensin homologue-induced putative kinase 1
PINK1-AS:	Antisense lncRNA of PINK1
SNCA:	α-synuclein
SNP:	Single nucleotide polymorphisms
SOX2:	SRY-related HMG-box 2 gene
SOX2-OT:	Overlapping transcript of the SOX2
UCHL1:	Ubiquitin carboxy-terminal hydrolase L1
UCHL1-AS:	Antisense lncRNA of the UCHL1.

Authors' Contributions

Sándor Márki, and Anikó Göblös, contributed equally to the manuscript.

Nikoletta Nagy, and Márta Széll, contributed equally to the manuscript.

Acknowledgments

Funding of the study reported in the paper was provided by the Hungarian Brain Research Program (Grant no. KTIA_13_NAP-A-II/15), the Social Renewal Operational Programme (TÁMOP-4.2.2.A-11/1/KONV-2012-0052 and TÁMOP-4.2.2.A-11/1/KONV-2012-0035), and the National Research Development and Innovation Office (GINOP-2.3.2-15-2016-00039). Sándor Márki was supported by the Szeged Scientist Academy (EMMI, TSZ:34232-3/2016/INTFIN) and by the New National Excellence Program by the Hungarian Ministry of Human Capacities (UNKP-17-2). The authors are grateful to the patients and their clinicians and healthy volunteers for providing samples. The authors would like to thank Eszter Hidas, Csilla Hornyák, Csaba Jónás, Tibor Kovács, and Lajos Varannai for patient recruitment.

References

[1] J. Massano and K. P. Bhatia, "Clinical approach to Parkinson's disease: features, diagnosis, and principles of management," *Cold Spring Harbor Perspectives in Medicine*, vol. 2, no. 6, p. a008870, 2012.

[2] S. Fahn, "Description of Parkinson's disease as a clinical syndrome," *Annals of the New York Academy of Sciences*, vol. 991, pp. 1–14, 2003.

[3] R. B. Postuma, D. Berg, M. Stern et al., "MDS clinical diagnostic criteria for Parkinson's disease," *Movement Disorders*, vol. 30, no. 12, pp. 1591–1601, 2015.

[4] L. Soreq, A. Guffanti, N. Salomonis et al., "Long non-coding RNA and alternative splicing modulations in Parkinson's leukocytes identified by RNA sequencing," *PLoS Computational Biology*, vol. 10, no. 3, p. e1003517, 2014.

[5] D. G. Hernandez, X. Reed, and A. B. Singleton, "Genetics in Parkinson disease: Mendelian versus non-Mendelian inheritance," *Journal of Neurochemistry*, vol. 139, no. 1, pp. 59–74, 2016.

[6] M. Ferreira and J. Massano, "An updated review of Parkinson's disease genetics and clinicopathological correlations," *Acta Neurologica Scandinavica*, vol. 135, no. 3, pp. 273–284, 2016.

[7] K. Kumar, A. Djarmati-Westenberger, and A. Grünewald, "Genetics of Parkinson's disease," *Seminars in Neurology*, vol. 31, no. 5, pp. 433–440, 2011.

[8] C. M. Lill, J. T. Roehr, M. B. McQueen et al., "Comprehensive research synopsis and systematic meta-analyses in Parkinson's disease genetics: the PDGene database," *PLoS Genetics*, vol. 8, no. 3, p. e1002548, 2012.

[9] M. A. Nalls, N. Pankratz, C. M. Lill et al., "Large-scale meta-analysis of genome-wide association data identifies six new risk loci for Parkinson's disease," *Nature Genetics*, vol. 46, no. 9, pp. 989–993, 2014.

[10] C. M. Lill, J. Hansen, J. H. Olsen, H. Binder, B. Ritz, and L. Bertram, "Impact of Parkinson's disease risk loci on age at onset," *Movement Disorders*, vol. 30, no. 6, pp. 847–850, 2015.

[11] R. Török, D. Zádori, N. Török, É. Csility, L. Vécsei, and P. Klivényi, "An assessment of the frequency of mutations in the GBA and VPS35 genes in Hungarian patients with sporadic Parkinson's disease," *Neuroscience Letters*, vol. 610, pp. 135–138, 2016.

[12] P. J. Batista and H. Y. Chang, "Long noncoding RNAs: cellular address codes in development and disease," *Cell*, vol. 152, no. 6, pp. 1298–1307, 2013.

[13] M. Sun and W. L. Kraus, "From discovery to function: the expanding roles of long noncoding RNAs in physiology and disease," *Endocrine Reviews*, vol. 36, no. 1, pp. 25–64, 2015.

[14] P. Wu, X. Zuo, H. Deng, X. Liu, L. Liu, and A. Ji, "Roles of long noncoding RNAs in brain development, functional diversification and neurodegenerative diseases," *Brain Research Bulletin*, vol. 97, pp. 69–80, 2013.

[15] M. Chiba, H. Kiyosawa, N. Hiraiwa, N. Ohkohchi, and H. Yasue, "Existence of Pink1 antisense RNAs in mouse and their localization," *Cytogenetic and Genome Research*, vol. 126, no. 3, pp. 259–270, 2009.

[16] C. Carrieri, A. R. R. Forrest, C. Santoro et al., "Expression analysis of the long non-coding RNA antisense to Uchl1 (AS Uchl1) during dopaminergic cells' differentiation in vitro and in neurochemical models of Parkinson's disease," *Frontiers in Cellular Neuroscience*, vol. 9, p. 114, 2015.

[17] W. Chen, W. Böcker, J. Brosius, and H. Tiedge, "Expression of neural BC200 RNA in human tumours," *Journal of Pathology*, vol. 183, no. 3, pp. 345–351, 1997.

[18] E. Mus, P. R. Hof, and H. Tiedge, "Dendritic BC200 RNA in aging and in Alzheimer's disease," *Proceedings of the National Academy of Sciences*, vol. 104, no. 25, pp. 10679–10684, 2007.

[19] D. Lin, T. V. Pestova, C. U. T. Hellen, and H. Tiedge, "Translational control by a small RNA: dendritic BC1 RNA targets the eukaryotic initiation factor 4A helicase mechanism," *Molecular and Cellular Biology*, vol. 28, no. 9, pp. 3008–3019, 2008.

[20] I. Arisi, M. D'Onofrio, R. Brandi et al., "Gene expression biomarkers in the brain of a mouse model for Alzheimer's disease: mining of microarray data by logic classification and feature selection," *Journal of Alzheimer's Disease*, vol. 24, pp. 721–738, 2011.

[21] A. Tolosa, J. Sanjuán, C. Leal, J. Costas, M. D. Moltó, and R. de Frutos, "Rapid evolving RNA gene HAR1A and schizophrenia," *Schizophrenia Research*, vol. 99, no. 1–3, pp. 370–372, 2008.

[22] E. Pasmant, I. Laurendeau, D. Héron, M. Vidaud, D. Vidaud, and I. Bièche, "Characterization of a germ-line deletion, including the entire INK4/ARF locus, in a melanoma-neural system tumor family: identification of ANRIL, an antisense noncoding RNA whose expression coclusters with ARF," *Cancer Research*, vol. 67, no. 8, pp. 3963–3969, 2007.

[23] M. T. Maurano, R. Humbert, E. Rynes et al., "Systematic localization of common disease-associated variation in regulatory DNA," *Science*, vol. 337, no. 6099, pp. 1190–1195, 2012.

[24] T. Tsunoda and T. Takagi, "Estimating transcription factor bindability on DNA," *Bioinformatics*, vol. 15, no. 7-8, pp. 622–630, 1999.

[25] W. J. Kent, C. W. Sugnet, T. S. Furey et al., "The human genome browser at UCSC," *Genome Research*, vol. 12, no. 6, pp. 996–1006, 2002.

[26] J. A. Santiago and J. A. Potashkin, "Network-based meta-analysis identifies HNF4A and PTBP1 as longitudinally dynamic biomarkers for Parkinson's disease," *Proceedings of the National Academy of Sciences*, vol. 112, no. 7, pp. 2257–2262, 2015.

[27] B. V. Skryabin, J. Kremerskothen, D. Vassilacopoulou et al., "The BC200 RNA gene and its neural expression are conserved in Anthropoidea (Primates)," *Journal of Molecular Evolution*, vol. 47, no. 6, pp. 677–685, 1998.

[28] P. Sosińska, J. Mikuła-Pietrasik, and K. Książek, "The double-edged sword of long non-coding RNA: the role of human brain-specific BC200 RNA in translational control, neurodegenerative diseases, and cancer," *Mutation Research/Reviews in Mutation Research*, vol. 766, pp. 58–67, 2015.

[29] A. Ludwig, T. S. Rozhdestvensky, V. Y. Kuryshev, J. Schmitz, and J. Brosius, "An unusual primate locus that attracted two independent Alu insertions and facilitates their transcription," *Journal of Molecular Biology*, vol. 350, no. 2, pp. 200–214, 2005.

[30] T. Khanam, T. S. Rozhdestvensky, M. Bundman, et al., "Two primate-specific small non-protein-coding RNAs in transgenic mice: neuronal expression, subcellular localization and binding partners," *Nucleic Acids Research*, vol. 35, no. 2, pp. 529–539, 2006.

[31] T. Arendt and M. K. Brückner, "Linking cell-cycle dysfunction in Alzheimer's disease to a failure of synaptic plasticity," *Biochimica et Biophysica Acta (BBA)-Molecular Basis of Disease*, vol. 1772, no. 4, pp. 413–421, 2007.

[32] M. A. Faghihi, F. Modarresi, A. M. Khalil et al., "Expression of a noncoding RNA is elevated in Alzheimer's disease and drives rapid feed-forward regulation of beta-secretase," *Nature Medicine*, vol. 14, no. 7, pp. 723–730, 2008.

[33] E. P. Booy, E. K. McRae, R. Howard et al., "The RNA helicase RHAU (DHX36) interacts with the 3' tail of the long non-coding RNA BC200 (BCYRN1)," *Journal of Biological Chemistry*, vol. 291, no. 10, pp. 5355–5372, 2016.

[34] H. Tiedge, W. Chen, and J. Brosius, "Primary structure, neural-specific expression, and dendritic location of human BC200 RNA," *Journal of Neuroscience*, vol. 13, no. 6, pp. 2382–2390, 1993.

[35] M. Halvorsen, J. S. Martin, S. Broadaway, and A. Laederach, "Disease-associated mutations that alter the RNA structural ensemble," *PLoS Genetics*, vol. 6, no. 8, p. e1001074, 2010.

[36] O. Wapinski and H. Y. Chang, "Long noncoding RNAs and human disease," *Trends in Cell Biology*, vol. 21, no. 6, pp. 354–361, 2011.

[37] T. R. Mercer, M. E. Dinger, S. M. Sunkin, M. F. Mehler, and J. S. Mattick, "Specific expression of long noncoding RNAs in the mouse brain," *Proceedings of the National Academy of Sciences*, vol. 105, no. 2, pp. 716–721, 2008.

[38] K. L. Yap, S. Li, A. M. Muñoz-Cabello et al., "Molecular interplay of the noncoding RNA ANRIL and methylated histone H3 lysine 27 by polycomb CBX7 in transcriptional silencing of INK4a," *Molecular Cell*, vol. 38, no. 5, pp. 662–674, 2010.

[39] C. E. Burd, W. R. Jeck, Y. Liu, H. K. Sanoff, Z. Wang, and N. E. Sharpless, "Expression of linear and novel circular forms of an INK4/ARF-associated non-coding RNA correlates with atherosclerosis risk," *PLoS Genetics*, vol. 6, no. 12, p. e1001233, 2010.

24

Parkinson's Disease and Cognitive Impairment

Yang Yang,[1,2] **Bei-sha Tang,**[1,2,3,4] **and Ji-feng Guo**[1,2,3,4]

[1]*Department of Neurology, Xiangya Hospital, Central South University, Changsha, Hunan 410008, China*
[2]*Key Laboratory of Hunan Province in Neurodegenerative Disorders, Central South University, Changsha, Hunan 410008, China*
[3]*State Key Laboratory of Medical Genetics, Changsha, Hunan 410008, China*
[4]*Neurodegenerative Disorders Research Center, Central South University, Changsha, Hunan 410008, China*

Correspondence should be addressed to Ji-feng Guo; guojifeng2003@163.com

Academic Editor: Yuan-Han Yang

Parkinson's disease (PD) is a progressive neurodegenerative disease primarily characterized by the hallmarks of motor symptoms, such as tremor, bradykinesia, rigidity, and postural instability. However, through clinical investigations in patients and experimental findings in animal models of Parkinson's disease for years, it is now well recognized that Parkinson's disease is more than just a motor-deficit disorder. The majority of Parkinson's disease patients suffer from nonmotor disabilities, for instance, cognitive impairment, autonomic dysfunction, sensory dysfunction, and sleep disorder. So far, anti-PD prescriptions and surgical treatments have been mainly focusing on motor dysfunctions, leaving cognitive impairment a marginal clinical field. Within the nonmotor symptoms, cognitive impairment is one of the most common and significant aspects of Parkinson's disease, and cognitive deficits such as dysexecutive syndrome and visuospatial disturbances could seriously affect the quality of life, reduce life expectancy, prolong the duration of hospitalization, and therefore increase burdens of caregiver and medical costs. In this review, we have done a retrospective study of the recent related researches on epidemiology, clinical manifestation and diagnosis, genetics, and potential treatment of cognitive deficits in Parkinson's disease, aiming to provide a summary of cognitive impairment in Parkinson's disease and make it easy for clinicians to tackle this challenging issue in their future practice.

1. Introduction

In developed countries, nearly one out of 100 people older than 60 years old are affected by Parkinson's disease [1]. Cognitive impairment in Parkinson's disease, characterized by predominant executive deficits, visuospatial dysfunction, and relatively unaffected memory, ranges from Parkinson's disease mild cognitive impairment (PD-MCI) to Parkinson's disease dementia (PDD), the former of which could only be detected by various means of comprehensive neuropsychological observations and normally does not affect the patients' daily operations whereas the latter hits more than one area of cognition and is severe enough to impair social or working functions. Moreover, longitudinal studies of long-term clinical investigations suggested that the majority of PD or PD-MCI patients develop dementia as disease deteriorates into the late stage [2–4], and Parkinson's disease dementia is a critically influential factor for the reduced life expectancy in patients with Parkinson's disease [5]. Movement disorder has long been addressed to be burdensome in Parkinson's disease and the development of relatively effective restoration of dopamine by pharmaceutical treatment also contributes to the success of management of motor symptoms, leaving the treatment of nonmotor deficits an unmet clinical need. Furthermore, the aggravation of cognitive disturbances might also be strongly predicted by neuropsychological testing in the early stage of disease with or without timely medical treatment [5–8].

In this review, we illustrate the demographic and clinical symptoms potentially assessed as risk factors for nonmotor deficits in Parkinson's disease and discuss the underlying mechanisms of these symptoms with evidence from genetic studies, with primary focus on the clinical manifestations and diagnosis supported by neuropsychology research, neuroimaging, pharmacology, and molecular genetics. At last, we probe into the clinical pharmacological and nonpharmacological management for Parkinson's disease patients in the light of its heterogeneous nature.

2. Epidemiology

PD is one of the most common neurodegenerative disorders, whose incidence is second only to Alzheimer disease. According to a 5-year follow-up study by Broeders and a Norwegian ParkWest study by Pedersen, 25% to 50% of patients with Parkinson disease develop PD-MCI or PDD or progress from PD-MCI to PDD within 5 years of diagnosis [9, 10]. Studies that followed patients prospectively diagnosed PD with normal cognition and discovered the incidence of cognitive impairment are few till now. However, according to the available evidence, the progression of cognitive impairment was very common and comparatively quick. For instance, one study exhibited that the cumulative incidence of developing cognitive impairment was 8.5% within 1-year follow-up and up to 47.4% within 6-year follow-up [11]. In other studies, the incidence of cognitive impairments in PD patients varied from 48% to 60% by 12–15 years of retrospective follow-up [12, 13]. In addition, the community-based studies indicated that 20–35% of PD population would develop PD-MCI and up to 10% would develop PDD per year [14, 15]. Nonetheless, it is difficult to compare the results of all studies mentioned above, due to differences in sample sizes and statistical methods used. Furthermore, one designed study also clarified that the onset of dementia in PD patients is approximately 70-year-old no matter when the onset of PD is [16].

Not only does the incidence of cognitive impairment in PD patients vary, but also the risk factors for PD-MCI and PDD vary. Pigott et al. claimed that increased baseline Hoehn & Yahr Scale score and Unified PD Rating Scale motor score, and decreased baseline Dementia Rating Scale (DRS-2) scores are powerful predictors of early cognitive deficits [17]. It is widely accepted that DRS-2 might be effective and adequate for predicting cognitive disturbance and could be used as a reference method to test comprehensive cognitive function [16, 18].

3. Etiology

In this part, we mainly focus on the genetics of PD. 18 PD-specific chromosomal loci are named PARK and numbered chronologically, nine of which have been identified and confirmed by linkage analysis or exome sequencing [19–33]. Eight of these loci were identified by linkage analysis, functional candidate gene approach or GWAS studies, and are deemed as susceptibility loci as risk factors [34–39]. And still one of them is supposed to be erroneous locus found to be identical with PARK1 [40]. Within the nine confirmed disease-causing genes, SNCA, LRRK, and VPS35 exhibit an autosomal dominant hereditary pattern while other six genes, Parkin, PINK1, DJ-1, ATP13A2, PLA2G6, and FBX07, display an autosomal recessive hereditary pattern. Besides, some other genes, such as GIGYF2, were reported to be susceptible to PD with specific variants in different ethnic populations [41]. The mutated genes involved in PD cause brain dysfunction through various molecular mechanisms, including disturbance of presynaptic vesicle recycling and dopamine transmission, toxicity from aggregation of mutant proteins, degeneration of dopaminergic axon in substantia nigra, instability or mislocation of certain kinases, overactivation of ubiquitin kinase activities, and decreased efficiencies of ubiquitin degradation pathways [42–52]. Although only 10–15% of PD cases are familial and studies related to the pathogenic mechanisms on the confirmed disease-causing genes or susceptible loci of PD are far from being complete, the discovery of PD-related genes is a critical step for us to unravel the mysteries behind neurodegeneration in PD. Up to date, there is limited research specifically dedicated to the study of the relationship between the genetic classifications of PD and molecular mechanisms of cognitive impairment in PD. However, some negative results indicated some distinctive genetic features of cognitive decline in PD could be differentiated from other neurodegenerative disorders with cognitive disturbances [53, 54]. Furthermore, the filamentous Lewy body formation could be observed in early onset of PDD carrying SNCA mutations and Dementia with Lewy bodies (DLB) [42, 55], and the aggregation of α-synuclein could be detected in substantia nigra as well as cortex in idiopathic PD patients, which suggests that the accumulation of α-synuclein could be the presynaptic dysfunction attributed to neuronal toxicity caused by various genetic or nongenetic risk factors. It is also found that the frequency of glucocerebrosidase mutations is increased in postmortem samples from PD patients who had positive α-synuclein inclusions [56, 57], and the BDNF (Met/Met) homozygotes demonstrate dramatically worse cognitive impairment in PD patients compared to noncarriers [58].

4. Clinical Characteristics and Diagnosis

There is dramatic heterogeneity in clinical definition and correlation of cognitive impairment in PD, ranging from mild cognitive impairment to dementia [18, 59, 60]. It has been a long time that the definition and characteristics of PD-MCI and PDD exist as a controversial issue, until the Movement Disorder Society (MDS) took the initiative to conduct a Task Force to systematically review the most representative literatures. They evaluated the incidences and characteristics of PD-MCI, as well as its relationship with dementia and its inclination of progressing to dementia [61]. For PD-MCI, the Movement Disorder Society (MDS) finally selected a total of 8 articles (6 cross-sectional studies and 2 longitudinal studies) from 1156 articles (874 for Parkinson & cognitive impairment and 172 for Parkinson & MCI) [18, 59, 62–67], in which the study design, population studied, methodology for statistical analysis, and criteria for PD-MCI/PDD definition vary considerably. On the other hand, publications related to PDD are much more available than those to PD-MCI. The MDS also reviewed the previous publications of dementia in PD excluding the cases of Dementia with Lewy Bodies (DLB) in terms of the "1-year rule," characterized the clinical manifestations, and used these results to illustrate the criteria of probable and possible PDD based on the consensus from experts [68].

The criteria of both PD-MCI and PDD are defined by clinical, cognitive, and functional aspects. As more time and effort have been devoted to the study of PDD, the criteria for

PDD were established first, which also profoundly influenced the proposed criteria for PD-MCI [68, 69]. Similar to the practicality of diagnosis in PDD criteria, a two-level operational schema on the thorough basis of neuropsychological testing is also applied in PD-MCI criteria [69]. Level I is a practical set which could be utilized easily by physicians and needs no neuropsychological testing from neurological or psychological experts, whereas Level II is documented in much more detail and is more favorable for researchers to conduct longitudinal studies.

In a brief assessment of Level I, clinical diagnosis of PD based on Queen's Square Brain Bank criteria for PD must be established for both PD-MCI and PDD [70, 71]. For PD-MCI, cognitive capability is declined slowly which might be described by caregivers or patients or observed by clinicians from testing results. On the other hand, cognitive impairment caused by the clinical manifestations of parkinsonism other than idiopathic PD, other primary possibilities for cognitive disturbances, and other PD-associated comorbid circumstances that could significantly influence the outcome of cognitive testing should be excluded from PD-MCI [68]. The most important point to differentiate PDD from DLB is that PD symptoms should develop prior to the onset of dementia, which could be obtained by clinicians, gathered from the patient him/herself, informant or follow-up records/past medical history [69]. As PD-MCI is a prestage of PDD and progresses to PDD in most cases, the cognitive deficits scaled by a global cognitive ability test or at least two of neuropsychological tests for the five cognitive domains (to erase the limitation of a single neuropsychological test) in PD-MCI should be subtle on complex functional task and not be sufficient to interfere significantly with functional independence [68]. However, the cognitive impairment, which can be examined by global cognitive ability tests (e.g., MMSE below 26 [72]) and by at least two of the neuropsychological tests (months reversed [73] or seven backward [72], lexical fluency or clock drawing [74], MMSE pentagons [72], and 3-word recall [72]), is supposed to be severe enough to impair daily living activities, which could be assessed by a list of simple tasks. And the cognitive impairment should be assessed without administration of antiparkinsonian drugs and not be attributed to other categories of abnormalities such as autonomic or motor symptoms caused by PDD [69].

Once the diagnosis of cognitive impairment, including PD-MCI or PDD, is established, specifying the subtypes of cognitive deficiency and evaluating the severity of disease are quite beneficial for research, clinical practicing and monitoring, and even standardized pharmacological interventions. For PD-MCI diagnosis by Level II criteria, at least two of neuropsychological tests examining each of the five cognitive domains are recommended by MDS. Performance of patients between 1 and 2 standard deviations (SD) below individual variation adjustment showing predominant impairment or premorbid levels may be demonstrated in PD-MCI. But patients within 1 SD below normalization tested by a serial of neuropsychological measurements or who reported significantly cognitive decline over time are also accredited to diagnose PD-MCI [75]. For PD-MCI subtyping, to differentiate PD-MCI as single or multiple domains, at least two

neuropsychological tests in each cognitive domain should be conducted. Impaired performance of two tests in the same one cognitive domain without impairment in other cognitive domains demonstrates the single-domain subtype. On the other hand, impaired performance of at least one test in no less than two cognitive domains indicates the multiple-domain type [76–91]. However, for PDD Level II testing, assessments of severity using quantitative measurements do not have upper limit scores in diagnosis. The goal of Level II testing, for one thing, is to confirm the uncertain PDD diagnosis when the clinical manifestations of cognitive impairment are not obvious or relatively confused. It also serves to depict the individual characteristic of PDD and as an indicator of pharmacological responsiveness. In PDD, there are five cognitive domains involved in Level II testing: global cognitive efficiency, executive functions, memory, instrumental functions, and neuropsychiatric functions, in which executive functions and memory are classified as subcorticofrontal functions and instrumental functions are believed to be cortically mediated [92].

5. Treatment

Abnormal activities of various subtypes of neurons have been involved in the cognitive impairment of PD, including the dysregulation of dopaminergic, cholinergic, and probably glutamatergic or noradrenergic neurons [93, 94].

Cholinesterase inhibitors, such as rivastigmine, have been proved beneficial to the improvement of global cognition and clinical manifestations as well as neuropsychiatric testing (especially for attention and executive functioning amelioration) by several large-scale multicenter randomized placebo-controlled trials [95–98]. However, Donepezil, also a cholinesterase inhibitor, was not effective for global cognitive improvement or other neuropsychiatric symptoms in PD-MCI or PDD in a large randomized controlled study [99, 100], although its beneficial effect was reported in some small placebo-controlled studies [99].

Partial NMDA-receptor antagonist has been used as a therapeutic option to treat PD patients with cognitive defects in several placebo-controlled trails [101–104]. However, the results of studies were not consistent or notable; only one trial showed statistical differences in the improvement of global cognition [102], whereas most of trials suggested no pharmacological effects of partial NMDA-receptor antagonist on neuropsychiatric symptoms or improvement of daily life [105].

Atomoxetine, a noradrenergic reuptake inhibitor, and clozapine, an inhibitor of serotonin and dopamine receptors, as well as second-generation tricyclic antidepressant (TCA) nortriptyline and pramipexole, have been shown to be beneficial for the regulation of attention, psychosis, and depression, respectively, by evidence from several placebo-controlled trials [93, 106, 107].

Dysexecutive profile, which is known as the most predominant component of cognitive deficits in PD-MCI and PDD, has been substantiated to be improved with levodopa treatment [6, 93]. Levodopa was found to act on some aspects of cognition such as flexibility and working memory without beneficial changes of other functions like visuospatial recognition, verbal ability, or associative learning [6, 93]. For patients with nondopaminergic antiparkinsonian administration, antagonists of the NMDA-type glutamate receptor, amantadine, for instance, could slow down the progressive transition from PD-MCI to PDD, via increasing dopamine release and blocking dopamine reuptake [108].

Subthalamic deep brain stimulation, which is commonly conducted on PD patients with motor complications that are resistant to antiparkinsonian medication, was claimed to be harmful for semantic and verbal fluency as well as executive profiles by a meta-analysis [109]. In the meantime, this invasive procedure, with the possibility of causing damage to the vital brain regions in charge of advanced cognitive functions, has been related to significant exacerbation of dysexecutive profile that is not observed in most desirable pharmacological treatments [110].

Neuroprotective agents aiming to interrupt α-synuclein aggregation or to restore neuronal integrity are currently not available, whereas some cognitive interventions that are helpful in Alzheimer's disease have been identified to have positive results in the early stage of randomized clinical studies [111, 112].

While deep brain stimulation (DBS) is effective for the motor deficits of Parkinson's disease (PD) that is well documented, cognitive and psychiatric benefits and side effects from the subthalamic nucleus (STN) and globus pallidus interna (GPi) DBS for PD are increasingly recognized. On one hand, it has been reported that DBS could significantly improve immediate verbal memory and reduce anxiety symptoms [113]; on the other hand, it is also investigated that certain types of impaired domain such as attention impairment predicted more detrimental results after DBS [114]. Therefore, the improvements of cognitive symptoms from DBS require further studies and warrant the precise cognitive tests that stratify the relative risks and benefits of surgery.

6. Conclusion

Cognitive impairment in PD, as in other neurodegenerative diseases, demonstrates the common role of neurodegeneration as well as the PD-featured damage in certain advanced cognitive brain regions accompanied with characterized clinical manifestations. The treatments for cognitive deficits in PD remain limited and inadequate since the disturbances of neuronal network involved in the process are still obscure and elusive. As the population ages, the increasing burden for both patients and caregivers from PD-MCI and PDD makes it urgent to approach to the pathogenic mechanisms and therapeutic targets of cognitive deficits in PD, as well as to research and develop novel pharmacological treatments and other interventions that could potentially be used in PD cognitive impairment.

References

[1] I. Litvan, K. P. Bhatia, D. J. Burn et al., "SIC task force appraisal of clinical diagnostic criteria for parkinsonian disorders," *Movement Disorders*, vol. 18, no. 5, pp. 467–486, 2003.

[2] T. C. Buter, A. van den Hout, F. E. Matthews, J. P. Larsen, C. Brayne, and D. Aarsland, "Dementia and survival in Parkinson disease: a 12-year population study," *Neurology*, vol. 70, no. 13, pp. 1017–1022, 2008.

[3] M. A. Hely, W. G. J. Reid, M. A. Adena, G. M. Halliday, and J. G. L. Morris, "The Sydney multicenter study of Parkinson's disease: the inevitability of dementia at 20 years," *Movement Disorders*, vol. 23, no. 6, pp. 837–844, 2008.

[4] D. Aarsland, K. Andersen, J. P. Larsen, A. Lolk, and P. Kragh-Sørensen, "Prevalence and characteristics of dementia in Parkinson disease: an 8-year prospective study," *Archives of Neurology*, vol. 60, no. 3, pp. 387–392, 2003.

[5] G. Levy, M.-X. Tang, E. D. Louis et al., "The association of incident dementia with mortality in PD," *Neurology*, vol. 59, no. 11, pp. 1708–1713, 2002.

[6] D. Weintraub, S. Mavandadi, E. Mamikonyan et al., "Atomoxetine for depression and other neuropsychiatric symptoms in Parkinson disease," *Neurology*, vol. 75, no. 5, pp. 448–455, 2010.

[7] E. Sinforiani, L. Banchieri, C. Zucchella, C. Pacchetti, and G. Sandrini, "Cognitive rehabilitation in Parkinson's disease," *Archives of gerontology and geriatrics. Supplement*, no. 9, pp. 387–391, 2004.

[8] A. P. París, H. G. Saleta, M. de la Cruz Crespo Maraver et al., "Blind randomized controlled study of the efficacy of cognitive training in Parkinson's disease," *Movement Disorders*, vol. 26, no. 7, pp. 1251–1258, 2011.

[9] M. Broeders, D. C. Velseboer, R. de Bie et al., "Cognitive change in newly-diagnosed patients with Parkinson's disease: a 5-year follow-up study," *Journal of the International Neuropsychological Society*, vol. 19, no. 6, pp. 695–708, 2013.

[10] K. F. Pedersen, J. P. Larsen, O.-B. Tysnes, and G. Alves, "Prognosis of mild cognitive impairment in early Parkinson disease: the Norwegian ParkWest study," *JAMA Neurology*, vol. 70, no. 5, pp. 580–586, 2013.

[11] L. A. Hershey and G. M. Peavy, "Cognitive decline in Parkinson disease: how steep and crowded is the slope?" *Neurology*, vol. 85, no. 15, pp. 1268–1269, 2015.

[12] M. A. Hely, J. G. L. Morris, W. G. J. Reid, and R. Trafficante, "Sydney multicenter study of Parkinson's disease: non-L-dopa-responsive problems dominate at 15 years," *Movement Disorders*, vol. 20, no. 2, pp. 190–199, 2005.

[13] T. C. Buter, A. Van Den Hout, F. E. Matthews, J. P. Larsen, C. Brayne, and D. Aarsland, "Dementia and survival in Parkinson disease: A 12-year Population Study," *Neurology*, vol. 70, no. 13, pp. 1017–1022, 2008.

[14] D. Aarsland, K. Andersen, J. P. Larsen, A. Lolk, H. Nielsen, and P. Kragh-Sørensen, "Risk of dementia in Parkinson's disease: a community-based, prospective study," *Neurology*, vol. 56, no. 6, pp. 730–736, 2001.

[15] P. Hobson, J. Gallacher, and J. Meara, "Cross-sectional survey of Parkinson's disease and parkinsonism in a rural area of the United Kingdom," *Movement Disorders*, vol. 20, no. 8, pp. 995–998, 2005.

[16] W. G. J. Reid, M. A. Hely, J. G. L. Morris, C. Loy, and G. M. Halliday, "Dementia in Parkinson's disease: a 20-year neuropsychological study (Sydney Multicentre Study)," *Journal*

of Neurology, Neurosurgery and Psychiatry, vol. 82, no. 9, pp. 1033–1037, 2011.

[17] K. Pigott, J. Rick, S. X. Xie et al., "Longitudinal study of normal cognition in Parkinson disease," *Neurology*, vol. 85, no. 15, pp. 1276–1282, 2015.

[18] D. Aarsland, K. Bronnick, C. Williams-Gray et al., "Mild cognitive impairment in Parkinson disease: a multicenter pooled analysis," *Neurology*, vol. 75, no. 12, pp. 1062–1069, 2010.

[19] J. H. Bower, D. M. Maraganore, B. J. Peterson, S. K. McDonnell, J. E. Ahlskog, and W. A. Rocca, "Head trauma preceding PD: A Case-control Study," *Neurology*, vol. 60, no. 10, pp. 1610–1615, 2003.

[20] H. Braak and E. Braak, "Pathoanatomy of Parkinson's disease," *Journal of Neurology, Supplement*, vol. 247, no. 2, pp. 3–10, 2000.

[21] A. Di Fonzo, M. C. J. Dekker, P. Montagna et al., "FBXO7 mutations cause autosomal recessive, early-onset parkinsonian-pyramidal syndrome," *Neurology*, vol. 72, no. 3, pp. 240–245, 2009.

[22] A. Di Fonzo, C. F. Rohé, J. Ferreira et al., "A frequent LRRK2 gene mutation associated with autosomal dominant Parkinson's disease," *Lancet*, vol. 365, no. 9457, pp. 412–415, 2005.

[23] A. Elbaz, J. H. Bower, D. M. Maraganore et al., "Risk tables for parkinsonism and Parkinson's disease," *Journal of Clinical Epidemiology*, vol. 55, no. 1, pp. 25–31, 2002.

[24] M. Farrer, P. Chan, R. Chen et al., "Lewy bodies and parkinsonism in families with parkin mutations," *Annals of Neurology*, vol. 50, no. 3, pp. 293–300, 2001.

[25] T. Foroud, S. K. Uniacke, L. Liu et al., "Heterozygosity for a mutation in the parkin gene leads to later onset Parkinson disease," *Neurology*, vol. 60, no. 5, pp. 796–801, 2003.

[26] M. Funayama, K. Hasegawa, H. Kowa, M. Saito, S. Tsuji, and F. Obata, "A new locus for Parkinson's Disease (PARK8) maps to chromosome 12p11.2-q13.1," *Annals of Neurology*, vol. 51, no. 3, pp. 296–301, 2002.

[27] W. P. Gilks, P. M. Abou-Sleiman, S. Gandhi et al., "A common LRRK2 mutation in idiopathic Parkinson's disease," *The Lancet*, vol. 365, no. 9457, pp. 415–416, 2005.

[28] S. Goldwurm, M. Zini, L. Mariani et al., "Evaluation of LRRK2 G2019S penetrance: relevance for genetic counseling in Parkinson disease," *Neurology*, vol. 68, no. 14, pp. 1141–1143, 2007.

[29] D. G. Healy, M. Falchi, S. S. O'Sullivan et al., "Phenotype, genotype, and worldwide genetic penetrance of LRRK2-associated Parkinson's disease: a case-control study," *The Lancet Neurology*, vol. 7, no. 7, pp. 583–590, 2008.

[30] A. J. Hughes, Y. Ben-Shlomo, S. E. Daniel, and A. J. Lees, "What features improve the accuracy of clinical diagnosis in Parkinson's disease: a clinicopathologic study," *Neurology*, vol. 57, no. 10, pp. S34–S38, 2001.

[31] A. J. Hughes, S. E. Daniel, Y. Ben-Shlomo, and A. J. Lees, "The accuracy of diagnosis of parkinsonian syndromes in a specialist movement disorder service," *Brain*, vol. 125, no. 4, pp. 861–870, 2002.

[32] M. M. Hulihan, L. Ishihara-Paul, J. Kachergus et al., "LRRK2 Gly2019Ser penetrance in Arab-Berber patients from Tunisia: a case-control genetic study," *The Lancet Neurology*, vol. 7, no. 7, pp. 591–594, 2008.

[33] C. Klein, K. Lohmann-Hedrich, E. Rogaeva, M. G. Schlossmacher, and A. E. Lang, "Deciphering the role of heterozygous mutations in genes associated with parkinsonism," *The Lancet Neurology*, vol. 6, no. 7, pp. 652–662, 2007.

[34] A. A. Hicks, H. Pétursson, T. Jónsson et al., "A susceptibility gene for late-onset idiopathic Parkinson's disease," *Annals of Neurology*, vol. 52, no. 5, pp. 549–555, 2002.

[35] B. Giovannone, E. Lee, L. Laviola, F. Giorgino, K. A. Cleveland, and R. J. Smith, "Two novel proteins that are linked to insulin-like growth factor (IGF-I) receptors by the Grb10 adapter and modulate IGF-I signaling," *Journal of Biological Chemistry*, vol. 278, no. 34, pp. 31564–31573, 2003.

[36] P. D. Smith, S. J. Crocker, V. Jackson-Lewis et al., "Cyclin-dependent kinase 5 is a mediator of dopaminergic neuron loss in a mouse model of Parkinson's disease," *Proceedings of the National Academy of Sciences of the United States of America*, vol. 100, no. 23, pp. 13650–13655, 2003.

[37] K. M. Strauss, L. M. Martins, H. Plun-Favreau et al., "Loss of function mutations in the gene encoding Omi/HtrA2 in Parkinson's disease," *Human Molecular Genetics*, vol. 14, no. 15, pp. 2099–2111, 2005.

[38] J. Simón-Sánchez, C. Schulte, J. M. Bras et al., "Genome-wide association study reveals genetic risk underlying Parkinson's disease," *Nature Genetics*, vol. 41, no. 12, pp. 1308–1312, 2009.

[39] M.-C. Chartier-Harlin, J. C. Dachsel, C. Vilariño-Güell et al., "Translation initiator EIF4G1 mutations in familial parkinson disease," *The American Journal of Human Genetics*, vol. 89, no. 3, pp. 398–406, 2011.

[40] N. Ostrerova, L. Petrucelli, M. Farrer et al., "α-Synuclein shares physical and functional homology with 14-3-3 proteins," *Journal of Neuroscience*, vol. 19, no. 14, pp. 5782–5791, 1999.

[41] Y. Zhang, Q.-Y. Sun, R.-H. Yu, J.-F. Guo, B.-S. Tang, and X.-X. Yan, "The contribution of GIGYF2 to Parkinson's disease: a meta-analysis," *Neurological Sciences*, vol. 36, no. 11, pp. 2073–2079, 2015.

[42] M. G. Spillantini, M. L. Schmidt, V. M.-Y. Lee, J. Q. Trojanowski, R. Jakes, and M. Goedert, "α-synuclein in Lewy bodies [8]," *Nature*, vol. 388, pp. 839–840, 1997.

[43] T. F. Outeiro and S. Lindquist, "Yeast cells provide insight into alpha-synuclein biology and pathobiology," *Science*, vol. 302, no. 5651, pp. 1772–1775, 2003.

[44] M. R. Cookson, "The role of leucine-rich repeat kinase 2 (LRRK2) in Parkinson's disease," *Nature Reviews Neuroscience*, vol. 11, no. 12, pp. 791–797, 2010.

[45] H. Plun-Favreau, K. Klupsch, N. Moisoi et al., "The mitochondrial protease HtrA2 is regulated by Parkinson's disease-associated kinase PINK1," *Nature Cell Biology*, vol. 9, no. 11, pp. 1243–1252, 2007.

[46] I. E. Clark, M. W. Dodson, C. Jiang et al., "*Drosophila pink1* is required for mitochondrial function and interacts genetically with *parkin*," *Nature*, vol. 441, no. 7097, pp. 1162–1166, 2006.

[47] A. H. Schapira, "Mitochondria in the aetiology and pathogenesis of Parkinson's disease," *The Lancet Neurology*, vol. 7, no. 1, pp. 97–109, 2008.

[48] C. B. Lücking, A. Dürr, V. Bonifati et al., "Association between early-onset Parkinson's disease and mutations in the parkin gene," *New England Journal of Medicine*, vol. 342, no. 21, pp. 1560–1567, 2000.

[49] K. K. K. Chung, Y. Zhang, K. L. Lim et al., "Parkin ubiquitinates the α-synuclein-interacting protein, synphilin-1: implications for Lewy-body formation in Parkinson disease," *Nature Medicine*, vol. 7, no. 10, pp. 1144–1150, 2001.

[50] V. Bonifati, P. Rizzu, M. J. Van Baren et al., "Mutations in the DJ-1 gene associated with autosomal recessive early-onset parkinsonism," *Science*, vol. 299, no. 5604, pp. 256–259, 2003.

[51] P. M. Abou-Sleiman, D. G. Healy, N. Quinn, A. J. Lees, and N. W. Wood, "The role of pathogenic DJ-1 mutations in Parkinson's disease," *Annals of Neurology*, vol. 54, no. 3, pp. 283–286, 2003.

[52] R. Bandopadhyay, A. E. Kingsbury, M. R. Cookson et al., "The expression of DJ-1 (PARK7) in normal human CNS and idiopathic Parkinson's disease," *Brain*, vol. 127, no. 2, pp. 420–430, 2004.

[53] Z. Liu, J. Guo, Y. Wang et al., "Lack of association between IL-10 and IL-18 gene promoter polymorphisms and Parkinson's disease with cognitive impairment in a Chinese population," *Scientific Reports*, vol. 6, Article ID 19021, 2016.

[54] Y. Q. Wang, B. S. Tang, Y. Yang et al., "Relationship between Alzheimer's disease GWAS-linked top hits and risk of Parkinson's disease with or without cognitive decline: a Chinese population-based study," *Neurobiology of Aging*, vol. 39, pp. 217.e9–217.e11, 2016.

[55] H. Okazaki, L. E. Lipkin, and S. M. Aronson, "Diffuse intracytoplasmic ganglionic inclusions (lewy type) associated with progressive dementia and quadriparesis in flexion," *Journal of Neuropathology and Experimental Neurology*, vol. 20, no. 2, pp. 237–244, 1961.

[56] J. Neumann, J. Bras, E. Deas et al., "Glucocerebrosidase mutations in clinical and pathologically proven Parkinson's disease," *Brain*, vol. 132, no. 7, pp. 1783–1794, 2009.

[57] E. Sidransky, M. A. Nalls, J. O. Aasly et al., "Multicenter analysis of glucocerebrosidase mutations in Parkinson's disease," *New England Journal of Medicine*, vol. 361, no. 17, pp. 1651–1661, 2009.

[58] F. R. Guerini, E. Beghi, G. Riboldazzi et al., "BDNF Val66Met polymorphism is associated with cognitive impairment in Italian patients with Parkinson's disease," *European Journal of Neurology*, vol. 16, no. 11, pp. 1240–1245, 2009.

[59] I. Litvan, D. Aarsland, C. H. Adler et al., "MDS task force on mild cognitive impairment in Parkinson's disease: critical review of PD-MCI," *Movement Disorders*, vol. 26, no. 10, pp. 1814–1824, 2011.

[60] Y.-Q. Wang, B.-S. Tang, X.-X. Yan et al., "A neurophysiological profile in Parkinson's disease with mild cognitive impairment and dementia in China," *Journal of Clinical Neuroscience*, vol. 22, no. 6, pp. 981–985, 2015.

[61] D. Muslimović, B. Post, J. D. Speelman, and B. Schmand, "Cognitive profile of patients with newly diagnosed Parkinson disease," *Neurology*, vol. 65, no. 8, pp. 1239–1245, 2005.

[62] T. Foltynie, C. E. G. Brayne, T. W. Robbins, and R. A. Barker, "The cognitive ability of an incident cohort of Parkinson's patients in the UK. The CamPaIGN Study," *Brain*, vol. 127, no. 3, pp. 550–560, 2004.

[63] S. Hoops, S. Nazem, A. D. Siderowf et al., "Validity of the MoCA and MMSE in the detection of MCI and dementia in Parkinson disease," *Neurology*, vol. 73, no. 21, pp. 1738–1745, 2009.

[64] E. Mamikonyan, P. J. Moberg, A. Siderowf et al., "Mild cognitive impairment is common in Parkinson's disease patients with normal Mini-Mental State Examination (MMSE) scores," *Parkinsonism and Related Disorders*, vol. 15, no. 3, pp. 226–231, 2009.

[65] M.-C. Pai and S.-H. Chan, "Education and cognitive decline in parkinson's disease: a study of 102 patients," *Acta Neurologica Scandinavica*, vol. 103, no. 4, pp. 243–247, 2001.

[66] C. C. Janvin, J. P. Larsen, D. Aarsland, and K. Hugdahl, "Subtypes of mild cognitive impairment in Parkinson's disease: progression to dementia," *Movement Disorders*, vol. 21, no. 9, pp. 1343–1349, 2006.

[67] C. H. Williams-Gray, T. Foltynie, C. E. G. Brayne, T. W. Robbins, and R. A. Barker, "Evolution of cognitive dysfunction in an incident Parkinson's disease cohort," *Brain*, vol. 130, no. 7, pp. 1787–1798, 2007.

[68] M. Emre, D. Aarsland, R. Brown et al., "Clinical diagnostic criteria for dementia associated with Parkinson's disease," *Movement Disorders*, vol. 22, no. 12, pp. 1689–1707, 2007.

[69] B. Dubois, D. Burn, C. Goetz et al., "Diagnostic procedures for parkinson's disease dementia: recommendations from the movement disorder society task force," *Movement Disorders*, vol. 22, no. 16, pp. 2314–2324, 2007.

[70] W. R. G. Gibb and A. J. Lees, "The relevance of the Lewy body to the pathogenesis of idiopathic Parkinson's disease," *Journal of Neurology, Neurosurgery and Psychiatry*, vol. 51, no. 6, pp. 745–752, 1988.

[71] A. J. Hughes, S. E. Daniel, S. Blankson, and A. J. Lees, "A clinicopathologic study of 100 cases of Parkinson's disease," *Archives of Neurology*, vol. 50, no. 2, pp. 140–148, 1993.

[72] M. F. Folstein, S. E. Folstein, and P. R. McHugh, ""Mini-mental state". A practical method for grading the cognitive state of patients for the clinician," *Journal of Psychiatric Research*, vol. 12, no. 3, pp. 189–198, 1975.

[73] D. H. K. Shum, K. A. McFarland, and J. D. Bain, "Construct validity of eight tests of attention: comparison of normal and closed head injured samples," *Clinical Neuropsychologist*, vol. 4, no. 2, pp. 151–162, 1990.

[74] T. Sunderland, J. L. Hill, A. M. Mellow et al., "Clock drawing in Alzheimer's disease: a novel measure of dementia severity," *Journal of the American Geriatrics Society*, vol. 37, no. 8, pp. 725–729, 1989.

[75] N. S. Jacobson and P. Truax, "Clinical significance: a statistical approach to defining meaningful change in psychotherapy research," *Journal of Consulting and Clinical Psychology*, vol. 59, no. 1, pp. 12–19, 1991.

[76] B. Pillon, B. Deweer, Y. Agid, and B. Dubois, "Explicit memory in Alzheimer's, Huntington's, and Parkinson's diseases," *Archives of Neurology*, vol. 50, no. 4, pp. 374–379, 1993.

[77] D. Weintraub, K. A. Oehlberg, I. R. Katz, and M. B. Stern, "Test characteristics of the 15-item geriatric depression scale and Hamilton depression rating scale in Parkinson disease," *The American Journal of Geriatric Psychiatry*, vol. 14, no. 2, pp. 169–175, 2006.

[78] A. M. Owen, M. Beksinska, M. James et al., "Visuospatial memory deficits at different stages of Parkinson's disease," *Neuropsychologia*, vol. 31, no. 7, pp. 627–644, 1993.

[79] J. A. Cooper, H. J. Sagar, N. Jordan, N. S. Harvey, and E. V. Sullivan, "Cognitive impairment in early, untreated Parkinson's disease and its relationship to motor disability," *Brain*, vol. 114, no. 5, pp. 2095–2122, 1991.

[80] K. A. Flowers and C. Robertson, "The effect of Parkinson's disease on the ability to maintain a mental set," *Journal of Neurology Neurosurgery and Psychiatry*, vol. 48, no. 6, pp. 517–529, 1985.

[81] F. Lhermitte, B. Pillon, and M. Serdaru, "Human autonomy and the frontal lobes. Part I: imitation and utilization behavior: a neuropsychological study of 75 patients," *Annals of Neurology*, vol. 19, no. 4, pp. 326–334, 1986.

[82] S. E. Starkstein, H. S. Mayberg, T. J. Preziosi, P. Andrezejewski, R. Leiguarda, and R. G. Robinson, "Reliability, validity, and clinical correlates of apathy in Parkinson's disease," *Journal of Neuropsychiatry and Clinical Neurosciences*, vol. 4, no. 2, pp. 134–139, 1992.

[83] J. L. Cummings, M. Mega, K. Gray, S. Rosenberg-Thompson, D. A. Carusi, and J. Gornbein, "The neuropsychiatric inventory: comprehensive assessment of psychopathology in dementia," *Neurology*, vol. 44, no. 12, pp. 2308–2314, 1994.

[84] E. Grober and H. Buschke, "Genuine memory deficits in dementia," *Developmental Neuropsychology*, vol. 3, no. 1, pp. 13–36, 1987.

[85] M. C. Tierney, A. Nores, W. G. Snow, R. H. Fisher, M. L. Zorzitto, and D. W. Reid, "Use of the Rey Auditory Verbal Learning Test in differentiating normal aging from Alzheimer's and Parkinson's dementia," *Psychological Assessment*, vol. 6, no. 2, pp. 129–134, 1994.

[86] U. P. Mosimann, G. Mather, K. A. Wesnes, J. T. O'Brien, D. J. Burn, and I. G. McKeith, "Visual perception in Parkinson disease dementia and dementia with Lewy bodies," *Neurology*, vol. 63, no. 11, pp. 2091–2096, 2004.

[87] C. Janvin, D. Aarsland, J. P. Larsen, and K. Hugdahl, "Neuropsychological profile of patients with Parkinson's disease without dementia," *Dementia and Geriatric Cognitive Disorders*, vol. 15, no. 3, pp. 126–131, 2003.

[88] A. L. Benton, P. J. Eslinger, and A. R. Damasio, "Normative observations on neuropsychological test performances in old age," *Journal of Clinical Neuropsychology*, vol. 3, no. 1, pp. 33–42, 1981.

[89] D. Aarsland, K. Brønnick, U. Ehrt et al., "Neuropsychiatric symptoms in patients with Parkinson's disease and dementia: frequency, profile and associated care giver stress," *Journal of Neurology, Neurosurgery and Psychiatry*, vol. 78, no. 1, pp. 36–42, 2007.

[90] A. F. G. Leentjens, F. R. J. Verhey, R. Lousberg, H. Spitsbergen, and F. W. Wilmink, "The validity of the Hamilton and Montgomery-Åsberg depression rating scales as screening and diagnostic tools for depression in Parkinson's disease," *International Journal of Geriatric Psychiatry*, vol. 15, no. 7, pp. 644–649, 2000.

[91] M. Visser, A. F. G. Leentjens, J. Marinus, A. M. Stiggelbout, and J. J. van Hilten, "Reliability and validity of the Beck depression inventory in patients with Parkinson's disease," *Movement Disorders*, vol. 21, no. 5, pp. 668–672, 2006.

[92] F. S. Ertan, T. Ertan, G. Kiziltan, and H. Uyguçgil, "Reliability and validity of the Geriatric Depression Scale in depression in Parkinson's disease," *Journal of Neurology, Neurosurgery and Psychiatry*, vol. 76, no. 10, pp. 1445–1447, 2005.

[93] D. Brandstaedter, S. Spieker, G. Ulm et al., "Development and evaluation of the Parkinson Psychosis Questionnaire: a screening-instrument for the early diagnosis of drug-induced psychosis in Parkinson's disease," *Journal of Neurology*, vol. 252, no. 9, pp. 1060–1066, 2005.

[94] A. A. Kehagia, R. A. Barker, and T. W. Robbins, "Neuropsychological and clinical heterogeneity of cognitive impairment and dementia in patients with Parkinson's disease," *The Lancet Neurology*, vol. 9, no. 12, pp. 1200–1213, 2010.

[95] J. C. Klein, C. Eggers, E. Kalbe et al., "Neurotransmitter changes in dementia with Lewy bodies and Parkinson disease dementia in vivo," *Neurology*, vol. 74, no. 11, pp. 885–892, 2010.

[96] M. Rolinski, C. Fox, I. Maidment, and R. McShane, "Cholinesterase inhibitors for dementia with Lewy bodies, Parkinson's disease dementia and cognitive impairment in Parkinson's disease," *Cochrane Database of Systematic Reviews*, vol. 3, Article ID CD006504, 2012.

[97] M. Emre, D. Aarsland, A. Albanese et al., "Rivastigmine for dementia associated with Parkinson's disease," *The New England Journal of Medicine*, vol. 351, no. 24, pp. 2509–2518, 2004.

[98] W. Poewe, E. Wolters, M. Emre et al., "Long-term benefits of rivastigmine in dementia associated with Parkinson's Disease: an active treatment extension study," *Movement Disorders*, vol. 21, no. 4, pp. 456–461, 2006.

[99] I. McKeith, T. Del Ser, P. Spano et al., "Efficacy of rivastigmine in dementia with Lewy bodies: a randomised, double-blind, placebo-controlled international study," *The Lancet*, vol. 356, no. 9247, pp. 2031–2036, 2000.

[100] T. Van Laar, P. P. De Deyn, D. Aarsland, P. Barone, and J. E. Galvin, "Effects of cholinesterase inhibitors in Parkinson's disease dementia: a review of clinical data," *CNS Neuroscience and Therapeutics*, vol. 17, no. 5, pp. 428–441, 2011.

[101] B. Dubois, E. Tolosa, J. Kulisevsky, P. Barone, and E. J. Galvin, "Efficacy and safety of donepezil in the treatment of Parkinsons disease patients with dementia," in *Proceedings of the 8th International Conference on Alzheimers and Parkinsons Diseases*, 2007.

[102] I. Leroi, R. Overshott, E. J. Byrne, E. Daniel, and A. Burns, "Randomized controlled trial of memantine in dementia associated with Parkinson's disease," *Movement Disorders*, vol. 24, no. 8, pp. 1217–1221, 2009.

[103] D. Aarsland, C. Ballard, Z. Walker et al., "Memantine in patients with Parkinson's disease dementia or dementia with Lewy bodies: a double-blind, placebo-controlled, multicentre trial," *The Lancet Neurology*, vol. 8, no. 7, pp. 613–618, 2009.

[104] M. Emre, M. Tsolaki, U. Bonuccelli et al., "Memantine for patients with Parkinson's disease dementia or dementia with Lewy bodies: a randomised, double-blind, placebo-controlled trial," *The Lancet Neurology*, vol. 9, no. 10, pp. 969–977, 2010.

[105] W. G. Ondo, L. Shinawi, A. Davidson, and D. Lai, "Memantine for non-motor features of Parkinson's disease: a double-blind placebo controlled exploratory pilot trial," *Parkinsonism and Related Disorders*, vol. 17, no. 3, pp. 156–159, 2011.

[106] V. Larsson, K. Engedal, D. Aarsland, C. Wattmo, L. Minthon, and E. Londos, "Quality of life and the effect of memantine in dementia with Lewy bodies and Parkinson's disease dementia," *Dementia and Geriatric Cognitive Disorders*, vol. 32, no. 4, pp. 227–234, 2011.

[107] K. Seppi, D. Weintraub, M. Coelho et al., "The movement disorder society evidence-based medicine review update: treatments for the non-motor symptoms of Parkinson's disease," *Movement Disorders*, vol. 26, supplement 3, pp. S42–S80, 2011.

[108] J. A. Cooper, H. J. Sagar, S. M. Doherty, N. Jordan, P. Tidswell, and E. V. Sullivan, "Different effects of dopaminergic and anticholinergic therapies on cognitive and motor function in Parkinson's disease follow-up study of untreated patients," *Brain*, vol. 115, no. 6, pp. 1701–1725, 1992.

[109] R. Inzelberg, U. Bonuccelli, E. Schechtman et al., "Association between amantadine and the onset of dementia in Parkinson's disease," *Movement Disorders*, vol. 21, no. 9, pp. 1375–1379, 2006.

[110] K. Witt, C. Daniels, P. Krack et al., "Negative impact of borderline global cognitive scores on quality of life after subthalamic nucleus stimulation in Parkinson's disease," *Journal of the Neurological Sciences*, vol. 310, no. 1-2, pp. 261–266, 2011.

[111] C. Daniels, P. Krack, J. Volkmann et al., "Risk factors for executive dysfunction after subthalamic nucleus stimulation in Parkinson's disease," *Movement Disorders*, vol. 25, no. 11, pp. 1583–1589, 2010.

[112] L. Bäckman, L. Nyberg, A. Soveri et al., "Effects of working-memory training on striatal dopamine release," *Science*, vol. 333, no. 6043, 2011.

[113] V. Tang, C. X. L. Zhu, D. Chan et al., "Evidence of improved immediate verbal memory and diminished category fluency following STN-DBS in Chinese-Cantonese patients with idio-pathic Parkinson's disease," *Neurological Sciences*, vol. 36, no. 8, pp. 1371–1377, 2015.

[114] H. Abboud, D. Floden, N. R. Thompson et al., "Impact of mild cognitive impairment on outcome following deep brain stimulation surgery for Parkinson's disease," *Parkinsonism and Related Disorders*, vol. 21, no. 3, pp. 249–253, 2015.

25

Meta-Analysis of the Relationship between the *APOE* Gene and the Onset of Parkinson's Disease Dementia

Suisui Pang, Jia Li⑩, Yingyu Zhang, and Jiajun Chen⑩

Department of Neurology, China Japan Union Hospital of Jilin University, No. 126, Xian Tai Road, Changchun, Jilin 130033, China

Correspondence should be addressed to Jiajun Chen; cjj@jlu.edu.cn

Academic Editor: Yuan-Han Yang

Purpose. To clarify the relationship between certain genotypes or alleles of the *APOE* gene and the onset risk of Parkinson's disease dementia (PDD). *Methods.* The PubMed, Cochrane, Embase, CBM, CNKI, and Wanfang databases were searched to identify all case-control studies and cohort studies published before October 30, 2017, that investigated the association between the *APOE* gene and the onset of PDD. Manual information retrieval was also performed. All studies that met the quality requirements were included in a meta-analysis performed using RevMan 5.3 software. *Results.* The meta-analysis included 17 studies, with a total of 820 patients in the PDD group and 1,922 in the non-PDD group. The influence of the *APOE* gene on PDD onset was analyzed from three aspects: five genotypes vs. $\varepsilon 3/3$, $\varepsilon 2+/\varepsilon 4+$ vs. $\varepsilon 3/3$, and $\varepsilon 4+$ vs. $\varepsilon 4-$. The risk factors for PDD may include the genotypes $\varepsilon 3/4$ (OR 1.47, 95% CI 1.14–1.89) and $\varepsilon 4/4$ (OR 2.93, 95% CI 1.20–7.14). In patients with PDD, there was no significant difference in the distribution of $\varepsilon 2+$ vs. $\varepsilon 3/3$ (OR 1.35, 95% CI 0.97–1.87, $P = 0.07$). The risk of PDD was 1.61 times greater in $\varepsilon 4+$ compared with $\varepsilon 3/3$ (OR 1.61, 95% CI 1.24–2.08, $P = 0.0003$). As the results indicated that $\varepsilon 2+$ did not play a role as a risk factor or a protective factor, we divided the population into $\varepsilon 4+$ and $\varepsilon 4$ for the meta-analysis and found that, among patients with Parkinson's disease, the dementia risk of those with $\varepsilon 4+$ was 1.72 times greater than that of those with $\varepsilon 4$ (OR 1.72, 95% CI 1.41–2.10, $P < 0.00001$). Subgroup analysis in accordance with different geographical regions revealed that $\varepsilon 4+$ was a risk factor for PDD in people from all regions. *Conclusions.* Among the *APOE* genotypes, $\varepsilon 2+$ is neither a risk factor nor a protective factor for PDD, while $\varepsilon 4+$ is a risk factor for PDD. The present results are applicable to Asian, European, and American patients with Parkinson's disease. Regarding the single *APOE* genotypes, $\varepsilon 3/4$ and $\varepsilon 4/4$ may be risk factors for PDD; however, further studies with large sample sizes are needed to verify this.

1. Introduction

Parkinson's disease (PD) is a common neurodegenerative disease among middle-aged and older adults. The major clinical features of PD include motor symptoms (such as static tremor, bradykinesia, myotonia, and postural balance disturbance), as well as nonmotor symptoms (such as disturbances of olfactory sensation and other senses, sleep disorders, autonomic dysfunction, and cognitive disorders). Parkinson's cognitive disorders are a common nonmotor symptom of PD, and these can be divided into mild cognitive impairment and Parkinson's disease dementia (PDD). An epidemiological investigation performed in 2005 showed that dementia develops in 24–31% of patients with PD and

that PDD accounts for 3-4% of patients with all types of dementia [1]. PDD can have a strong impact on the quality of life and social function of patients and can increase the mortality and disability rates [2]; this increases the burden of carers, prolongs the duration of hospitalization, increases hospitalization costs, and causes substantial burdens to family and society.

The clinical features of PDD include insidious onset and slowly developed deficits of attention, executive function, visual spatial function, and memory, accompanied by illusion, delusion, indifference, and other spiritual and emotional changes [3]. The pathogenesis is still unclear; however, PDD may be caused by various pathologic changes, such as an increase in the number of Lewy bodies in brain tissue, neurofibrillary tangles, senile plaque formation, microvascular lesions, and the presence of argyrophilic inclusion bodies [4–8]. The risk factors for PDD are also diverse and may include demographic characteristics and living habits such as advanced age, lower educational level, and smoking; the risk of PDD may also be increased in those with akinetic-rigid motor symptoms, those with nonmotor symptoms like mild cognitive impairment, rapid eye movement sleep behavior disorder, and illusion, and those with changes in biologic tumor markers such as low serum epidermal growth factor and low uric acid [9]. With technological developments, researchers have begun to explore the risk factors for PDD at a genetic level, and the *APOE*, *MAPT*, *SNCA*, *GBA*, *LRRK2*, and *COMT* genes have been found to play a role in the onset and development of PDD [10].

The risk factors for the onset of PDD are likely to be related with the presence of specific genes, and the presence of a certain genotype or an allele may predict whether the risk of PDD is increased in patients with PD. This would enable the risk factors for the onset of PDD to be predicted through testing for related genes, and people identified as being at high risk of PDD could promptly commence tracking and prevention therapies to prevent PDD and suspend its progress. Regarding the research into various genes related to the risk factors for the onset of PDD, a greater number of studies have evaluated the *APOE* gene than any other gene, and the *APOE* gene is generally regarded as the gene that has the largest influence on dementia and a stronger predictability compared with other genes.

The *APOE* gene has ε2, ε3, and ε4 alleles, which can be classified into six different genotypes: ε2/ε2, ε2/ε3, ε2/ε4, ε3/ε3, ε3/ε4, and ε4/ε4. These genotypes can be divided into the E2 phenotype (ε2/2 and ε3/2), E3 phenotype (ε3/3), and E4 phenotype (ε4/3, ε4/2, and ε4/4), among which the E3 phenotype is the most common and is referred to as the wild type [11]. These three phenotypes correspond to their respective protein isoforms (E2, E3, and E4) [12], and these three protein isoforms are collectively called apolipoprotein E (*APOE*) [13]. In the central nervous system, *APOE* can influence cholesterol/lipid homeostasis, synaptic function, glycometabolism, neurogenesis, mitochondrial function, tau protein phosphorylation, neuron atrophy, neuroinflammation, and the metabolic and gathering pathways of β-amyloid protein (Aβ) [14–16]. *APOE* can also protect the central nervous system by reducing its oxidative stress and inflammatory response level, resulting in cerebral protection [17]. Furthermore, *APOE* can stimulate neural stem cells to enhance their survival through the conduction path of the extracellular-signal-regulated kinase signal [18]. Different genes may lead to different *APOE* functions, affecting the abovementioned biochemical reaction processes and causing cognition impairment.

At present, it is widely believed that the *APOEε2* allele protects the central nervous system, and a longitudinal study found that *APOEε2* effectively reduces damage to the parts of the brain that control daily function and episodic memory [19]. In contrast, *APOEε4* causes damage to the central nervous system that can increase the risk of cognitive

disorder and is one of the major risk factors for dementia [20]. Many studies have investigated the effect of the *APOE* gene on the risk of onset of PDD. A case-control study investigating the relationships between PDD and different *APOE* genotypes found no obvious differences in *APOE* genotypes and gene frequency between patients with versus without PDD [21]. In contrast, one study reported that *APOEε2+* and ε4+ might carry a higher risk of PDD [22], while another study verified that *APOEε4* increases the risk of PDD and that ε2 has no relationship with dementia development in patients with PD [23]. The conclusions of other studies vary due to differences in race, age, and sex; furthermore, the study results are also influenced by research techniques, diagnostic criteria, and sample size. Hence, there is a need for an objective quantitative synthesis of the currently available research results to further define whether the *APOE* gene is related to the risk factors for the onset of PDD and to define its risk level.

The present meta-analysis was performed to make a quantitative synthesis and comprehensive assessment of published materials on the association between the *APOE* gene and the onset of PDD. The aim of the present meta-analysis was to provide a more objective evidence-based medicine foundation for the relationship between different *APOE* genotypes and the risk factors for the onset of PDD.

2. Materials and Methods

2.1. Data Retrieval. A method combining subject and free terms was applied to comprehensively and systematically search the PubMed, Cochrane, Embase, CBM, CNKI, and Wanfang databases for case-control studies and cohort studies published before October 30, 2017, that investigated the relationship between the *APOE* gene and the onset of PDD. The references of retrieved articles, conference literature, and gray literature were also searched manually. The search words were Parkinson disease, Parkinson's disease, primary parkinsonism, parkinsonism, primary, paralysis agitans, Parkinson's disease, Parkinson dementia complex, apolipoprotein E, apoprotein E, APOE, APO-E, APO E, AD2, LPG, LDLCQ5, dementia, cognition disorders, cognitive defect, dementias, demention, amentia, amentias, case-control study, and cohort studies.

2.2. Inclusion and Exclusion Criteria. Inclusion criteria were as follows: (1) observational study investigating the relationship between the *APOE* gene and the onset of PDD; (2) explicit clinical diagnosis of PD (made using the diagnostic criteria of PD from UK Brain Bank, Calne criteria, or diagnostic criteria of the First National Symposium on Extrapyramidal Diseases in China) or pathological diagnosis; (3) *APOE* genotype recorded; (4) at least one method used to assess dementia; (5) complete description of the results, and the odds ratio (OR) and 95% confidence interval (CI) of the case and control groups could be obtained either directly or indirectly; (6) case-control study or cohort study; (7) published in Chinese or English; (8) full text could be obtained, or the authors could provide the requisite information and data; and (9) published or unpublished materials before October 30, 2017. Exclusion criteria were as follows: (1) failure to match the research aim (study did not include patients with PD, or the investigated gene was not *APOE*); (2) diagnostic criteria of PD were not stated clearly, or unspecialized diagnostic criteria were used; (3) incomplete gene detection records; (4) the method used to assess dementia was not described; (5) abstract, literature review, case report, seminar, or repetitively published literature; for repetitively published literature, the most recent article or the article with most complete data was selected; and (6) full text could not be obtained, or sample data were not complete or clear and requisite information and data could not be acquired after contacting the author.

2.3. Literature Quality Assessment.
The Newcastle-Ottawa Scale was used to assess the methodological quality of the included studies [24]. For case-control studies, this comprised the determination of (1) adequate case definition, (2) representativeness of cases, (3) selection of control, (4) definition of control, (5) comparability of case and control groups, (6) exposure, (7) whether there were identical exposure methods for cases and controls, and (8) nonresponse rate. For cohort studies, this comprised the determination of (1) representativeness of the exposed cohort, (2) selection of the unexposed cohort, (3) determination of exposure, (4) whether the study subjects had an ending event that occurred before the study began, (5) comparability of the cohorts, (6) evaluation of the ending event, (7) whether follow-up was sufficient, and (8) integrality of follow-up examinations.

Exposure was defined as the allele or genotype of the *APOE* gene, and the exposure assessment method was defined as the method used to detect the gene. Each item that met one of the abovementioned criteria was represented by *, and each * was equivalent to 1 point, giving a potential total of 9 points. Higher scores indicated higher quality studies; studies with a score of 6 points or higher were included in the present meta-analysis.

2.4. Data Extraction.
The following data were extracted and tabulated: first author, publication date, country of the study population, race, age, diagnostic criteria of PD, diagnostic criteria of dementia, study design, sample capacity, and genotype distributions of the case and control groups. The literature screening, quality assessment, and data extraction were completed by two researchers, and disagreements were resolved via discussion with a third researcher.

2.5. Statistical Analysis.
RevMan 5.3 software was used to analyze the relationship between the *APOE* gene and the onset of PDD and to calculate the OR and 95% CI for the analyses of the five genotypes (ε2/ε2, ε2/ε3, ε2/ε4, ε3/ε4, and ε3/ε4) vs. ε3/3, ε2+/ε4+ vs. ε3/3, and ε4+ vs. ε4−. The Q value and I^2 were used to test the heterogeneity. $P < 0.10$ was considered to indicate heterogeneity between combined studies. I^2 values of 0–25% indicated no heterogeneity,

25–50% indicated mild heterogeneity, 50–75% indicated moderate heterogeneity, and 75–100% indicated major heterogeneity [25, 26]. The statistical analysis method was selected in accordance with the heterogeneity results; when there was no heterogeneity, the Mantel–Haenszel fixed-effect model [27] was used for data consolidation analysis, while the DerSimonian–Laird random-effect model [28] was used in other cases. Z was used to test and calculate the significance of the OR value and was the criterion used to evaluate risk correlation. The applied inspection level was $a = 0.05$, and $P < 0.05$ was considered to indicate a significant difference. Heterogeneity tests were initially done within each group; when heterogeneity was detected, the source of the heterogeneity was investigated via subgroup analysis. The single removal method was applied in the sensitivity analysis to test the stability of the results. Funnel plots were used to test for publication bias.

3. Results

3.1. Data Retrieval.
There were 426 articles retrieved; screening of the titles and abstracts resulted in the exclusion of 62 articles that were repeated literature, six that were conference literature, and 316 that were incompatible with the research contents of the present analysis. Of the remaining 42 articles, the original text of one article could not be obtained, two articles reported the same experiment (the one with more complete data was included), the experimental grouping in five articles differed from that used in the present meta-analysis, five articles had used undefined or incorrect diagnostic criteria for PD, four articles had no cognitive evaluation criteria, four articles had incomplete or irrelevant data, and the quality assessment score of five articles was less than 6 points. A final total of 17 articles were included in the meta-analysis (the retrieval process is shown in Figure 1).

3.2. Essential Features of the Included Studies.
All 17 included studies investigated the relationship between dementia in patients with PD who carried the ε4 genotype (ε4+) and those without the ε4 genotype (ε4−) [4, 21–23, 30–42]. Only 10 included studies comprehensively evaluated the relationships between all six genotypes of the *APOE* gene and PDD [21–23, 30–36]. Relevant data are shown in Table 1.

3.3. Meta-Analysis Results

3.3.1. Risk Factors for the Onset of PDD for Each Genotype.
In the 10 included studies that investigated all genotypes of the *APOE* gene, the frequencies of some genotypes were low and the event counts were 0, and thus, it was impossible to calculate the OR values separately. Therefore, we calculated OR values and 95% CIs for the five genotypes (ε2/ε2, ε2/ε3, ε2/ε4, ε3/ε4, and ε4/ε4) vs. ε3/3. As shown in Figure 2, compared with patients with PD who had the ε3/3 genotype, there was a significantly greater risk of dementia in those with genotypes ε3/4 (OR 1.47, 95% CI 1.14–1.89) and ε4/4 (OR 2.93 95% CI 1.20–7.14), while there was no difference in

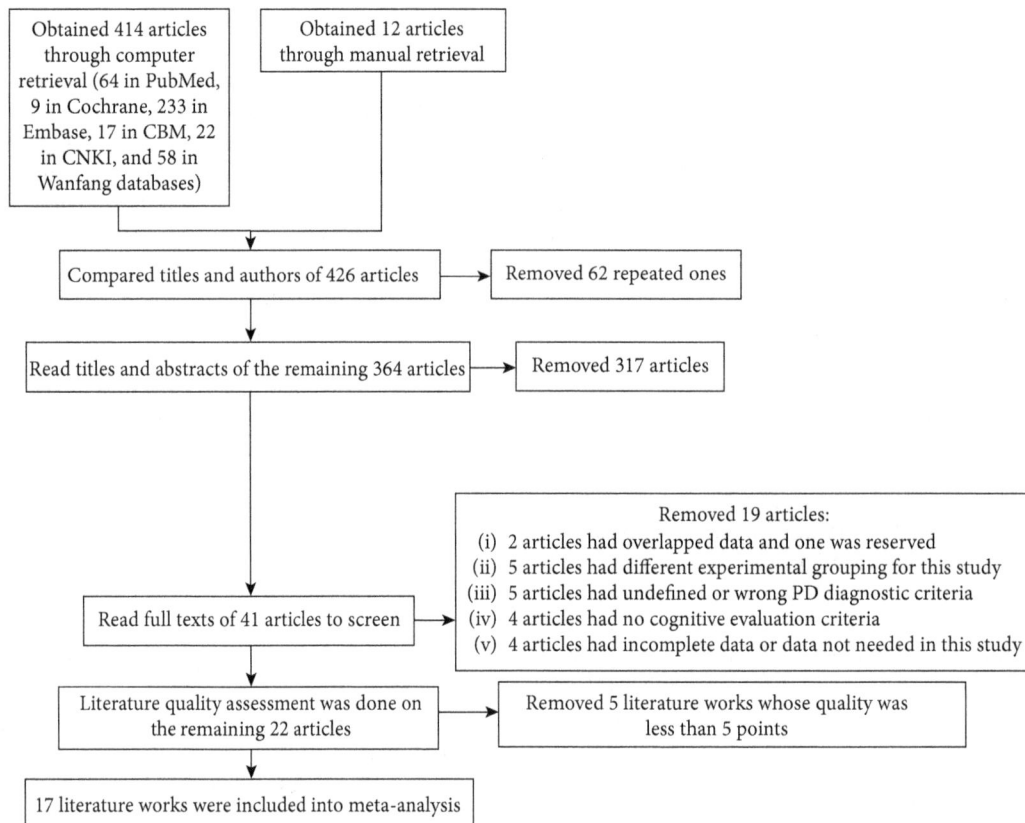

FIGURE 1: Flow chart of the study retrieval process.

the risk of PDD between those with the ε3/3 genotype and those with the genotypes ε2/2 (OR 1.07, 95% CI 0.33–3.48), ε2/3 (OR 1.17, 95% CI 0.85–1.61), and ε2/4 (OR 1.25, 95% CI 0.63–2.47).

3.3.2. Risk Factors for the Onset of PDD for ε2+ and ε4+. The OR and 95% CI for ε2+/ε4+ vs. ε3/3 in 10 included studies are shown in Figures 3 and 4, respectively. There was no obvious heterogeneity (*Q* testing, *P* > 0.10), and so the fixed-effect model was selected. The combined OR value in Figure 4 shows that the risk of PDD development in ε4+ patients was 1.61 times greater than that in those with the ε3/3 genotype (OR 1.61, 95% CI 1.24–2.08, *P* = 0.0003). Figure 3 shows that those with the ε3/3 genotype had a similar risk of PDD development compared with ε2+ patients (OR 1.35, 95% CI 0.97–1.87, *P* = 0.07).

3.3.3. PDD Onset Risk of ε4+ versus ε4– Patients. This part of the meta-analysis included 17 studies, and the OR and 95% CI for ε4+ vs. ε4– are shown in Figure 5. As heterogeneity = 0.16 and I^2 = 25%, the fixed-effect model was used. The combined OR value in Figure 5 shows that the risk of PDD onset in ε4+ patients was 1.72 times greater than that in ε4– patients (OR 1.72, 95% CI 1.41–2.10, *P* < 0.00001), indicating that carrying the ε4 genotype was a significant risk factor for the development of PDD.

3.4. Subgroup Analysis. To determine whether there were regional differences in the influence of the *APOE* gene on the risk of PDD onset, we performed a subgroup analysis in accordance with the regional distributions of patients.

3.4.1. Influence of Regional Distribution on PDD Onset Risk of ε2+/ε4+. In accordance with the geographic distribution of the study populations, the 10 studies were divided into five studying Asian patients (Chinese), four studying European patients, and one studying American patient. In both Asian and European patients, ε2+ was not a risk factor for PDD development compared with patients carrying the ε3/3 genotype (Figure 6). However, for Asian patients, the risk of PDD was 1.89 times greater in ε4+ compared with ε3/3 (OR 1.89, 95% CI 1.23–2.90, *P* = 0.003); for Europeans, the risk of PDD was 1.53 times greater in ε4+ compared with ε3/3 (OR 1.53, 95% CI 1.08–2.16, *P* = 0.002). All subgroups had no heterogeneity (Figure 7).

3.4.2. Differences in PDD Onset Risk between ε4+ and ε4– Patients in Different Regions. In accordance with the geographic distribution of the study populations, the 17 studies were divided into five studying Asian patients (Chinese), six studying European patients, and six studying American patients. Figure 8 shows that, in Asia, Europe, and America, carrying the ε4 genotype was a risk factor for PDD development, but the degree of risk varied in different regions; the

TABLE 1: Data extraction table.

Researcher	Time	Country	Experimental group (PDD group)						Control group (PDND group)						Experimental group		Control group		PDD diagnostic criteria	Dementia evaluation method	Experimental method	Sample capacity (experimental group and control group ≥ 50)	Patient source	Average age	Literature quality
			2/2	2/3	2/4	3/3	3/4	4/4	2/2	2/3	2/4	3/3	3/4	4/4	ε4+	ε4−	ε4+	ε4−							
Koller et al. [21]	1995	America	1	6	3	29	12	1	0	6	2	38	14	1	16	36	17	44	Calne criteria	DRS	Case-control study	Yes	Research center	PD67.4, PDD74.7	8
Harhangi et al. [22]	2000	Netherlands	1	8	1	7	9	0	0	14	2	51	13	1	10	16	16	65	Calne criteria	DSM	Cohort study	No	Community	PD75.8, PDD82.1	7
Wang et al. [30]	2001	China	0	1	0	6	4	0	0	1	0	35	4	0	4	7	4	36	Diagnostic criteria of National Symposium on Extrapyramidal Diseases in 1984	DSM	Case-control study	No	Hospital	PD66.13, PDD71.09	6
Zhou et al. [31]	2004	China	0	1	0	10	3	1	2	3	0	24	6	1	4	11	7	29	Diagnostic criteria of National Symposium on Extrapyramidal Diseases in 1984	DSM	Case-control study	No	Hospital	平均 Averagely 67.4	6
Camicioli et al. [37]	2005	Canada													9	19	3	16	Pathology	DSM	Cohort study	No	Hospital	PD77.5, PDD78.1	7
Pankratz et al. [38]	2006	America													19	31	62	212	UK Brain Bank	MMSE	Case-control study	No	Community	Averagely 60.9	7
Troster et al. [39]	2006	America													9	11	11	31	Calne criteria	DRS	Case-control study	Yes	Research center	Averagely 68.6	7
Blazquez et al. [40]	2006	Spain													6	25	25	220	UK Brain Bank	MMSE	Case-control study	No	Hospital	Averagely 71.1	7
Ma [23]	2007	China	0	9	2	48	19	3	1	17	2	96	16	1	24	57	19	114	UK Brain Bank	DSM	Case-control study	No	Hospital	PD68.38, PDD69.72	8
Jasinska-Myga et al. [32]	2007	Poland	1	11	3	56	24	3	1	8	7	56	25	3	30	68	35	65	UK Brain Bank	DSM, MMSE	Case-control study	Yes	Hospital	PD61.7, PDD71.4	8
Tong [33]	2008	China	0	4	0	13	3	0	0	3	0	52	12	0	3	17	12	55	UK Brain Bank	DSM, MMSE	Case-control study	Yes	Hospital	PD70.35, PDD75.44	7
Ezquerra et al. [34]	2008	Spain	0	7	1	57	20	1	0	11	0	101	26	0	22	64	26	112	UK Brain Bank	PDD diagnostic criteria	Case-control study	No	Hospital	PD56, PDD58.3	7
Williams-Gray et al. [41]	2009	America													8	11	23	65	UK Brain Bank	DSM, MMSE	Cohort study	Yes	Community	Unknown	7
Irwin et al. [4]	2012	America													40	49	4	38	UK Brain Bank	DSM	Case-control study	No	Research center	PD80, PDD79	7
Wang [35]	2014	China	1	8	0	70	17	1	0	18	3	116	20	0	18	79	23	134	UK Brain Bank	PDD diagnostic criteria	Case-control study	No	Hospital	PD65.20, PDD67.95	8
Mengel et al. [36]	2016	Germany	0	12	3	34	22	1	5	56	9	222	81	2	26	46	92	283	UK Brain Bank	MDS-TFC	Case-control study	Yes	Research center	Averagely 66.7	6
Nicoletti et al. [42]	2016	Italy													13	12	12	12	UK Brain Bank	MMSE	Case-control study	Yes	Unknown	Averagely 64.7	8

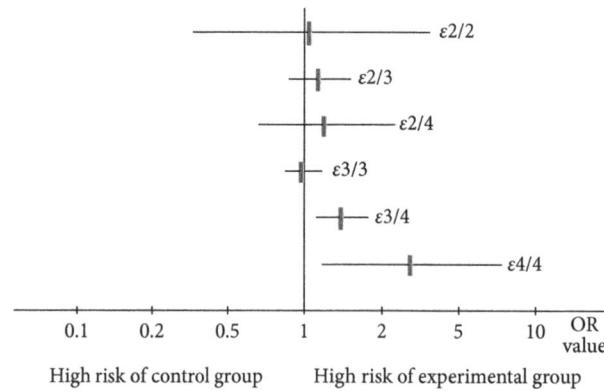

FIGURE 2: Risk of Parkinson's disease dementia in those with the five *APOE* genotypes compared with the ε3/3 genotype (assessed in 10 studies).

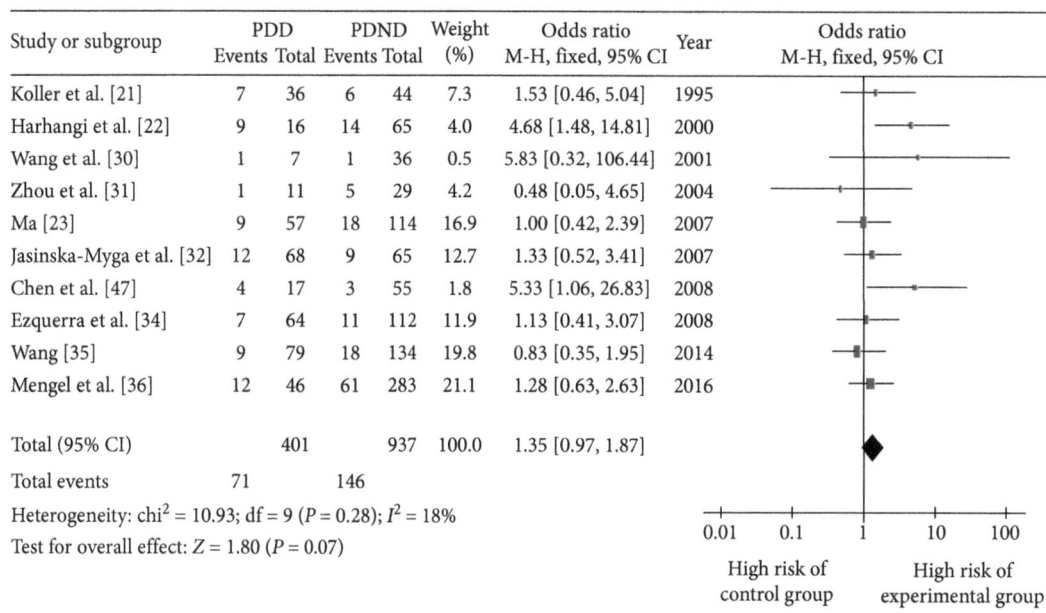

Study or subgroup	PDD Events	Total	PDND Events	Total	Weight (%)	Odds ratio M-H, fixed, 95% CI	Year	Odds ratio M-H, fixed, 95% CI
Koller et al. [21]	7	36	6	44	7.3	1.53 [0.46, 5.04]	1995	
Harhangi et al. [22]	9	16	14	65	4.0	4.68 [1.48, 14.81]	2000	
Wang et al. [30]	1	7	1	36	0.5	5.83 [0.32, 106.44]	2001	
Zhou et al. [31]	1	11	5	29	4.2	0.48 [0.05, 4.65]	2004	
Ma [23]	9	57	18	114	16.9	1.00 [0.42, 2.39]	2007	
Jasinska-Myga et al. [32]	12	68	9	65	12.7	1.33 [0.52, 3.41]	2007	
Chen et al. [47]	4	17	3	55	1.8	5.33 [1.06, 26.83]	2008	
Ezquerra et al. [34]	7	64	11	112	11.9	1.13 [0.41, 3.07]	2008	
Wang [35]	9	79	18	134	19.8	0.83 [0.35, 1.95]	2014	
Mengel et al. [36]	12	46	61	283	21.1	1.28 [0.63, 2.63]	2016	
Total (95% CI)		401		937	100.0	1.35 [0.97, 1.87]		
Total events	71		146					

Heterogeneity: chi^2 = 10.93; df = 9 (P = 0.28); I^2 = 18%
Test for overall effect: Z = 1.80 (P = 0.07)

FIGURE 3: Forest plot for the risk of Parkinson's disease dementia onset in ε2+ patients assessed in 10 studies.

risk of PDD onset in ε4+ patients compared with ε4− patients was increased by a factor of 1.46 in Asian patients (OR 1.76, 95% CI 1.17–2.65, P = 0.007), a factor of 1.41 in European patients (OR 1.41, 95% CI 1.05–1.89, P = 0.02), and a factor of 2.32 in American patients (OR 2.32, 95% CI 1.61–3.35, P < 0.00001).

3.5. Sensitivity Analysis. In Section (3.4), we performed analyses of ε2+ vs. ε3/3, ε4+ vs. ε3/3, and ε4+ vs. ε4−. After removing the studies included in the analyses of ε4+ vs. ε3/3 and ε4+ vs. ε4−, we performed a meta-analysis of the remaining studies; there were no obvious changes in the combined OR values, and all had statistical significance. Moreover, we did not identify any individual studies that had brought significant heterogeneity into the analysis of various studies. Removing the study published by Wang in 2014 [35] from the analysis of ε2+ vs. ε3/3 changed the result

from having no statistical significance (OR 1.35, 95% CI 0.97–1.87, P = 0.07) to having statistical significance (OR 1.48, 95% CI 1.04–2.11, P = 0.03); however, the quality of this study was high, the diagnosis and gene detection methods were standard, the experiment design was reasonable, and the results were reliable [35], and so we concluded that this study should not be removed blindly. We considered that the reason that this study made such an impact on the stability of the analysis was that it had a large sample size and thus its proportion of the overall result was large, which led to a change in the overall result after its removal. To evaluate the influence of sample size, we performed separate meta-analyses on the large sample size group (experimental and control groups both >50) and small sample size group (experimental or control groups <50) and found that the result of the large sample size group was stable and had no statistical significance or heterogeneity (OR 1.04, P = 0.87, P for heterogeneity = 0.90, I^2 = 0%).

Study or subgroup	PDD Events	Total	PDND Events	Total	Weight (%)	Odds ratio M-H, fixed, 95% CI	Year	Odds ratio M-H, fixed, 95% CI
Koller et al. [21]	13	42	15	53	10.2	1.14 [0.47, 2.75]	1995	
Harhangi et al. [22]	9	16	14	65	2.7	4.68 [1.48, 14.81]	2000	
Wang et al. [30]	4	10	4	39	1.1	5.83 [1.14, 29.90]	2001	
Zhou et al. [31]	4	14	7	31	3.5	1.37 [0.33, 5.75]	2004	
Ma [23]	22	70	17	113	9.9	2.59 [1.26, 5.33]	2007	
Jasinska-Myga et al. [32]	27	83	28	84	20.9	0.96 [0.51, 1.84]	2007	
Chen et al. [47]	3	16	12	64	4.3	1.00 [0.25, 4.07]	2008	
Ezquerra et al. [34]	21	78	26	127	16.1	1.43 [0.74, 2.77]	2008	
Wang [35]	18	88	20	136	13.9	1.49 [0.74, 3.01]	2014	
Mengel et al. [36]	23	57	83	305	17.4	1.81 [1.01, 3.25]	2016	
Total (95% CI)		474		1017	100.0	1.61 [1.24, 2.08]		
Total events	144		226					

Heterogeneity: chi^2 = 11.18; df = 9 (P = 0.26); I^2 = 20%
Test for overall effect: Z = 3.63 (P = 0.0003)

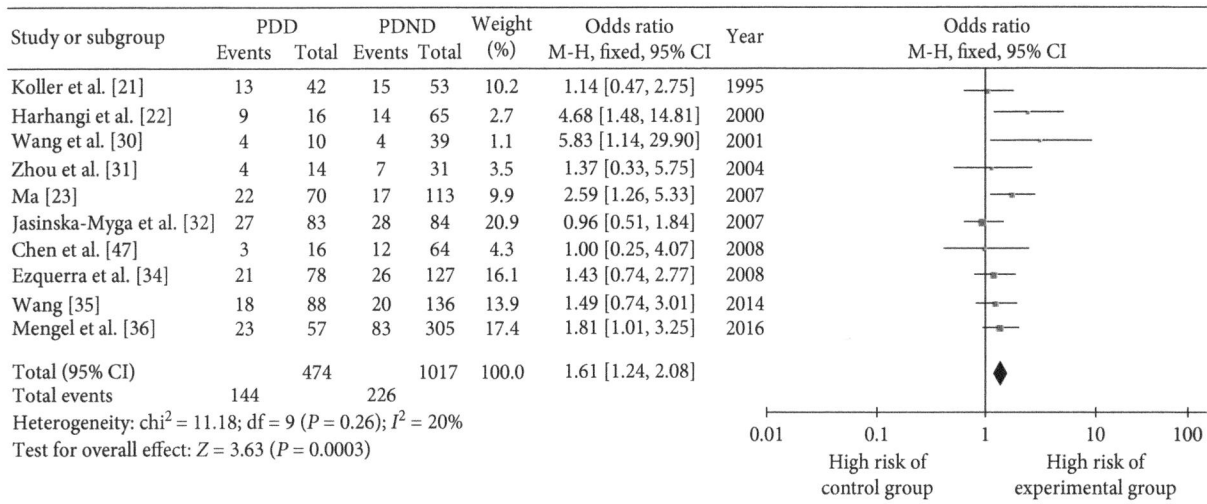

FIGURE 4: Forest plot for the risk of Parkinson's disease dementia onset in ε4+ patients assessed in 10 studies.

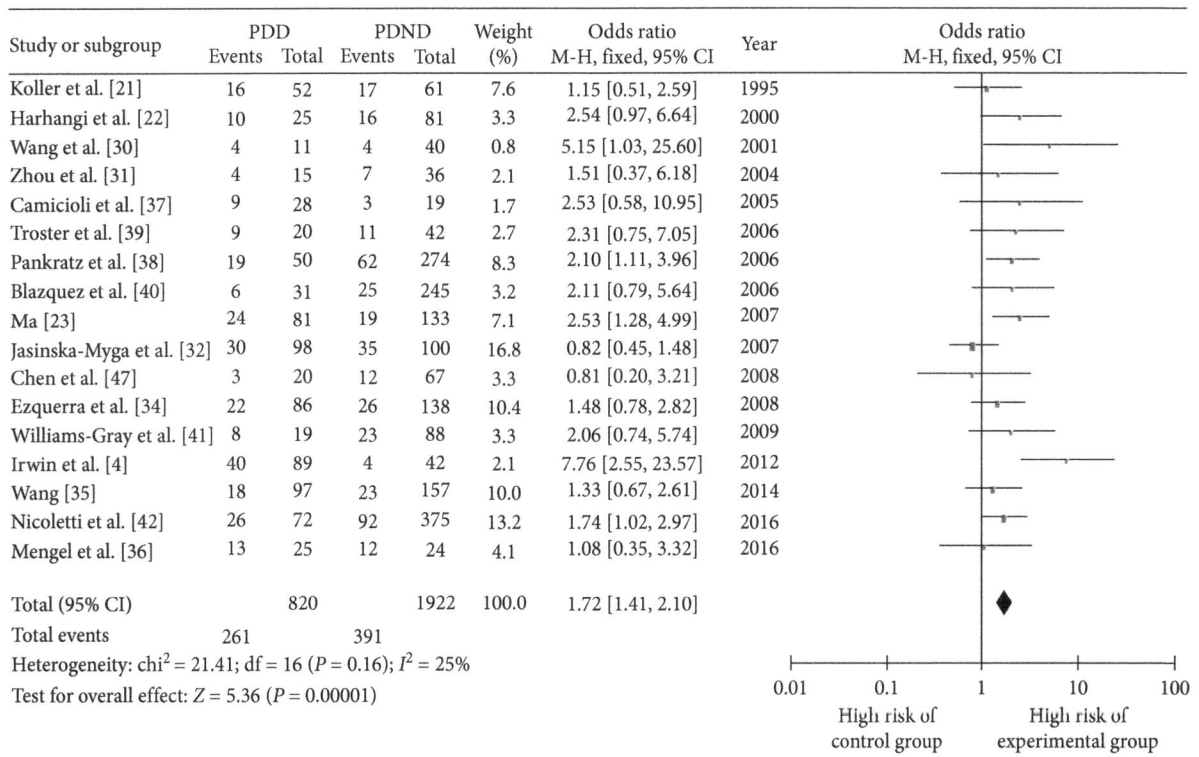

Study or subgroup	PDD Events	Total	PDND Events	Total	Weight (%)	Odds ratio M-H, fixed, 95% CI	Year	Odds ratio M-H, fixed, 95% CI
Koller et al. [21]	16	52	17	61	7.6	1.15 [0.51, 2.59]	1995	
Harhangi et al. [22]	10	25	16	81	3.3	2.54 [0.97, 6.64]	2000	
Wang et al. [30]	4	11	4	40	0.8	5.15 [1.03, 25.60]	2001	
Zhou et al. [31]	4	15	7	36	2.1	1.51 [0.37, 6.18]	2004	
Camicioli et al. [37]	9	28	3	19	1.7	2.53 [0.58, 10.95]	2005	
Troster et al. [39]	9	20	11	42	2.7	2.31 [0.75, 7.05]	2006	
Pankratz et al. [38]	19	50	62	274	8.3	2.10 [1.11, 3.96]	2006	
Blazquez et al. [40]	6	31	25	245	3.2	2.11 [0.79, 5.64]	2006	
Ma [23]	24	81	19	133	7.1	2.53 [1.28, 4.99]	2007	
Jasinska-Myga et al. [32]	30	98	35	100	16.8	0.82 [0.45, 1.48]	2007	
Chen et al. [47]	3	20	12	67	3.3	0.81 [0.20, 3.21]	2008	
Ezquerra et al. [34]	22	86	26	138	10.4	1.48 [0.78, 2.82]	2008	
Williams-Gray et al. [41]	8	19	23	88	3.3	2.06 [0.74, 5.74]	2009	
Irwin et al. [4]	40	89	4	42	2.1	7.76 [2.55, 23.57]	2012	
Wang [35]	18	97	23	157	10.0	1.33 [0.67, 2.61]	2014	
Nicoletti et al. [42]	26	72	92	375	13.2	1.74 [1.02, 2.97]	2016	
Mengel et al. [36]	13	25	12	24	4.1	1.08 [0.35, 3.32]	2016	
Total (95% CI)		820		1922	100.0	1.72 [1.41, 2.10]		
Total events	261		391					

Heterogeneity: chi^2 = 21.41; df = 16 (P = 0.16); I^2 = 25%
Test for overall effect: Z = 5.36 (P = 0.00001)

FIGURE 5: Forest plot for the risk of Parkinson's disease dementia onset in ε4+ versus ε4− patients assessed in 17 studies.

3.6. Publication Bias Analysis. Visual inspection revealed that the funnel plots of ε2+ vs. ε3/3 and ε4+ vs. ε3/3 were basically symmetrical, with all points evenly dispersed on both sides of the central line and basically located within the 95% CI and no unfilled corners. Hence, we considered that the possibility of bias was not large. Inspection of the funnel plot of ε4+ vs. ε4− revealed that the symmetry was good, but that two studies were located outside the 95% CI, indicating that there might be a degree of bias; however, separate

removal of these two studies showed that their removal exerted no influence on the result (Figure 9).

4. Discussion

The present meta-analysis included 17 studies, comprising 820 patients in the experimental group (PDD group) and 1,922 in the control group (non-PDD group). The PDD onset risks of patients with different genotypes of the *APOE*

Study or subgroup	PDD Events	PDD Total	PDND Events	PDND Total	Weight (%)	Odds ratio M-H, fixed, 95% CI	Year
Asian (Chinese)							
Wang et al. [30]	1	7	1	36	1.1	5.83 [0.32, 106.44]	2001
Zhou et al. [31]	1	11	5	29	9.7	0.48 [0.05, 4.65]	2004
Ma [23]	9	57	18	114	39.2	1.00 [0.42, 2.39]	2007
Chen et al. [47]	4	17	3	55	4.2	5.33 [1.06, 26.83]	2008
Wang [35]	9	79	18	134	45.9	0.83 [0.35, 1.95]	2014
Subtotal (95% CI)		171		368	100.0	1.11 [0.65, 1.88]	
Total events	24		45				

Heterogeneity: chi^2 = 5.91; df = 4 (P = 0.21); I^2 = 32%
Test for overall effec: Z = 0.37 (P = 0.71)

European							
Harhangi et al. [22]	9	16	14	65	8.1	4.68 [1.48, 14.81]	2000
Jasinska-Myga et al. [32]	12	68	9	65	25.5	1.33 [0.52, 3.41]	2007
Ezquerra et al. [34]	7	64	11	112	24.0	1.13 [0.41, 3.07]	2008
Mengel et al. [36]	12	46	61	283	42.4	1.28 [0.63, 2.63]	2016
Subtotal (95%CI)		194		525	100.0	1.54 [0.98, 2.40]	
Total events	40		95				

Heterogeneity: chi^2 = 4.29; df = 3 (P = 0.23); I^2 = 30%
Test for overall effect: Z = 1.88 (P = 0.06)

Test for subgroup differences: chi^2 = 0.87; df = 1 (P = 0.35); I^2 = 0%

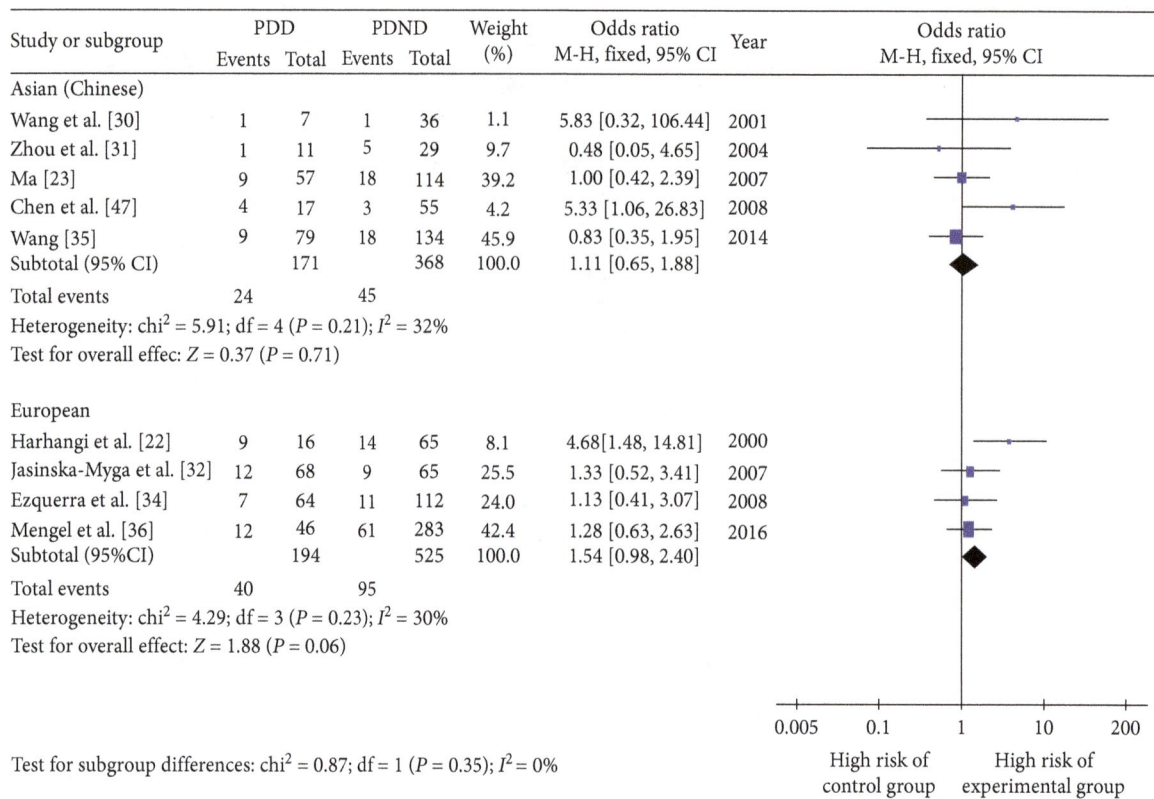

FIGURE 6: Forest plot for the influence of regional distribution on Parkinson's disease dementia onset risk of ε2+ patients.

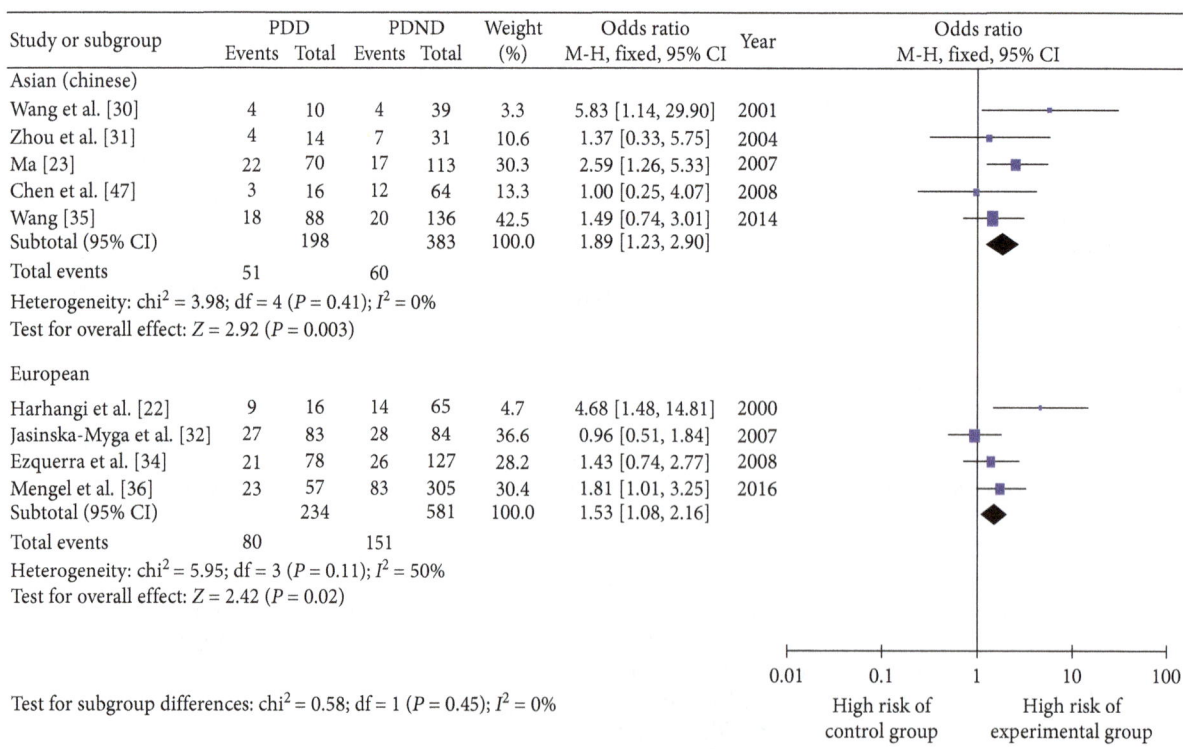

Study or subgroup	PDD Events	PDD Total	PDND Events	PDND Total	Weight (%)	Odds ratio M-H, fixed, 95% CI	Year
Asian (chinese)							
Wang et al. [30]	4	10	4	39	3.3	5.83 [1.14, 29.90]	2001
Zhou et al. [31]	4	14	7	31	10.6	1.37 [0.33, 5.75]	2004
Ma [23]	22	70	17	113	30.3	2.59 [1.26, 5.33]	2007
Chen et al. [47]	3	16	12	64	13.3	1.00 [0.25, 4.07]	2008
Wang [35]	18	88	20	136	42.5	1.49 [0.74, 3.01]	2014
Subtotal (95% CI)		198		383	100.0	1.89 [1.23, 2.90]	
Total events	51		60				

Heterogeneity: chi^2 = 3.98; df = 4 (P = 0.41); I^2 = 0%
Test for overall effect: Z = 2.92 (P = 0.003)

European							
Harhangi et al. [22]	9	16	14	65	4.7	4.68 [1.48, 14.81]	2000
Jasinska-Myga et al. [32]	27	83	28	84	36.6	0.96 [0.51, 1.84]	2007
Ezquerra et al. [34]	21	78	26	127	28.2	1.43 [0.74, 2.77]	2008
Mengel et al. [36]	23	57	83	305	30.4	1.81 [1.01, 3.25]	2016
Subtotal (95% CI)		234		581	100.0	1.53 [1.08, 2.16]	
Total events	80		151				

Heterogeneity: chi^2 = 5.95; df = 3 (P = 0.11); I^2 = 50%
Test for overall effect: Z = 2.42 (P = 0.02)

Test for subgroup differences: chi^2 = 0.58; df = 1 (P = 0.45); I^2 = 0%

FIGURE 7: Forest plot for the influence of regional distribution on Parkinson's disease dementia onset risk of ε4+ patients.

Study or subgroup	PDD Events	Total	PDND Events	Total	Weight (%)	Odds ratio M-H, fixed, 95% CI	Year	Odds ratio M-H, fixed, 95% CI
Asian (Chinese)								
Wang et al. [30]	4	11	4	40	3.3	5.14 [1.03, 25.60]	2001	
Zhou et al. [31]	4	15	7	36	9.19	1.51 [0.37, 6.18]	2004	
Ma [23]	24	81	19	133	30.5	2.53 [1.28, 4.99]	2007	
Chen et al. [47]	3	20	12	67	14.1	0.81 [0.20, 3.21]	2008	
Wang [35]	18	97	23	157	43.0	1.33 [0.67, 2.61]	2014	
Subtotal (95% CI)		224		433	100.0	1.76 [1.17, 2.65]		
Total events	53		65					

Heterogeneity: chi^2 = 4.74; df = 4 (P = 0.32); I^2 = 16%
Test for overall effect: Z = 2.71 (P = 0.007)

European								
Harhangi et al. [22]	10	26	16	81	6.6	2.54 [0.97, 6.64]	2000	
Blazquez et al. [40]	6	31	25	245	6.2	2.11 [0.79, 5.64]	2006	
Jasinska-Myga et al. [32]	30	98	35	100	32.9	0.82 [0.45, 1.48]	2007	
Ezquerra et al. [34]	22	86	26	138	20.3	1.48 [0.78, 2.82]	2008	
Mengel et al. [36]	26	72	92	375	25.9	1.74 [1.02, 2.97]	2016	
Nicoletti et al. [42]	13	25	12	24	8.0	1.08 [0.35, 3.32]	2016	
Subtotal (95% CI)		338		963	100.0	1.41 [1.05, 1.89]		
Total events	107		206					

Heterogeneity: chi^2 = 6.12; df = 5 (P = 0.29); I^2 = 18%
Test for overall effect: Z = 2.27 (P = 0.02)

American								
Koller et al. [21]	16	52	17	61	29.5	1.15 [0.51, 2.59]	1995	
Camicioli et al. [37]	9	28	3	19	6.6	2.53 [0.58, 10.95]	2005	
Troster et al. [39]	9	20	11	42	10.6	2.31 [0.75, 7.05]	2006	
Pankratz et al. [38]	19	50	62	274	32.3	2.10 [1.11, 3.96]	2006	
Williams-Grey et al. [41]	8	19	23	88	12.9	2.06 [0.74, 5.74]	2009	
irwin et al. [4]	40	89	4	42	8.1	7.76 [2.55, 23.57]	2012	
Subtotal (95% CI)		258		526	100.0	2.32 [1.61, 3.35]		
Total events	101		120					

Heterogeneity: chi^2 = 7.56; df = 5 (P = 0.18); I^2 = 34%
Test for overall effect: Z = 4.51 (P < 0.00001)

Test for subgroup differences: chi^2 = 4.40; df = 2 (P = 0.11); I^2 = 54.4 = 5%

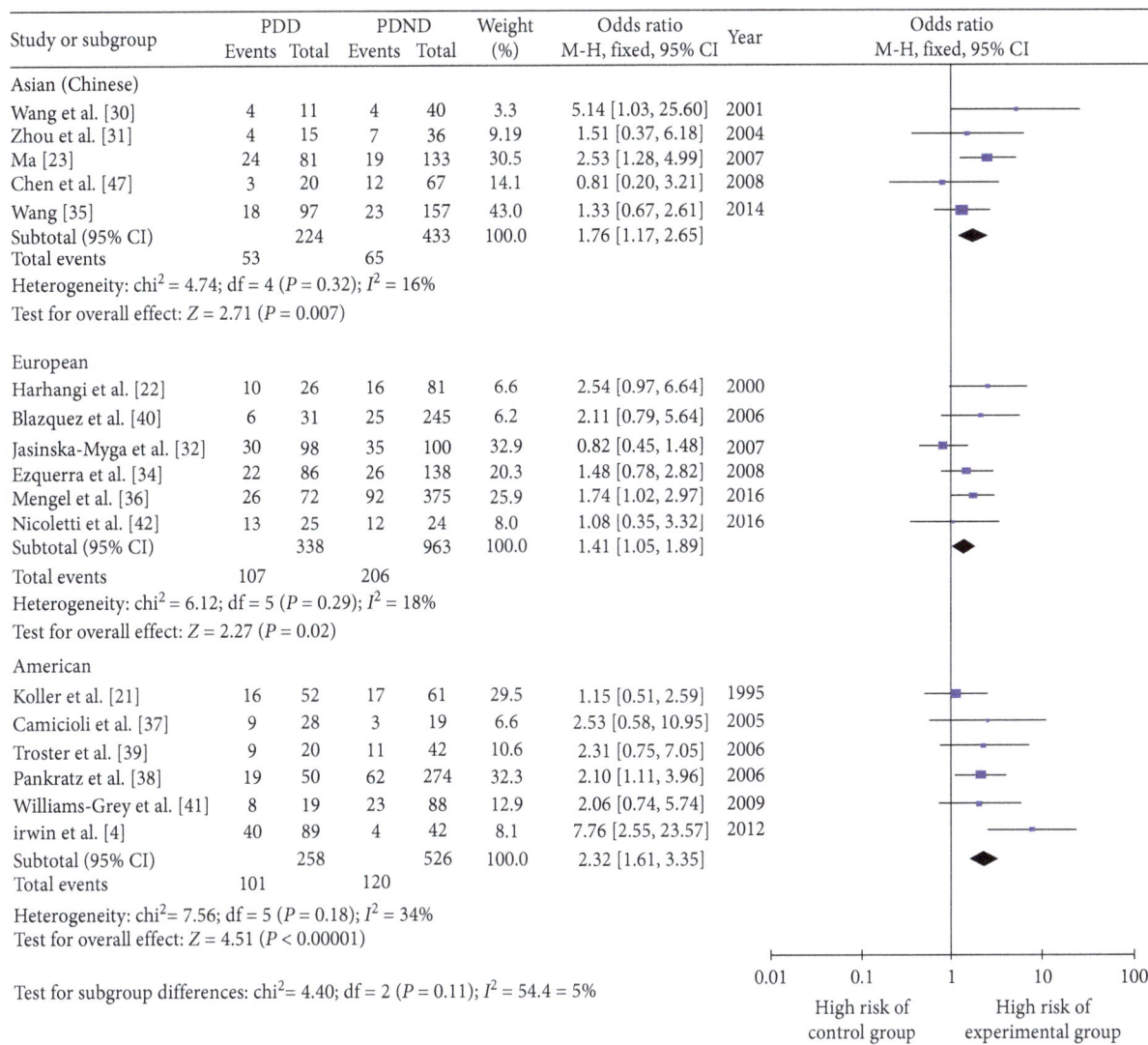

FIGURE 8: Forest plot for the influence of geographical distribution on Parkinson's disease dementia onset risk of ε4+ patients compared with ε4− patients.

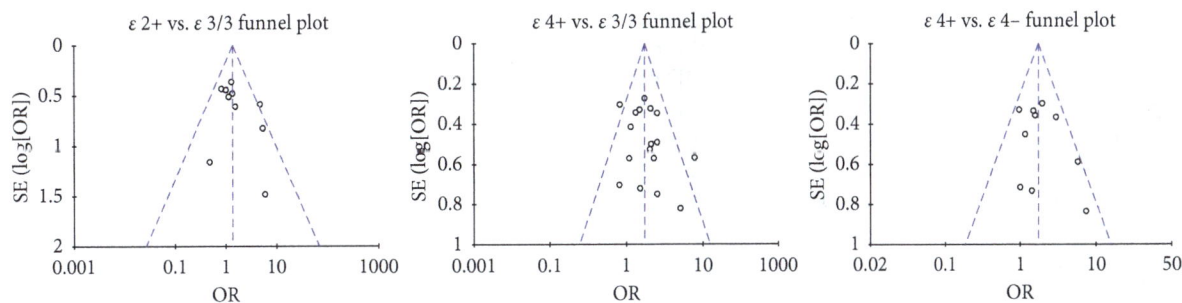

FIGURE 9: Funnel plots of ε2+ vs. ε3/3, ε4+ vs. ε3/3, and ε4+ vs. ε4−.

gene were analyzed from three aspects: five genotypes vs. ε3/3, ε2+/ε4+ vs. ε3/3, and ε4+ vs. ε4−. It was revealed that the ε3/4 and ε4/4 genotypes may be risk factors for PDD. ε2+ was neither a risk factor nor a protective factor for the development of PDD compared with the ε3/3 genotype, and the distribution of ε2+ was similar in the PDD and non-PDD groups. The incidence of ε4+ was significantly greater in the

PDD group than the non-PDD group, suggesting that ε4+ was a risk factor for PDD onset. As ε2+ had no role as a risk factor or a protective factor in the development of PDD, we divided the patients into ε4+ and ε4− for the meta-analysis, which revealed that the risk of PDD onset was 1.72 times greater in patients who are ε4+ compared with ε4− patients, but the risks varied slightly in accordance with the geographical region; the increased risk of PDD onset in those who were ε4+ compared with those who were ε4– was the highest in American patients (2.32 times greater), while it was 1.76 times greater in Asian patients and 1.41 times greater in European patients.

The mechanism by which different *APOE* genotypes influence dementia development in patients with PD is still unclarified, although many studies have investigated the mechanism by which *APOEε4* leads to dementia. *APOEε4* participates in the mechanism of dementia via the following four aspects: first, Aβ retention can form age pigmentation and vascular amyloidosis and thus lead to dementia. *APOE* adjusts the combination of Aβ through lipidation [43], and it combines with Aβ in the form of a molecular chaperone to influence the elimination of Aβ. The ability of ε4+ to eliminate Aβ is weaker than that of ε3/3 [44]. Second, tau albumen participates in normal apoptosis and maintains the stability of the cell, and the impairment of the microtubule assembly ability of unusually phosphorylated tau albumen can lead to the destruction of nerve cells. The albumens in the E3 and E2 phenotypes combine with tau albumen through the Cys residue to form stable compounds, protecting the structure of tau albumen and preventing it from undergoing abnormal phosphorylation; however, the residue in the E4 phenotype is minimal, and its ability to combine with tau albumen is weak, leading to abnormal phosphorylation [45]. Third, different phenotypes of the *APOE* gene can participate in the immune adjustment of the central nervous system; the immune response of the central nervous system in ε4+ is stronger than that in ε3+, and excessively strong immune responses can lead to brain injury and dementia [46]. Fourth, the *APOE* gene subtype can play a regulatory effect in the injury and repair of synapses, and a decline in the number of dendrites in the hippocampus of ε4+ may be related to dementia [47].

The present meta-analysis revealed that *APOEε4* is one of the risk factors for PDD, and this information can be used to guide the therapeutic direction in patients with PD. Detection of the *APOE* gene can predict the risk of PDD onset; high-risk patients can then be more closely monitored, intervening measures (such as controlling the risk factors) can be implemented to prevent PDD, and PDD can be diagnosed and treated in the early stage so that the disease progression can be postponed, patients' quality of life can be improved, social and family burdens can be relieved, and the mortality rate can be lowered. It is already known that the onset of Alzheimer's disease (AD) is related to the *APOE* gene, and the present results indicate that this gene is also a risk factor for the onset of PDD, suggesting that the pathogeneses of PDD and AD may be similar. Although there are only few studies on PDD, we may be able to use the relatively better understood pathogenesis and treatment of AD as a reference to provide ideas for research on PDD. In addition, as the pathogenic factors of AD and PDD may be similar, it is possible that the treatment methods used for AD are applicable to PDD. These theories should be investigated in subsequent studies, for which the results of the present meta-analysis can provide theoretical foundations.

Compared with two previous meta-analyses [41, 48], the present meta-analysis used stricter criteria concerning the inclusion, exclusion, and quality of studies. We also included new studies that had not been published when the previous meta-analyses were performed and excluded studies with poor experimental designs, Newcastle-Ottawa Scale scores of less than 6 points, and no definite diagnostic descriptions of PD and PDD. The present meta-analysis also had some limitations. First, although the diagnostic criteria of PD and PDD have been refined, the diagnostic criteria have not been unified; for example, various studies used only the PD diagnostic criteria of the UK Brain Bank or used PDD criteria to directly assess cognitive disorders. Second, the occurrence and severity of cognitive disorder can be influenced by age, education level, smoking history, living habits, and the presence of other genes that may cause dementia; however, no original data have been studied comprehensively, and thus, subgroup analysis or metaregression analysis cannot be performed. Third, the sample size of some included studies was small, and the event counts of many genotypes with small occurrence frequencies were 0, so the OR values of each genotype could not be calculated; therefore, sensitivity analysis and heterogeneity testing could not be conducted, and the results could not be systematically assessed. Hence, the risk of PDD in patients with certain genotypes should be predicted from the combined sample. Fourth, there were fewer community-based control studies and more hospital-based studies; thus, the samples may not be representative of the general population of patients with PD.

The present meta-analysis investigated the risk of PDD onset in relation to the presence of the *APOE* gene and revealed some limitations that may provide future research directions. A reasonable PDD diagnostic method is urgently required, as no studies have investigated the effectiveness of the currently available diagnostic criteria for PDD, so many studies have used unsuitable criteria such as the diagnostic and statistical manual of mental disorders (DSM) and the mini-mental state examination. In addition, future studies should enhance the representativeness and credibility of sample populations, adopt multicenter, multiracial, and larger sample sized community-based control or cohort studies, and further evaluate the link between the *APOE* gene and the risk of PDD onset among people of different ages and education levels.

5. Conclusions

Among the *APOE* genotypes, ε2+ is neither a risk factor nor a protective factor for PDD onset, while ε4+ is a risk factor for PDD. The present findings are especially applicable to Asian, European, and American patients with PD. Regarding single *APOE* genotypes, ε3/4 and ε4/4 may be risk factors of PDD, but studies with large sample sizes are needed to verify this.

References

[1] D. Aarsland, J. Zaccai, and C. Brayne, "A systematic review of prevalence studies of dementia in parkinson's disease," *Movement Disorders*, vol. 20, no. 10, pp. 1255–1263, 2005.

[2] G. Levy, M. X. Tang, E. D. Louis et al., "The association of incident dementia with mortality in PD," *Neurology*, vol. 59, no. 11, pp. 1708–1713, 2002.

[3] M. Emre, D. Aarsland, R. Brown et al., "Clinical diagnostic criteria for dementia associated with parkinson's disease," *Movement Disorders*, vol. 22, no. 12, pp. 1689–1707, 2007.

[4] D. J. Irwin, M. T. White, J. B. Toledo et al., "Neuropathologic substrates of parkinson disease dementia," *Annals of Neurology*, vol. 72, no. 4, pp. 587–598, 2012.

[5] K. Del Tredici and H. Braak, "Dysfunction of locus coeruleus-norepinephrine system and related circuitry in parkinson's disease-related dementia," *Journal of Neurology, Neurosurgery and Psychiatry*, vol. 84, no. 7, pp. 774–783, 2013.

[6] J. Horvath, F. R. Herrmann, P. R. Burkhard, C. Bouras, and E. Kovari, "Neuropathology of dementia in a large cohort of patients with parkinson's disease," *Parkinsonism and Related Disorders*, vol. 19, no. 10, pp. 864–868, 2013.

[7] G. M. Halliday, J. B. Leverenz, J. S. Schneider, and C. H. Adler, "The neurobiological basis of cognitive impairment in parkinson's disease," *Movement Disorders*, vol. 29, no. 5, pp. 634–650, 2014.

[8] J. E. Galvin, J. Pollack, and J. C. Morris, "Clinical phenotype of parkinson disease Dementia," *Neurology*, vol. 67, no. 9, pp. 1605–1611, 2006.

[9] Y. Xu and H. Shang, "Research progress of PDD risk factor," *Chinese Journal of Geriatrics Research (Electronic Edition)*, vol. 3, no. 1, pp. 21–25, 2016.

[10] E. S. Fagan and L. Pihlstrøm, "Genetic risk factors for cognitive decline in parkinson's disease: a review of literature," *European Journal of Neurology*, vol. 24, no. 4, pp. 561–e20, 2017.

[11] J. A. Hubacek, V. Adamkova, and Z. Skodova, "Rare variant of apolipoprotein E(Arg136→Ser) in two normolipidemic individuals," *Physiological Research*, vol. 54, no. 5, pp. 573–575, 2005.

[12] P. S. Hauser, V. Narayanaswami, and R. O. Ryan, "Apolipoprotein E: from lipid transport to neurobiology," *Progress in Lipid Research*, vol. 50, no. 1, pp. 62–74, 2011.

[13] H. Zhu, H. Xue, H. Wang, Y. Ma, J. Liu, and Y. Chen, "The association of apolipoprotein E (*APOE*) gene polymorphisms with atherosclerosis susceptibility: a meta-analysis," *Minerva Cardioangiologica*, vol. 64, no. 1, pp. 47–54, 2016.

[14] L. M. Tai, R. Thomas, F. M. Marottoli et al., "The role of *APOE* in cerebrovascular dysfunction," *Acta Neuropathologica*, vol. 131, no. 5, pp. 709–723, 2016.

[15] D. Seripa, F. Panza, M. Franceschi et al., "Non-apolipoprotein E and apolipoprotein E genetics of sporadic alzheimer's disease," *Ageing Research Reviews*, vol. 8, no. 3, pp. 214–236, 2009.

[16] P. K. Namboori, K. V. Vineeth, V. Rohith et al., "The *APOE* gene of alzheimer's disease (AD)," *Functional and Integrative Genomics*, vol. 11, no. 4, pp. 519–522, 2011.

[17] S. Ghura, L. Tai, M. Zhao et al., "arabidopsis thaliana extracts optimized for polyphenols production as potential therapeutics for *APOE*-modulated neuroinflammation characteristic of alzheimer's disease in vitro," *Scientific Reports*, vol. 6, no. 1, 2016.

[18] H. T. Gan, M. Tham, S. Hariharan et al., "Identification of APOE as an autocrine/paracrine factor that stimulates neural stem cell survival via MAPK/ERK signaling pathway," *Journal of Neurochemistry*, vol. 117, no. 3, pp. 565–578, 2011.

[19] A. Bonner-Jackson, O. Okonkwo, and G. Tremont, "Apolipoprotein E epsilon2 and functional decline in amnestic mild cognitive impairment and alzheimer disease," *American Journal of Geriatric Psychiatry*, vol. 20, no. 7, pp. 584–593, 2012.

[20] T. G. Nock, R. Chouinard-Watkins, and M. Plourde, "Carriers of an apolipoprotein E epsilon 4 allele are more vulnerable to a dietary deficiency in omega-3 fatty acids and cognitive decline," *Biochimica et Biophysica Acta (BBA)-Molecular and Cell Biology of Lipids*, vol. 1862, no. 10, pp. 1068–1078, 2017.

[21] W. C. Koller, S. L. Glatt, J. P. Hubble et al., "Apolipoprotein E genotypes in parkinson's disease with and without dementia," *Annals of neurology*, vol. 37, no. 2, pp. 242–245, 1995.

[22] B. S. Harhangi, M. C. de Rijk, C. M. van Duijn, C. Van Broeckhoven, A. Hofman, and M. M. Breteler, "APOE and risk of PD with or without dementia in a population-based study," *Neurology*, vol. 54, no. 6, pp. 1272–1276, 2000.

[23] A. Ma, *Relevant Study on PDD and Alzheimer Disease*, Tianjin Medical University, Tianjin, China, 2007.

[24] G. Wells, B. Shea, D. O'Connell et al., *The Newcastle-Ottawa Scale (NOS) for Assessing Quality of Nonrandomized Studies in Meta-analyses*, Ottawa Health Research Institute, Ottawa, Canada, 2000, http://www.ohri.ca/programs/clinical_epidemiology/oxford.asp.

[25] W. G. Cochran, "The combination of estimates from different experiments," *Biometrics*, vol. 10, no. 1, pp. 101–129, 1954.

[26] J. P. Higgins and S. G. Thompson, "Quantifying heterogeneity in a meta-analysis," *Statistics in Medicine*, vol. 21, no. 11, pp. 1539–1558, 2002.

[27] N. Mantel and W. Haenszel, "Statistical aspects of analysis of data from retrospective studies of disease," *Journal of the National Cancer Institute*, vol. 22, no. 4, pp. 719–748, 1959.

[28] R. DerSimonian, "Meta-analysis in design and monitoring of clinical trials," *Statistics in Medicine*, vol. 15, no. 12, pp. 1237–1248, 1996.

[29] P. G. Anthopoulos, S. J. Hamodrakas, and P. G. Bagos, "Apolipoprotein E polymorphisms and type 2 diabetes: a meta-analysis of 30 studies including 5423 cases and 8197 controls," *Molecular Genetics and Metabolism*, vol. 100, no. 3, pp. 283–291, 2010.

[30] F. Wang, M. Li, and Z. Yang, "An analysis on correlation between polymorphism of apolipoprotein E gene and dementia for patients with parkinson's disease," *Modern Rehabilitation*, vol. 5, no. 2, pp. 50-51, 2001.

[31] C. Zhou, J. Xu, J. Gui et al., "On correlation between polymorphism of apolipoprotein E gene and parkinson's disease," *Carcinogenesis, Teratogenesis and Mutagenesis*, vol. 16, no. 1, pp. 21–23, 2004.

[32] B. Jasinska-Myga, G. Opala, C. G. Goetz et al., "Apolipoprotein E gene polymorphism, total plasma cholesterol level, and parkinson disease dementia," *Archives of Neurology*, vol. 64, no. 2, pp. 261–265, 2007.

[33] C. Tong, "A study on cognition impairment of parkinson's disease and related genetic factors," Doctoral dissertation, PLA Postgraduate Medical School, Beijing, China, 2008.

[34] M. Ezquerra, J. Campdelacreu, C. Gaig et al., "Lack of association of APOE and tau polymorphisms with dementia in parkinson's disease," *Neuroscience Letters*, vol. 448, no. 1, pp. 20–23, 2008.

[35] Y. Wang, *A Study on Cognition Impairment and Genetic Predisposition of Parkinson's Disease*, Central South University, Changsha, China, 2014.

[36] D. Mengel, J. Dams, J. Ziemek et al., "Apolipoprotein E epsilon4 does not affect cognitive performance in patients with parkinson's disease," *Parkinsonism and Related Disorders*, vol. 29, pp. 112–116, 2016.

[37] R. Camicioli, A. Rajput, M. Rajput et al., "Apolipoprotein E ε4 and catechol-O-methyltransferase alleles in autopsy-proven parkinson's disease: relationship to dementia and hallucinations," *Movement Disorders*, vol. 20, no. 8, pp. 989–994, 2005.

[38] N. Pankratz, L. Byder, C. Halter et al., "Presence of an APOE4 allele results in significantly earlier onset of parkinson's disease and a higher risk with dementia," *Movement Disorders*, vol. 21, no. 1, pp. 45–49, 2006.

[39] A. I. Troster, J. A. Fields, A. M. Paolo, and W. C. Koller, "Absence of apolipoprotein E epsilon4 allele is associated with working memory impairment in parkinson's disease," *Journal of the Neurological Sciences*, vol. 248, no. 1-2, pp. 62–67, 2006.

[40] L. Blazquez, D. Otaegui, A. Saenz et al., "Apolipoprotein E epsilon4 allele in familial and sporadic parkinson's disease," *Neuroscience Letters*, vol. 406, no. 3, pp. 235–239, 2006.

[41] C. H. Williams-Gray, A. Goris, M. Saiki et al., "Apolipoprotein E genotype as a risk factor for susceptibility to and dementia in parkinson's disease," *Journal of Neurology*, vol. 256, no. 3, pp. 493–398, 2009.

[42] G. Nicoletti, D. N. Manners, F. Novellino et al., "Voxel-based morphometry to detect effect of APOE on brain gray matter changes in parkinson's disease," *Psychiatry Research: Neuroimaging*, vol. 254, pp. 177–179, 2016.

[43] V. Hirsch-Reinshagen, B. L. Burgess, and C. L. Wellington, "Why lipids are important for alzheimer disease?," *Molecular and Cellular Biochemistry*, vol. 326, no. 1-2, pp. 121–129, 2009.

[44] A. J. Hanson, S. Craft, and W. A. Banks, "The APOE genotype: modification of therapeutic responses in alzheimer's disease," *Current Pharmaceutical Design*, vol. 21, no. 1, pp. 114–120, 2015.

[45] Y. Huang, "Abeta-independent roles of apolipoprotein E4 in the pathogenesis of alzheimer's disease," *Trends in Molecular Medicine*, vol. 16, no. 6, pp. 287–294, 2010.

[46] C. D. Keene, E. Cudaback, X. Li et al., "Apolipoprotein E isoforms and regulation of the innate immune response in brain of patients with alzheimer's disease," *Current Opinion in Neurobiology*, vol. 21, no. 6, pp. 920–928, 2011.

[47] Y. Chen, M. S. Durakoglugil, X. Xian, and J. Herz, "APOE4 reduces glutamate receptor function and synaptic plasticity by selectively impairing APOE receptor recycling," *Proceedings of the National Academy of Sciences*, vol. 107, no. 26, pp. 12011–12016, 2010.

[48] X. Huang, P. Chen, D. I. Kaufer, A. I. Troster, and C. Poole, "Apolipoprotein E and dementia in parkinson disease: a meta-analysis," *Archives of Neurology*, vol. 63, no. 2, pp. 189–193, 2006.

26

Effect of a Traditional Chinese Herbal Medicine Formulation on Cell Survival and Apoptosis of MPP$^+$-Treated MES 23.5 Dopaminergic Cells

Shuifen Ye,[1,2] **Ho Kee Koon,**[3] **Wen Fan,**[1,4] **Yihui Xu,**[1,5] **Wei Wei,**[1,6] **Chuanshan Xu,**[3,7] **and Jing Cai**[1]

[1]*Department of Integrative Medicine, Fujian University of Traditional Chinese Medicine, Fuzhou 350122, China*
[2]*Longyan First Hospital Affiliated to Fujian Medical University, Longyan 364000, China*
[3]*School of Chinese Medicine, Faculty of Medicine, The Chinese University of Hong Kong, Shatin, Hong Kong*
[4]*Xiamen Haicang Hospital, Xiamen 361026, China*
[5]*Second People's Hospital, Fujian University of Traditional Chinese Medicine, Fuzhou 350003, China*
[6]*No. 477 Hospital of Chinese People's Liberation Army, Xiangyang 441000, China*
[7]*Shenzhen Research Institute, The Chinese University of Hong Kong, Shenzhen 518057, China*

Correspondence should be addressed to Jing Cai; caij1@163.com

Academic Editor: Cristine Alves da Costa

Progressive degeneration of dopaminergic neurons in the substantia nigra (SN) is implicated in Parkinson's disease (PD). The efficacy of these currently used drugs is limited while traditional Chinese medicine (TCM) has been used in the management of neurodegenerative diseases for many years. This study was designed to evaluate the effect of a modified traditional Chinese herbal medicine decoction, Cong Rong Jing (CRJ), on cell survival and apoptosis of 1-methyl-4-phenylpyridinium- (MPP$^+$-) treated MES23.5 dopaminergic cells. CRJ was prepared as a decoction from three Chinese herbs, namely, *Herba Cistanches*, *Herba Epimedii*, and *Rhizoma Polygonati*. We reported here that CRJ significantly enhanced the cell survival of MES23.5 cells after the exposure of MPP$^+$ and inhibited the production of intracellular reactive oxygen species (ROS) induced by MPP$^+$. CRJ also prevented the MPP$^+$-treated MES23.5 cells from apoptosis by reducing the externalization of phosphatidylserine and enhancing the Bcl-2/Bax protein expression ratio. Signaling proteins such as JAK2, STAT3, and ERK1/2 were also involved in the action of CRJ. Taken together, these results provide a preliminary mechanism to support clinical application of the TCM formulation in PD and possibly other neurodegenerative diseases associated with ROS injury and apoptosis.

1. Introduction

Parkinson's disease (PD) is a neurodegenerative disorder due to the progressive and selective degeneration of dopaminergic neurons in the substantia nigra (SN), leading to the depletion of dopamine in striatum [1, 2]. Although the biochemical and molecular pathogenesis of the loss of dopaminergic neurons in PD has not yet been fully understood, it is believed that the pathogenesis is multifactorial which includes oxidative stress, mitochondrial dysfunction, and glutamate-mediated excitotoxicity and inflammation [3, 4]. Emerging evidence also shows that apoptotic pathways are probably involved in the death of dopaminergic neurons in PD [5, 6]. Prevention of the dopaminergic neurons from proceeding apoptosis would be useful in the treatment of PD.

Traditional Chinese medicine (TCM) has been shown to reduce the progression of the symptoms of PD for many years [7–10]. It exerts therapeutic effect in controlling the progression of the disease and reducing the dosage of dopamine for treatment [10]. We have previously tested five Chinese herbs (*Fructus Ligustri Lucidi*, *Herba Cistanches*, *Herba Epimedii Rhizoma Polygonati*, and *Semen Cuscutae*) with "kidney-tonifying" properties according to the theories of TCM and found that some of the herbs showed better neuroprotective effects in PD mouse model [11] and H_2O_2-injured MES23.5 cell model [12] as compared to selegiline, a monoamine oxidase inhibitor which is used to reduce early symptoms of PD. These herbs demonstrated differential neuroprotective effects by (1) increasing the neurotropic factors such as nerve growth factor (NGF), brain-derived neurotrophic factor (BDNF), and glial cell line-derived neurotrophic factor (GDNF) [11, 12], (2) reducing neuronal apoptosis through the inhibition of proapoptotic FasL and caspase-3 expression and enhancement of antiapoptotic Bcl-2 expression [11, 12], and (3) increasing tyrosine hydroxylase (TH) activity [11]. As the pathogenesis of PD is complex, it is expected that the herbal formulations may probably provide broader neuroprotective effects due to the multitargeted actions [13, 14]. Therefore, in the present study we selected three Chinese herbs (*Herba Cistanches*, *Herba Epimedii*, and *Rhizoma Polygonati*) from our previous findings to prepare a TCM formulated decoction, namely, Cong Rong Jing (CRJ), to further investigate the effect of the herbal formulation on cell survival and apoptosis of MPP^+-treated MES23.5 cells.

2. Materials and Methods

2.1. Materials. Fetal bovine serum (FBS) and cell culture medium Dulbecco's modified Eagles' medium Nutrient Mixture-F12 (DMEM/F12) were purchased from Life Technologies (Waltham, MA, USA). AG490 (JAK2 inhibitor), PD98059 (ERK inhibitor), 3-(4,5-dimethylthiazol-2-yl)-2,5-diphenyltetrazolium bromide (MTT), 1-methyl-4-phenyl-pyridiniuiodide (MPP^+), and 2′,7′-Dichlorofluorescin diacetate (DCFH-DA) were purchased from Sigma (St. Louis, MO, USA). Annexin V apoptosis detection kit was purchased from KeyGEN biotech (Nanjing, China). Antibodies of phospho-JAK2 (p-JAK2), JAK2, phospho-STAT3 (p-STAT3), STAT3, phospho-ERK1/2 (p-ERK1/2), ERK1/2, Bcl-2, Bax, and β-actin were purchased from Cell Signaling Technology (Beverly, MA, USA).

2.2. Preparation of the Aqueous Extract. The traditional Chinese medicinal herbs, *Herba Cistanches* (Rou Cong Rong), *Herba Epimedii* (Yin Yang Huo), and *Rhizoma Polygonati* (Huang Jing), were purchased from Fujian Pharmaceutical Co. Ltd. (Fuzhou, China) and were carefully authenticated by Laboratory of Pharmacognosy and Chinese Medicine according to the Chinese pharmacopoeia (The Pharmacopoeia Commission of People's Republic of China, 2005). To prepare CRJ aqueous extract, *Herba Cistanches* (50 g), *Herba Epimedii* (50 g), and *Rhizoma Polygonati* (90 g) were mixed and ground. The raw herbal powder was immersed in a total volume of 10 times (w/v) that of distilled water for 1 hour and then boiled for 2 hours. The solution was filtered and the filtrate was collected. The entire residue was collected and further boiled with a total volume of 8 times (w/v) that of distilled water for 2 hours. The solution was filtered and the two filtrates were combined, concentrated, and freeze-dried. The yield of the final dried extract was 25% (w/w) of the starting raw herbal materials and the resulting extract was stored at −20°C until used. The concentration of CRJ in

this study was calculated according to the starting raw herbal materials. The stock solution CRJ (10 mg/mL) was prepared by dissolving CRJ in PBS, followed by sonication, sterilization at 100°C, and filtration.

2.3. Cell Culture. MES23.5 cells, which were originally established and developed by Dr. Weidong Le at Baylor College of Medicine, USA, were cultured as described in Li et al.'s report [15]. Briefly, MES23.5 cells were maintained in DMEM/F12 culture medium supplemented with 5% FBS (Life Technologies, Waltham, MA, USA), 1% L-glutamine (Sigma, St. Louis, MO, USA), 2% of 50x Sato's solution [12, 16], 100 U/mL of penicillin, and 0.1 mg/mL of streptomycin (Life Technologies, Waltham, MA, USA). The cells were maintained and incubated in a humidified 5% CO_2 incubator at 37°C.

2.4. MPP^+ and CRJ Treatment. MES23.5 cells were seeded in poly-D-lysine (PDL) coated 96-well plate at a density of 1 × 10^5 cells per well. Different concentrations of MPP^+ were administered to the cells for 24 or 48 hours to optimize the experimental condition. To evaluate the neuroprotective effect of CRJ, MPP^+ containing medium was removed after 24 hours of incubation and then further treated with different concentrations of CRJ for 24 or 48 hours. The cells in the control were only treated by culture medium not containing CRJ and MPP^+.

2.5. Cell Viability Assay. Cell viability was detected by MTT assay. After the indicated time of treatment, 20 μL of MTT solution (5 mg/mL) was added to the cells and further incubated for 4 hours at dark environment. After that, the supernatant was removed and 150 μL of DMSO was added to each well of the plate. The plate was further shaken for 10 min to dissolve the formazan crystal. Optical density of each well was measured by spectrophotometer (BIO-TEK ELX 800, BioTek Instruments, Inc., Vermont, USA). Freshly prepared DMEM/F12 culture medium was used as a negative control.

2.6. Detection of Intracellular ROS Production. Intracellular ROS level was examined using flow cytometry with H2DCF-DA staining as described by Wang et al. [17]. Briefly, the treated cells were washed with serum-free medium followed by incubation of DCFH-DA in the absence of light for 30 min at 37°C. Cells were then washed, centrifuged, and resuspended in PBS. The cells were analyzed by FACSVerse™ flow cytometer (Becton Dickinson, New Jersey, USA) with the excitation wavelength of 488 nm and the fluorescent signals were acquired by the FL-1 channel. Data were analyzed by the CellQuest software.

2.7. Apoptosis Detection. The percentage of apoptosis was detected using flow cytometry with Annexin V-fluorescein isothiocyanate (FITC) Apoptosis Detection Kit (NanJing KeyGen Biotech Co., Ltd, Nanjing, China) according to the manufacturer's instructions. Briefly, the treated cells were harvested and collected by EDTA-free trypsin. The action of trypsin was neutralized by serum-containing culture medium. At least 1×10^5 cells were collected and washed once with cold PBS after the centrifugation. The cells were then suspended in 500 μL binding buffer followed by the addition of staining (Annexin-V-FITC) reagent and propidium iodide (PI). After incubation in the dark at room temperature for 10 min, the cells were analyzed by BD FACSVerse flow cytometer (Becton Dickinson, New Jersey, USA). The results were further analyzed using Cell Quest software.

2.8. Western Blot Analysis. Control or treated MES23.5 cells were lysed in RIPA lysis buffer (Beyotime Co., Shanghai, China) containing 50 mM Tris-HCl (pH 7.4), 150 mM NaCl, 1% Triton X-100, 1% sodium deoxycholate, 0.1% sodium dodecyl sulfate (SDS), protease inhibitor (sodium orthovanadate, sodium fluoride, EDTA, and leupeptin), and phenylmethylsulfonyl fluoride (PMSF, 1 mM). Protein concentration of the cell lysates was measured by BCA assay. Cell lysates (50 μg) were then loaded and separated by 10% SDS gel and then transferred to polyvinylidene difluoride (PVDF) membrane. Blots were probed with p-JAK2, JAK2, p-STAT3, STAT3, p-ERK1/2, ERK1/2, Bcl-2, Bax, and β-actin (1 : 1000) at 4°C overnight. After washing with TBST, the membrane was incubated with an appropriately diluted secondary antibody (1 : 5000) conjugated with horseradish peroxidase for 1 hour at room temperature. Chemiluminescence was detected using the Western blotting substrate (ECL) and visualized on an X-ray film. ImageJ software was used to measure the densitometry of bands generated from Western blot analysis.

2.9. Statistical Analysis. Each experiment was performed at least three times and data were expressed as mean ± SEM and analyzed using Graphpad prism v.6.0. Time course changes in protein expression were analyzed by unpaired Student's t-test. One-way analysis of variance (ANOVA) followed by Turkey's multiple comparison post hoc test was used to compare the differences between groups. A value of $P < 0.05$ was considered to be statistically significant.

3. Results

3.1. CRJ Enhanced Cell Survival of MPP+-Treated MES23.5 Cells. The concentrations of MPP+ and CRJ for the treatment of MES23.5 dopaminergic cells were optimized for the present study using MTT assay. CRJ treatment alone showed no significant cytotoxicity effect on MES23.5 cells at the concentration of 250 μg/mL. MPP+ treatment demonstrated dose- and time-dependent cytotoxicity to MES23.5 cells at the concentrations of 12.5 to 800 μM (Figure 1(a)). The treatment of different concentrations of CRJ (100, 200, and 250 μg/mL) significantly increased the cell survival of MPP+-treated MES23.5 cells from 65% to 91% and from 40% to 56% at 24 hours (Figure 1(b)) and 48 hours (Figure 1(c)), respectively ($P < 0.001$).

3.2. CRJ Reduced ROS Production in MES23.5 Cells after MPP+ Treatment. MPP+ is well known to induce the production of ROS and cause neurotoxicity [18, 19]. To evaluate whether the rescue of MPP+-treated MES23.5 cells by CRJ

is associated with the level of intracellular ROS, an indirect measurement of ROS using fluorescence method was adopted. Figure 2 shows a significant increase in ROS level in MPP+-treated MES23.5 cells as compared to the control ($P < 0.001$). However, the treatment of CRJ significantly reduced the generation of intracellular ROS level after MPP+ treatment, as compared to MPP+-treated cells alone ($P < 0.001$). This indicated that CRJ may exhibit the neuroprotective effect in MPP+-treated MES23.5 via the removal of intracellular ROS.

3.3. CRJ Reduced MPP+-Induced Apoptosis in MES23.5 Cells. Phosphatidylserine is a phospholipid located at inner plasma membrane. During the early apoptosis, phosphatidylserine will translocate to the outer plasma membrane [20]. The externalization of phosphatidylserine indicates the early event of apoptosis and could be revealed by the binding of Annexin V-FITC. PI counterstain was used to detect cells undergoing necrosis or late apoptosis. In this study, MPP+-treated MES23.5 cells were positively stained with Annexin V-FITC after 24 hours, indicating that MPP+ triggered the apoptotic process. In the presence of CRJ, the percentage of Annexin V-FITC positively stained cells significantly decreased ($P < 0.05$) in the dose-dependent manner (Figure 3), indicating that CRJ treatment reduced MPP+-induced apoptosis in MES23.5 cells.

3.4. CRJ Increased the Ratio of Bcl-2/Bax in the MPP+-Treated MES23.5 Cells. To further confirm the mode of cell protection of CRJ in MPP+-induced neurocytotoxicity in MES23.5 cells, the expression of the ratio of Bcl-2 and Bax proteins was determined by Western blot analysis. It is well known that Bcl-2 is the antiapoptotic protein while Bax is the proapoptotic protein [18]. The decrease of the ratio of Bcl-2/Bax could favour the process of intrinsic mitochondria-mediated apoptosis [21, 22]. In this study, MPP+ downregulated the protein expression of Bcl-2 while upregulating the expression of Bax in MES23.5 cells (Figure 4(a)). The treatment of CRJ increased the expression of Bcl-2 while decreasing the expression of Bax in MPP+-treated MES23.5 cells in the dose-dependent manner, resulting in a significant increase ($P < 0.05$) of the overall ratio of Bcl-2/Bax (Figure 4(b)).

3.5. Modulation of the Expression of JAK2/STAT3 and ERK1/2 by CRJ in Untreated or MPP+-Treated MES23.5 Cells. JAK2/STAT3 and/or survival signaling pathway have been reported to associate with the expression of Bcl-2 and Bax [23, 24]. Therefore, we attempted to further investigate the effect of CRJ treatment on the expression of JAK2/STAT3 and ERK1/2 signaling proteins in our model. Untreated MES23.5 cells were pretreated with either AG490 (JAK2 inhibitor) or PD98059 (ERK1/2 inhibitor) for 1 hour, followed by treatment of CRJ for 24 hours. Total cell lysates were then collected and the phosphorylation states of JAK2 (p-JAK2), STAT3 (p-STAT3), and ERK1/2 (p-ERK1/2) were determined by Western blot analysis (Figures 5(a) and 5(b)). The results showed that p-JAK2, p-STAT3, and p-ERK1/2 were found

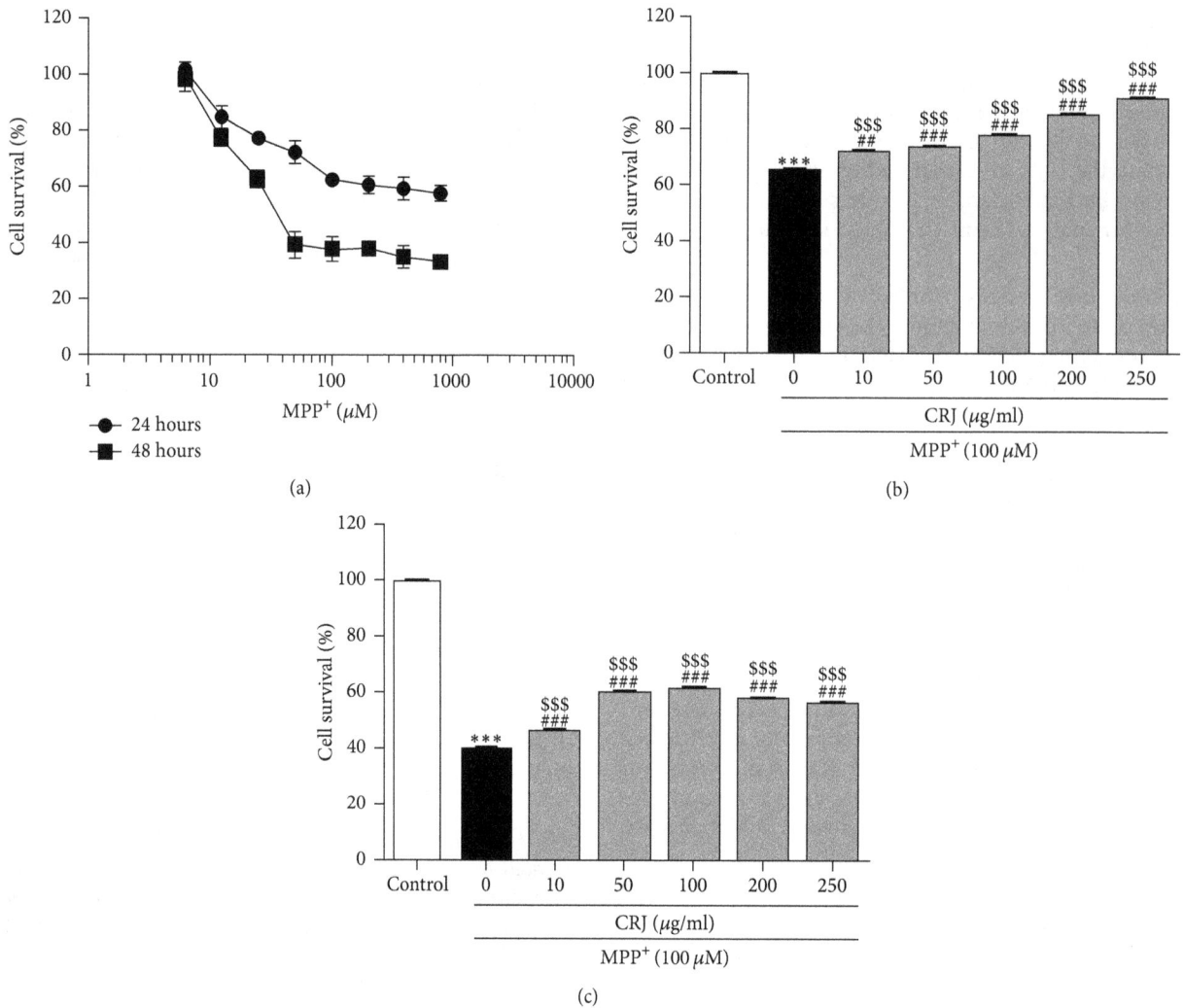

(a)

(b)

(c)

Figure 1: Effect of CRJ on the cell survival in MPP$^+$-treated MES23.5 dopaminergic neurons. (a) Exposure of MPP$^+$ alone for 24 or 48 hours resulted in the decrease of cell survival in MES23.5 cells. Posttreatment of different concentration of CRJ for (b) 24 or (c) 48 hours in MPP$^+$-treated MES23.5 cells enhanced the cell survival as compared to the MPP$^+$ treatment group without CRJ treatment. Data were represented as mean ± SEM in three independent experiments. ***$P < 0.001$, MPP$^+$-treated cells as compared to control. ##$P < 0.01$, ###$P < 0.001$, CRJ + MPP$^+$ groups as compared to MPP$^+$-treated cells. $$$$$$P < 0.001$, CRJ + MPP$^+$ groups as compared to control.

to be expressed in the untreated MES23.5 cells. Treatment of CRJ could further increase the expression of p-JAK2, p-STAT3, and p-ERK1/2 in MES23.5 cells. The activation of p-JAK2, p-STAT3, and p-ERK1/2 by CRJ was partially inhibited by AG490 and PD98059, respectively. The results suggested that CRJ was involved in the upregulation of the expression of p-JAK2, p-STAT3, and p-ERK1/2 signaling proteins.

We further tested the effect of CRJ treatment on the p-JAK2, p-STAT3, and p-ERK1/2 signaling proteins in MES23.5 cells after 24-hour treatment with MPP$^+$ (100 μM). We found that the treatment of CRJ (250 μg/mL) in the first 30 min and 60 min after MPP$^+$ treatment significantly activated the expression of p-JAK2 and p-STAT3 ($P < 0.05$) and slightly increased p-ERK1/2 ($P = 0.05$) (Figures 5(c) and 5(d)). This indicated that further upregulation of the p-JAK2, p-STAT3, and probably p-ERK1/2 protein expressions in MPP$^+$-treated MES23.5 cells would be associated with the treatment of CRJ.

4. Discussion

Currently, dopamine replacement therapy is the first-line clinical management to control the motor symptoms in PD patients. However, the treatment could only be maintained for few years due to the development of the end-of-dose and on-off phenomenon [25]. Neuroprotection has emerged as one of the main interests in PD researches [26]. Identification of drugs that lead to preventing the dopaminergic neurons from apoptosis and oxidative stress may probably help reduce the dosage and side effects of dopamine replacement therapy. Accelerating evidences show that some active ingredients of *Cistanches Herba* and *Herba Epimedii* such as phenylethanoid glycosides, echinacoside, and icariin exhibit antioxidant and neuroprotective activities [27–29]. Our previous studies showed that the decoction of different "kidney-tonifying" Chinese herbs regulated the expression of apoptotic-related

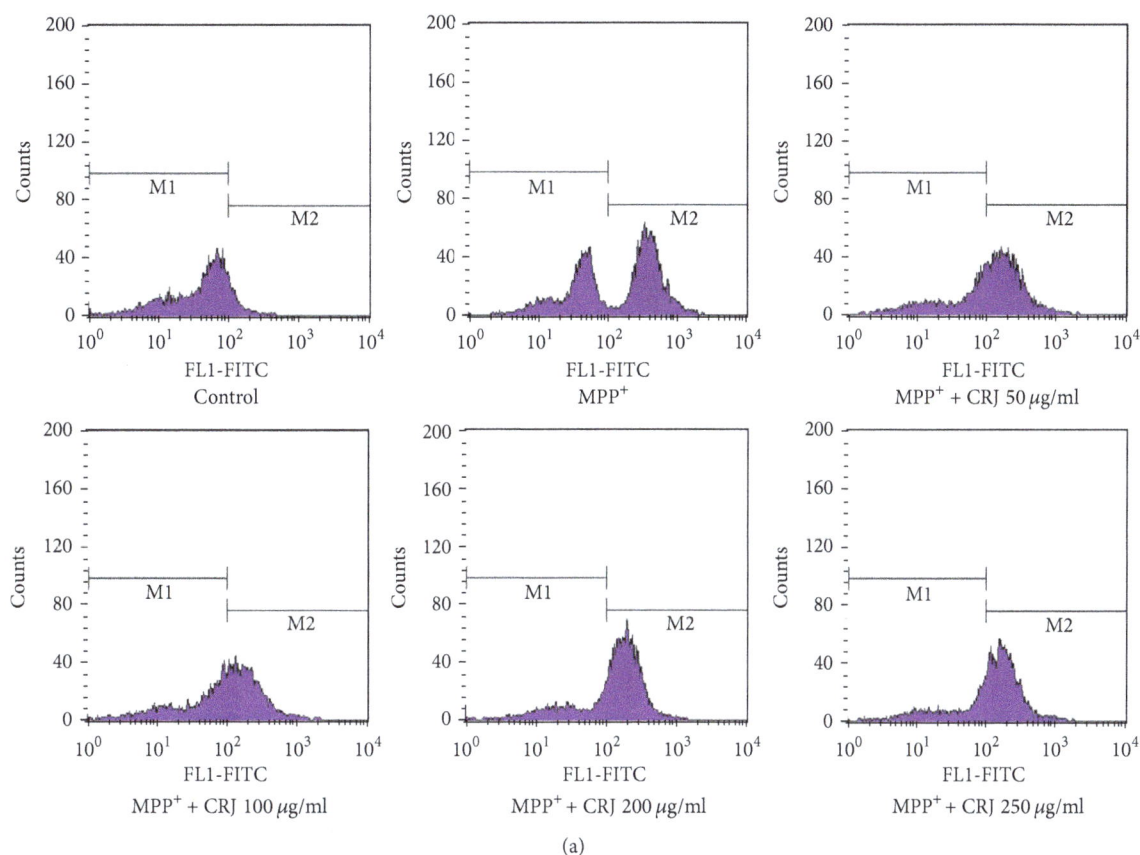

(a)

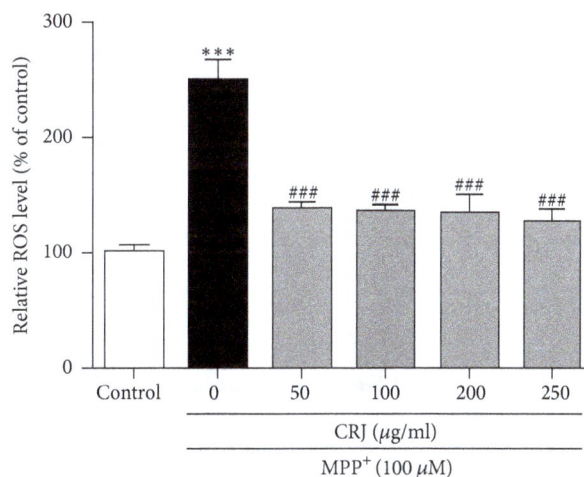

(b)

FIGURE 2: Detection of ROS in MES23.5 cells using flow cytometric analysis. MES23.5 cells were treated with MPP$^+$ (100 μM) for 24 hours, followed by the posttreatment of CRJ for another 24 hours. MPP$^+$ (100 μM) increased the production of ROS in MES23.5 cells. Posttreatment of CRJ resulted in the decrease of ROS production in MPP$^+$-treated MES23.5 cells. Fluorescence intensity of control group was set as 100%. Data were represented as mean ± SEM in three independent experiments. $^{***}P < 0.001$, MPP$^+$-treated cells as compared to control. $^{###}P < 0.001$, CRJ + MPP$^+$ groups as compared to MPP$^+$-treated cells.

factors and also neurotrophic factors in PD cell and animal models [11, 12]. Since the pathological pathways of PD are multifactorial and complex, the neuroprotective actions of a single herbal medicine are limited. For example, in the PD mouse model, *Herba Epimedii* prevented the loss of TH activity but not Bcl-2, while *Rhizoma Polygonati* was able to reduce the expression of apoptosis-promoting factors in the model but had no effect on the TH activity [11]. Therefore, in this study, we aimed at evaluating the therapeutic actions of CRJ, a TCM formulation comprising three selected Chinese herbal medicines (*Herba Cistanches*, *Herba Epimedii*, and *Rhizoma Polygonati*) instead of single Chinese herbs, in a

(a)

(b)

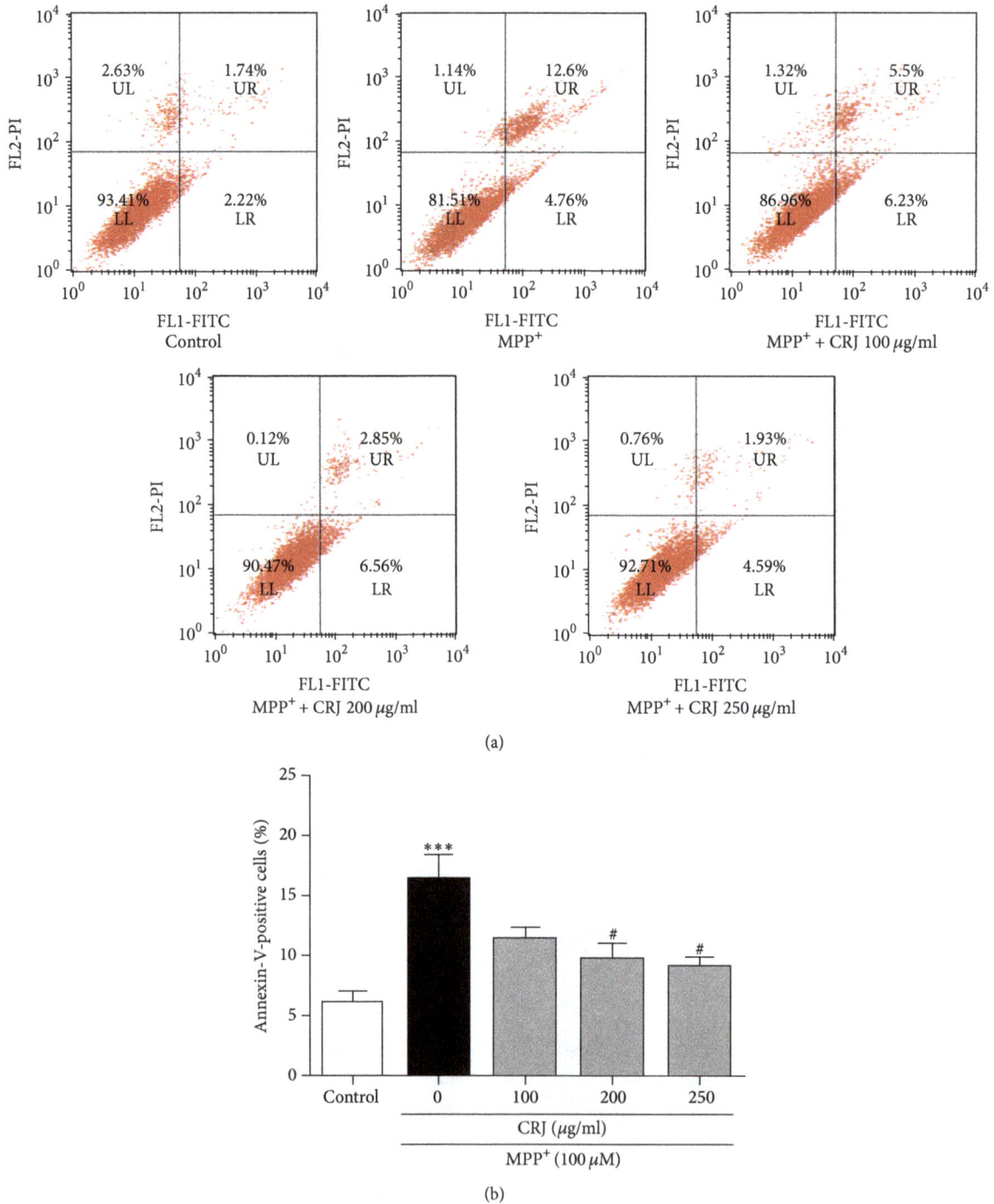

FIGURE 3: Percentage of Annexin-V-positive cells was analyzed by flow cytometry. MES23.5 cells were treated as described in Figure 2. MPP$^+$ (100 μM) increased the percentage of Annexin-V-positive MES23.5 cells. Posttreatment of CRJ resulted in the decrease of Annexin-V-positive MES23.5 cells after the exposure of MPP$^+$. Data were represented as mean ± SEM in three independent experiments. $^{***}P < 0.001$, MPP$^+$-treated cells as compared to control. $^\#P < 0.05$, CRJ + MPP$^+$ groups as compared to MPP$^+$-treated cells.

MPP$^+$-injured dopaminergic cell model. We observed that CRJ could exhibit multiple significant protective effects.

MPP$^+$ has been demonstrated as a neurotoxin that inhibits complex I of the mitochondrial electron-transport chain, which leads to oxidative stress and mitochondrial dysfunction in MES23.5 cells and other neuronal cell types

[30–32]. In this study, CRJ was found to partially abolish the ROS in MES23.5 cells after MPP$^+$ treatment. It is a crucial observation as the dopaminergic neurons keep generating ROS including hydrogen peroxide and hydroxyl radicals during the dopamine metabolism [33, 34]. It is believed that the dopaminergic neurons would be less vulnerable

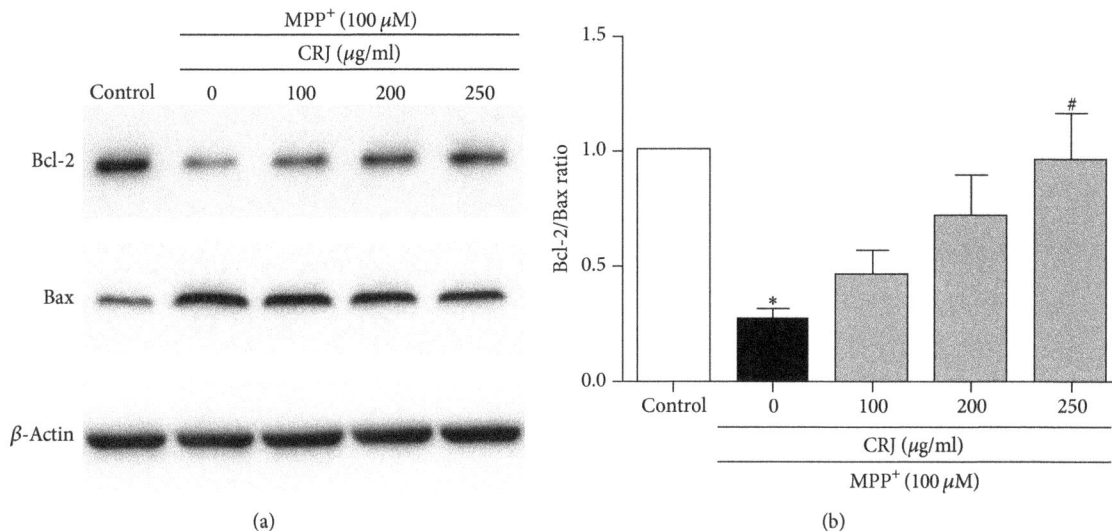

(a)   (b)

FIGURE 4: Effects of CRJ on the Bcl-2/Bax ratio in MPP$^+$-treated MES23.5 cells. MES23.5 cells were treated as described in Figure 2. (a) Expression of antiapoptotic (Bcl-2) and proapoptotic (Bax) proteins. β-Actin was used as protein loading control. (b) The Bcl-2/Bax ratio was determined by densitometric analysis of bands from Western blot. Data were represented as mean $\pm$ SEM in three independent experiments. $^*P < 0.05$, compared to control. $^\#P < 0.05$, compared to MPP$^+$-treated cells.

to oxidative injury in the presence of CRJ. Another common consequence of mitochondrial dysfunction would be the initiation of intrinsic mitochondrion-mediated apoptotic pathway. The externalization of phosphatidylserine at inner plasma membrane and the alternation of the balance between antiapoptotic and proapoptotic Bcl-2 family proteins would finally lead to the downstream cascades of intrinsic apoptotic cell death [20]. Our study showed that CRJ might play a central role in the prevention of apoptotic cell death induced by MPP$^+$ through the modulation of Bcl-2 and Bax proteins and prevention of the externalization of phosphatidylserine.

JAK/STAT signaling pathway has been recognized as a conserved signaling pathway involved in both physiological and pathological cellular events such as proliferation [35], differentiation [36], and survival [37, 38]. Blockage of the JAK2/STAT3 pathway using pharmacological inhibitor AG490 has been shown to reduce the neuronal survival [38] and abolish the neuroprotective effect of neuroprotectants [39, 40]. In the present study, significant upregulation of p-JAK2 and p-STAT3 was observed. The neuroprotective effect of CRJ in MPP$^+$-treated MES23.5 cells was likely associated with the phosphorylation of JAK2 and STAT3, resulting in the reduction of apoptosis.

ERK is another important signaling pathway which mediates cell survival. Many neuroprotectants are found to protect neuronal cell death via the activation of ERK signaling pathway. Activation of ERK pathways by long-term administration of valproic acid (VPA) enhanced neurite growth, cell survival in SH-SY5Y cells [41], ERK-dependent gene expression of Bcl-2, and neurogenesis in mice embryonic cortical neurons and adult hippocampus [42]. Ginsenoside Rb1 prevents MPP$^+$-induced apoptosis in PC12 cells through the activation of ERK/Akt pathways and inhibition of SAPK/JNK and p38 MAPK pathways [43]. In this study, the

treatment of CRJ did not significantly increase the expression of ERK in MPP$^+$-treated MES23.5 cells but it upregulated the expression of ERK in untreated MES23.5 cells and also showed nonsignificant trend of transient activation of ERK in MPP$^+$-treated cells. It may be implicated that CRJ would probably induce the cell survival pathways in MES23.5 cells, leading to the reduction of MPP$^+$-induced apoptosis.

5. Conclusion

In summary, the present study has demonstrated significant protective actions of a TCM formulation, CRJ, which includes the Chinese herbs Herba Cistanches, Herba Epimedii, and Rhizoma Polygonati, on MPP$^+$-treated MES23.5 dopaminergic cells. It is believed that the neuroprotection of the Chinese herbal formulation is "multitargeted." Based on the preclinical findings in this study, it is speculated that the CRJ formulation would be a potential candidate for the management of PD or possibly other neurodegenerative diseases that involve oxidative injury and neuronal apoptosis.

Authors' Contributions

Jing Cai contributed to the design of the thesis, directed graduated students to complete the experiment, and made the payment. Shuifen Ye, Wen Fan, Yihui Xu, and Wei Wei completed the experiment. Ho Kee Koon wrote the essay. Chuanshan Xu helped confirm the experimental results and shared responsibility as cocorresponding author.

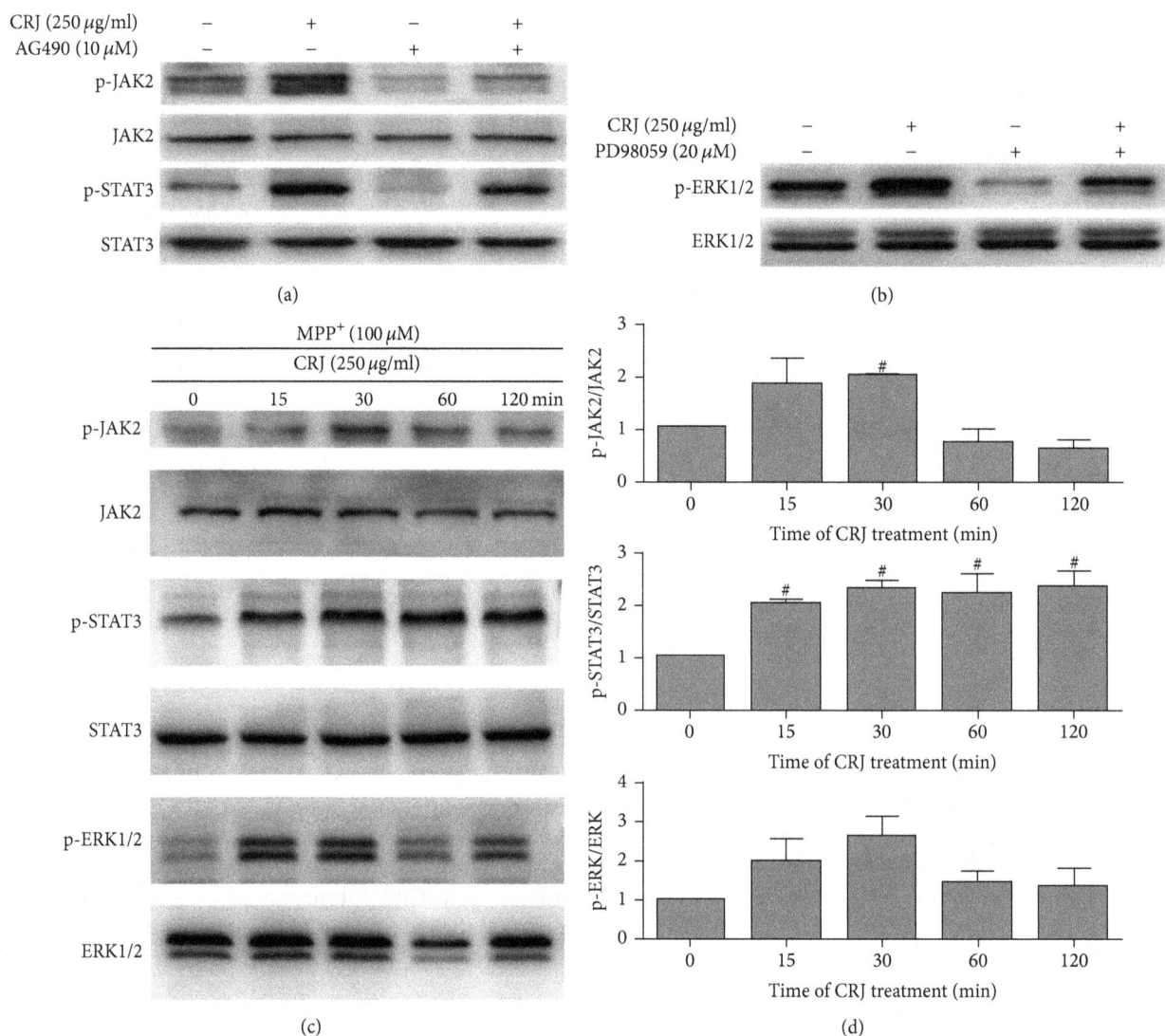

(a)

(b)

(c)

(d)

FIGURE 5: Protein expression of p-JAK2, p-STAT3, and p-ERK1/2 in MES23.5 cells and MPP$^+$-treated MES23.5 cells. ((a) and (b)) MES23.5 cells were pretreated with AG490 (JAK inhibitor) or PD98059 (ERK1/2 inhibitor) for 1 hour, followed by CRJ (250 μg/mL) incubation for 24 hours. CRJ alone enhanced the expression of (a) p-JAK2 and p-STAT3 and (b) p-ERK1/2 in MES23.5 cells. The effect could be inhibited by the corresponding pharmacological inhibitors. ((c) and (d)) Time courses of the changes of protein levels of p-JAK2, p-STAT3, and p-ERK1/2 in MPP$^+$-treated MES23.5 cells after the posttreatment of CRJ (250 μg/mL). Densitometric analysis of protein expression was determined. Data were represented as mean ± SEM in three independent experiments. Total form of each of the phosphorylated proteins was used as protein loading control. $^#P < 0.05$, compared to MPP+-treated cells 0 min after the posttreatment of CRJ.

Acknowledgments

This work was supported by Guiding project of Science and Technology Department, Fujian Province (2017 Y 0053). The authors express their thanks to Professor Biao Chen, Director, Department of Neurology, Xuanwu Hospital, Capital Medical University, for the support of their study.

References

[1] N. I. Bohnen and R. L. Albin, "The cholinergic system and Parkinson disease," *Behavioural Brain Research*, vol. 221, no. 2, pp. 564–573, 2011.

[2] P. Calabresi, B. Picconi, L. Parnetti, and M. Di Filippo, "A convergent model for cognitive dysfunctions in Parkinson's disease: the critical dopamine-acetylcholine synaptic balance," *Lancet Neurology*, vol. 5, no. 11, pp. 974–983, 2006.

[3] J. C. Martinez-Castrillo, L. Vela, J. Del Val, and A. Alonso-Canovas, "Nonmotor disorders and their correlation with dopamine: can they be treated by currently available methods?" *Neurologist*, vol. 17, supplement 1, no. 6, pp. S9–s17, 2011.

[4] S. Mullin and A. H. V. Schapira, "Pathogenic mechanisms of neurodegeneration in parkinson disease," *Neurologic Clinics*, vol. 33, no. 1, pp. 1–17, 2015.

[5] W. G. Tatton, R. Chalmers-Redman, D. Brown, and N. Tatton, "Apoptosis in Parkinson's disease: signals for neuronal degradation," *Annals of Neurology*, vol. 53, supplement 3, pp. S61–S72, 2003.

[6] S. Singh and M. Dikshit, "Apoptotic neuronal death in Parkinson's disease: involvement of nitric oxide," *Brain Research Reviews*, vol. 54, no. 2, pp. 233–250, 2007.

[7] L. W. Chen, Y. Q. Wang, L. C. Wei, M. Shi, and Y. S. Chan, "Chinese herbs and herbal extracts for neuroprotection of dopaminergic neurons and potential therapeutic treatment of Parkinson's disease," *CNS and Neurological Disorders: Drug Targets*, vol. 6, no. 4, pp. 273–281, 2007.

[8] M. Li, M.-H. Yang, Y. Liu, X.-D. Luo, J.-Z. Chen, and H.-J. Shi, "Analysis of clinical evaluation of response to treatment of Parkinson's disease with integrated Chinese and Western medicine therapy," *Chinese Journal of Integrative Medicine*, vol. 21, no. 1, pp. 17–21, 2015.

[9] J. Zhang, Y.-Z. Ma, and X.-M. Shen, "Evaluation on the efficacy and safety of Chinese herbal medication Xifeng Dingchan Pill in treating Parkinson's disease: Study protocol of a multicenter, open-label, randomized active-controlled trial," *Journal of Chinese Integrative Medicine*, vol. 11, no. 4, pp. 285–290, 2013.

[10] Q. Li, D. Zhao, and E. Bezard, "Traditional Chinese medicine for Parkinson's disease: a review of Chinese literature," *Behavioural Pharmacology*, vol. 17, no. 5-6, pp. 403–410, 2006.

[11] J. Cai, Y. Tian, R. Lin, X. Chen, Z. Liu, and J. Xie, "Protective effects of kidney-tonifying Chinese herbal preparation on substantia nigra neurons in a mouse model of Parkinson's disease," *Neural Regeneration Research*, vol. 7, no. 6, pp. 413–420, 2012.

[12] S. Lin, S. Ye, J. Huang et al., "How do Chinese medicines that tonify the kidney inhibit dopaminergic neuron apoptosis?" *Neural Regeneration Research*, vol. 8, no. 30, pp. 2820–2826, 2013.

[13] J.-X. Song, S. C.-W. Sze, T.-B. Ng et al., "Anti-Parkinsonian drug discovery from herbal medicines: what have we got from neurotoxic models?" *Journal of Ethnopharmacology*, vol. 139, no. 3, pp. 698–711, 2012.

[14] X.-Z. Li, S.-N. Zhang, S.-M. Liu, and F. Lu, "Recent advances in herbal medicines treating Parkinson's disease," *Fitoterapia*, vol. 84, no. 1, pp. 273–285, 2013.

[15] X.-P. Li, W.-J. Xie, Z. Zhang, S. Kansara, J. Jankovic, and W.-D. Le, "A mechanistic study of proteasome inhibition-induced iron misregulation in dopamine neuron degeneration," *NeuroSignals*, vol. 20, no. 4, pp. 223–236, 2012.

[16] J. E. Bottenstein and G. H. Sato, "Growth of a rat neuroblastoma cell line in serum-free supplemented medium," *Proceedings of the National Academy of Sciences of the United States of America*, vol. 76, no. 1, pp. 514–517, 1979.

[17] J. Wang, X.-X. Du, H. Jiang, and J.-X. Xie, "Curcumin attenuates 6-hydroxydopamine-induced cytotoxicity by anti-oxidation and nuclear factor-kappaB modulation in MES23.5 cells," *Biochemical Pharmacology*, vol. 78, no. 2, pp. 178–183, 2009.

[18] J. Lotharius, L. L. Dugan, and K. L. O'Malley, "Distinct mechanisms underlie neurotoxin-mediated cell death in cultured dopaminergic neurons," *The Journal of Neuroscience*, vol. 19, no. 4, pp. 1284–1293, 1999.

[19] N. A. Simonian and J. T. Coyle, "Oxidative stress in neurodegenerative diseases," *Annual Review of Pharmacology and Toxicology*, vol. 36, no. 1, pp. 83–106, 1996.

[20] S. Elmore, "Apoptosis: a review of programmed cell death," *Toxicologic Pathology*, vol. 35, no. 4, pp. 495–516, 2007.

[21] Y. Shi, "A structural view of mitochondria-mediated apoptosis," *Nature Structural & Molecular Biology*, vol. 8, no. 5, pp. 394–401, 2001.

[22] R. J. Youle and A. Strasser, "The BCL-2 protein family: opposing activities that mediate cell death," *Nature Reviews Molecular Cell Biology*, vol. 9, no. 1, pp. 47–59, 2008.

[23] G. Badr, M. Mohany, and F. Abu-Tarboush, "Thymoquinone decreases F-actin polymerization and the proliferation of human multiple myeloma cells by suppressing STAT3 phosphorylation and Bcl2/Bcl-XL expression," *Lipids in Health and Disease*, vol. 10, article 236, 2011.

[24] C. X. Wang, J. H. Song, D. K. Song, V. W. Yong, A. Shuaib, and C. Hao, "Cyclin-dependent kinase-5 prevents neuronal apoptosis through ERK-mediated upregulation of Bcl-2," *Cell Death and Differentiation*, vol. 13, no. 7, pp. 1203–1212, 2006.

[25] R. D. Sweet and F. H. McDowell, "Plasma dopa concentrations and the "on-off" effect after chronic treatment of parkinson's disease," *Neurology*, vol. 24, no. 10, pp. 953–956, 1974.

[26] M.-C. Boll, M. Alcaraz-Zubeldia, and C. Rios, "Medical management of parkinson's disease: focus on neuroprotection," *Current Neuropharmacology*, vol. 9, no. 2, pp. 350–359, 2011.

[27] Z. Li, H. Lin, L. Gu, J. Gao, and C.-M. Tzeng, "Herba Cistanche (Rou Cong-Rong): One of the best pharmaceutical gifts of traditional Chinese medicine," *Frontiers in Pharmacology*, vol. 7, article 41, 2016.

[28] M. Chen, J. Wu, Q. Luo et al., "The anticancer properties of herba epimedii and its main bioactive componentsicariin and icariside II," *Nutrients*, vol. 8, no. 9, article 563, 2016.

[29] A. L. Xu, M. C. Jiang, X. H. Chen, and W. F. Chen, "Icariin protects against MPP(+)-induced neurotoxicity in MES23.5 cells," *Sheng Li Xue Bao*, vol. 68, no. 5, pp. 585–591, 2016.

[30] T. W. Jung, J. Y. Lee, W. S. Shim et al., "Rosiglitazone protects human neuroblastoma SH-SY5Y cells against MPP+ induced cytotoxicity via inhibition of mitochondrial dysfunction and ROS production," *Journal of the Neurological Sciences*, vol. 253, no. 1-2, pp. 53–60, 2007.

[31] W.-B. Liu, J. Zhou, Y. Qu et al., "Neuroprotective effect of osthole on MPP$^+$-induced cytotoxicity in PC12 cells via inhibition of mitochondrial dysfunction and ROS production," *Neurochemistry International*, vol. 57, no. 3, pp. 206–215, 2010.

[32] H. Xu, H. Jiang, J. Wang, and J. Xie, "Rg1 protects the MPP+-treated MES23.5 cells via attenuating DMT1 up-regulation and cellular iron uptake," *Neuropharmacology*, vol. 58, no. 2, pp. 488–494, 2010.

[33] K. Zhang, Z. Ma, J. Wang, A. Xie, and J. Xie, "Myricetin attenuated MPP$^+$-induced cytotoxicity by anti-oxidation and inhibition of MKK4 and JNK activation in MES23.5 cells," *Neuropharmacology*, vol. 61, no. 1-2, pp. 329–335, 2011.

[34] J. Lotharius and P. Brundin, "Pathogenesis of Parkinson's disease: dopamine, vesicles and alpha-synuclein," *Nature Reviews. Neuroscience*, vol. 3, no. 12, pp. 932–942, 2002.

[35] M. Tsuda, Y. Kohro, T. Yano et al., "JAK-STAT3 pathway regulates spinal astrocyte proliferation and neuropathic pain maintenance in rats," *Brain*, vol. 134, no. 4, pp. 1127–1139, 2011.

[36] Y. H. Kim, J.-I. Chung, H. G. Woo et al., "Differential regulation of proliferation and differentiation in neural precursor cells by the Jak pathway," *Stem Cells*, vol. 28, no. 10, pp. 1816–1828, 2010.

[37] R. K. Monroe and S. W. Halvorsen, "Cadmium blocks receptor-mediated Jak/STAT signaling in neurons by oxidative stress," *Free Radical Biology and Medicine*, vol. 41, no. 3, pp. 493–502, 2006.

[38] A. Yadav, A. Kalita, S. Dhillon, and K. Banerjee, "JAK/STAT3 pathway is involved in survival of neurons in response to insulin-like growth factor and negatively regulated by suppressor of cytokine signaling-3," *Journal of Biological Chemistry*, vol. 280, no. 36, pp. 31830–31840, 2005.

[39] H. M. Yu, J. L. Zhi, Y. Cui et al., "Role of the JAK-STAT pathway in protection of hydrogen peroxide preconditioning against apoptosis induced by oxidative stress in PC12 cells," *Apoptosis*, vol. 11, no. 6, pp. 931–941, 2006.

[40] A. Kretz, C. J. Happold, J. K. Marticke, and S. Isenmann, "Erythropoietin promotes regeneration of adult CNS neurons

via Jak2/Stat3 and PI3K/AKT pathway activation," *Molecular and Cellular Neuroscience*, vol. 29, no. 4, pp. 569–579, 2005.

[41] P.-X. Yuan, L.-D. Huang, Y.-M. Jiang, J. S. Gutkind, H. K. Manji, and G. Chen, "The mood stabilizer valproic acid activates mitogen-activated protein kinases and promotes neurite growth," *Journal of Biological Chemistry*, vol. 276, no. 34, pp. 31674–31683, 2001.

[42] Y. Hao, T. Creson, L. Zhang et al., "Mood stabilizer valproate

promotes ERK pathway-dependent cortical neuronal growth and neurogenesis," *Journal of Neuroscience*, vol. 24, no. 29, pp. 6590–6599, 2004.

[43] R. Hashimoto, J. Yu, H. Koizumi, Y. Ouchi, and T. Okabe, "Ginsenoside Rb1 prevents MPP$^+$-induced apoptosis in PC12 cells by stimulating estrogen receptors with consequent activation of ERK1/2, Akt and inhibition of SAPK/JNK, p38 MAPK," *Evidence-Based Complementary and Alternative Medicine*, vol. 2012, Article ID 693717, 8 pages, 2012.

27

Systematic Review and Critical Analysis of Cost Studies Associated with Parkinson's Disease

Tânia M. Bovolenta,[1] Sônia Maria Cesar de Azevedo Silva,[2] Roberta Arb Saba,[3] Vanderci Borges,[3] Henrique Ballalai Ferraz,[3] and Andre C. Felicio[4]

[1]Programa de Pós-Graduação, Hospital Israelita Albert Einstein, São Paulo, SP, Brazil
[2]Movement Disorders Department in Neurology, Universidade Federal de São Paulo (UNIFESP), São Paulo, SP, Brazil
[3]Universidade Federal de São Paulo (UNIFESP), São Paulo, SP, Brazil
[4]Neurology Program, Hospital Israelita Albert Einstein, São Paulo, SP, Brazil

Correspondence should be addressed to Andre C. Felicio; cf.andre@gmail.com

Academic Editor: Antonio Pisani

Parkinson's disease (PD) is the second most prevalent neurodegenerative disease worldwide, affecting more than four million people. Typically, it affects individuals above 45, when they are still productive, compromising both aging and quality of life. Therefore, the cost of the disease must be identified, so that the use of resources can be rational and efficient. Additionally, in Brazil, there is a lack of research on the costs of neurodegenerative diseases, such as PD, a gap addressed in this study. This systematic review critically addresses the various methodologies used in original research around the world in the last decade on the subject, showing that costs are hardly comparable. Nonetheless, the economic and social impacts are implicit, and important information for public health agents is provided.

1. Introduction

Health and the economy are related intrinsically. The purpose of the studies on the costs of diseases is describing them, estimating costs, comparing established programs, and projecting these costs based on clinical, demographic, epidemiological, and technological factors. In fact, over the past decade, there has been a growing number of studies, which are presumed to be valuable decision tools, because the limited amount of resources must be used rationally and efficiently as not to miss opportunities to improve overall population health [1].

In neurodegenerative diseases, such as Parkinson's disease (PD), whose prevention is still impossible, the burden borne by society, whether it is financial, social, or even psychological, is often heavy. Being the second most prevalent neurodegenerative disease worldwide, it generally affects individuals between 40 and 50 (late-onset PD) [2, 3], compromising their productive life and aging. As such, research needs to be directed to reducing their costs.

Studies on disease costs may have several approaches, such as economic assessment, epidemiological design, or even type of cost involved, as well as the viewpoint of defining resource use strategies. The diversity in methods is a significant factor why cost estimates differ between studies, opening the discussion about which public policies are most appropriate for PD.

This systematic review provides introductory concepts on the types of studies on costs and analyzes results in selected articles critically, highlighting the benefits and limitations of their methods. Moreover, this study identifies the most common studies regarding DP costs worldwide over the past 10 years, showing possibilities for studies being carried out in Brazil, where there is a lack of this type of analysis because most studies only involve the clinical aspects of the disease.

2. Methodology

In March 2016, two *online* bibliographic information services were accessed—SCOPUS and PubMed—with the aim of

TABLE 1: Types of economic evaluation and their main characteristics.

Type of economic analysis	Costs	Advantages	Disadvantages
Cost minimization (CMA)	Monetary	This technique only measures costs	It does not describe results, and it has little applicability to health
Cost-effectiveness (CEA)	Monetary	It allows comparisons between health programs	Difficulty in comparison of results
Cost-benefit (CBA)	Monetary	This analysis allows comparisons between strategies because it works with the same monetary unit	Difficulty of valuing human life
Cost-utility (CUA)	Monetary	This analysis considers the level of well-being and preferences of the individual	The scales of measurement of quality are arbitrary

selecting original articles about the cost of PD over the past decade.

The following terms were used for access: *(parkinson disease) AND TITLE-ABS-KEY (economics) OR TITLE-ABS-KEY (costs of illness) OR TITLE-ABS-KEY (health expenditures) OR TITLE-ABS-KEY (cost effectiveness analysis) OR TITLE-ABS-KEY (cost benefit analysis) OR TITLE-ABS - CUT (cost utility analysis) OR TITLE-ABS-KEY (cost minimization analysis) OR TITLE-ABS-KEY (direct costs) OR TITLE-ABS-KEY (CB costs) OR TITLE-ABS-KEY (out of pockets) AND DOCTYPE (air OR re) AND PUBYEAR > 2004 AND (LIMIT-TO (LANGUAGE, "English")) AND (LIMIT-TO (DOCTYPE, "air")).*

This method identified 522 papers. The inclusion criterion was that articles refer to costs related to this disease in general and/or regarding the use of medication. Papers that compared procedures and/or medicines, dealt with specific therapies, as well as PD surgeries, or were related to patient caregivers or already selected papers but were neither applicable to the research nor available to access were excluded. Revisions were also not selected (380 papers were excluded because of the title, for not being compatible, having been duplicated, and/or being reviews). Once the first levels of inclusion were satisfied, 142 papers were selected for reading the *abstract*. Although 35 of these had a suggestive title, that is, they did not tackle general costs of disease exclusively, 107 were separated for complete reading, and 30 met the criteria for research (Figure 1).

2.1. Basic Concepts of Health Studies.
The determination of the costs of a disease facilitates learning what its burden to society is, assessing its degree of efficiency, and understanding how the market tends to organize itself regarding certain values [4].

2.1.1. Economic Assessment.
The basic function of any economic assessment is to identify, measure, value, and compare the costs and consequences of alternative proposals [4–8].

In this case, four techniques are possible (Table 1):

(1) Cost-Minimization. Cost-minimization is the least used technique, because it only compares costs of interventions that produce the same outcomes with different costs. For chronic diseases, such as PD, there are no studies using this type of analysis.

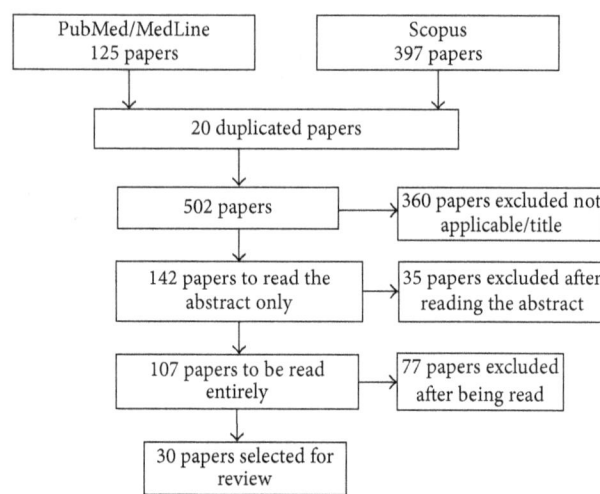

FIGURE 1: Search, selection, and inclusion of papers for critical analysis of studies on economic PD evaluation in *online* platforms.

(2) Cost-Effectiveness. Cost-effectiveness is the technique most used in literature, which assesses the impact of different alternatives that bring better results with lower costs; these are always comparative and explicit and designed to select the best option to achieve what is perceived in clinical practice.

(3) Cost-Benefit. This analysis determines whether a new health technology or intervention generates net benefits to society. However, due to its difficulty, complexity, and controversies in valuing human life and certain health conditions in monetary terms, this analysis is rarely found in the literature.

(4) Cost-Utility. This analysis assesses the impacts on survival and quality of life, which are determining criteria to judge the effects of strategies in health care, that is, the level of well-being and preferences of the individual.

2.1.2. Study Designs.
The epidemiological study designs define how the research will be performed in relation to adopted method [9–13]. The most discussed study designs in PD research are as follows (Table 2).

(1) Prevalence and Incidence. The prevalence estimates the number of deaths, hospitalizations, prevention, and research attributable to a disease in a given period (usually a year),

TABLE 2: Main study designs on costs.

Approaches	Description	Advantages	Disadvantages
Prevalence	Frequency measure It evaluates all existing cases in a given period	Ample results Specific policy planning Fast study and recommended for chronic diseases	Considered weak at estimating the risk of developing disease
Incidence	Frequency measure Assesses the number of new cases in a given period	Implementation of measures to reduce new cases It is used more for acute diseases, since it estimates the risk of developing the disease	Not recommended for chronic diseases
Top-down	It measures the proportion of a disease attributed to several risk factors. It involves a study directed from total to lower levels	When the scope of study is well understood	More comprehensive, it hampers the study on the details of the disease
Bottom-up	Related to the unit costs of inputs used. It involves the study directed from individual levels to the total.	More detailed	Risk of double counting
Prospective	Temporal study, performed during disease. Probes the effect through the cause	Used in chronic diseases	Time-consuming and expensive
Retrospective	Temporal study performed with preexisting data. Probes the cause through the effect	Quick and cheaper	Risk of memory bias
Econometric	Comparison of groups	Minor amount of data required Cost difference between the two populations	Long study, requiring that the control group be paired to the study group
Markov models	Stochastic process Used in prospective studies. Patients stratified in stages of disease	Dynamic model aiming at studying the transition from one stage to another, evaluating the costs of each step	Transition of stages is independent, without considering the previous one

to subsequently estimate the costs incurred by these consequences. Incidence refers to the number of new cases in a predefined period, and it foresees the associated costs from the onset of the disease until its disappearance (usually cure or death), through a rough projection of the flow of these values.

Studies on prevalence display greater results than incidence ones, for diseases are usually long-term sequelae, as is the case of PD, and they are of great importance in planning specific policies on certain diseases when their economic burden was underestimated. Therefore, they can identify the main components of current expenses and uncharged resources.

(2) Top-Down and Bottom-Up. *Top-down* approaches are normally used in prevalence studies, when the expenses of a disease are widely known from national or regional statistics. In *bottom-up* studies, cost estimates are more detailed. The data depend on the scope of the study, and they are intrinsically related to the unit costs of inputs used, through interviews, questionnaires or chart review, and assessment of individual cost. The average cost per person is then obtained by means of the number of times the service was used and the number of people with the disease. Although *bottom-up* studies are more complete when it comes to resources and more precise

regarding patient selection, they run a high risk of double counting costs (e.g., if a patient has more than one disease and costs of comorbidities are confused and/or grouped). The majority of studies with PD adopt this approach.

(3) Prospective and Retrospective Approaches. There is a temporal relationship, where in prospective studies the relevant events have not happened yet, that is, studying the patient over time, formalizing a system of data collection focused on the purpose of the research, such as questionnaires designed specifically for patients and/or their caregivers, where everything is recorded in "real time." In retrospective studies, all events had already occurred when the study was initiated. They are usually employed in long-term chronic diseases, as is the case of PD. In this case, research efficiency can only be possible with enough observational datasets. It would be best if the data were stored electronically to minimize memory bias due to omission of facts or values.

(4) Econometric Approaches. Econometric approaches estimate differences between groups. One of the groups has the disease and the other does not; however, both have the same characteristics, which are assessed by several regression analyses involving demographic factors such as sex, age, marital

TABLE 3: Classification of costs.

Types of costs	Description
Direct medical	Directly related to the disease. Hospitalization, medication, medical appointments, treatments, laboratory tests, and diagnosis
Direct nonmedical	Directly related to the disease. Transport, domestic modifications, food
Indirect	Loss of productivity: partial, temporary, or permanent They may affect the patient and/or caregiver Early retirement
Intangible	Psychological and psychosocial and costs, difficult measurement
Personal	Costs incurred by the patient and/or their family, when there is no support from private and/or public health care. Private consultations, medication, treatments, and domestic modifications. Linked with direct costs

status, ethnicity, relationship between patient and caregiver, housing, and duration of the disease.

(5) Markov Models. Markov models are used in several studies of chronic diseases, when patients are studied over time, and they are stratified according to disease scale. In the case of PD, the scale of Hoehn and Yahr (it assesses the degree of disability due to the disease in scores) is key to building this model. These are typically prospective studies, proposing cost increases with disease severity.

Several approaches may be featured in the same study; that is, we may have a retrospective, prevalent, and *bottom-up* study, for instance, because its purpose, most of the time, is to maximize the content of information, contributing to enriching knowledge.

2.1.3. Classification of Costs. The costs of a disease are typically stratified as follows [4, 7, 10, 14] (Table 3).

(1) Direct Costs. Direct costs are related to the disease and its equation; their charges may concern public administration, insurance companies, the patient, the patient's family, or even a combination of all or some of these determinants. The estimates of direct costs associated with chronic diseases are higher than those associated with acute and communicable diseases, on the condition that better treatments and methods of prevention are adopted. This group can be divided into direct medical costs and nonmedical ones, although not all studies adopt this division.

(2) Indirect Costs. Indirect costs refer to the loss of income and/or productivity; they are caused by disease. Additionally, they can incur costs to both the patient and the employer. Depending on the disease, this loss may be partial, temporary, or permanent, and it may be restricted to the patient and/or caregiver (as in the case of advanced stage PD), frequently leading to early retirement. If there is a possibility of returning to regular activities, this disease may not occur on the same productivity level as before, or lead to frequent absences (absenteeism), incurring additional costs, such as loss of promotions.

(3) Intangible Costs. Intangible costs are virtually impossible to measure, since they incur psychological and psychosocial

costs imposed to the patients, their family, and acquaintances due to the disease, as well as pain, behavioral changes, and everyday activities. They depend on the perception that the patient's health problems lead to social consequences, such as isolation.

(4) Personal Costs. Personal costs are the costs borne by the patient and/or their family and friends due to consultations with health professionals, medication, laboratory tests, domestic adjustments, locomotion resources, and the need for home care. Depending on the country, these costs, also called copayments, are borne by the government, health insurance, or religious or private health institutions. Sometimes, these payments are also designated as direct costs because they are associated with the disease. They may be redeemable or not, implying an additional expense to the patient, who has to spend a certain amount of money in advance.

2.1.4. Perspectives. Who bears the costs related to the program defines which costs are included for analysis [6, 7, 10] (Table 4).

(1) Industry (Human Capital). The industry bears the costs due to absenteeism or loss of productivity, and early retirement due to the disease.

(2) Society. A more comprehensive perspective considers all costs related to the program, regardless of who will pay the expenses (patient, government, or insurance companies). This approach is thought to be the most appropriate to support health-related decisions. Most research on PD addresses this perspective, although some studies include more than one viewpoint.

(3) Patients and Their Family. Costs are borne by the patient concerning appointments, transport used for his treatment, purchase of medication, expenses with caregivers, domestic changes, and so on.

(4) Programs, Public Health, and/or Insurance Companies. When there is a need to identify all the inputs related to the disease, for which monetary value explains the base period and the form of assessment used should be assigned, this

TABLE 4: Description of the main perspectives used in cost studies.

Perspective	Description
Industry	Related to human capital. Considers the individual as an investment target
Society	More common in the literature. It is comprehensive and based on health-related decisions. It represents the public interest
Patient/family	Less common, only addresses the patient's and their family's costs
Public/private health care	To identify and quantify all inputs used in the production of the service/procedure. Important to form the cost of illness

perspective is highly likely to underestimate the cost of disease, especially when greater profit or lower production costs are targeted.

2.2. Studies on the Socioeconomic Impact of PD. Although PD affects more than four million people worldwide [15], little is known about their progression rates, the costs of medical care, and the management of resources specific to this disease [16]. In Brazil, although its notification is not compulsory, unofficial data estimate 220,000 PD sufferers. Considering local records of patients with PD, in a study conducted in the city of Bambuí, Minas Gerais, it was found that 3% of the population above 64 had the disease, a result similar to the prevalence rates found in elderly studies in European and American countries and slightly above the rates in Eastern countries [17].

PD was considered among the most prevalent and costly diseases of the brain, being the fourth most expensive second study in 28 European countries [18]. However, the level of socioeconomic development, budget availability of health systems, and culture of each country or region determine research methodologies, which are directed to a subset of expenses, using only a few components and all expenditure resulting from a disease, which would be practically impossible. Therefore, there is no one method more or less appropriate for this type of study, as the costs of PD in all countries involved cannot be compared and the information cannot be simply transferred from one country to another without having any evidence to support the use of the data.

Over the past decade, there has been a significant increase in the number of papers related to costs of diseases. Figure 2 shows the evolution for PD, between 2005 and February 2016, with a higher concentration between 2011 and 2013, triggered by the need to investigate the values involved in the cost of this disease. The demographic transition is a reality, and health managers need data that can enable their strategies towards public policies. The graph shows the 522 identified papers (125 Pubmed, 397 Scopus) and the 30 selected among them for this review.

3. Discussion

The papers selected for this review are summarized in Table 5. The PD cost may be very different from one country to another. Nonetheless, the monetary value of the year in which the study happened should be considered. All values were converted to US dollars ($) and daily, quarterly, or half-yearly

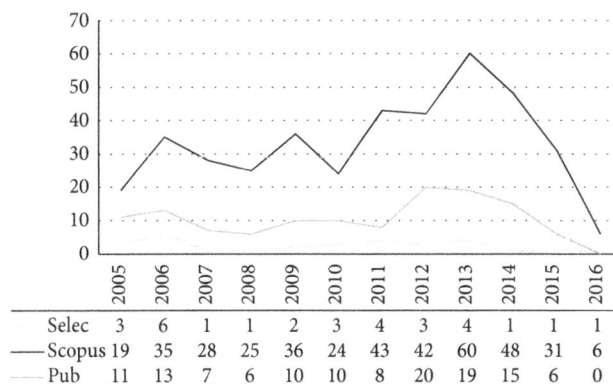

	2005	2006	2007	2008	2009	2010	2011	2012	2013	2014	2015	2016
Selec	3	6	1	1	2	3	4	3	4	1	1	1
Scopus	19	35	28	25	36	24	43	42	60	48	31	6
Pub	11	13	7	6	10	10	8	20	19	15	6	0

FIGURE 2: Number of publications on PD costs over the past 10 years. Scopus = 397 papers; Pubmed = 125 papers; Selected = 30.

results were converted to annual. Only one article had values by period of life [19], and another took into consideration those 40 to 79 years of age [20].

Practically, all articles used the general costs of the disease, without naming the type of economic evaluation. Only one article [21] referred to the burden of disease as DALY (disability-adjusted life in years), suggesting the use of cost-utility.

Because there is no way of implementing measures so as to reduce new cases, the most appropriate model for PD costs may be developed from prevalence studies. They are conducted when diagnosis has already been established, obtaining ample results, and are to conduct than incidence ones, which demand rigorous criteria for diagnosis. In this review, we identified 20 papers that followed this line of research (see Table 4).

The use of questionnaires, suggesting a bottom-up approach, is common practice found in the research reviewed here, although not all of them described the design. The unit value of the inputs used is more easily acquired than full reports obtained from large databases in top-down approaches, although at least six papers suggest the use of this approach for studying large samples [22–27].

Since it is a disease with long survival, retrospective studies are the most common for PD, despite the bias of memory that can be generated depending on the retroactive period. In reviewed articles, 12 authors (see Table 4) opted for a prospective study with patient monitoring. Despite being

TABLE 5: Comparison of findings on costs of PD in selected studies.

Author	Country/Region	Year	n	Design	Costs studied	Perspective	Value/year US$	Comments
Yoritaka et al. [40]	Japan	2016	715	SPO	D	S	5,828	Direct cost
Martínez-Martin et al., [44]	Spain	2015	174	PO/BU	D/I	S	13,720.24/year 4	Magnitude of disease and quality of life
Tamás et al. [39]	Hungary	2014	110	PE/BU	D/I/OOP	S/CH	6,831	Costs of illness and quality of life
Kowal et al. [22]	USA	2013	630,000	PE	D/I	S	22,800	Economic load current and projected (by 2050) in the USA
Zhao et al. [19]	Singapore	2013	195	PE/MK/BU	D/I	S	68,519 (over the lifetime period)	Cost of illness
Johnson et al. [41]	USA	2013	1,151	RE	D/I	CS	43,506 PDINST (cohort)	Cost of illness x several cohorts
Bhattacharjee and Sambamoorthi [29]	USA	2013	350	RE	D/OOP	S	15,404	Cost of illness/over expenditure associated with PD
Kaltenboeck et al. [23]	USA	2012	25,577	RE	D	G	78,042 (ambulatory pac. PD)	Survival rates and costs of patients of health programs
Bach et al. [43]	Germany	2012	1,449	PE	D/I	G	6.00 (2190) to 12.69 (4631.85)	Cost of illness/drugs/comorbidities
Lökk et al. [25]	Sweden	2012	4,163	PE/RE	D	S	9,333	Cost of illness/drugs
Johnson et al. [20]	USA	2011	278	PO	I	S/CH/CS	569,393 (45 years), 188,590 (55), 35,496 (65), 2,451 (75) (from 40 to 79 years)	Indirect costs
Jennum et al. [26]	Denmark	2011	13,400	RE/PO	D/I	S	7,763	Cost of illness
Zhao et al. [38]	Singapore	2011	195	PE/BU	D/I/OOP	S	10,129	Cost of illness
von Campenhausen et al. [45]	Europe (6 countries)	2011	486	PE/RE/BU	D/I/OOP	S	2,968 to 11,124	Cost of illness
Winter et al. [30]	Italy	2010	70	PO/BU	D/I/OOP	S	19,574	Cost of illness/drugs
Winter et al. [46]	Germany	2010	145	PO/PE/BU	D/I/OOP	G	22,763	Cost of illness
Winter et al. [47]	Germany	2010	145/133	PE/RE	D/I	S	21,138 to 35,864	Cost of illness
Winter et al. [32]	Czech Rep.	2009	100	PE/RE/BU	D/I	S/CH/P	12,483	Cost of illness
Winter et al. [37]	Russia	2009	100	PE/PO/BU	D/I	S/CH	5,935	Cost of illness
Vargas et al. [42]	Brazil	2008	144	PE/PO/BU	IN	NA	NA	Resource use X incapacity
McCrone et al. [33]	UK	2007	175	PE/RE	D/OOP	CS/P	19,861	Cost of illness
Leibson et al. [35]	USA	2006	92	PE/RE	D	NA	Unclear	Cost of illness per groups
Ragothaman et al. [36]	India	2006	175	PE/PO	D	S	707	Cost of illness/direct costs
Wang et al. [48]	China	2006	190	PE/RE/BU	D/I	S	925	Cost of illness

TABLE 5: Continued.

Author	Country/Region	Year	n	Design	Costs studied	Perspective	Value/year US$	Comments
Vossius et al. [31]	Germany/Norway	2006	438	PE/RE/PO	D	S	2,389 (Germany), 1,620 (Norway)	Cost of PD drugs
Noyes et al. [27]	USA	2006	717	PE/RE	D/OOP	S/P	18,528	Cost of illness/drugs/medicare
Cordato et al. [28]	Australia	2006	12	PE/PO	D/I	S	5,380	Cost of illness
Huse et al. [24]	USA	2005	20,016	PE/RE	D	CS	10,037	Cost of illness
Spottke et al. [34]	Germany	2005	145	PE/PO	D/I/OOP	S/G/P	22,723 ± 28,297	Cost of illness
Cubo et al. [21]	Spain	2005	23,417	RE	Int.	G	NA	Years of life lost

Notes: SPO = semiprospective; PO = prospective; BU = bottom-up; PE = prevalent; PE = prevalent, MK = Markov; RE = retrospective; D = direct cost; I = indirect cost; OOP = out-of-pocket; Int. = intangible; S = society; CH = human capital; CS = insurance companies; G = government; NA = not applicable; P = patient; PDINST = patients with PD institutionalized; Medicare = USA health care.

lengthy and expensive, some studies used Markov models [19] or econometric studies [28, 29] with cohorts, for example.

The aforementioned chosen variables are related to the purpose of the study, but, in general, we observed that 20 (see Table 4) out of 30 papers opted for the total cost of the disease, including direct, indirect, and/or personal costs. In one of the studies [20], however, indirect costs were only considered, from the perspective of insurance companies and human capital, whereas, in another [21], the aim was to evaluate intangible costs alone through lost years of life. Similarly, three studies concentrated only on medication costs [25, 30, 31].

Among direct costs, the most common variables analyzed in most studies were medication, hospitalizations, outpatient visits, auxiliary treatments, home care, transport, and special equipment. Not all studies divided the direct costs into medical and nonmedical (Table 3). In one of the studies, even dental care provided to patients was assessed [29].

Regarding indirect costs, most studies are related to the patient and/or the caregiver in terms of loss of productivity, early retirement, and sick leaves (medical certificates). As for personal costs, they consider informal care, copayment treatments, drugs, and equipment.

The society costs are the most studied, the society being the most affected regarding allocation of resources. Only four studies assessed this prospect from the patient's point of view [27, 32–34].

Clarity is needed in the way data and/or results are expressed, which may generate uncertainty or confusion in the conclusion of a study. For instance, one of the studies [35] does not provide a clear cost of PD, and groups are very stratified and only the differences between them are highlighted. Moreover, albeit the many variables analyzed, important components were not assessed, such as auxiliary treatments. On the other hand, another study [20] does not enlist which direct cost components were used. As such, statistical analyses must be well established, so that other studies can be replicated if necessary. In this review, some studies did not provide that [25, 31, 36].

Many authors have chosen to direct certain types of costs towards one category, which reinforces the uniqueness of each study. One author [37] argued that informal care should be placed with indirect costs, but with direct nonmedical ones, based on the fact that if home care is not provided by the family, professional care would be needed.

The fact that the same cost component is classified in different categories can have a strong influence on the final results, not considering the values set by the inputs in each country. In a study conducted in Russia [37], for example, direct costs accounted for 67% of total costs, while indirect ones accounted for 33%. Besides, in a study in Singapore [38], direct costs were 38.5% and indirect ones 61.5% of the total cost. Another author states [39] that costs were distributed as 35.7% direct, 29.4% as direct nonmedical costs and 34.9% as indirect. In this study, we have verified that the value of consultation with a specialist in the Hungarian public health care system costs around $7, while in the UK [33] this value is approximately $225.

Issues related to health insurance also influence the comparison of studies greatly and must be considered. For example, in India, a study [36] revealed that only 7.4% of patients are covered by health insurance, and, unlike most studies reviewed, the cost of PD treatment is very low, at around $707 per year, since most of the expenses are covered by the patients and their family. Conversely, in the UK [33], maintaining virtually the same research approach, a final value of around $20,000 a year was calculated. In Japan, on the other hand [40], a study found a value of around $6,000 per PD patient, where the health insurance covers 100% of the population. Depending on the patient's income or age, he/she contributes 10% to 30% to medical costs.

There are some other factors that certainly affect the results obtained: samples ranged from small cohorts ($n = 12$) [28] to large populations ($n = 630,000$) [22], some studies [41, 42] have excluded from their samples patients with advanced PD (Hoehn & Yahr 5), and others [19, 43] assessed not only PD, but also its complications and/or comorbidities.

Finally, with regard to the revised articles of this manuscript, we could suggest an instrument as a guideline to determine PD-related costs even though several methodologies and different variables could be taken into account for each particular scenario. Therefore, prospective studies would be the ideal methodology, but cross-sectional, retrospective ones, with a bottom-up approach from the perspective of society, could be more feasible. The questionnaire to obtain data could be divided into the following parts:

(1) Clinical, social, demographic, and economic issues of the patient;

(2) Medical and nonmedical direct costs;

(3) Indirect costs;

(4) Personal costs (including caregivers).

The most common variables found in the literature used to determine the costs of PD, depending on the scope of the study, are shown in Table 6.

4. Conclusion

The concepts mentioned in this review do not aim to finalize the discussion on health economics tackling the costs of neurodegenerative diseases, such as PD, but only to allow access to introductory concepts of these assessments, so that the reader can contextualize the articles analyzed here.

The very definition of studies on costs of disease suggests limitations, as the articles here reviewed display methodological heterogeneity regarding PD costs, and this variation is an important factor that should receive more attention in literature. Unlike Alzheimer's disease, which has a validated instrument to determine the costs of illness [49], PD presents considerable problems in its analysis, since evaluations and comparisons are made between individual studies. If there were a standardized and validated instrument, the data costs would be more reliable and transparent and there would be rational allocation of resources and better collection of data for cost analysis and efficacy.

We observed that there is no standardization of terminology used for the definition of costs, or even unanimity in the

TABLE 6: Most common variables found in the cost studies of Parkinson's disease.

Patient/disease	Direct medical cost	Direct nonmedical cost	Indirect cost	Out-of-pockets
Age	Hospitalization	Ancillary therapy/rehabilitation	Retirement	Transportation*
Gender	Pharmacotherapy (PD and comorbidities)	Home Care*	Retirement premature	Special food
Marital status	Outpatient visit	Transportation*	Sick leave	Laundry
Instruction	Diagnostics	Special equipment*	Working days loss of the patient	Home Care*
Working status	Nursing home	Home modification*	Working days loss of the caregivers	Caregivers
Duration of PD		Copayments*	Productivity loss	Special equipment*
Comorbidities			Loss of leisure time	Home modification*
H & Y stage[1]				Private health plans
UPDRS[2]				Copayments*
PQD-39[3]				
MMSE[4]				

[1]Hoehn & Yahr scale of disability/[2]Unified Parkinson's Disease Rating Scale/[3]Parkinson's Disease Questionnaire–39 (quality of life)/[4]Mini-Mental State Examination.
*Variables that may be in more than one cost type.

identification of categories because a variable can be found in different classifications, depending on the criterion used by the researcher, which may underestimate the total cost of the disease.

On the other hand, there is no one perfect research methodology covering a single answer for all solutions. Sometimes, certain types of studies are more appropriate than others. There are several limitations that must be discussed and related to, such as the methodological problems, and the validity of their assumptions can differ because they may introduce bias in analysis in favor of a variable, lack of interest in its assessment, or even lack of information. Therefore, researchers must be careful with the source of their data and the method used for performing the calculations, so that their research can be replicated and validated, since there is no specific instrument for the assessment of PD costs. A limitation also deals with the funding sources of studies, which may be from government sources, insurance companies, or pharmaceutical industries, for example, generating important biases that also need to be addressed. It is necessary to define useful metrics for public health and private ones for managers of health, employers, insurance companies, and even patients themselves, because, without this agreement, the work of researchers and the funds invested shall remain uncertain and inconsistent.

Nevertheless, if the evidence obtained is of good quality in terms of transparency, there is quality and credibility in the data completeness of the documentation. Overall, if they are relevant to health care [50], these studies contribute to a better allocation of resources that are not related to savings but evaluate the efficiency, effectiveness, and safety of interventions.

The age group that the PD affects, if well attended to, can experience "healthy aging," with a good quality of life and preserve its autonomy for longer, thus reducing its cost to the state and society.

References

[1] F. Catalá-López, A. García-Altés, E. Alvarez-Martín, R. Gènova-Maleras, C. Morant-Ginestar, and A. Parada, "Burden of disease and economic evaluation of healthcare interventions: are we investigating what really matters?" BMC health services research, vol. 11, article 75, 2011.

[2] S.-Y. Liu, J.-J. Wu, J. Zhao et al., "Onset-related subtypes of Parkinson's disease differ in the patterns of striatal dopaminergic dysfunction: a positron emission tomography study," Parkinsonism and Related Disorders, vol. 21, no. 12, pp. 1448–1453, 2015.

[3] X. Guo, W. Song, K. Chen et al., "Gender and onset age-related features of non-motor symptoms of patients with Parkinson's disease—a study from Southwest China," Parkinsonism & Related Disorders, vol. 19, no. 11, pp. 961–965, 2013.

[4] C. R. D. Nero, "What is health economics?" in Health Economics: Concepts and Contributions to Health Management, S. F. Piola and S. M. Vianna, Eds., chapter I, pp. 5–23, Ipea, Brasília, Brazil, 2002.

[5] T. Vanni, P. M. Luz, R. A. Ribeiro, H. M. D. Novaes, and C. A. Polanczyk, "Economic evaluation in health: applications in infectious diseases," Cadernos de saúde pública, vol. 25, no. 12, 2009.

[6] Brazil Ministry of Health, Methodological Guidelines: Economic Evaluation of Health Technologies, Brazil Ministry of Health, Brasília, Brazil, 2009, http://bvsms.saude.gov.br/bvs/publicacoes/avaliacao_economica_tecnologias_saude_2009.pdf.

[7] E. Moraes, G. M. Campos, N. B. Figlie, R. R. Laranjeira, and M. B. Ferraz, "Introductory concepts of health economics and the social impact of alcohol abuse," Revista Brasileira de Psiquiatria, vol. 28, no. 4, pp. 321–325, 2006.

[8] S. R. Secoli, M. E. Nita, S. K. Ono-Nita, and M. Nobre, "Health technology assessment. II. Cost effectiveness analysis," *Arquivos de Gastroenterologia*, vol. 47, no. 4, pp. 329–333, 2010.

[9] J.-E. Tarride, G. Blackhouse, M. Bischof et al., "Approaches for economic evaluations of health care technologies," *Journal of the American College of Radiology*, vol. 6, no. 5, pp. 307–316, 2009.

[10] C. Jo, "Cost-of-illness studies: concepts, scopes, and methods," *Clinical and Molecular Hepatology*, vol. 20, no. 4, pp. 327–337, 2014.

[11] D. P. Rice, "Cost of illness studies: what is good about them?" *Injury Prevention*, vol. 6, no. 3, pp. 177–179.

[12] R. Tarricone, "Cost-of-illness analysis. What room in health economics?" *Health Policy*, vol. 77, no. 1, pp. 51–63, 2006.

[13] A. Gustavsson, M. Svensson, F. Jacobi et al., "Cost of disorders of the brain in Europe 2010," *European Neuropsychopharmacology*, vol. 21, no. 10, pp. 718–779, 2011.

[14] Organização Mundial da Saúde, *Financing Health Systems: The Road to Universal Coverage*, Organização Mundial da Saúde, Genebra, Switzerland, 2010, http://www.who.int/eportuguese/publications/WHR2010.pdf?ua=1.

[15] E. R. Dorsey, R. Constantinescu, J. P. Thompson et al., "Projected number of people with Parkinson disease in the most populous nations, 2005 through 2030," *Neurology*, vol. 68, no. 5, pp. 384–386, 2007.

[16] M. E. Morris, J. J. Watts, R. Iansek et al., "Quantifying the profile and progression of impairments, activity, participation, and quality of life in people with Parkinson disease: protocol for a prospective cohort study," *BMC Geriatrics*, vol. 9, no. 1, article no. 2, 2009.

[17] M. T. Barbosa, P. Caramelli, D. P. Maia et al., "Parkinsonism and Parkinson's disease in the elderly: a community-based survey in Brazil (the Bambuí Study)," *Movement Disorders*, vol. 21, no. 6, pp. 800–808, 2006.

[18] P. Andlin-Sobocki, B. Jönsson, H. U. Wittchen, and J. Olesen, "Cost of disorders of the brain in Europe," *European Journal of Neurology*, vol. 12, supplement 1, pp. 1–27, 2005.

[19] Y. J. Zhao, L. C. S. Tan, W. L. Au et al., "Estimating the lifetime economic burden of Parkinson's disease in Singapore," *European Journal of Neurology*, vol. 20, no. 2, pp. 368–374, 2013.

[20] S. Johnson, M. Davis, A. Kaltenboeck et al., "Early retirement and income loss in patients with early and advanced Parkinsons disease," *Applied Health Economics and Health Policy*, vol. 9, no. 6, pp. 367–376, 2011.

[21] E. Cubo, E. Alvarez, C. Morant et al., "Burden of disease related to Parkinson's disease in Spain in the year 2000," *Movement Disorders*, vol. 20, no. 11, pp. 1481–1487, 2005.

[22] S. L. Kowal, T. M. Dall, R. Chakrabarti, M. V. Storm, and A. Jain, "The current and projected economic burden of Parkinson's disease in the United States," *Movement Disorders*, vol. 28, no. 3, pp. 311–318, 2013.

[23] A. Kaltenboeck, S. J. Johnson, M. R. Davis et al., "Direct costs and survival of medicare beneficiaries with early and advanced parkinson's disease," *Parkinsonism and Related Disorders*, vol. 18, no. 4, pp. 321–326, 2012.

[24] D. M. Huse, K. Schulman, L. Orsini, J. Castelli-Haley, S. Kennedy, and G. Lenhart, "Burden of illness in Parkinson's disease," *Movement Disorders*, vol. 20, no. 11, pp. 1449–1454, 2005.

[25] J. Lökk, S. Borg, J. Svensson, U. Persson, and G. Ljunggren, "Drug and treatment costs in Parkinson's disease patients in Sweden," *Acta Neurologica Scandinavica*, vol. 125, no. 2, pp. 142–147, 2012.

[26] P. Jennum, M. Zoetmulder, L. Korbo, and J. Kjellberg, "The health-related, social, and economic consequences of parkinsonism: A Controlled National Study," *Journal of Neurology*, vol. 258, no. 8, pp. 1497–1506, 2011.

[27] K. Noyes, H. Liu, Y. Li, R. Holloway, and A. W. Dick, "Economic burden associated with Parkinson's disease on elderly Medicare beneficiaries," *Movement Disorders*, vol. 21, no. 3, pp. 362–372, 2006.

[28] D. J. Cordato, R. Schwartz, E. Abbott, R. Saunders, and L. Morfis, "A comparison of health-care costs involved in treating people with and without Parkinson's disease in Southern Sydney, New South Wales, Australia," *Journal of Clinical Neuroscience*, vol. 13, no. 6, pp. 655–658, 2006.

[29] S. Bhattacharjee and U. Sambamoorthi, "Co-occurring chronic conditions and healthcare expenditures associated with Parkinson's disease: a propensity score matched analysis," *Parkinsonism and Related Disorders*, vol. 19, no. 8, pp. 746–750, 2013.

[30] Y. Winter, S. Von Campenhausen, J. P. Reese et al., "Costs of Parkinson's disease and antiparkinsonian pharmacotherapy: an Italian cohort study," *Neurodegenerative Diseases*, vol. 7, no. 6, pp. 365–372, 2010.

[31] C. Vossius, M. Gjerstad, H. Baas, and J. P. Larsen, "Drug costs for patients with Parkinson's disease in two different European countries," *Acta Neurologica Scandinavica*, vol. 113, no. 4, pp. 228–232, 2006.

[32] Y. Winter, S. von Campenhausen, H. Brozova et al., "Costs of Parkinson's disease in Eastern Europe: a Czech cohort study," *Parkinsonism and Related Disorders*, vol. 16, no. 1, pp. 51–56, 2010.

[33] P. McCrone, L. M. Allcock, and D. J. Burn, "Predicting the cost of Parkinson's disease," *Movement Disorders*, vol. 22, no. 6, pp. 804–812, 2007.

[34] A. E. Spottke, M. Reuter, O. Machat et al., "Cost of illness and its predictors for Parkinson's disease in Germany," *PharmacoEconomics*, vol. 23, no. 8, pp. 817–836, 2005.

[35] C. L. Leibson, K. Hall Long, D. M. Maraganore et al., "Direct medical costs associated with Parkinson's disease: a population-based study," *Movement Disorders*, vol. 21, no. 11, pp. 1864–1871, 2006.

[36] M. Ragothaman, S. T. Govindappa, R. Rattihalli, D. K. Subbakrishna, and U. B. Muthane, "Direct costs of managing Parkinson's disease in India: concerns in a developing country," *Movement Disorders*, vol. 21, no. 10, pp. 1755–1758, 2006.

[37] Y. Winter, S. V. Campenhausen, G. Popov et al., "Costs of illness in a Russian cohort of patients with parkinsons disease," *PharmacoEconomics*, vol. 27, no. 7, pp. 571–584, 2009.

[38] Y. J. Zhao, L. C. S. Tan, S. C. Li et al., "Economic burden of Parkinson's disease in Singapore," *European Journal of Neurology*, vol. 18, no. 3, pp. 519–526, 2011.

[39] G. Tamás, L. Gulácsi, D. Bereczki et al., "Quality of life and costs in Parkinson's disease: a cross sectional study in Hungary," *PLoS ONE*, vol. 9, no. 9, Article ID e107704, 2014.

[40] A. Yoritaka, J. Fukae, T. Hatano, E. Oda, and N. Hattori, "The direct cost of Parkinson disease at Juntendo medical university hospital, Japan," *Internal Medicine*, vol. 55, no. 2, pp. 113–119, 2016.

[41] S. J. Johnson, A. Kaltenboeck, M. Diener et al., "Costs of parkinson's disease in a privately insured population," *PharmacoEconomics*, vol. 31, no. 9, pp. 799–806, 2013.

[42] A. P. Vargas, F. J. Carod-Artal, S. S. Nunes, and M. Melo, "Disability and use of healthcare resources in Brazilian patients

with Parkinson's disease," *Disability and Rehabilitation*, vol. 30, no. 14, pp. 1055–1062, 2008.

[43] J.-P. Bach, O. Riedel, J. Klotsche, A. Spottke, R. Dodel, and H.-U. Wittchen, "Impact of complications and comorbidities on treatment costs and health-related quality of life of patients with Parkinson's disease," *Journal of the Neurological Sciences*, vol. 314, no. 1-2, pp. 41–47, 2012.

[44] P. Martínez-Martin, C. Rodriguez-Blazquez, S. Paz et al., "Parkinson symptoms and health related quality of life as predictors of costs: A Longitudinal Observational Study with Linear Mixed Model Analysis," *PLOS ONE*, vol. 10, no. 12, Article ID e0145310, 2015.

[45] S. von Campenhausen, Y. Winter, A. Rodrigues e Silva et al., "Costs of illness and care in Parkinson's disease: an evaluation in six countries," *European Neuropsychopharmacology*, vol. 21, no. 2, pp. 180–191, 2011.

[46] Y. Winter, M. Balzer-Geldsetzer, A. Spottke et al., "Longitudinal study of the socioeconomic burden of Parkinson's disease in Germany," *European Journal of Neurology*, vol. 17, no. 9, pp. 1156–1163, 2010.

[47] Y. Winter, M. Balzer-Geldsetzer, S. von Campenhausen et al., "Trends in resource utilization for Parkinson's disease in Germany," *Journal of the Neurological Sciences*, vol. 294, no. 1-2, pp. 18–22, 2010.

[48] G. Wang, Q. Cheng, R. Zheng et al., "Economic burden of Parkinson's disease in a developing country: a retrospective cost analysis in Shanghai, China," *Movement Disorders*, vol. 21, no. 9, pp. 1439–1443, 2006.

[49] R. Dodel, B. Jönsson, J. P. Reese et al., "Measurement of costs and scales for outcome evaluation in health economic studies of Parkinson's disease," *Movement Disorders*, vol. 29, no. 2, pp. 169–176, 2014.

[50] A. Langer, "A framework for assessing Health Economic Evaluation (HEE) quality appraisal instruments," *BMC health services research*, vol. 12, article no. 253, 2012.

28

An Integrated Review of Psychological Stress in Parkinson's Disease: Biological Mechanisms and Symptom and Health Outcomes

Kim Wieczorek Austin,[1] Suzanne Weil Ameringer,[1] and Leslie Jameleh Cloud[2]

[1]*Virginia Commonwealth University School of Nursing, 1100 East Leigh Street, Richmond, VA 23219, USA*
[2]*Virginia Commonwealth University Parkinson's and Movement Disorders Center and VCU Health Neuroscience, Orthopaedic, and Wellness Center, 11958 West Broad Street, Richmond, VA 23233, USA*

Correspondence should be addressed to Kim Wieczorek Austin; kim@kwaustin.net

Academic Editor: Elka Stefanova

Parkinson's disease (PD) is characterized by complex symptoms and medication-induced motor complications that fluctuate in onset, severity, responsiveness to treatment, and disability. The unpredictable and debilitating nature of PD and the inability to halt or slow disease progression may result in psychological stress. Psychological stress may exacerbate biological mechanisms believed to contribute to neuronal loss in PD and lead to poorer symptom and health outcomes. The purpose of this integrated review is to summarize and appraise animal and human research studies focused on biological mechanisms, symptom, and health outcomes of psychological stress in PD. A search of the electronic databases PubMed/Medline and CINAHL from 1980 to the present using the key words *Parkinson's disease and stress, psychological stress, mental stress, and chronic stress* resulted in 11 articles that met inclusion criteria. The results revealed significant associations between psychological stress and increased motor symptom severity and loss of dopamine-producing neurons in animal models of PD and between psychological stress and increased symptom severity and poorer health outcomes in human subjects with PD. Further research is needed to fully elucidate the underlying biological mechanisms responsible for these relationships, for the ultimate purpose of designing targeted interventions that may modify the disease trajectory.

1. Introduction

Parkinson's disease (PD) is characterized by complex symptom patterns that fluctuate in onset, severity, responsiveness to treatment, and associated level of disability. The classic motor symptoms of tremor, rigidity, bradykinesia, and postural instability are compounded by nonmotor symptoms such as depression, cognitive impairments, sleep disturbances, fatigue, pain, and autonomic dysfunction. Many of these nonmotor symptoms respond poorly to available treatment options and significantly contribute to poorer quality of life and increased functional disability [1]. Early in the course of the disease, medications for PD typically improve motor symptoms. However, as the disease progresses, higher medication doses become necessary which can then cause

debilitating dystonia and dyskinesia [2]. Reductions in medication dosages are often required to lessen the severity of these complications, resulting in breakthrough primary motor symptomology. Further complicating the illness experience, prolonged and/or high dose treatment with PD medications has been associated with on-off phenomena, which leads to unpredictable motor symptom exacerbations and periods of immobility. The ability to reduce these medication-induced complications while still achieving motor symptom benefits becomes more difficult as the disease progresses, leading to greater functional disability and poorer quality of life.

The unpredictable and debilitating nature of the symptoms associated with PD combined with the inability to halt or slow disease progression has the potential to result in psychological stress. Psychological stress is a complex phenomenon that involves cognitive, emotional, behavioral, and biological responses to events or experiences that are perceived as threatening [3]. An individual's ability to cope with and adapt to psychological stress can be influenced by the number and significance of stressful events experienced within a given period of time, the degree to which stressors are perceived as threatening or harmless, and biological responses designed to promote adaptation [4, 5]. The inability to cope with or adapt to psychological stress has been associated with poorer symptom and health outcomes that may be relevant in PD. For example, in non-PD populations, significant relationships have been demonstrated between psychological stress and increased motor symptomology [6], pain [7, 8], fatigue, [6, 8], cognitive decline [9], and functional disability [9, 10].

Biological responses of the neuroendocrine and immune systems represent plausible mechanisms that may explain relationships between psychological stress and poorer symptom and health outcomes. A complex network of bidirectional links between the neuroendocrine and immune systems serve as major regulatory mechanisms for mounting effective biological responses to psychological stress [11]. The hypothalamic-pituitary-adrenal axis (HPAA) coordinates these responses by stimulating the release of cortisol in humans and corticosterone in humans and rodents. Glucocorticoids play an important role in mediating immunological responses to psychological stress by regulating microglial activation and proinflammatory cytokine and transcription factor expression and release [12]. Stress-induced dysregulation of relationships between the neuroendocrine and immune systems has been associated with neuroinflammation, oxidative stress, and loss of dopamine (DA) producing neurons within the central nervous system [13–18]. Prolonged exposure to psychological stress has also been shown to sensitize the neuroendocrine and immune systems to the detrimental effects of future insults, thereby exaggerating inflammatory responses, oxidative stress, and neuronal loss [14, 19, 20].

Based upon work in non-PD animal models, a number of underlying biological mechanisms have been implicated in stress-induced neuroinflammation, oxidative stress, and neuronal loss to include microglial activation, upregulation of proinflammatory cytokines, transcription factors, and isoenzymes, increased production of reactive oxygen species (ROS), and imbalances in the production of ROS and antioxidant reduction. Table 1 summarizes the literature on these biological mechanisms. Specifically, studies have demonstrated that both stress and the administration of exogenous corticosterone increase microglial activation, reactivity, and proliferation [14, 16, 20]. Under normal conditions, microglia cells, which are found in particularly high concentrations in the substantia nigra, exist in a resting state. Once activated, microglia provide the first line of immune defense by releasing immune mediators that coordinate innate and adaptive immune responses within the central nervous system to include the expression and release of proinflammatory cytokines and transcription factors [21, 22]. Whereas acute activation of microglia facilitates tissue repair, prolonged or

exaggerated responses result in increased neuroinflammation and oxidative stress, both of which have been associated with dopaminergic neurotoxicity [14, 21–23]. Dopaminergic neurons are particularly vulnerable to neuroinflammatory and oxidative processes due to the high rate of oxygen consumption and limited antioxidant defenses within the central nervous system [24].

The upregulation of proinflammatory cytokines and transcription factors may further perpetuate stress-induced neuroinflammation and oxidative stress within the central nervous system. Cytokines play an important role in stimulating and coordinating the cellular interactions necessary for mounting effective immune responses to infection, injury, and disease [25]. Psychological stress has been associated with significant elevations in tumor necrosis factor alpha (TNF-α), interleukin-1 (IL-1), and interleukin-6 (IL-6), proinflammatory cytokines that have been implicated in oxidative stress and apoptosis within the central nervous system [26–29]. Proinflammatory cytokines also stimulate activation of nuclear transcription factor-kappa B (NF-kB) pathways [30, 31], which have been implicated in apoptosis of nigral dopaminergic neurons in animal models of PD [17, 32]. Activation of NF-kB pathways also results in the production of cyclooxygenase-2 (COX-2), an enzyme involved in prostaglandin mediated inflammatory responses [33]. While COX-2 is normally expressed in relatively constant amounts within the central nervous system, stress-induced upregulation of COX-2 has been associated with increased generation of ROS, oxidative stress, neurotoxicity, and apoptosis within the central nervous system [30, 34, 35].

Stress-induced oxidative mechanisms have also been associated with neuronal loss within the central nervous system. Oxidation, and the subsequent production of ROS, occurs normally throughout the body as a result of aerobic metabolism. The greatest concentrations of ROS are found within mitochondria, the main site of adenosine triphosphate (ATP) production [36]. Under normal conditions, ROS are maintained at relatively constant levels as a result of balances between the rate of ROS production and removal by antioxidant substrates [37]. Oxidative stress occurs as a result of imbalances in the production of ROS and antioxidant reduction, resulting in excessive lipid peroxidation and tissue injury within the central nervous system. Psychological stress has been associated with increased mitochondrial production of ROS [38] and increased production of nicotinamide adenine dinucleotide phosphate (NADPH) oxidase, a membrane-bound enzyme involved in neutrophil respiratory bursts [39]. Normally, NADPH remains latent in neutrophils and is tightly regulated by hormones, cytokines, and a variety of other mechanisms. Stress-induced activation of NADPH has been associated with increased production of ROS, neuroinflammation, and degeneration of dopaminergic and nondopaminergic neurons [39]. Psychological stress has also been associated with decreased expression and release of antioxidants [38, 40]. Dysregulation of the antioxidant system, coupled with increased ROS production, has been shown to perpetuate oxidative stress, lipid peroxidation, and tissue damage within the central nervous system [26, 38, 41].

TABLE 1: Overview of potential biological mechanisms of psychological stress-induced neuroinflammation, oxidative stress, and neuronal loss in non-PD animal models.

Study author/date	Major study findings
Lucca et al., 2009 [38]	Chronic mild psychological stress resulted in significant elevations in superoxide, a reactive oxygen species, in the submitochondrial particles of the prefrontal cortex, cortex, and hippocampus in subjects when compared to controls. The results also demonstrated significant elevations in TBARS, a measure of lipid peroxidation, in the cortex of stressed subjects.
De Pablos et al., 2006 [14]	Induction of chronic variate psychological stress enhanced LPS-induced neuroinflammation in the PFC of stressed subjects when compared to nonstressed LPS-induced subjects and controls. Significant findings included increased microglial activation, levels of DA and its metabolite DOPAC, expression of proinflammatory cytokine mRNA (TNF-α, IL-1β, and IL-6), activation of MAP kinases, and loss of NeuN-positive neurons in the PFC.
Munhoz et al., 2006 [18]	Chronic, unpredictable psychological stress potentiated NF-κB binding activity in the frontal cortex and hippocampus and proinflammatory gene expression of IL-β, TNF-α, and NOS-2 as mediated by elevated GC levels in LPS-induced subjects when compared to controls.
Kim et al., 2005 [41]	Acute psychological stress resulted in elevated BH4 and DA levels in striatal tissues and led to greater lipid peroxidation, protein-bound quinone, neuromelanin, and antioxidant enzyme activities, markers of oxidative stress, in the substantia nigra and striatum of subjects when compared to controls. Furthermore, in subjects exposed to stress, TH-immunoreactive DA neurons demonstrated strong Fluoro-Jade staining, indicating selective degeneration of dopaminergic neurons. In contrast, no Fluoro-Jade staining was identified in controls.
Munhoz et al., 2004 [26]	Repeated psychological stress was associated with time-dependent markers of oxidative stress in brain tissue to include increase in Ca²⁺-independent NOS-2 activity, lipid peroxidation, TNF-α, and TACE activity in subjects when compared to controls.
Madrigal et al., 2003 [33]	Acute psychological stress was associated with higher levels of PGE₂, a marker of COX-2 neuronal activity, MDA and oxidized glutathione, markers of lipid peroxidation, and NOS-2 in the cortex of subjects when compared to controls.
Madrigal et al., 2002 [30]	Acute psychological stress induced the expression of iNOS in the brain cortex, which was preceded by increased expression of TACE and the subsequent release of TNF-α in subjects as compared to controls. Furthermore, the results demonstrated that increased production of TNF-α was involved in stress-induced expression of iNOS as mediated by activation of NF-κB.

TBARS, thiobarbituric acid reactive species; LPS, lipopolysaccharide; PFC, prefrontal cortex; DA, dopamine; DOPAC, 3,4-dihydroxyphenylacetic; mRNA, messenger ribonucleic acid; TNF-α, tumor necrosis factor alpha; IL-1β, interleukin-1 beta; IL-6, interleukin-6; MAP, mitogen-activated protein; NeuN-positive, neuronal nuclei positive; GC, glucocorticoids; BH4, tetrahydrobiopterin; TH-immunoreactive, tyrosine hydroxylase; Ca²⁺, calcium²⁺; NOS-2, inducible nitric oxide synthase; TACE, TNF-α converting enzyme; iNOS, inducible nitric oxide synthase; PGE₂, prostaglandin E2; COX-2, cyclooxygenase-2; MDA, malondialdehyde.

TABLE 2: Potential biological mechanisms of neuroinflammation and oxidative stress associated with neurodegeneration in PD.

Study author/date	Major study findings
	Microglia activation
Gerhard et al., 2006 [43]	In vivo PET imaging revealed widespread and longitudinal microglial activation in subjects with PD when compared to controls
Ouchi et al., 2005 [44]	Microglial activation was associated with damage in nigrostriatal pathway in drug-naïve subjects with PD when compared to controls
Depino et al., 2003 [45]	Induction of PD in animals (6-OHDA model) resulted in increased microglial activation and atypical production of proinflammatory cytokine mRNA when compared to controls
	Proinflammatory cytokine production
Lindqvist et al., 2012 [54]	Serum levels of IL-6 significantly higher in subjects with PD than controls
Scalzo et al., 2010 [46]	Serum levels of IL-6 significantly higher in subjects with PD than controls
Reale et al., 2009 [47]	Basal and bacterial LPS-induced production of IL-1β, TNF-α, and IFN-Y significantly higher in subjects with PD than controls
	Proinflammatory transcription pathway activation
Tobón-Velasco et al., 2013 [48]	Induction of PD in animals (6-OHDA model) resulted in enhanced NF-κB activation which was associated with increased TNF-α and COX-2 levels when compared to controls
Liang et al., 2007 [32]	Induction of PD in animals (6-OHDA model) resulted in activation of NF-κB pathways which contributed to oxidative stress-induced degeneration of dopaminergic neurons when compared to controls
	Proinflammatory isoenzyme production
Hernandes et al., 2013 [50]	Induction of PD in animals (6-OHDA) demonstrated that NDAPH oxidases contribute to dopaminergic neurodegeneration in the nigrostriatal pathway
Teismann et al., 2003 [49]	Brain tissue samples of subjects with and animal models of PD (6-OHDA) demonstrated increased COX-2 upregulation in dopaminergic neurons when compared to controls
	Oxidative stress
Lin et al., 2012 [51]	Induction of PD in animals (rotenone model) associated with significantly higher levels of oxidative proteins in the striatum leading to greater levels of apoptotic cell death of dopaminergic neurons within the nigrostriatal system when compared to controls
Seet et al., 2010 [52]	Biomarkers of oxidative stress (F_2-isoprostanes, hydroxyeicosatetraenoic acid products, 7B- and 27-hydroxycholesterol, 7-ketocholesterol, neuroprostanes, and urinary 8-hydroxy-2'deoxyguanosine) significantly higher in subjects with PD when compared to controls
Keeney et al., 2006 [53]	Misassembled mitochondrial complex I as reflected by significant loss of its 8 kDa subunits associated with oxidative damage in brain tissue of subjects with PD when compared to controls

PET, position emission tomography; PD, Parkinson's disease; 6-OHDA, 6-hydroxydopamine; mRNA, messenger ribonucleic acid; IL-6, interleukin-6; LPS, lipopolysaccharide; IL-1β, interleukin-1 beta; TNF-α, tumor necrosis factor alpha; IFN-Y, interferon gamma; NF-κB, nuclear factor-kappa-light-chain-enhancer of activated B cells; COX-2, cyclooxygenase-2; NDAPH oxidase, nicotinamide adenine dinucleotide phosphate oxidase.

Stress-induced dysregulation of the neuroendocrine and immune systems may play an important role in symptom and health outcomes in PD. While the exact cause remains unknown, progressive loss of dopaminergic neurons within the substantia nigra pars compacta (SNc) and nondopaminergic neurons within the central, peripheral, and autonomic nervous systems are believed to contribute to symptom and disease progression [42]. As briefly summarized in Table 2, a considerable body of research exists to suggest that biological mechanisms associated with neuroinflammation and oxidative stress contribute to the loss of dopaminergic neurons in PD. These biological mechanisms include but are not limited to increased microglial activation [43–45], atypical production of select proinflammatory cytokines (IL-1β, IL-6, TNF-α, and IFN-γ) [41, 46, 47], enhanced activation of NF-κB pathways [32, 48], increased upregulation of COX-2 [49] and NDAPH oxidases [50], and increased production of

select biomarkers of oxidative stress [51–53]. As such, stress-induced neuroendocrine and immune system dysregulation may exacerbate pathogenic mechanisms in PD, resulting in poorer symptom and health outcomes. The purpose of this integrated review is to summarize and critically appraise the current state of the science regarding biological mechanisms and symptom and health outcomes of psychological stress in individuals with and animal models of PD. Limitations of the existing literature as well as directions for future research will also be discussed.

2. Methods

An integrated review was conducted to examine human and animal research studies that focused on biological mechanisms and symptom and health outcomes of psychological stress in PD. A title search of the electronic databases

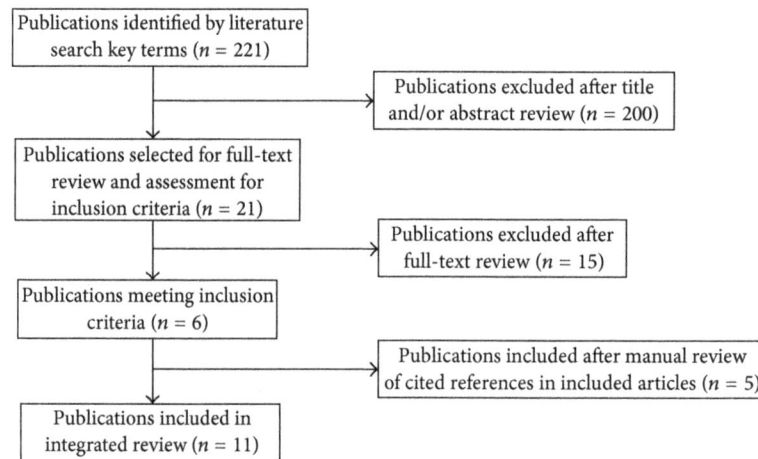

FIGURE 1: Literature review process.

PubMed/Medline and CINAHL was conducted from 1980 to the present using the key words *Parkinson's disease and stress, psychological stress, mental stress, and chronic stress.* A total of 221 articles were identified (Figure 1). Articles were reviewed based on the following inclusion criteria: (1) research studies involved human subjects with PD or animal models of PD with a primary aim of examining the effects of psychological stress on biological mechanisms and symptom and health outcomes; (2) animal studies reported using a recognized model of PD to include 1-methyl-4-phenyl-1,2,3,6-tetrahydropyridine (MPTP), 6-hydroxydopamine (6-OHDA), or rotenone induction; (3) animal studies involved the induction of psychological stress; (4) human studies involved the induction of psychological stress and/or quantified psychological stress levels; and (5) the study was written in English. Based on these inclusion criteria, a title/abstract review resulted in the exclusion of 200 articles, the majority of which focused on oxidative, nitrosative, and/or endoreticulum stress ($n = 171$) or caregiver stress ($n = 9$) in PD. Full-text review and assessment for inclusion criteria was conducted on the remaining 21 articles. An additional 15 articles were excluded, the majority of which were literature reviews and involved biological mechanisms of psychological stress in non-PD animal models or case-studies that did not involve the induction of psychological stress and/or quantify psychological stress levels. The remaining six articles met the above identified inclusion criteria and were included in this review. An additional five articles were identified after a manual review of the references cited in the included articles and excluded articles that underwent a full-text review. A total of eleven articles met the inclusion criteria and were included in this review.

3. Results and Discussion

Of the 11 studies included in this review, seven examined biological mechanisms of psychological stress that contribute to pathophysiological processes and symptom outcomes in animal models of PD [55–61]. In contrast, the remaining four

studies focused on biological mechanisms, symptom, and/or health outcomes of psychological stress that may modify the illness trajectory in human subjects with PD [62–65]. Each of these studies is further discussed below.

3.1. Biological Mechanisms of Psychological Stress That Contribute to Pathophysiological Processes and Symptom Outcomes in Animal Models of PD. Seven of the studies included in this review examined biological mechanisms and symptom outcomes of psychological stress in animal models of PD [55–61]. Health outcomes of psychological stress were not examined in these studies. Biological mechanisms in the reviewed studies included biomarkers of dopamine production and metabolism [55, 56, 58–61], serotonin (5-HT) [55], norepinephrine [61], and/or dopaminergic neurodegeneration [57, 58]. In addition, two studies examined biological mechanisms associated with stress responses of the neuroendocrine system, specifically the effects of corticosterone administration [57] and norepinephrine levels [61] on motor symptom outcomes. Of particular importance, one study [55] examined the effects of psychological stress on the expression of α-synuclein, a misfolded protein complex that is recognized as a pathological hallmark of PD. All of the animal studies included in this review examined symptom outcomes specific to the motor manifestations of PD [55–61]. Only one study examined the effects of psychological stress on behaviors associated with depression, a common nonmotor symptom in PD [55]. In addition, one study focused on the effects of psychological stress on the neuroprotective effects of voluntary exercise on symptom and biological outcomes [58]. These studies are further discussed below and summarized in Table 3.

Using a MPTP/probenecid (MPTP/p) animal model of PD, researchers examined the effects of chronic mild psychological stress on biological mechanisms involving DA and 5-HT levels and the expression of dopaminergic markers of the nigrostriatal (substantia nigra and striatum) and nonnigrostriatal (hippocampus, cortex, and cerebellum) systems and symptom outcomes specific to depression [55]. Symptom

TABLE 3: Biological mechanisms of psychological stress that contribute to pathophysiological processes and symptom outcomes in animal models of PD.

Study author & date	Study purpose & sample	Method(s) of psychological stress induction	Measures of biological mechanisms & symptom outcomes	Major study findings
Janakiraman et al., 2016 [55]	*Purpose*: to examine the effects of psychological stress on symptom outcomes of depression and biological mechanisms of DA, 5-HT, and α-synuclein. *Sample*: male C57BL/6 mice (n = 72); MPTP/probenecid induction	"Cage tilting, damp sawdust, placement in empty cage, group housing, placement in empty cage with water on the bottom, placement of a foreign object in cage, inversion of light/dark cycle, food or water deprivation, lights on for a short period of time during the dark phase, and switching cages" (p. 3)	*Biological mechanisms*: DA, 5-HT, TH, DAT, VMAT-2, α-synuclein levels in nigrostriatal (substantia nigra and striatum) and nonnigrostriatal tissues (hippocampus, cortex, and cerebellum) *Symptom outcomes*: depression as measured by behavioral deficits and anhedonia using the (a) open filed test; (b) narrow beam walking test; and (c) sucrose intake test	*Biological mechanisms*: increased depletion of DA, 5-HT, TH, DAT, and VMAT-2 was identified in stress-treated lesioned subjects. Stress exaggerated the expression of nigrostriatal and nonnigrostriatal α-synuclein. *Symptom outcomes*: stress increased behavioral deficits and anhedonia in stress-treated lesioned subjects.
Hemmerle et al., 2014 [56]	*Purpose*: to examine the effects of psychological stress on motor symptom outcomes and biological mechanisms associated with loss of DA neurons *Sample*: rats (sample size/gender not provided); 6-OHDA induction	Chronic variable stress (protocol not provided)	*Biological mechanisms*: TH cell counts in the SNc *Symptom outcomes*: forelimb asymmetry tests (not defined)	*Biological mechanisms*: stress was associated with significantly lower TH cell counts in the SNc in lesioned subjects. *Symptom outcomes*: stress was associated with significant forelimb asymmetry in lesioned subjects.
Smith et al., 2008 [57]	*Purpose*: to examine the effects of psychological stress and corticosterone administration on motor symptom outcomes and biological mechanisms of DA neurodegeneration *Sample*: female rats (n = 71); 6-OHDA induction	Restraint in Plexiglas tubes	*Biological mechanisms*: plasma concentrations of corticosterone and TH positive cells, Fluoro-Jade B cells, and GFAP immunoreactivity in the MTA, VTA, and SNc *Symptom outcomes*: skilled forelimb reaching, skilled walking, open field behavior, and apomorphine-induced rotations	*Biological mechanisms*: in stress- and corticosterone-treated lesioned subjects, the loss of TH positive cells was associated with significant increases in Fluor-Jade B cells in the SNc. Significant reductions in Nissl-positive cells in the VTA and SNc and enhanced GFAP immunoreactivity in the SNc were also demonstrated in stress-and corticosterone-treated lesioned subjects. *Symptom outcomes*: stress and elevated corticosterone levels impaired skilled limb reaching and limb coordination, impeded spontaneous recovery, and altered exploratory behavior in lesioned subjects.
Howells et al., 2005 [58]	*Purpose*: to examine the effects of psychological stress on the neuroprotective effects of voluntary exercise on motor symptom outcomes and biological mechanisms of dopaminergic neurodegeneration *Sample*: male rats (n = 31); 6-OHDA induction	Running wheel immobilization and shifting light/dark cycles	*Biological mechanisms*: TH positive cells in the SNc *Symptom outcomes*: number of running wheel revolutions and apomorphine-induced rotations	*Biological mechanisms*: stressed runners demonstrated lower TH positive cells in the SNc. *Symptom outcomes*: stressed runners demonstrated a significant increase in rotational behavior.

TABLE 3: Continued.

Study author & date	Study purpose & sample	Method(s) of psychological stress induction	Measures of biological mechanisms & symptom outcomes	Major study findings
Keefe et al., 1990 [59]	*Purpose:* to examine the extent to which psychological stress affects motor symptom outcomes and biological mechanisms specific to DA concentrations *Sample:* male rats (sample size not provided); 6-OHDA	Tail-shock stress	*Biological mechanisms:* extracellular striatal DA, DOPAC, and HVA levels in vivo and in brain tissue specimens *Symptom outcomes:* akinesia defined as latency to move all four paws when placed on a flat surface within 120 seconds and catalepsy defined as latency to return all four paws to table surface within 120 seconds	*Biological mechanisms:* subjects exposed to tail-shock stress demonstrated significantly increased striatal extracellular DA, DOPAC, and HVA levels. In all but one subject, these levels did not reach levels comparable to those demonstrated in nonlesioned animals following tail-shock stress. *Symptom outcomes:* no consistent pattern was demonstrated between stress and akinetic and cataleptic motor behaviors. A significant negative correlation was shown between poststress latencies for catalepsy and extracellular DA concentrations, with a similar trend identified for akinesia.
Urakami et al., 1988 [60]	*Purpose:* to examine the effects of psychological stress on motor symptom outcomes and biological mechanisms involving DA *Sample:* male rats (*n* = 20); MPTP induction	Immobilization in water kept at 25°C for 15 consecutive hours	*Biological mechanisms:* striatal DA content, DOPAC and HVA levels, and DA indices (DOPAC + HVA/DA) in brain tissue specimens *Symptom outcomes:* locomotor activity (not defined)	*Biological mechanisms:* striatal DA content was significantly lower in stress-treated lesioned subjects. Striatal DA indices were significantly elevated in both the stress-treated lesioned and control groups. No significant difference was demonstrated in the DA metabolites DOPAC or HVA. *Symptom outcomes:* in lesioned subjects, stress was associated with more pronounced but transient decreases in locomotor activity.
Snyder et al., 1985 [61]	*Purpose:* to examine the effects of psychological stress on motor symptom outcomes of akinesia and biological mechanisms involving DA and norepinephrine levels *Sample:* male rats (*n* = 194); 6-OHDA induction	Glucodeprivation while withholding food, osmotic diuresis while withholding water, cold exposure, and tail shock	*Biological mechanisms:* DA and norepinephrine content in brain tissue specimens *Symptom outcomes:* akinesia defined as latency to move of greater than 60 seconds during the following two tests: (a) movement of all four paws when placed on a flat surface and (b) return of front or rear paws to the ground after being elevated on a Styrofoam block	*Biological mechanisms:* stress was associated with DA deficiencies in the striatum. *Symptom outcomes:* striatal DA deficiencies were more predictive of stress-induced akinesias than in other areas of the brain. There was no consistent relationship between hippocampal norepinephrine levels and stress-induced akinesia.

MPTP, 1-methyl-4-phenyl-1,2,3,6-tetrahydropyridine; DA, dopamine; 5-HT, serotonin; TH, tyrosine hydroxylase; DAT, dopamine transporter; VMAT-2, vesicular monoamine transporters; 6-OHDA, 6-hydroxydopamine; SNc, substantia nigra pars compacta; MTA, medial tegmental area; VTA, ventral tegmental area; GFAP, glial fibrillary acidic protein; DOPAC, dihydroxyphenylacetic acid; HVA, homovanillic acid.

outcomes of depression included measures of locomotion, activity, and anhedonia. Subjects were randomly assigned to a saline-treated control group, MPTP/p group, stress group, MPTP/p followed by stress group, stress followed by MPTP/p group, and stress before and after MPTP/p group. Both the before and after MPTP/p stress groups demonstrated greater DA depletion in all studied brain regions when compared to the stress or MPTP/p alone groups, with greater levels of DA depletion identified in the MPTP/p followed by stress group. Serotonin levels were also decreased in both the stress and MPTP/p groups, with the greatest reduction identified in all studied brain regions in the MPTP/p followed by stress group. In the MPTP/p followed by stress group, greater reductions in tyrosine hydroxylase (TH), dopamine transporter (DAT), and vesicular monoamine transporters (VMAT-2) expression were identified in all studied brain regions, suggesting that stress affects the biosynthesis and transport of DA. In stress-treated MPTP/p subjects, stress exaggerated the expression of nigrostriatal and nonnigrostriatal α-synuclein, which plays a major role in the development and progression of PD. While no significant changes were identified in locomotion, activity, and anhedonia in the stress or MPTP/p groups, greater behavioral changes in all parameters were identified in the MPTP/p followed by stress group. Cumulatively, these findings provide important evidence to suggest that psychological stress may contribute to biological mechanisms, symptom outcomes, and disease progression in PD.

In a 6-OHDA animal model of PD, researchers examined the effects of chronic variable psychological stress on biological mechanisms involving DA as measured by TH cell counts and motor symptom outcomes [56]. Subjects were assigned to 6-OHDA lesioned stressed and nonstressed groups, a sham-lesioned group, and a control group. Both 6-OHDA groups demonstrated impaired contralateral forelimb use when compared to the sham-lesioned group. However, following four weeks of chronic, variable stress, the 6-OHDA lesioned group demonstrated significantly more forelimb asymmetry when compared to the 6-OHDA lesioned nonstressed group. Significantly lower TH cell counts were identified in the SNc of stressed 6-OHDA subjects when compared to nonstressed 6-OHDA subjects. These findings suggest chronic variable stress may exacerbate motor symptom outcomes as a result of biological mechanisms associated with dopamine deficiencies in PD.

In a 6-OHDA animal model of PD, researchers examined the effects of restraint stress and corticosterone administration on biological mechanisms associated with dopaminergic neurodegeneration and motor symptom outcomes [57]. The results revealed psychological stress and elevated corticosterone levels in lesioned subjects impaired skilled limb reaching and limb coordination, impeded spontaneous recovery and compensation, and altered exploratory behavior. Fluoro-Jade positive cells, a biomarker of neuronal degeneration, were detected earlier in stress-treated lesioned subjects than controls. In stress- and corticosterone-treated lesioned subjects, the loss of TH positive cells, a biomarker of dopamine-producing cells, was associated with a significant increase in Fluoro-Jade positive cells in the SNc. Stress- and corticosterone-treated lesioned subjects

demonstrated significant reductions in Nissl-positive cells in the ventral tegmental area (VTA) and SNc, suggesting greater neurodegeneration in these areas when compared to controls. Stress- and corticosterone-treated lesioned subjects also demonstrated enhanced glial fibrillary acidic protein (GFAP) immunoreactivity in the SNc when compared to controls, indicating greater reactive gliosis in the central nervous system. In stress-treated lesioned subjects, motor impairments were associated with higher numbers of Fluoro-Jade positive cells in the SNc and VTA. Cumulatively, these findings provide important evidence to suggest that psychological stress and stress-response hormones may contribute to pathogenic mechanisms involved in motor symptom outcomes in PD as a result of biological mechanisms associated with dopaminergic neurodegeneration.

Using a 6-OHDA animal model of PD, researchers examined the effects of psychological stress on the neuroprotective effects of voluntary exercise to include motor symptom outcomes as measured by rotational behavior and biological mechanisms associated with dopaminergic neurodegeneration [58]. Subjects were randomly assigned to one of three groups: runners or stressed runners, both of which had free access to running wheels, or nonrunners who had immobilized running wheels. Nonrunners demonstrated significantly higher numbers of apomorphine-induced contralateral rotations, a measure indicative of DA depletions exceeding 80%, when compared to stressed and nonstressed runners. This finding suggests voluntary exercise exerted neuroprotective effects on dopaminergic neurons in both stressed and nonstressed runners. The administration of apomorphine resulted in a significant increase in rotational behavior in stressed runners when compared to nonstressed runners, suggesting that stress may ameliorate the neuroprotective effects of voluntary exercise. Nonstressed runners demonstrated a nonsignificant decrease in the percentage of dopaminergic neurons lost when compared to both the stressed runners (4%) and nonrunners (14%). Significant differences were also identified in the number of baseline wheel rotations and the amount of DA destruction in the stressed runners and between the stressed and nonstressed runners. Significant group differences were found in the number of apomorphine-induced rotations and loss of DA between the stressed and nonstressed runners, the stressed runners and nonrunners, and all three groups. These findings suggest psychological stress may cancel the neuroprotective effects of voluntary exercise and contribute to greater DA deficiencies and poorer motor symptom outcomes.

In a 6-OHDA animal model of PD, researchers examined the extent to which motor symptom outcomes as measured by akinetic and cataleptic behaviors and biological mechanisms specific to DA concentrations were affected by psychological stress [59]. Biological mechanisms investigated in this study included the extent to which nigrostriatal DA neurons were capable of responding to the additional demand for DA during tail-shock stress and relationships between extracellular striatal DA concentrations and motor symptom outcomes before and after psychological stress exposures. When compared to baseline, subjects exposed to tail-shock stress demonstrated significantly increased striatal extracellular DA, dihydroxyphenylacetic acid (DOPAC), and homovanillic acid (HVA) levels. These findings suggest residual nigrostriatal DA neurons are capable of producing DA in response to psychological stress. However, in all but one subject, these levels did not reach levels comparable to those demonstrated in nonlesioned animals following tail-shock stress. While no consistent pattern was demonstrated between stress and akinetic and cataleptic motor behaviors, a significant negative correlation was shown between poststress latencies for catalepsy and extracellular DA concentrations, with a similar trend identified for akinesia. These findings suggest psychological stress may lead to poorer motor symptom outcomes as a consequence of lower than normal DA responsiveness in the striatum.

In a MPTP animal model of PD, researchers examined the effects of immersion immobilization stress on motor symptom outcomes associated with locomotor activity and biological mechanisms involving DA content, metabolites (DOPAC and HVA), and indices (DOPAC + HVA/DA) [60]. Subjects were allocated to one of four subgroups: MPTP-treated group, saline-treated group, MPTP and stress-treated group, or saline and stress-treated group. The results revealed the induction of psychological stress in the MPTP-treated group was associated with a more pronounced but transient decrease in locomotor activity when compared to the stress-treated saline group. Striatal DA content was significantly lower in the stress-treated MPTP group when compared to the MPTP-treated group. Striatal DA indices were significantly elevated in both the MPTP- and saline-treated stress groups, indicating increased DA turnover. There was no significant difference in the striatal DA metabolites DOPAC or HVA between the two MPTP-treated groups or the two saline-treated groups. These findings provide evidence to suggest that psychological stress may contribute to motor symptom outcomes and biological mechanisms associated with dopamine deficiencies in PD.

Finally, in a 6-OHDA animal model of PD, researchers examined the effects of psychological stress on biological mechanisms involving DA and norepinephrine that may contribute to motor symptom outcomes of akinesia [61]. The results revealed the induction of acute psychological stress precipitated the development of transient akinesia in all lesioned subjects but had no effect on controls. Dopamine deficiencies in the striatum were more predictive of stress-induced akinesias than in other areas of the brain. While some subjects demonstrated moderate depletion in hippocampal norepinephrine levels, there was no consistent relationship with stress-induced akinesia. These findings suggest DA deficiencies may affect the ability to maintain normal motor function under conditions of psychological stress.

Collectively, these studies suggest important relationships exist between psychological stress and biological mechanisms that contribute to pathophysiological processes and symptom outcomes in animal models of PD. Specifically, significant relationships have been demonstrated between psychological stress and increased motor symptom severity [55–61] and depression [55] as well as dopamine deficiencies [55, 56, 58–61], dopaminergic neurodegeneration [55, 57], and the

expression of α-synuclein [55]. One study demonstrated significant relationships between corticosterone administration, a key mediator of neuroendocrine stress responses, and increased motor symptoms and loss of dopaminergic neurons [57]. However, another study failed to demonstrate a significant relationship between hippocampal norepinephrine levels, another biomarker of neuroendocrine-mediated stress responses, and stress-induced akinesia [61], suggesting additional research is needed in order to fully elucidate the role the neuroendocrine system plays in biological mechanisms and symptom outcomes of psychological stress in PD. None of the reviewed studies examined underlying biological mechanisms of neuroinflammation and oxidative stress that may contribute to symptom and health outcomes in PD.

3.2. Symptom and Health Outcomes of Psychological Stress That May Modify the Illness Trajectory in Human Subjects with PD. The remaining four studies in this review examined symptom and health outcomes of psychological stress that may modify the illness trajectory in human subjects with PD [62–65]. Three of these studies focused on symptom outcomes of psychological stress to include freezing of gait (FoG) [63], the ability to experience pleasure, reach-to-grasp movements [64], and nonmotor symptom frequencies [65]. One study examined relationships between psychological stress and health outcomes [65]. In contrast to research in animal models of PD, only one study examined biological outcomes of psychological stress, specifically sympathetic skin responses (SSR), a biomarker of sympathetic cholinergic sudomotor function associated with autonomic dysfunction [62]. Each of these studies is further discussed below and summarized in Table 4.

In subjects with PD ($n = 29$) and controls ($n = 27$), researchers examined the effects of psychological stress on biological mechanisms of autonomic dysfunction, specifically SSR [62]. SSR is a noninvasive biomarker of sympathetic cholinergic sudomotor function associated with autonomic dysfunction. Autonomic dysfunction is common in PD and can result in nonmotor symptoms such as diaphoresis, hypotension, and urinary and gastrointestinal dysfunction. In this study, SSR onset latencies, peak-to-peak, and amplitude recordings were obtained before and after a series of mental stressors designed to induce psychological stress. The results revealed no significant difference in SSR parameters before or after mental stress between subjects with PD and controls. However, the exclusion of subjects presenting with clinical autonomic dysfunction may explain the lack of significant findings in this study.

In a cross-sectional study, researchers examined factors that influence symptom outcomes of FoG in subjects with PD ($n = 130$) [63]. FoG, a common motor symptom of PD, results in a sudden and transient inability to walk typically in response to obstacles or situations that affect visual or proprioceptive input. Early in the disease, FoG is often triggered when initiating walking or by turning, confined spaces, rushed situations, or approaching a destination. As the disease progresses, FoG begins to occur in the absence of these triggers, perpetuating the unpredictability of this

TABLE 4: Symptom and health outcomes of psychological stress that may modify the illness trajectory in human subjects with PD.

Study author & date	Study purpose & sample	Method(s) of psychological stress induction	Measures of biological mechanisms, symptom, and health outcomes	Major study findings
Giza et al., 2012 [62]	*Purpose*: to examine the effects of psychological stress on biological mechanisms of autonomic dysfunction, specifically SSR parameters. *Sample*: male and female subjects with PD and controls (n = 56)	Arithmetic calculations using the WAIS-R arithmetic subscale	*Biological mechanisms*: 4-channel Nihon Kohen Neuropack S/MFrB 5504K used to record SSR in accordance with International Federation of Clinical Neurophysiology Guidelines	*Biological mechanisms*: no significant differences in SSR parameters were demonstrated between subjects or controls before or after the induction of psychological stress.
Rahman et al., 2008 [63]	*Purpose*: to examine factors that influence symptom outcomes of FoG in subjects with PD. *Sample*: male and female subjects with PD (n = 130)	Not applicable	*Symptom outcomes*: factors influencing walking/freezing questionnaire (tool not specified)	*Symptom outcomes*: stress was identified as a trigger of FoG by 53.1% of subjects.
Macht et al., 2007 [64]	*Purpose*: to examine the effects of psychological stress on symptom outcomes, specifically goal directed movements and hedonic responsiveness. *Sample*: male and female subjects with PD and controls (n = 38)	Arithmetic calculations while listening to loud music (protocol not specified)	*Symptom outcomes*: Eshkol and Wachman coding system for reach-to-grasp movements, duration of forward and backward movements, and emotional state questionnaire (tool not specified)	*Symptom outcomes*: stress was associated with significant deteriorations in mood and reduced hedonistic responsiveness in subjects with PD. Stress did not result in significant differences in each-to-grasp movements between subjects and controls.
Macht et al., 2005 [65]	*Purpose*: to examine patterns of psychological problems in subjects with PD to include symptom frequencies and health outcomes. *Sample*: male and female subjects with PD (n = 3075)	Not applicable	*Symptoms outcomes*: Inventory of Psychosocial Stress in PD. *Health outcomes*: Inventory of Psychosocial Stress in PD and benefits of social support questionnaire (tool not specified)	*Symptom outcomes*: Symptom increases with even small amounts of stress were reported by approximately two-thirds of subjects. Higher stress levels were associated with greater frequencies in depressive moods, sleep disturbances, anxiety, sexual problems, and communication difficulties. *Health outcomes*: higher stress was associated with greater difficulties coping with PD, worsening social relationships, less enjoyment of life, and the need for more psychological support.

PD, Parkinson's disease; FoG, freezing of gait; WAIS-R, Wechsler Adult Intelligence Scale-Revised; SSR, sympathetic skin responses.

symptom. While turning around and fatigue were the most prevalent factors cited as contributing to FoG, 53.1% of subjects (n = 105) cited being in a stressful situation as a significant trigger of FoG.

In subjects with PD (n = 19) and matched controls (n = 19), researchers examined the effects of psychological stress on symptom outcomes, specifically goal directed movements and hedonic responsiveness [64]. Impaired goal directed movements and reduced hedonic responsiveness, defined in this study as impaired reach-to-grasp movements and decreased ability to experience physical or social pleasure, respectively, are two common symptoms in PD. Subjective ratings of mood state and pleasure associated with eating as well as reach-to-grasp movement measurements were obtained at baseline and after the induction of emotional stress. Deterioration in mood and reduction in hedonic responsiveness following the induction of psychological stress were significantly more pronounced in subjects with PD than controls. Psychological stress did not result in significant differences in reach-to-grasp movements between subjects and controls. However, the majority of subjects in this study were receiving treatment with a combination of dopamine replacement therapy and dopamine agonists, which may have ameliorated the effects of psychological stress on motor symptoms.

In a cross-sectional study, researchers examined patterns of psychological problems in subjects with PD (n = 3075) to include symptom and health outcomes of psychological stress [65]. Cluster analysis revealed four patterns of psychological problems: general low stress, general high stress, sexual and social problems, and nonsocial problems. Approximately two-thirds of the total subjects (69% of women; 67% of men) reported symptom increases with even small amounts of stress. Subjects with high stress reported greater frequencies of depressive moods, sleep disturbances, anxiety, sexual problems, and communications difficulties. Subjects with high stress also reported a greater frequency of symptom increases with even small amounts of stress as well as poorer health outcomes to include greater difficulty coping with PD, poorer social relationships, less enjoyment of life, and needing more psychological support.

These studies provide preliminary evidence to support relationships between psychological stress and poorer symptom and health outcomes in individuals with PD. Significant relationships were demonstrated between psychological stress and symptom outcomes to include increased FoG [63], decreased ability to experience pleasure [64], and increased symptom frequencies for select nonmotor symptoms such as depressive mood, sleep disturbances, anxiety, sexual problems, and communication difficulties [65]. Psychological stress was not associated with significant differences in reach-to-grasp movements between subjects and controls [64]. Greater psychological stress was also associated with poorer health outcomes such as difficulty coping with PD, poorer social relationships, less enjoyment of life, and the need for more psychological support [65]. Evidence is lacking regarding biological mechanisms of psychological stress that may contribute to symptom and health outcomes in human subjects with PD.

4. Conclusion

This integrated review supports the notion that psychological stress affects biological mechanisms and symptom and health outcomes in PD. Evidence in animal models has demonstrated that significant relationships exist between psychological stress and poorer symptom outcomes to include increased motor symptom severity and behaviors associated with depression. Significant relationships have also been demonstrated between psychological stress and biological mechanisms involving biomarkers of dopamine production and metabolism, serotonin, and dopaminergic neurodegeneration. Specifically, the evidence suggests psychological stress in animal models of PD results in greater DA depletions in the nigrostriatal and nonnigrostriatal systems, exaggerated expression of nigrostriatal and nonnigrostriatal α-synuclein, increased neurodegeneration of dopaminergic neurons as indicated by increased Fluoro-Jade positive cells and GFAP in the SNc, and decreased 5-HT levels. These findings suggest the induction of psychological stress in animal models of PD contributes to poorer motor symptom outcomes by exacerbating underlying pathogenic features associated with PD.

Preliminary evidence also exists to suggest psychological stress may play a role in symptom and health outcomes in individuals with PD. In human subjects with PD, evidence supports relationships between psychological stress and increased symptom severity and poorer health outcomes. Significant relationships have been demonstrated between psychological stress and poorer symptom outcomes to include increased FoG, depressive moods, sleep disturbances, anxiety, sexual problems, and communication difficulties and decreased hedonic responsiveness. Greater levels of psychological stress have also been associated with poorer health outcomes such as difficulty coping with PD, poorer social relationships, less enjoyment of life, and the need for more social support. Evidence is lacking regarding underlying biological mechanisms of psychological stress that contribute to these findings in human subjects with PD.

Cumulatively, the studies included in this review provide evidence of the potential importance of psychological stress to biological mechanisms and symptom and health outcomes in PD. It should be noted however that many of the reviewed studies demonstrated limitations that may affect the validity and generalizability of these findings. These limitations include issues associated with translating experimental outcomes in animal models to human populations, key differences in the primary outcomes examined, methods for inducing psychological stress, and underlying stress paradigms and study design and methodologies issues.

A number of limitations exist when attempting to translate outcomes of animal experimentation to human populations. Routine laboratory procedures and conditions, such as artificial and restricted housing environments, noise, human handling, and contagious anxiety, have been associated with elevations in stress-related biomarkers, factors that may confound experimental results [66, 67]. The complexity of human diseases is often difficult to replicate, resulting in discrepancies between animal models of select diseases and actual human conditions [66–68]. Animal models involve the induction of diseases in healthy, homogenous subjects that lack the many predisposing factors and comorbidities that contribute to disease development and progression in human populations [67, 68]. Differences in physiology, behavior, pharmacokinetics, and genetics may limit the ability to generalize experimental data from animal models to human populations [66, 67]. Experimental animal studies often lack fundamental aspects of study design that are required in human clinical trials, specifically randomization, blinding of research personnel, and sample size calculations, which may result in overestimated outcome effects [67, 68]. Furthermore, the small sample sizes typically used in animal experimentation often lead to underpowered studies, which may increase the risk of erroneously detecting treatment effects [67, 68]. Each of these issues confounds the ability to translate findings in experimental models to human populations with PD.

Key differences were identified in the primary outcomes examined in the reviewed studies. The majority of the animal studies included in this review focused on the effects of psychological stress on biological mechanisms that may contribute to pathophysiological processes in PD whereas the studies involving human subjects focused on the effects of psychological stress on symptom and health outcomes that may modify the illness trajectory. Extreme caution should be exercised when attempting to extrapolate biological outcomes in animal models as a means of explaining factors that modify symptom and health outcomes in those living with PD. As such, this highlights the need for additional research that focuses on biological mechanisms of psychological stress specific to underlying pathophysiological processes that may modify symptom and health outcomes in human populations with PD.

Important differences were demonstrated in the manner in which psychological stress was induced in animal models of and human subjects with PD. In the reviewed studies, the induction of psychological stress in individuals with PD involved performing strenuous mental tasks [62, 64]. In contrast, the induction of psychological stress in animal models of PD involved physiological insults such as glucodeprivation, osmotic diuresis, hypothermia, and painful stimuli [59–61]. Stress induction techniques used in animal models may result in the activation of biological pathways unrelated to psychological stress responses. For example, the dopaminergic system has been implicated in biological responses associated with pain perception and processing variability as well as central control of thermoregulation [69, 70]. Activation of these pathways may have confounded the ability to interpret outcomes of psychological stress in animal models of PD. Furthermore, the induction of stress in animal models of PD does not adequately reflect the multidimensional and dynamic nature of stress experiences in individuals living with PD. Each of these factors necessitates the use of caution when attempting to translate these findings to human populations with PD.

Key differences in acute versus chronic stress paradigms are important to consider when evaluating the studies included in this review. The underlying stress paradigms in the majority of the reviewed studies focused on the implementation of acute psychological stressors that varied in timing and type so as to limit predictability [55, 57–62, 64]. Only one study specifically focused on chronic variable stress [56]. Important differences exist in biological mechanisms responsible for mediating physiological responses to acute versus chronic psychological stressors. For example, activation of the HPAA and the release of glucocorticoids in response to acute psychological stress have been associated with transient immunosuppressive effects [22, 71, 72]. In contrast, sustained activation of the HPAA and release of glucocorticoids, as seen with chronic psychological stress, have been associated with exaggerated inflammatory responses, cell damage, and death [18, 22, 73]. Chronic psychological stress has also been associated with dysregulation of glucocorticoid feedback mechanisms. Under normal circumstances, transient increases in circulating glucocorticoids exert inhibitory effects on further HPAA stimulation. Dysregulation of these feedback mechanisms, as seen with chronic psychological stress, has been associated with increased expression and release of glucocorticoids [18]. Furthermore, the increased energy demands needed to respond to chronic psychological stress have been associated with increased production of ROS, oxidative stress, lipid peroxidation, and tissue damage within the central nervous system [14, 26, 38, 74]. Given that individuals with PD often face a variety of stressors across the illness trajectory, additional research is needed that considers differences in biological mechanisms, symptoms, and health outcomes associated with acute versus chronic stress paradigms.

A number of design and methodological issues were identified in the reviewed studies. For instance, between-subject procedural variability [61], the introduction of potential confounders [58, 61], and inadequately operationalized key variables/procedures [56, 59, 60] were identified in several of the reviewed animal studies. With regard to the human studies, the limited number of studies and relatively small sample sizes in all but one study represent limitations to the generalizability of these findings. In several studies, inadequate operationalization of key variables and/or unknown psychometric properties for the measurement tools that were utilized may have affected the validity and reliability of the results [62–65]. The operationalization of hedonistic responsiveness as pleasurable food experiences in one study may also present a potential limitation given individuals with PD often experience loss of taste and swallowing difficulties, factors that were not controlled for and may have confounded differences in hedonistic responsiveness between subjects and controls [64]. Finally, in another study, advertising the study as a mobility study may have led to the overrepresentation of subjects with mobility problems [63].

As this review has demonstrated, significant gaps exist in our understanding of biological mechanisms and symptom and health outcomes of psychological stress in individuals living with PD. Much of what is currently known about biological mechanisms and symptom outcomes of psychological stress in PD has been conducted in animal models of PD and/or predicated on research in non-PD animal models. While important, this knowledge may not adequately reflect these constructs in individuals living with the disease, particularly given the multifaceted nature of stress in human populations and similarities in key pathogenic features of PD that may be exacerbated by underlying biological mechanisms of psychological stress. As a result, additional research is needed in order to further elucidate underlying biological mechanisms and symptom and health outcomes of psychological stress in PD. Psychoneuroimmunological frameworks provide an important opportunity for gaining insight into plausible biological mechanisms of the neuroendocrine and immune systems that may contribute to stress-induced neuroinflammation, oxidative stress, and loss of dopaminergic neurons in PD, which may lead to poorer symptom and health outcomes [11]. Rigorously designed studies that provide a deeper understanding of these relationships would provide the foundation for designing interventions specifically targeted to biological mechanisms and symptom and health outcomes of psychological stress in PD.

Healthcare providers need to be aware of multifaceted factors that may contribute to symptom and health outcomes in PD. Given the progressive and unpredictable nature of PD, individuals living with the disease must cope with and adapt to a variety of stressors over a protracted period of time. The cumulative costs of psychological stressors may further exacerbate pathogenic mechanisms in PD thereby perpetuating neuronal loss within the central nervous system. Consideration of these factors in the design of future research studies as well as the clinical care of individuals with PD represents an important opportunity to improve symptom and health outcomes in those living with the disease.

Disclosure

The development of this manuscript was not associated with any specific grant funding from any funding agency in the public, commercial, or not-for-profit sectors.

References

[1] A. Antonini, P. Barone, R. Marconi et al., "The progression of non-motor symptoms in Parkinsons disease and their contribution to motor disability and quality of life," *Journal of Neurology*, vol. 259, pp. 2621–2631, 2012.

[2] C. C. Aquino and S. H. Fox, "Clinical spectrum of levodopa-induced complications," *Movement Disorders*, vol. 30, no. 1, pp. 80–89, 2015.

[3] M. S. Clark, M. J. Bond, and J. R. Hecker, "Environmental stress, psychological stress and allostatic load," *Psychology, Health and Medicine*, vol. 12, no. 1, pp. 18–30, 2007.

[4] T. H. Holmes and R. H. Rahe, "The social readjustment rating scale," *Journal of Psychosomatic Research*, vol. 11, no. 2, pp. 213–218, 1967.

[5] J. K. Kiecolt-Glaser, L. McGuire, T. F. Robles, and R. Glaser, "Emotions, morbidity, and mortality: new perspectives from psychoneuroimmunology," *Annual Review of Psychology*, vol. 53, pp. 83–107, 2002.

[6] M. Sorenson, L. Janusek, and H. Mathews, "Psychological stress and cytokine production in multiple sclerosis: correlation with disease symptomatology," *Biological Research for Nursing*, vol. 15, no. 2, pp. 226–233, 2013.

[7] M. C. Davis, A. J. Zautra, and J. W. Reich, "Vulnerability to stress among women in chronic pain from fibromyalgia and osteoarthritis," *Annals of Behavioral Medicine*, vol. 23, no. 3, pp. 215–226, 2001.

[8] A. W. M. Evers, E. W. M. Verhoeven, H. Van Middendorp et al., "Does stress affect the joints? Daily stressors, stress vulnerability, immune and HPA axis activity, and short-term disease and symptom fluctuations in rheumatoid arthritis," *Annals of the Rheumatic Diseases*, vol. 73, no. 9, pp. 1683–1688, 2014.

[9] T. E. Seeman, B. H. Singer, J. W. Rowe, R. I. Horwitz, and B. S. McEwen, "Price of adaptation—allostatic load and its health consequences," *Archives of Internal Medicine*, vol. 157, no. 19, pp. 2259–2268, 1997.

[10] J. Kulmala, M. B. von Bonsdorff, S. Stenholm et al., "Perceived stress symptoms in midlife predict disability in old age: a 28-year prospective cohort study," *The Journals of Gerontology Series A: Biological Sciences and Medical Sciences*, vol. 68, no. 8, pp. 984–991, 2013.

[11] N. L. McCain, D. P. Gray, J. M. Walter, and J. Robins, "Implementing a comprehensive approach to the study of health dynamics using the psychoneuroimmunology paradigm," *Advances in Nursing Science*, vol. 28, no. 4, pp. 320–332, 2005.

[12] F. S. Dhabhar, "Enhancing versus suppressive effects of stress on immune function: implications for immunoprotection and immunopathology," *NeuroImmunoModulation*, vol. 16, no. 5, pp. 300–317, 2009.

[13] C. J. Barnum, T. W. W. Pace, F. Hu, G. N. Neigh, and M. G. Tansey, "Psychological stress in adolescent and adult mice increases neuroinflammation and attenuates the response to LPS challenge," *Journal of Neuroinflammation*, vol. 9, article 9, 2012.

[14] R. M. De Pablos, R. F. Villarán, S. Argüelles et al., "Stress increases vulnerability to inflammation in the rat prefrontal cortex," *Journal of Neuroscience*, vol. 26, no. 21, pp. 5709–5719, 2006.

[15] M. G. Frank, M. V. Baratta, D. B. Sprunger, L. R. Watkins, and S. F. Maier, "Microglia serve as a neuroimmune substrate for stress-induced potentiation of CNS pro-inflammatory cytokine responses," *Brain, Behavior, and Immunity*, vol. 21, no. 1, pp. 47–59, 2007.

[16] M. G. Frank, B. M. Thompson, L. R. Watkins, and S. F. Maier, "Glucocorticoids mediate stress-induced priming of microglial pro-inflammatory responses," *Brain, Behavior, and Immunity*, vol. 26, no. 2, pp. 337–345, 2012.

[17] J. L. M. Madrigal, B. García-Bueno, J. R. Caso, B. G. Pérez-Nievas, and J. C. Leza, "Stress-induced oxidative changes in brain," *CNS and Neurological Disorders—Drug Targets*, vol. 5, no. 5, pp. 561–568, 2006.

[18] C. D. Munhoz, L. B. Lepsch, E. M. Kawamoto et al., "Chronic unpredictable stress exacerbates lipopolysaccharide-induced activation of nuclear factor-κB in the frontal cortex and hippocampus via glucocorticoid secretion," *The Journal of Neuroscience*, vol. 26, no. 14, pp. 3813–3820, 2006.

[19] J. B. Buchanan, N. L. Sparkman, J. Chen, and R. W. Johnson, "Cognitive and neuroinflammatory consequences of mild

repeated stress are exacerbated in aged mice," *Psychoneuroendocrinology*, vol. 33, no. 6, pp. 755–765, 2008.

[20] M. G. Frank, S. A. Hershman, M. D. Weber, L. R. Watkins, and S. F. Maier, "Chronic exposure to exogenous glucocorticoids primes microglia to pro-inflammatory stimuli and induces NLRP3 mRNA in the hippocampus," *Psychoneuroendocrinology*, vol. 40, no. 1, pp. 191–200, 2014.

[21] M. L. Block, L. Zecca, and J.-S. Hong, "Microglia-mediated neurotoxicity: uncovering the molecular mechanisms," *Nature Reviews Neuroscience*, vol. 8, no. 1, pp. 57–69, 2007.

[22] H. A. Jurgens and R. W. Johnson, "Dysregulated neuronal–microglial cross-talk during aging, stress and inflammation," *Experimental Neurology*, vol. 233, no. 1, pp. 40–48, 2012.

[23] H.-M. Gao, J. Jiang, B. Wilson, W. Zhang, J.-S. Hong, and B. Liu, "Microglial activation-mediated delayed and progressive degeneration of rat nigral dopaminergic neurons: relevance to parkinson's disease," *Journal of Neurochemistry*, vol. 81, no. 6, pp. 1285–1297, 2002.

[24] G. Lucca, C. M. Comim, S. S. Valvassori et al., "Increased oxidative stress in submitochondrial particles into the brain of rats submitted to the chronic mild stress paradigm," *Journal of Psychiatric Research*, vol. 43, no. 9, pp. 864–869, 2009.

[25] J. S. Myers, "Proinflammatory cytokines and sickness behavior: implications for depression and cancer-related symptoms," *Oncology Nursing Forum*, vol. 35, no. 5, pp. 802–807, 2008.

[26] C. Munhoz, J. L. M. Madrigal, B. García-Bueno et al., "TNF-α accounts for short-term persistence of oxidative status in rat brain after two weeks of repeated stress," *European Journal of Neuroscience*, vol. 20, no. 4, pp. 1125–1130, 2004.

[27] J.-P. Gouin, R. Glaser, W. B. Malarkey, D. Beversdorf, and J. Kiecolt-Glaser, "Chronic stress, daily stressors, and circulating inflammatory markers," *Health Psychology*, vol. 31, no. 2, pp. 264–268, 2012.

[28] S. Holmin and T. Mathiesen, "Intracerebral administration of interleukin-1β and induction of inflammation, apoptosis, and vasogenic edema," *Journal of Neurosurgery*, vol. 92, no. 1, pp. 108–120, 2000.

[29] D. Zhou, A. W. Kusnecov, M. R. Shurin, M. DePaoli, and B. S. Rabin, "Exposure to physical and psychological stressors elevates plasma interleukin 6: Relationship to the activation of hypothalamic-pituitary-adrenal axis," *Endocrinology*, vol. 133, no. 6, pp. 2523–2530, 1993.

[30] J. L. M. Madrigal, O. Hurtado, M. A. Moro et al., "The increase in TNF-α levels is implicated in NF-κB activation and inducible nitric oxide synthase expression in brain cortex after immobilization stress," *Neuropsychopharmacology*, vol. 26, no. 2, pp. 155–163, 2002.

[31] A. Bierhaus, J. Wolf, M. Andrassy et al., "A mechanism converting psychosocial stress into mononuclear cell activation," *Proceedings of the National Academy of Sciences of the United States of America*, vol. 100, no. 4, pp. 1920–1925, 2003.

[32] Z.-Q. Liang, Y.-L. Li, X.-L. Zhao et al., "NF-κB contributes to 6-hydroxydopamine-induced apoptosis of nigral dopaminergic neurons through p53," *Brain Research*, vol. 1145, no. 1, pp. 190–203, 2007.

[33] J. L. M. Madrigal, M. A. Moro, I. Lizasoain et al., "Induction of cyclooxygenase-2 accounts for restraint stress-induced oxidative status in rat brain," *Neuropsychopharmacology*, vol. 28, no. 9, pp. 1579–1588, 2003.

[34] S. Vesce, D. Rossi, L. Brambilla, and A. Volterra, "Glutamate release from astrocytes in physiological conditions and in neurodegenerative disorders characterized by neuroinflammation," *International Review of Neurobiology*, vol. 82, pp. 57–71, 2007.

[35] K. Yamagata, K. I. Andreasson, W. E. Kaufmann, C. A. Barnes, and P. F. Worley, "Expression of a mitogen-inducible cyclooxygenase in brain neurons: regulation by synaptic activity and glucocorticoids," *Neuron*, vol. 11, no. 2, pp. 371–386, 1993.

[36] S. R. Subramaniam and M.-F. Chesselet, "Mitochondrial dysfunction and oxidative stress in Parkinson's disease," *Progress in Neurobiology*, vol. 106-107, pp. 17–32, 2013.

[37] M. Valko, D. Leibfritz, J. Moncol, M. T. D. Cronin, M. Mazur, and J. Telser, "Free radicals and antioxidants in normal physiological functions and human disease," *The International Journal of Biochemistry & Cell Biology*, vol. 39, no. 1, pp. 44–84, 2007.

[38] G. Lucca, C. M. Comim, S. S. Valvassori et al., "Effects of chronic mild stress on the oxidative parameters in the rat brain," *Neurochemistry International*, vol. 54, no. 5-6, pp. 358–362, 2009.

[39] H.-M. Gao, H. Zhou, and J.-S. Hong, "NADPH oxidases: novel therapeutic targets for neurodegenerative diseases," *Trends in Pharmacological Sciences*, vol. 33, no. 6, pp. 295–303, 2012.

[40] I. Paduraru, O. Paduraru, G. Manolidis, W. Bild, and I. Haulica, "Antioxidant activity in rat models of nociceptive stress," *Revista medico-chirurgicala a Societații de Medici si Naturalisti din Iasi*, vol. 114, no. 1, pp. 175–179, 2010.

[41] S. T. Kim, J. H. Choi, J. W. Chang, S. W. Kim, and O. Hwang, "Immobilization stress causes increases in tetrahydrobiopterin, dopamine, and neuromelanin and oxidative damage in the nigrostriatal system," *Journal of Neurochemistry*, vol. 95, no. 1, pp. 89–98, 2005.

[42] D. T. Dextera and P. Jenner, "Parkinson disease: from pathology to molecular disease mechanisms," *Free Radical Biology and Medicine*, vol. 62, pp. 132–144, 2013.

[43] A. Gerhard, N. Pavese, G. Hotton et al., "In vivo imaging of microglial activation with [^{11}C](R)-PK11195 PET in idiopathic Parkinson's disease," *Neurobiology of Disease*, vol. 21, no. 2, pp. 404–412, 2006.

[44] Y. Ouchi, E. Yoshikawa, Y. Sekine et al., "Microglial activation and dopamine terminal loss in early Parkinson's disease," *Annals of Neurology*, vol. 57, no. 2, pp. 168–175, 2005.

[45] A. M. Depino, C. Earl, E. Kaczmarczyk et al., "Microglial activation with atypical proinflammatory cytokine expression in a rat model of Parkinson's disease," *European Journal of Neuroscience*, vol. 18, no. 10, pp. 2731–2742, 2003.

[46] P. Scalzo, A. Kümmer, F. Cardoso, and A. L. Teixeira, "Serum levels of interleukin-6 are elevated in patients with Parkinson's disease and correlate with physical performance," *Neuroscience Letters*, vol. 468, no. 1, pp. 56–58, 2010.

[47] M. Reale, C. Iarlori, A. Thomas et al., "Peripheral cytokines profile in Parkinson's disease," *Brain, Behavior, and Immunity*, vol. 23, no. 1, pp. 55–63, 2009.

[48] J. C. Tobón-Velasco, J. H. Limón-Pacheco, M. Orozco-Ibarra et al., "6-OHDA-induced apoptosis and mitochondrial dysfunction are mediated by early modulation of intracellular signals and interaction of Nrf2 and NF-κB factors," *Toxicology*, vol. 304, pp. 109–119, 2013.

[49] P. Teismann, K. Tieu, D.-K. Choi et al., "Cyclooxygenase-2 is instrumental in Parkinson's disease neurodegeneration," *Proceedings of the National Academy of Sciences of the United States of America*, vol. 100, no. 9, pp. 5473–5478, 2003.

[50] M. S. Hernandes, C. C. Café-Mendes, and L. R. G. Britto, "NADPH oxidase and the degeneration of dopaminergic neurons in Parkinsonian mice," *Oxidative Medicine and Cellular Longevity*, vol. 2013, Article ID 157857, 13 pages, 2013.

[51] T.-K. Lin, C.-H. Cheng, S.-D. Chen, C.-W. Liou, C.-R. Huang, and Y.-C. Chuang, "Mitochondrial dysfunction and oxidative stress promote apoptotic cell death in the striatum via cytochrome c/caspase-3 signaling cascade following chronic rotenone intoxication in rats," *International Journal of Molecular Sciences*, vol. 13, no. 7, pp. 8722–8739, 2012.

[52] R. C. S. Seet, C.-Y. J. Lee, E. C. H. Lim et al., "Oxidative damage in Parkinson disease: measurement using accurate biomarkers," *Free Radical Biology & Medicine*, vol. 48, no. 4, pp. 560–566, 2010.

[53] P. M. Keeney, J. Xie, R. A. Capaldi, and J. P. Bennett Jr., "Parkinson's disease brain mitochondrial complex I has oxidatively damaged subunits and is functionally impaired and misassembled," *The Journal of Neuroscience*, vol. 26, no. 19, pp. 5256–5264, 2006.

[54] D. Lindqvist, E. Kaufman, L. Brundin, S. Hall, Y. Surova, and O. Hansson, "Non-motor symptoms in patients with Parkinson's disease—correlations with inflammatory cytokines in serum," *PLoS ONE*, vol. 7, no. 10, Article ID e47387, 2012.

[55] U. Janakiraman, T. Manivasagam, A. J. Thenmozhi et al., "Influences of chronic mild stress exposure on motor, non-motor impairments and neurochemical variables in specific brain areas of mptp/probenecid induced neurotoxicity in mice," *PLoS ONE*, vol. 11, no. 1, Article ID e0146671, 2016.

[56] A. M. Hemmerle, J. W. Dickerson, J. P. Herman, and K. B. Seroogy, "Stress exacerbates experimental Parkinson's disease," *Molecular Psychiatry*, vol. 19, no. 6, pp. 638–640, 2014.

[57] L. K. Smith, N. M. Jadavji, K. L. Colwell, S. K. Perehudoff, and G. A. Metz, "Stress accelerates neural degeneration and exaggerates motor symptoms in a rat model of Parkinson's disease," *European Journal of Neuroscience*, vol. 27, no. 8, pp. 2133–2146, 2008.

[58] F. M. Howells, V. A. Russell, M. V. Mabandla, and L. A. Kellaway, "Stress reduces the neuroprotective effect of exercise in a rat model for Parkinson's disease," *Behavioural Brain Research*, vol. 165, no. 2, pp. 210–220, 2005.

[59] K. A. Keefe, E. M. Stricker, M. J. Zigmond, and E. D. Abercrombie, "Environmental stress increases extracellular dopamine in striatum of 6-hydroxydopamine-treated rats: in vivo microdialysis studies," *Brain Research*, vol. 527, no. 2, pp. 350–353, 1990.

[60] K. Urakami, N. Masaki, K. Shimoda, S. Nishikawa, and K. Takahashi, "Increase of striatal dopamine turnover by stress in MPTP-treated mice," *Clinical Neuropharmacology*, vol. 11, no. 4, pp. 360–368, 1988.

[61] A. M. Snyder, E. M. Stricker, and M. J. Zigmond, "Stress-induced neurological impairments in an animal model of parkinsonism," *Annals of Neurology*, vol. 18, no. 5, pp. 544–551, 1985.

[62] E. Giza, Z. Katsarou, G. Georgiadis, and S. Bostantjopoulou, "Sympathetic skin response in Parkinson's disease before and after mental stress," *Clinical Neurophysiology*, vol. 42, no. 3, pp. 125–131, 2012.

[63] S. Rahman, H. J. Griffin, N. P. Quinn, and M. Jahanshahi, "The factors that induce or overcome freezing of gait in Parkinson's disease," *Behavioural Neurology*, vol. 19, no. 3, pp. 127–136, 2008.

[64] M. Macht, S. Brandstetter, and H. Ellgring, "Stress affects hedonic responses but not reaching-grasping in Parkinson's disease," *Behavioural Brain Research*, vol. 177, no. 1, pp. 171–174, 2007.

[65] M. Macht, R. Schwarz, and H. Ellgring, "Patterns of psychological problems in Parkinson's disease," *Acta Neurologica Scandinavica*, vol. 111, no. 2, pp. 95–101, 2005.

[66] A. Akhtar, "The flaws and human harms of animal experimentation," *Cambridge Quarterly of Healthcare Ethics*, vol. 24, no. 4, pp. 407–419, 2015.

[67] D. G. Hachman, "Translating animal research into clinical benefit," *British Medical Journal*, vol. 334, article 163, 2007.

[68] M. I. Martić-Kehl, R. Schibli, and P. A. Schubiger, "Can animal data predict human outcome? Problems and pitfalls of translational animal research," *European Journal of Nuclear Medicine and Molecular Imaging*, vol. 39, no. 9, pp. 1492–1496, 2012.

[69] S. K. Jääskeläinen, P. Lindholm, T. Valmunen et al., "Variation in the dopamine D2 receptor gene plays a key role in human pain and its modulation by transcranial magnetic stimulation," *Pain*, vol. 155, no. 10, pp. 2180–2187, 2014.

[70] P. J. Schwartz and S. D. Erk, "Regulation of central dopamine-2 receptor sensitivity by a proportional control thermostat in humans," *Psychiatry Research*, vol. 127, no. 1-2, pp. 19–26, 2004.

[71] N. K. Leidy, "A physiologic analysis of stress and chronic illness," *Journal of Advanced Nursing*, vol. 14, no. 10, pp. 868–876, 1989.

[72] J. K. Kiecolt-Glaser, L. McGuire, T. F. Robles, and R. Glaser, "Psychoneuroimmunology: psychological influences on immune function and health," *Journal of Consulting and Clinical Psychology*, vol. 70, no. 3, pp. 537–547, 2002.

[73] A. M. Espinosa-Oliva, R. M. de Pablos, R. F. Villarán et al., "Stress is critical for LPS-induced activation of microglia and damage in the rat hippocampus," *Neurobiology of Aging*, vol. 32, no. 1, pp. 85–102, 2011.

[74] E. Izzo, P. P. Sanna, and G. F. Koob, "Impairment of dopaminergic system function after chronic treatment with corticotropin-releasing factor," *Pharmacology, Biochemistry, and Behavior*, vol. 81, no. 4, pp. 701–708, 2005.

29

Cost of Living with Parkinson's Disease over 12 Months in Australia: A Prospective Cohort Study

Shalika Bohingamu Mudiyanselage,[1] **Jennifer J. Watts,**[1] **Julie Abimanyi-Ochom,**[1] **Lisa Lane,**[1] **Anna T. Murphy,**[2,3] **Meg E. Morris,**[4,5] **and Robert Iansek**[2,3]

[1]*Centre for Population Health Research, School of Health & Social Development, Faculty of Health, Deakin University, Burwood, VIC 3125, Australia*
[2]*Clinical Research Centre for Movement Disorders and Gait, The National Parkinson Foundation Centre of Excellence, Kingston Centre, Monash Health, Cheltenham, VIC 3192, Australia*
[3]*School of Clinical Sciences Monash University, Clayton, VIC 3168, Australia*
[4]*Healthscope, Northpark Private Hospital, Plenty and Greenhills Roads, Bundoora, VIC 3083, Australia*
[5]*School of Allied Health, La Trobe University, Bundoora, VIC 3083, Australia*

Correspondence should be addressed to Jennifer J Watts; j.watts@deakin.edu.au

Academic Editor: Antonio Pisani

Background. Parkinson disease (PD) is a costly chronic condition in terms of managing both motor and nonmotor symptoms. The burden of disease is high for individuals, caregivers, and the health system. The aim of this study is to estimate the annual cost of PD from the household, health system, and societal perspectives. *Methods.* A prospective cohort study of newly referred people with PD to a specialist PD clinic in Melbourne, Australia. Participants completed baseline and monthly health resource use questionnaires and Medicare data were collected over 12 months. *Results.* 87 patients completed the 12-month follow-up assessments. The mean annual cost per person to the health care system was $32,556 AUD. The burden to society was an additional $45,000 per annum per person with PD. The largest component of health system costs were for hospitalisation (69% of total costs). The costs for people with moderate to severe disease were almost 4 times those with mild PD ($63,569 versus $17,537 $p < 0.001$). *Conclusion.* PD is associated with significant costs to individuals and to society. Costs escalated with disease severity suggesting that the burden to society is likely to grow with the increasing disease prevalence that is associated with population ageing.

1. Introduction

Parkinson's disease (PD) is a chronic and degenerative neurological condition that is associated with lifelong disability [1]. Movement disorders such as slowness, balance impairment, tremor, freezing, and rigidity are characteristic of PD and nonmotor symptoms such as anxiety, depression, fatigue, and cognitive impairment are common [2]. Modified Hoehn and Yahr (HY) score is the clinical rating method to determine the level/severity of motor function in people with PD [3]. Progression in HY stages correlates with deterioration in an individual's quality of life [4, 5]. As the disease progresses, people with PD become highly vulnerable to falls and fall-related injuries [6]. The range of symptoms associated with PD

means that the disease burden to the household (individual and family), health system, and society is usually significant.

Parkinson's disease is the second most common neurological disorder after Alzheimer's disease [1, 7]. The number of new cases of PD in Australia grew by 17% during the period 2005 to 2011 [8]. Average life expectancy after a diagnosis of PD is around 12 years although people can live more than 20 years with comprehensive care [9]. A European study of six countries highlighted that 160 in 100,000 people aged 65 years and older population have a diagnosis of PD and in future this will increase with rapid population aging [10].

A US study estimated that the annual health system cost of PD per person was in the range $1,750–$17,560 USD in

2002 [11] but in 2010 this was closer to $23,000 USD per person with the national burden of PD exceeding $14 billion USD [12]. In Australia the cost to the individual with PD was more than $15,000 per year in 2011 [8]. There was a significant burden to the health system ($8,000 per year in 2014 [8]) including hospitalisations and pharmaceutical and medical services. A recent prospective cohort study indicated that medication expenses contributed nearly 35% of total health system costs related to PD [13]. People with PD and their families also face significant out-of-pocket expenses for caregiving and loss of productivity [14].

A number of international and Australian studies have investigated the health-related quality of life (HRQOL) of people with PD [5, 15]. Several studies have evaluated the economic burden related to caring for people with PD [13, 16–18] and some have focused on the association between resource utilisation and disease severity [18].

Given the paucity of recent data on the costs of PD, the aim of this paper is to estimate the costs of PD over 12 months from the perspective of the household, the health system, and society. A secondary aim is to investigate the impact of disease severity on annual costs and resource use.

2. Methodology

2.1. Study Design. This was a prospective cohort study with a 12-month follow-up conducted in Melbourne, Australia.

2.2. Study Population. The target population were people with idiopathic PD who were newly referred to a specialist PD clinic in metropolitan Melbourne [19]. *Inclusion criteria* for the study were (i) confirmed diagnosis of idiopathic PD; (ii) informed consent to participate in the study; (iii) ability to attend assessment clinics; and (iv) ability to complete questionnaires over 12 months. *Exclusion criteria* were (i) coexisting neurological conditions and (ii) disease category of HY stage five. Participants were also asked to consent to retrieval of their data from Medicare Australia, but nonconsent did not preclude them from participating in this study.

2.3. Ethics Approval. Ethics approvals were obtained from the Southern Health Human Research Ethics Committee (HREC number 06107B) and Monash University Standing Committee on Ethics in Research Involving Humans (SCERH number 2006/728MCC).

2.4. Data Collection. Participant's health services resource utilisation over 12 months was assessed through a series of questionnaires administered monthly, at baseline, 3 months, and 12 months. The baseline and 3- and 12-month questionnaires assessed PD duration and severity. Home based care services and community services (informal care, formal care, and meal-on-wheels) were also collected at 3 and 12 months. Participants were assessed by a trained assessor at home, or outpatient clinic [19]. Data related to health service resource use were collected via the monthly questionnaires [19]. These included questions to assess hospital admissions (length of stay, name of hospital, and method of transport to hospital), medical services (general practitioner, medical specialist, imaging services, and pathologist), and allied health services (physiotherapy, podiatry, etc.). Monthly questionnaires were completed with the help of a project officer who met with participants. Where participants consented, individual data on medical services and pharmaceutical use over 12 months were obtained from the national insurer, Medicare Australia. Resources were categorised according to the perspective of the analysis: individual/household, health system, or limited societal (inclusive of informal care but not productivity losses). Table 1 shows the sources of data collection and perspective for cost estimates.

2.5. Cost Analysis. Costs were attributed to self-reported resource utilisation according to service category. Costs for Medicare Australia data were reported as the individual out-of-pocket component, government cost (benefit paid) and societal cost (out-of-pocket + government). All costs are reported in 2012 Australian dollars.

2.5.1. Hospitalisation. Hospitalisation data including number of admissions and total length of stay (LOS) over a 12-month period for both private and public hospitals for all causes were obtained from self-report via the monthly questionnaires. To estimate the cost of hospitalisation per participant, the mean cost of a hospital admission per day was calculated using the national average cost per weighted separation from the Independent Hospital Pricing Authority (IHPA) [21] and the average hospital length of stay from the Australian Institute of Health and Welfare (AIHW) [20] according to the formulas shown in Table 2. Where resource data were missing from the monthly questionnaires, data for the number of hospital admissions and total length of stay over 12 months were imputed based on a weighted average from the available data for each participant.

2.5.2. Medical Services and Pharmaceuticals. Medicare Australia data were obtained for consenting participants and used to determine the total charges and benefits paid for visits to general practitioners, medical specialists (including private hospital visits), pathology, imaging, and pharmaceuticals over 12 months. For participants who did not consent to Medicare data an imputation method was used to replace missing data based on disease severity according to HY score; less than 2.5 for mild disease and moderate to severe if HY was equal to or more than 2.5 [7].

2.5.3. Allied Health Services. The costs of physiotherapy and podiatry services were estimated from both Medicare data and self-reported data taken from resource use questionnaires. Where both sources of data overlapped, preference was given to Medicare data. Costs for occupational therapy, speech therapy, psychology, dietetics, chiropractor, and optometry services were analysed using self-reported data. "Other services" included remedial massage and naturopathy services. Cost of allied health services was calculated from the number of visits and unit cost (Table 2) for each health service (for self-reported data).

TABLE 1: Economic analysis perspectives and data collection sources.

	Perspective			Date source		
	Individual	Health system	Societal	Questionnaire at 3 and 12 months	Monthly questionnaire	Medicare Australia
Hospitalisations						
Public hospital	—	*	*	—	*	—
Private hospital	—	*	*	—	*	—
Hospital transport						
Ambulance (road and air)	—	*	*	—	*	—
Private car	*	—	*	—	*	—
Taxi	*	—	*	—	*	—
Medical services						
General practitioner	*	*	*	—	*	*
Medical specialist	*	*	*	—	*	*
Imaging	*	*	*	—	*	*
Pathology	*	*	*	—	*	*
Pharmaceuticals						
Medication	*	*	*	—	*	*
Allied health services						
Physiotherapist	*	*	*	—	*	*
Podiatrist	*	*	*	—	*	*
Occupational therapy	*	*	*	—	*	—
Speech therapy	*	*	*	—	*	—
Psychology	*	*	*	—	*	—
Dietetic	*	*	*	—	*	—
Chiropractic	*	*	*	—	*	—
Optometry	*	*	*	—	*	—
Other	*	*	*	—	*	—
Other medical services						
Dental	*	*	*	—	*	—
Home based care and community services						
Formal care, nurse	—	*	*	*	—	—
Formal care, PCA	—	*	*	*	—	—
Informal care	*	—	*	*	—	—
Meals on wheels	—	*	*	*	—	—

2.5.4. Other Medical Services. Cost of dental visits was analysed using unit costs from the Australian Government Department of Veterans Affairs and study data were gathered from self-reported data taken from resource use questionnaires.

2.5.5. Home Based Care and Community Services. Formal care included both personal care assistants (PCA) and home based nursing care. PCA and nurses helped with showering, dressing, and regular review. The resource use questionnaire included data on how often home carers visited (twice daily, daily, every second day, and other). It was assumed the duration of each visit was 1 hour and the cost for home based nursing was $27 per hour [22] and for PCA was $25 per hour [22] (Table 2). "Other community services" included

were the provision of meals by meal on wheels; the daily cost was assumed to be $16.50 [22]. The number of informal care hours per week was obtained from the self-reported questionnaires at 3 and 12 months. The total cost of informal care was estimated by multiplying total number of informal care hours over 12 months (multiplying weekly informal care hours by 52) by an hourly dollar value for informal care of $25 per hour [22] (Table 2).

3. Results

3.1. Participants. 198 people with PD attended the Victorian Comprehensive Parkinson's Programme (VCPP) and, of this population, 150 people who met the inclusion criteria were invited to participate in the study (Figure 1). From this

TABLE 2: Unit costs and assumptions for cost analysis.

Parameter	Unit cost ($)	Unit	Assumption/estimations	Data source
Hospitalisations				
Public hospital	1627.12	Per day	$\dfrac{NACWS*}{ALOS**}$	Australian hospital statistics 2011-12 [20] Independent Hospital Pricing Authority [21]
Private hospital	1334.24	Per day	$\dfrac{NACWS}{ALOS} \times 0.82$ Private hospital costs are weighted at 82% of public hospital costs to account for doctors charges which are included in Medicare data for private patients	Australian hospital statistics 2011-12 [20] Independent Hospital Pricing Authority [21]
Hospital transport				
Ambulance (road)	688.50	Per transport	Same average cost for both metropolitan and rural/remote region	Watts et al. (2013) [22]
Ambulance (air)	2682.30	Per transport	—	Victoria state government-Health [23]
Private car	0.66	Per kilometre	Average of 30 km for full journey and same average cost for all types of motor vehicles	Australian government taxation office- car expenses [24]
Taxi	5.54	Per kilometre	Average of 30 km for full journey	Taxi service commission [25]
Allied health services				
Physiotherapy	62.25	Per visit	85% covered by Medicare Out-of-pocket cost is $9.30	MBS item 10960 [26]
Podiatry	62.25	Per visit	85% covered by Medicare Out-of-pocket cost is $9.30	MBS item 10962 [26]
Occupational therapy	62.25	Per visit	85% covered by Medicare Out-of-pocket cost is $9.30	MBS item 10958 [26]
Speech therapy	62.25	Per visit	85% covered by Medicare Out-of-pocket cost is $9.30	MBS item 10970 [26]
Psychology	62.25	Per visit	85% covered by Medicare Out-of-pocket cost is $9.30	MBS item 10968 [26]
Dietetics	62.25	Per visit	85% covered by Medicare Out-of-pocket cost is $9.30	MBS item 10954 [26]
Chiropractic	62.25	Per visit	85% covered by Medicare Out-of-pocket cost is $9.30	MBS item 10964 [26]
Optometry	66.80	Per visit	For initial consultation	MBS item 10905 [26]
Remedial massage	55.92	Per visit	For initial consultation Total out-of-pocket cost	Worksafe Victoria item M600 [27]
Naturopathy	31.80	Per visit	Standard consultation Total out-of-pocket cost	Worksafe Victoria item N602 [28]
Other medical services				
Dental	53.55	Per visit	For a comprehensive oral examination Total out-of-pocket cost	Australian Government Department of Veterans Affairs-item D011 [29]
Home based care and community services				
Formal care, nurse	27.00	Per hour	Duration of formal nursing visit is equal to one hour	Watts et al. (2013) [22]
Formal care, PCA	25.00	Per hour	Duration of formal nursing visit is equal to one hour	Watts et al. (2013) [22]
Informal care	25.00	Per hour	—	Watts et al. (2013) [22]
Meals on wheels	16.50	Per day	Cost of meals per day is $16 for 2 meals and $16.50 for 3 meals	Watts et al. (2013) [22]

*NACWS = national average cost per weighted separation [20]

**ALOS = average length of stay [21].

TABLE 3: Population demographics.

	Mild n = 35	Moderate–severe n = 52	Study population
Mean age (years)	68.1	69.6	69.0
	SD 9.4	SD 9.7	SD 9.6
40–65 years (n)	12 (34%)	13 (25%)	25 (29%)
65+ years (n)	23 (66%)	39 (75%)	62 (71%)
Gender			
Female (n)	13 (37%)	23 (44%)	36 (42%)
Male (n)	22 (63%)	29 (56%)	51 (58%)
Mini mental state examination (mean)	28.7	26.7	27.5
	SD 1.9	SD 4.0	SD 3.4
Disease duration (years)	2.7	8.2	6.0
	SD 3.1	SD 5.4	SD 5.3
Disease severity (HY stage)	35 (40.2%)	52 (59.8%)	87 (100%)
Stage 1	22 (25.3%)	0	22 (25.3%)
Stage 1.5	2 (2.3%)	0	2 (2.3%)
Stage 2	11 (12.6%)	0	11 (12.6%)
Stage 2.5	0	26 (29.9%)	26 (29.9%)
Stage 3	0	16 (18.4%)	16 (18.4%)
Stage 4	0	10 (11.5%)	10 (11.5%)

population 100 people were willing to participate in the study. From the sample population (n = 100) 13 participants withdrew over the 12-month period due to coexisting neurological conditions (n = 6) and deceased (n = 2) and difficulties in further participation (n = 5). There were 87 participants who completed the study at 12 months.

The age of the study population ranged from 43 to 89 years with a mean age of 69 years. 71% of the study population were aged 65 years and older (Table 3). There were 36 females (42%) and 51 males (58%) who participated in the study. There were 52 (60%) who had moderate to severe PD (HY equal or more than 2.5) and 35 (40%) with mild disease (HY less than 2.5). Most of the participants were in HY stage 2.5 (n = 26, 30%) while HY stage 1.5 (n = 2, 2%) had the least number of participants.

3.2. Resource Utilisation and Cost Analysis

3.2.1. Hospitalisation. The study population had a mean number of hospital admissions per person of 1.01 (SD 1.31), with a mean total length of stay over 12 months of 7.1 (SD 9.11) days (Table 4). This differed by severity; for people with mild disease the mean annual number of days in hospital was 4 days compared to 20 days in the people with more severe PD (p < 0.001). Similarly the cost of all hospitalisations (public and private) over 12 months differed by severity with a mean annual cost of $6,160 (SD 9,292) in people with mild disease to $30,061 (SD 40,732) (p < 0.001) for those with more severe PD (Table 5). The mean cost of transport to hospital over 12 months including ambulance, taxi, or private vehicle was $362 (SD 799), of which the mean cost of ambulance was $338 (SD 791) per person. The single largest reason for hospital

admissions was to optimize/adjust Parkinson medications (42%), a further 21% of hospitalisations were directly or indirectly related to PD (falls injuries, pain management, deep brain stimulation and surgical procedures), and 17% of hospitalisations were for reasons not related to PD or an unknown reason. Two participants reported an admission for deep brain stimulation treatments, each with a LOS of 22 days.

3.2.2. Pharmaceuticals. The mean total cost of all prescribed medications was $3,644 (SD 2,240) for people with mild disease and $5,601 (SD 2,573) for more severe cases of PD over 12 months (p < 0.001) (Table 5). This comprised a mean benefit paid per person of $3,144 (SD 2,311) and $5,011 (SD 2,453) for mild and moderate to severe disease, respectively. Mean out-of-pocket charges were $490 (SD 195) for people with mild disease and $596 (SD 26) for people with more severe disease.

3.2.3. Medical Services and Allied Health Services. There was no difference in the annual number of visits to a general practitioner for people with mild and moderate to severe disease; however, people with moderate to severe disease had more than twice the number of visits to a medical specialist compared to those with mild disease (28.3 versus 12; p < 0.001) (Table 4). The mean annual cost of visits to a medical specialist was $4,272 (SD 6,251) for people with moderate to severe disease and $2,706 (SD 2,429) for people with mild disease (p = 0.08). The mean annual out-of-pocket cost for all medical services was $1,179 (SD 1,113) for people with mild disease and $1,464 (SD 2,309) for people with moderate disease (p = 0.25) (Table 5).

TABLE 4: Resource utilization related to Parkinson's disease over 12 months.

	Mild $n = 35$	Moderate–severe $n = 52$	p value
Hospitalisations			
Mean number of hospital admissions per person per year	0.60 SD 0.81	1.29 SD 1.29	<0.001
Public hospital	0.11 SD 0.32	0.62 SD 1.19	0.01
Private hospital	0.49 SD 0.74	0.67 SD 1.12	0.20
Mean hospital LOS (days) per person per year	4.43 SD 6.77	20.15 SD 26.20	<0.001
Public hospital LOS	0.86 SD 2.81	10.83 SD 24.06	<0.001
Private hospital LOS	3.57 SD 6.56	9.33 SD 16.58	0.02
Hospital transport (mean number times)			
Ambulance (road + air)	0.11 SD 0.32	0.58 SD 1.18	0.01
Private car	0.43 SD 0.65	0.98 SD 1.39	0.02
Taxi	0.09 SD 0.37	0.04 SD 0.19	0.22
Medical services (mean number of visits)			
General practice	10.17 SD 4.62	10.25 SD 4.35	0.47
Medical specialist Services	12.00 SD 9.66	28.32 SD 18.56	<0.001
Imaging	4.50 SD 1.90	2.98 SD 1.53	<0.001
Pathology	13.51 SD 5.70	18.58 SD 16.92	0.05
Allied health services (mean number of visits)			
Physiotherapy	7.11 SD 12.66	10.06 SD 12.99	0.15
Podiatry	1.06 SD 1.86	2.38 SD 3.09	0.01
Occupational therapy	0.34 SD 0.76	0.83 SD 1.69	0.06
Speech therapy	0.03 SD 0.17	0.56 SD 1.70	0.04
Psychology	0.03 SD 0.17	0.30 SD 0.82	0.04
Dietetics	0.00 SD 0.00	0.21 SD 1.07	0.12
Chiropractic	0.03 SD 0.17	0.44 SD 1.81	0.09
Optometry	0.06 SD 0.24	0.04 SD 0.20	0.34

TABLE 4: Continued.

	Mild n = 35	Moderate–severe n = 52	p value
Other	1 SD 1.96	1.02 SD 2.57	0.49
Other medical services (dental) (mean number of visits)	1.11 SD 4.15	0.25 SD 1.40	0.08
Home based care and community services (mean number of hours)			
Formal care hours, nurse	—	7.00 SD 30.94	—
Formal care hours, PCA	—	31.00 SD 80.60	—
Informal care hours	96.2 SD 354.53	775 SD 1492.37	0.01
Meals on wheels	11.89 SD 50.58	89.00 263.41	0.05

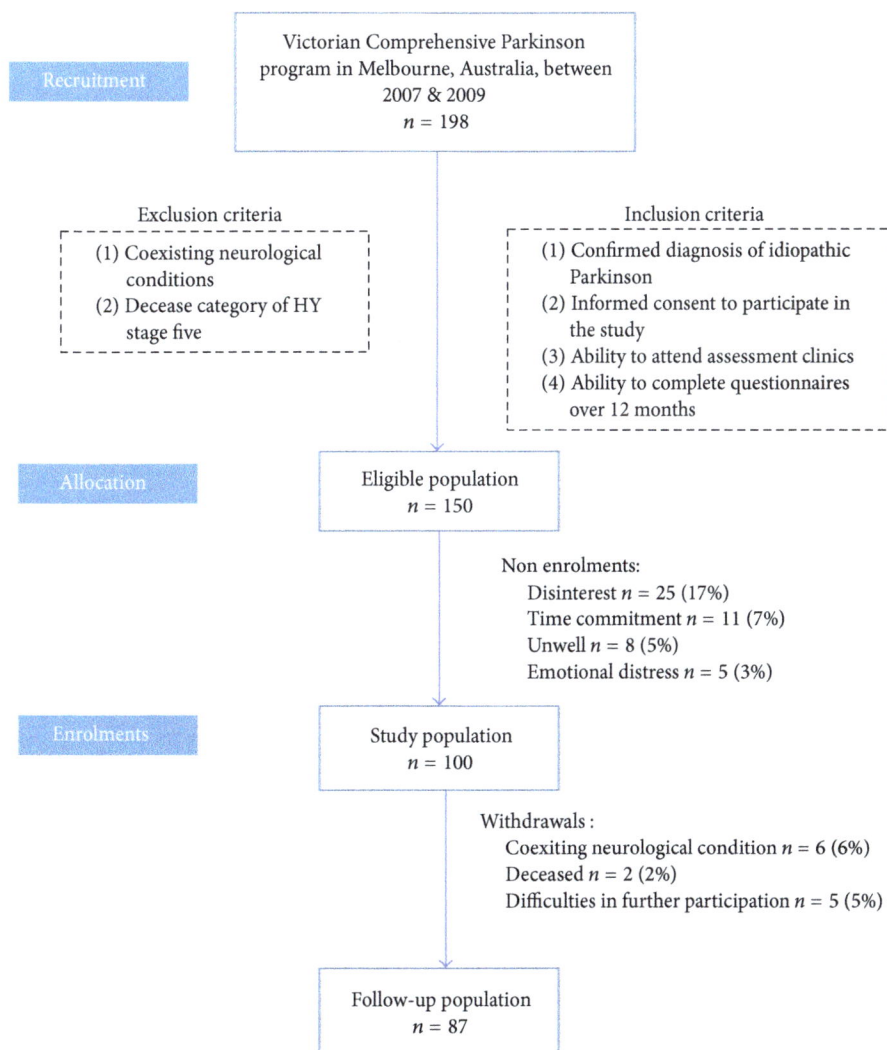

Recruitment
Victorian Comprehensive Parkinson program in Melbourne, Australia, between 2007 & 2009
n = 198

Exclusion criteria
(1) Coexisting neurological conditions
(2) Decease category of HY stage five

Inclusion criteria
(1) Confirmed diagnosis of idiopathic Parkinson
(2) Informed consent to participate in the study
(3) Ability to attend assessment clinics
(4) Ability to complete questionnaires over 12 months

Allocation
Eligible population
n = 150

Non enrolments:
Disinterest n = 25 (17%)
Time commitment n = 11 (7%)
Unwell n = 8 (5%)
Emotional distress n = 5 (3%)

Enrolments
Study population
n = 100

Withdrawals:
Coexiting neurological condition n = 6 (6%)
Deceased n = 2 (2%)
Difficulties in further participation n = 5 (5%)

Follow-up population
n = 87

FIGURE 1: Consort chart; study population.

TABLE 5: Mean annual cost per person with PD from individual, health system, and societal perspectives ($AUD).

Cost perspective	Mild n = 35			Moderate–severe n = 52			Total study population n = 87		
	Individual ($)	Health system ($)	Societal ($)	Individual ($)	Health system ($)	Societal ($)	Individual ($)	Health system ($)	Societal ($)
Hospitalisations	00 (SD 00)	6,160 (SD 9,292)	6,160 (SD 9,292)	00 (SD 00)	30,061 (SD 40,732)	30,061 (SD 40,732)	00 (SD 00)	20,446 (SD 34,014)	20,446 (SD 34,014)
Public hospital	00 (00)	1,395 (SD 4,571)	1,395 (SD 4,571)	00 (00)	17,617 (SD 39,153)	17,617 (SD 39,153)	00 (00)	11,091 (SD 31,326)	11,091 (SD 31,326)
Private hospital	00 (SD 00)	4,765 (SD 8,751)	4,765 (SD 8,751)	00 (SD 00)	12,444 (SD 22,117)	12,444 (SD 22,117)	00 (SD 00)	9,355 (SD 18,294)	9,355 (SD 18,294)
Hospital transport	23 (SD 61)	193 (SD 643)	215 (SD 643)	26 (SD 41)	436 (SD 870)	461 (SD 881)	25 (SD 50)	338 (SD 791)	362 (SD 799)
Ambulance (road + air)	00 (SD 00)	193 (SD 943)	193 (SD 943)	00 (SD 00)	436 (SD 870)	436 (SD 870)	00 (SD 00)	338 (SD 791)	338 (SD 791)
Private car	8 (SD 13)	00 (SD 00)	8 (SD 13)	19 (SD 28)	00 (SD 00)	19 (SD 28)	15 (SD 23)	00 (SD 00)	15 (SD 23)
Taxi	14 (SD 62)	00 (SD 00)	14 (SD 62)	6 (SD 32)	00 (SD 00)	6 (SD 32)	10 (SD 46)	00 (SD 00)	10 (SD 46)
Medical services	1,179 (SD 1,113)	3,217 (SD 1,533)	4,394 (SD 2,491)	1,464 (SD 2,309)	4,194 (SD 4,271)	5,664 (SD 6,470)	1,349 (SD 1,916)	3,793 (SD 3,460)	5,141 (SD 5,258)
General practitioner	40 (SD 63)	430 (SD 288)	469 (SD 293)	41 (SD 64)	371 (SD 397)	411 (SD 419)	41 (SD 63)	395 (SD 357)	434 (SD 372)
Medical specialist	929 (SD 1,020)	1,777 (SD 1,565)	2,706 (SD 2,429)	1,229 (SD 2,281)	3,043 (SD 4,088)	4,272 (SD 6,251)	1,108 (SD 1,876)	2,534 (SD 3,357)	2,883 (SD 3,593)
Imaging	144 (SD 132)	672 (SD 334)	815 (SD 413)	133 (SD 186)	469 (SD 271)	602 (SD 435)	137 (SD 166)	551 (SD 312)	688 (SD 437)
Pathology	67 (SD 80)	338 (SD 251)	404 (SD 315)	60 (SD 90)	298 (SD 204)	359 (SD 262)	63 (SD 86)	314 (SD 224)	377 (SD 284)
Pharmaceuticals	490 (SD 195)	3,144 (SD 2,311)	3,644 (SD 2,240)	596 (SD 26)	5,011 (SD 2,453)	5,601 (SD 2,573)	554 (SD 241)	4,260 (SD 2,555)	4,814 (SD 2,616)
Total allied health	544 (SD 824)	56 (SD 86)	564 (SD 833)	802 (SD 938)	171 (SD 245)	971 (SD 1,045)	698 (SD 898)	125 (SD 190)	807 (SD 981)
Dental services	60 (SD 222)	00 (SD 00)	60 (SD 222)	13 (SD 75)	00 (SD 00)	13 (SD 75)	32 (SD 153)	0.00 (SD 00)	32 (SD 153)
Home based care and community services	2,405 (SD 8,863)	95 (SD 405)	2,500 (SD 8,846)	19,375 (SD 37,309)	1,532 (SD 3,024)	20,908 (SD 37,024)	12,548 (SD 30,440)	954 (SD 2,448)	13,502 (SD 30,434)
Formal care, nurse	00 (SD 00)	00 (SD 00)	00 (SD 00)	00 (SD 00)	775 (SD 2,015)	775 (SD 2,015)	00 (SD 00)	463 (SD 1,598)	463 (SD 1,598)
Formal care, PCA	00 (SD 00)	00 (SD 00)	00 (SD 00)	00 (SD 00)	203 (SD 887)	203 (SD 887)	00 (SD 00)	121 (SD 698)	121 (SD 698)
Informal care	2,405 (SD 8,863)	00 (SD 00)	2,405 (SD 8,863)	19,375 (SD 37,309)	00 (SD 00)	19,375 (SD 37,309)	12,548 (SD 30,440)	00 (SD 00)	12,548 (SD 30,440)

TABLE 5: Continued.

Cost perspective	Mild n = 35			Moderate–severe n = 52			Total study population n = 87		
	Individual ($)	Health system ($)	Societal ($)	Individual ($)	Health system ($)	Societal ($)	Individual ($)	Health system ($)	Societal ($)
Meals on wheels	00	95	95	00	555	555	00	370	370
	SD 00	SD 405	SD 405	SD 00	SD 1,509	SD 1,509	SD 00	SD 1,211	SD 1,211
	4,701	12,865	17,537	22,277	41,396	63,659	15,137	29,916	45,104
Mean total cost	SD 9,425	SD 10,917	SD 17,397	SD 37,221	SD 42,862	SD 50,629	SD 30,546	SD 36,532	SD 46,446
	2,296	12,865	15,132	2,902	41,396	44,284	2,589	29,916	32,556
Mean total cost without informal care	SD 1,475	SD 10,917	SD 10,909	SD 2,530	SD 42,862	SD 42,794	SD 2,184	SD 36,532	SD 36,603

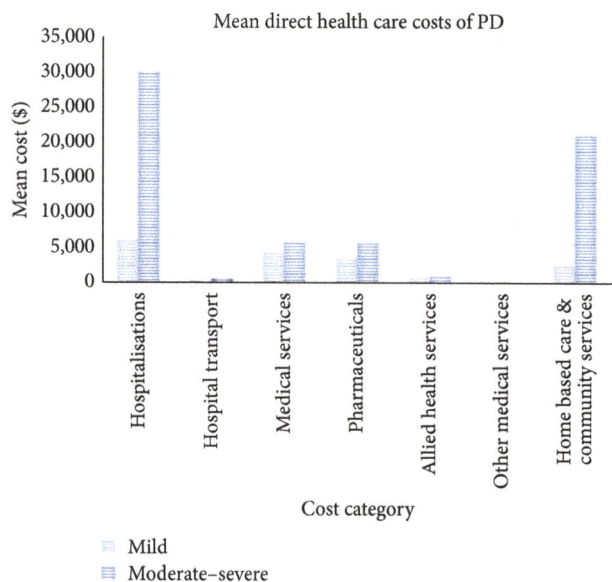

FIGURE 2: Cost of Parkinson's disease per year per person.

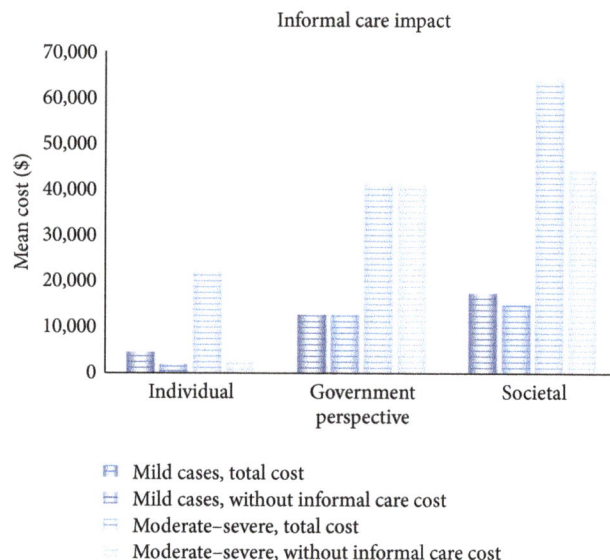

FIGURE 3: Cost impact of informal care.

In addition people with PD consulted a range of allied health practitioners over 12 months. For people with mild disease the mean total cost of all allied health was $564 of which $447 (79%) were for physiotherapy. For people with moderate to severe disease the total cost was $971 with $627 (65%) for physiotherapy and $148 (15%) for podiatry. For both groups 86% of allied health professional costs were paid out-of-pocket (Table 5).

3.2.4. Home Based Care, Community Services, and Informal Care. The study population had an average of 2 hours of nurse visits per week and 4 hours per week of PCA visits with a mean cost of $121 (SD 698) for nursing care and $463 (1,598) for PCA care per person per year (Tables 4 and 5). It was only people with moderate to severe disease who reported the use of community-based nursing care (Table 4). Informal care contributed to the largest economic burden in the PD population. Fifty-two percent of the study population relied on informal care and for most of them a family member who lived with them helped with their daily activities. The mean number of hours was 24 hours per week from the primary informal caregiver (Table 4). In addition to this, people with PD reported an average of 3 hours of help from an additional carer each week. Other community-based services reported were the provision of meals on a regular basis. Fourteen percent of the study population reported using this service at a mean cost of $370 (SD 1,233) per person annually.

3.2.5. Total Cost. Mean total cost per person from a societal perspective of living with PD over 12 months for the entire study population was $45,104 (SD 46,446) (Table 5). From this 66% of costs were attributed to the health system and 34% a burden to households and individuals. Mean total cost varies according to disease severity (Figure 2); for mild cases the mean total societal cost was $17,537 (SD 17,397) and for people with moderate to severe disease was $63,659 (SD

50,629). Informal care represented 28% of total costs and differed according to whether PD was mild (informal care 14%) or moderate to severe (informal care 30%) (Figures 2 and 3).

4. Discussion

The mean annual cost to the health system for this cohort of people with PD was $29,916 (SD 36,532) per person in 2012 AUD. In 2016 this is equivalent to $32,300 AUD or $24,600 USD. In addition annual out-of-pocket expenses were $15,137 (SD 30,546) per person. This is slightly higher than a European study that estimated that the total cost per person with PD was €11,153 per year in 2010 (2012 AUD $14,020). This represented €5,626 direct medical costs, €4,417 direct nonmedical cost, and €1,109 for indirect costs (2012 AUD comparison: $7,020; $5,552; and $1,496) [30]. This represents a significant burden to both individuals and households and to the health care system. In our study two-thirds of the burden to the health care system was related to hospitalisation, with medical services and pharmaceuticals a significant contributor to total costs. As disease severity increased, the burden to the health system was even greater at more than three times that for people with mild PD. The increase in costs as disease progresses is consistent with findings from other studies with one international study determining that the direct cost related to PD doubled when disease progressed from HY stages I to IV [12]. A European study found that a one-unit increase on the dyskinesia severity scale (Part IVa of the Unified Parkinson's Disease Rating Scale (UPDRS)) resulted in an additional mean total cost of €737 per patient over a 6-month period [31].

The study participants were admitted to both private and public hospitals during the study period. There was an average of one admission per person with PD over a 12-month period with an average annual length of stay of 13.5 days. This compares to the average number of admissions of 0.8 for the Australian population aged over 55 years in 2009/10 [32, 33].

The main reason reported for hospitalisation was to adjust PD medication since frequent changes in symptoms require alteration of drug dosage and frequency. Other reasons for admission were for secondary causes including falls (9%). Other studies have found a higher rate of admissions due to the complications of PD [8].

Although there was no difference in the number of GP medical services by disease severity, the number of specialist medical services for the moderate to severe group was more than double for people with mild disease. Other than ongoing management of disease symptoms, a contributing factor to this difference could be that medical specialist services provided in private hospitals as part of the inpatient admission are billed to the national insurer, Medicare Australia. Although the number of admissions are similar between the two groups, the moderate to severe groups have five times the number of days in hospital over 12 months compared to the participants with mild disease. People with moderate to severe PD are more likely to receive specialist doctor visits the more days they are in hospital.

Medication use in the management of PD is ongoing and costly. The cost of all medications was 11% of the total cost of PD over the study period. The total annual cost of medications in this cohort was $418,775, of which the government paid $370,616 (86% of the total) and the remainder formed out-of-pocket costs for people with PD. With disease progression, drug dosage and frequency are likely to increase [34] and people with PD may need to take other medications to control the side effects of the drugs (e.g., to relieve nausea and vomiting and gastric reflux).

Due to disability and progressively increasing mobility conditions associated with PD, people living with PD often require allied health services such as physiotherapy, podiatry, and speech therapy to manage their strength and motor symptoms and to improve their quality of life [9, 13, 15]. The mean number of physiotherapy services reported was just under 9 visits per person per year, which represents less than one service per month. Factors contributing to this relatively low number of reported services might be that physiotherapy services may be provided as part of the hospital episode and not reported separately. An alternative explanation is that allied health services are often not claimable through Medicare Australia; therefore people are likely to face high out-of-pocket charges over 12 months. In this study allied health visits represented 27% of the total annual costs of PD to the household, excluding the burden of informal care.

From the study population almost 60% had moderate or severe PD implying that they have disability that affects their daily living. Participants reported that they were regularly assisted by a family member, or friends as carers in their day to day life. The largest burden from the individual/household perspective was the cost of informal care, estimated at $12,548 per person over 12 months. This was based on the opportunity cost method for valuing informal care that is on the assumption that if a family member was not able to provide this care then it would be the cost of equivalent care provided by a nursing care attendant. People with moderate to severe disease reported an average of 775 informal care hours annually. Only 33% of study participants reported receiving carer payments from the Australian federal government for the informal care they provided. In addition to informal care, participants received home nursing care and other services such as meals. The mean total cost of home based community care services was $950 per person over 12 months. It has been reported that between 2005 and 2011 the cost of informal care for people with PD doubled ($5.4 million versus $11.2 million) [8]. This included income in a formal work environment foregone by carers [35]. The growth reflects the additional number of people with PD and higher average earnings in the workforce. A number of studies suggest that the largest component of household burden was due to providing informal care and the subsequent loss of earnings [12, 36, 37]. Studies highlight that family relationships can be affected in the early stage of disease and it is important to be referred early for home help and counselling and to PD support groups [38, 39].

The strength of this study is the detail provided in the resource use questionnaires about the range and costs of health and community services utilised by people with PD. Combining these data with Medicare and pharmaceutical use over 12 months and including the frequency of questionnaires have provided an accurate picture of the resources used by someone with PD from several perspectives. A limitation was that participants were referred to a specialist PD clinic and therefore may not be representative of the PD community. By separately analysing the cohort by disease severity it is likely that those with more severe disease are similar to the PD population with moderate to severe disease in terms of health care resource utilisation. We were not able to obtain case level hospital admission data; therefore, our cost estimates are based on an average day of stay in an Australian hospital, with no reference to reason for admission or comorbidities.

Our population cohort included two people who had had deep brain stimulation (DBS) so we were not able to comment on the increased costs likely to be associated with DBS [40]. As DBS and other device-aided therapies are likely to become more common therapy for people with PD it is expected that the direct costs of managing PD will be higher in the future. In addition an ageing population means that people with PD are likely to live longer with increased disease severity. The relationship that we have found between higher costs and advancing disease and others have found with increased disability (based on the UPDRS) [31] will be more apparent in future studies. We recommend that future studies should determine the relative contribution to costs of different movement disorders, such as dyskinesia, freezing, bradykinesia, and postural instability.

5. Conclusion

The annual costs to the health system for people with PD are high, with more than two-thirds attributed to hospitalisation. Individuals also face a high out-of-pocket burden for nonhospital related health services and households face a burden from providing informal care, which represents approximately 28% of total costs. The difference in total costs by disease severity suggests that the burden to society is likely to grow in the future with increasing prevalence of chronic diseases such as PD in an ageing population.

Acknowledgments

This project was funded by a National Parkinson Foundation Centre Research grant. Shalika Bohingamu Mudiyanselage was the recipient of a Deakin University School of Health and Social Development Writing Scholarship, 2014. The authors wish to acknowledge the valuable contributions and support of the participants and their caregivers, Ms. Romi Haas and Ms. Tracy Taylor for their management of this project, and the assessors throughout Melbourne and country Victoria who contributed to data collection.

References

[1] T. K. Khoo, A. J. Yarnall, G. W. Duncan et al., "The spectrum of nonmotor symptoms in early Parkinson disease," *Neurology*, vol. 80, no. 3, pp. 276–281, 2013.

[2] D. A. Gallagher and A. H. Schapira, "Non-motor symptoms and pre-motor diagnosis of Parkinson's disease," in *Non-motor Symptoms of Parkinson's Disease*, p. 10, Oxford University Press, Oxford, UK, 2014.

[3] R. Bhidayasiri and D. Tarsy, "Parkinson's disease: hoehn and yahr scale," in *Movement Disorders: A Video Atlas*, pp. 4–5, Springer, Berlin, Germany, 2012.

[4] L. Kadastik-Eerme, M. Rosenthal, T. Paju, M. Muldmaa, and P. Taba, "Health-related quality of life in Parkinson's disease: a cross-sectional study focusing on non-motor symptoms," *Health and Quality of Life Outcomes*, vol. 13, no. 1, article 83, 2015.

[5] J. M. T. van Uem, J. Marinus, C. Canning et al., "Health-Related Quality of Life in patients with Parkinson's disease—a systematic review based on the ICF model," *Neuroscience and Biobehavioral Reviews*, vol. 61, pp. 26–34, 2016.

[6] M. E. Morris, H. B. Menz, J. L. McGinley et al., "A randomized controlled trial to reduce falls in people with Parkinson's disease," *Neurorehabilitation and Neural Repair*, vol. 29, no. 8, pp. 777–785, 2015.

[7] C. J. Stam, "Modern network science of neurological disorders," *Nature Reviews Neuroscience*, vol. 15, no. 10, pp. 683–695, 2014.

[8] Deloitte Access Economics, *Living with Parkinson's Disease—Update*, Parkinson's Australia, 2011.

[9] M. A. Hely, W. G. J. Reid, M. A. Adena, G. M. Halliday, and J. G. L. Morris, "The Sydney multicenter study of Parkinson's disease: the inevitability of dementia at 20 years," *Movement Disorders*, vol. 23, no. 6, pp. 837–844, 2008.

[10] S. von Campenhausen, Y. Winter, A. Rodrigues e Silva et al., "Costs of illness and care in Parkinson's disease: an evaluation in six countries," *European Neuropsychopharmacology*, vol. 21, no. 2, pp. 180–191, 2011.

[11] D. M. Huse, K. Schulman, L. Orsini, J. Castelli-Haley, S. Kennedy, and G. Lenhart, "Burden of illness in Parkinson's disease," *Movement Disorders*, vol. 20, no. 11, pp. 1449–1454, 2005.

[12] S. L. Kowal, T. M. Dall, R. Chakrabarti, M. V. Storm, and A. Jain, "The current and projected economic burden of Parkinson's disease in the United States," *Movement Disorders*, vol. 28, no. 3, pp. 311–318, 2013.

[13] D. J. Cordato, R. Schwartz, E. Abbott, R. Saunders, and L. Morfis, "A comparison of health-care costs involved in treating people with and without Parkinson's disease in Southern Sydney, New South Wales, Australia," *Journal of Clinical Neuroscience*, vol. 13, no. 6, pp. 655–658, 2006.

[14] M. Krol, "Informal care costs have 'strong impact' on economic analyses," *PharmacoEconomics & Outcomes News*, vol. 715, no. 1, pp. 21–28, 2014.

[15] S.-E. Soh, J. L. McGinley, J. J. Watts et al., "Determinants of health-related quality of life in people with Parkinson's disease: a path analysis," *Quality of Life Research*, vol. 22, no. 7, pp. 1543–1553, 2013.

[16] C. Mateus and J. Coloma, "Health economics and cost of illness in Parkinson's disease," *European Neurological Review*, vol. 8, no. 1, pp. 6–9, 2013.

[17] R. Dodel, J.-P. Reese, M. Balzer, and W. H. Oertel, "The economic burden of Parkinson's disease," *European Neurological Review*, vol. 3, no. 2, supplement, pp. 11–14, 2008.

[18] L. Findley, M. Aujla, P. G. Bain et al., "Direct economic impact of Parkinson's disease: a research survey in the United Kingdom," *Movement Disorders*, vol. 18, no. 10, pp. 1139–1145, 2003.

[19] M. E. Morris, J. J. Watts, R. Iansek et al., "Quantifying the profile and progression of impairments, activity, participation, and quality of life in people with Parkinson disease: protocol for a prospective cohort study," *BMC Geriatrics*, vol. 9, no. 1, article 2, 2009.

[20] Australian Institute of Health and Welfare, "Australian hospital statistics 2011-2012," Health Services Series no. 50 Cat. no. HSE 134, AIHW, Canberra, Australia, 2013.

[21] Independent Hospital Pricing Authority (IHPA), *National Efficient Price Determination 2012-2013*, IHPA, Australian Government, 2012.

[22] J. J. Watts, J. Abimanyi-Ochom, and K. Sanders, *Osteoporosis Costing All Australians: A New Burden of Disease Analysis 2012–2022*, Osteoporosis Australia, Sydney, Australia, 2013.

[23] Ambulance Victoria, *Ambulance Fees 2016-2017*, Department of Health & Human Services, Victoria, Australia, 2016, https://www2.health.vic.gov.au/hospitals-and-health-services/patient-care/ambulance-and-nept/ambulance-fees/.

[24] Australian Taxation Office, "Car expenses," Commonwealth of Australia, 2016, https://www.ato.gov.au/Individuals/Income-and-deductions/Deductions-you-can-claim/Vehicle-and-travel-expenses/Car-expenses.

[25] Taxi Services Commission, "Taxi fares," 2016 http://taxi.vic.gov.au/passengers/taxi-passengers/taxi-fares.

[26] Medicare Benefits Schedule, *MBS Online*, Commonwealth of Australia, 2016, http://www.mbsonline.gov.au/internet/mbsonline/publishing.nsf/Content/Home.

[27] Worksafe Victoria, "Remedial Massage Service," 2016, http://www.worksafe.vic.gov.au/__data/assets/pdf_file/0010/194383/WS-Remedial-Massage-Fee-Sch.-20160701.pdf.

[28] Worksafe Victoria, "Naturopathy Service," 2016 http://www.worksafe.vic.gov.au/__data/assets/pdf_file/0006/194280/WS-Naturopathy-Fee-Sch.-20160701.pdf.

[29] Department of Veteran's Affairs, *Fee Schedule of Dental Services, Dentists and Dental Specialists*, Australian Government, Victoria, Australia, 2016, http://www.dva.gov.au/sites/default/files/files/providers/dental/DentalFeeSched.pdf.

[30] J. Olesen, A. Gustavsson, M. Svensson, H.-U. Wittchen, and B. Jönsson, "The economic cost of brain disorders in Europe," *European Journal of Neurology*, vol. 19, no. 1, pp. 155–162, 2012.

[31] M. Péchevis, C. E. Clarke, P. Vieregge et al., "Effects of dyskinesias in Parkinson's disease on quality of life and health-related costs: A Prospective European Study," *European Journal of Neurology*, vol. 12, no. 12, pp. 956–963, 2005.

[32] Australian Bureau of Statistics, *3101.0—Australian Demographic Statistics, Dec 2015*, Australian Government, 2016, http://www.abs.gov.au/ausstats/abs@.nsf/mf/3101.0.

[33] Australian Institute of Health and Welfare, "Australian hospital statistics 2009-2010," Health Services Series no. 40. Cat. no. HSE 107, AIHW, Canberra, Australia, 2011.

[34] A. H. V. Schapira, P. Barone, R. A. Hauser et al., "Patient-reported convenience of once-daily versus three-times-daily dosing during long-term studies of pramipexole in early and advanced Parkinson's disease," *European Journal of Neurology*, vol. 20, no. 1, pp. 50–56, 2013.

[35] N. Costa, L. Ferlicoq, H. Derumeaux-Burel et al., "Comparison of informal care time and costs in different age-related dementias: a review," *BioMed Research International*, vol. 2013, Article ID 852368, 15 pages, 2013.

[36] T. Keranen, S. Kaakkola, K. Sotaniemi et al., "Economic burden and quality of life impairment increase with severity of PD," *Parkinsonism & Related Disorders*, vol. 9, no. 3, pp. 163–168, 2003.

[37] Y. Winter, S. V. Campenhausen, G. Popov et al., "Costs of illness in a Russian cohort of patients with parkinsons disease," *PharmacoEconomics*, vol. 27, no. 7, pp. 571–584, 2009.

[38] L. D. Frazier, V. Cotrell, and K. Hooker, "Possible selves and illness: a comparison of individuals with Parkinson's disease, early-stage Alzheimer's disease, and healthy older adults," *International Journal of Behavioral Development*, vol. 27, no. 1, pp. 1–11, 2003.

[39] A. Schrag, A. Hovris, D. Morley, N. Quinn, and M. Jahanshahi, "Caregiver-burden in Parkinson's disease is closely associated with psychiatric symptoms, falls, and disability," *Parkinsonism & Related Disorders*, vol. 12, no. 1, pp. 35–41, 2006.

[40] T. Fundament, P. R. Eldridge, A. L. Green et al., "Deep brain stimulation for Parkinson's disease with early motor complications: a UK cost-effectiveness analysis," *PLoS ONE*, vol. 11, no. 7, Article ID e0159340, 2016.

30

Consensus on the Definition of Advanced Parkinson's Disease: A Neurologists-Based Delphi Study (CEPA Study)

Maria-Rosario Luquin,[1] Jaime Kulisevsky,[2,3] Pablo Martinez-Martin,[3,4] Pablo Mir,[3,5] and Eduardo S. Tolosa[5,6]

[1]Department of Neurology, Clínica Universidad de Navarra, Universidad de Navarra, Pamplona, Spain
[2]Department of Neurology, Movement Disorders Unit, Hospital de la Santa Creu i Sant Pau (IIB Sant Pau),
 Universitat Autònoma de Barcelona, Universitat Oberta de Catalunya (UOC), Barcelona, Spain
[3]Centro de Investigación Biomédica en Red sobre Enfermedades Neurodegenerativas (CIBERNED), Madrid, Spain
[4]Area of Applied Research, National Center of Epidemiology, Carlos III Institute of Health, Madrid, Spain
[5]Unidad de Trastornos del Movimiento, Servicio de Neurología y Neurofisiología Clínica, Instituto de Biomedicina de Sevilla,
 Hospital Universitario Virgen del Rocío/CSIC/Universidad de Sevilla, Seville, Spain
[6]Neurology Service, Hospital Clínic, IDIBAPS, Universitat de Barcelona, Barcelona, Spain

Correspondence should be addressed to Maria-Rosario Luquin; rluquin@unav.es

Academic Editor: Hélio Teive

To date, no consensus exists on the key factors for diagnosing advanced Parkinson disease (APD). To obtain consensus on the definition of APD, we performed a prospective, multicenter, Spanish nationwide, 3-round Delphi study (CEPA study). An ad hoc questionnaire was designed with 33 questions concerning the relevance of several clinical features for APD diagnosis. In the first-round, 240 neurologists of the Spanish Movement Disorders Group participated in the study. The results obtained were incorporated into the questionnaire and both, results and questionnaire, were sent out to and fulfilled by 26 experts in Movement Disorders. Review of results from the second-round led to a classification of symptoms as indicative of "definitive," "probable," and "possible" APD. This classification was confirmed by 149 previous participating neurologists in a third-round, where 92% completely or very much agreed with the classification. Definitive symptoms of APD included disability requiring help for the activities of daily living, presence of motor fluctuations with limitations to perform basic activities of daily living without help, severe dysphagia, recurrent falls, and dementia. These results will help neurologists to identify some key factors in APD diagnosis, thus allowing users to categorize the patients for a homogeneous recognition of this condition.

1. Introduction

Parkinson disease (PD) is the second most common age-related neurodegenerative disorder after Alzheimer's disease, affecting nearly 1% of the population over 60 years and 5% in subjects up to 85 years [1, 2], with high health, social, and economic impact [3].

While currently effective antiparkinsonian drugs are available, allowing patients to have an acceptable functional capacity during the early years of PD, as time goes by, motor and functional deterioration develop, partly due to the presence of motor and nonmotor complications, highly influencing patients' quality of life. At this stage, the conventional medication is unable to provide an adequate clinical control [4–6] and the term advanced PD is frequently used (APD).

However, the term APD is still controversial and is variably applied to patients with long disease duration or with motor fluctuations and severe or moderate dyskinesia, with disorders of gait and equilibrium, or with cognitive impairment or neuropsychiatric symptoms [4, 7, 8]. Many of these symptoms do not improve with conventional therapies, although for motor fluctuations and dyskinesias there are alternative treatments, so-called "advanced therapies," including deep brain stimulation (DBS), continuous subcutaneous apomorphine infusion, or the infusion of levodopa/carbidopa intestinal gel [9], to which the majority of patients can have a satisfactory response. Therefore, it is of interest to know the patients' clinical characteristics that can define APD and that make these patients eligible for advanced therapies.

In this context, the primary objective of this study was to reach a consensus on the definition of APD using three round questionnaires with Delphi methodology.

2. Methods

2.1. Study Design. This multicenter study was performed using Delphi method [10–12]. The study protocol was approved by the Ethics Committee of Hospital Clínic i Provincial de Barcelona (Spain) in May 2013.

2.2. Scientific Committee. Five neurologists from 5 different Spanish centers, experts in Movement Disorders and PD, formed the Scientific Committee. After a careful review of the literature [13], a questionnaire reflecting some of the proposed features defining APD (clinical characteristics and treatment) was created. The Scientific Committee validated the methodology, study design, and study protocol and prepared the questionnaire, analyzed the results of the two first rounds, and added the statistical analysis from the first-round to the second questionnaire. Based on the results of the two rounds, the Scientific Committee elaborated a list of clinical characteristics of APD, which was again sent to all participants (third-round) to reach a final consensus.

2.3. Questionnaires. The first-round questionnaire included a total of 33 items with a 0–4 scale: 0 (no determinant), 1 (little), 2 (some), 3 (sufficiently), and 4 (absolutely) (available at http://cepa.medynet.com/).

The selected questions assessed the significance of 7 different factors in the diagnosis and definition of APD (general characteristics of the disease, type and level of disability, presence and severity of motor fluctuations and dyskinesia induced by dopaminergic drugs, occurrence and severity of motor and nonmotor symptoms related to the disease, neuropsychiatric and cognitive manifestations, and response of symptoms to available therapies). In the second round questionnaire, the results obtained in the first-round questionnaire were incorporated.

2.4. Participant Groups. To obtain valid results, the Scientific Committee estimated the minimum number of participants as 150 neurologists in the first-round, 25 in the second-round, and 125 in the third-round, to obtain a confidence level of 90% and a margin of error of ±5.35% in the first-round and a confidence level of 95% and a margin of error of ±5% in the third-round.

Participants included in the three rounds were neurologists attending more than 10 PD patients per year (66% of participants attended more than 100 patients with PD/year) and with professional activity in Spain. In the first-round,

neurologists of the Movement Disorders Group of the Spanish Society of Neurology were included, while, in the second-round, neurologists with recognized expertise in PD (defined as working in specialized Movement Disorder Units), who also had participated in the first-round, were selected. Finally, neurologists of the first-round participated in the third-round again.

2.5. Delphi Methodology. The study was performed using a Delphi process, based on the anonymity for the individual responses, controlled opinion feedback, and statistical analysis of responses.

After fulfilling the first-round questionnaires, statistical analysis and conclusions were performed and incorporated to the second-round questionnaires, the results of which led to obtain the final conclusions, which were subsequently confirmed and assessed by the third-round experts.

According to the Delphi methodology [14, 15], consensus was established at percentages > 75% in one or two consecutive scores. Hence, symptoms were classified as (1) definitive for the diagnosis (considered as absolutely determinant by >75% of participants); (2) probable (considered as sufficient or absolute determinant by >75%); and (3) possible (considered as some, sufficiently, or absolutely determinant by >75%).

In the third-round, participants were asked about their level of agreement with the definition of APD, using the scores: 0 (no determinant), 1 (little), 2 (some), 3 (sufficiently), and 4 (absolutely).

2.6. Statistical Analysis. Results were expressed as a measure of central tendency and dispersion for continuous variables and as absolute numbers and relative frequencies for categorical variables. Comparisons in the clinical variables were performed using a Student's t-test or one-way ANOVA for continuous variables (normality assumption was previously confirmed) and Fisher exact test for categorical variables. Statistical significance was set at $p < 0.05$. The statistical analysis was performed using SAS v.9.1.3 (SAS Institute Inc., USA).

The minimum sample size ($n = 150$) was representative from the Spanish neurologists and was calculated to obtain a sample error of 0.0535, considering a maximum variability of $P = Q = 50\%$ and a confidence interval of 90%. The minimum sample size of the third-round ($n = 125$) was calculated to obtain a sample error of 0.05 at a confidence interval of 95%.

3. Results

3.1. Participants. The study was performed from May 2013 to April 2014. A total of 240 Spanish neurologists participated in the first-round and 26 in the second-round, and 149 neurologists of the first-round also participated in the third-round.

During the first-round, a total of 240 questionnaires were collected and 230 were considered valid (95.83%), from the 10 nonvalid questionnaires, 4 were incomplete, and 6 were completed by neurologists who attend less than 10 PD patients per year. Participants of the second-round attended more patients/year (65.38% attended >300 patients/year) than the first-round participants (26.52% attended >300 patients/year).

3.2. Determinant Factors for APD

3.2.1. General Characteristics. The majority of participants considered that disease duration was a determinant factor for the diagnosis of APD (86.10% in first-round and 92.31% in second-round considered it sufficiently or absolutely determinant). Participants considered a mean disease duration of 9.17 ± 1.95 years (median = 10.00 years) as determinant factor for APD.

3.2.2. Disability. In both rounds all participants considered that the type and level of disability were sufficiently (mean score = 3) or absolutely decisive (mean score = 4) for the diagnosis of APD. Second-round researchers considered that a minimum level of disability was required to establish the diagnosis of APD. 100% considered that patients have APD "when the patient requires help for the activities of daily living (such as communication, transportation, shopping, grooming, eating, or medication management)" while for 73.08% the fact that the patient has limitations to perform basic activities of daily living without help can be absolutely determinant to establish the diagnosis of APD.

3.2.3. Motor Symptoms Related to Dopaminergic Treatment. The presence of motor fluctuations was sufficiently or absolutely decisive for the diagnosis of APD for 68.30% of participants in the first-round and for 88.46% in the second-round (Table 1). All participants of the second-round who were in agreement with this statement ($n = 23$) also considered that the duration of *off* periods when the best conventional treatment has been prescribed was key for the diagnosis of APD. In addition, they considered a mean percentage of waking day in *off* situation of 24.13% ± 11.45 (median: 25.00%). "Any limitation to perform basic activities of daily living, with preservation of autonomy," and "requiring help for the activities of daily living" were also considered by 78.26% and 100%, respectively, the required level of disability during *off* periods.

88.70% of participants in the first-round and 76.92% in the second-round considered that the functional disability created by dyskinesia was sufficiently or absolutely crucial for APD diagnosis (Table 1). In the second-round, participants were asked to determine the mean percentage of daily *on* hours with dyskinesias, reporting a mean of 28.25% of the daily *on* hours with dyskinesia (median = 25.00%).

Those participants agreeing that functional disability created by dyskinesia was sufficiently or absolutely important for APD diagnosis also considered that the minimum level of disability due to dyskinesia for APD diagnosis was "requiring help for the activities of daily living" (100%) and "limitation to perform basic activities, but the patient can perform them without help" (90.00%).

3.2.4. Motor and Nonmotor Symptoms Related to the Disease. For 87.80% of participants of the first-round the presence of recurrent falls was sufficiently or absolutely decisive for APD diagnosis (sufficiently: 47.40%; absolutely: 40.4%) and in the second-round 100% of participants agreed (Table 1). Freezing of gait was also considered a key factor for the diagnosis for most neurologists both in first- (82.60%) and second-round (96.15%) (Table 1). For 88.70% of neurologists in the first-round and 92.31% of participants in the second-round, alterations of postural reflexes and equilibrium were quite or absolutely determinant (Table 1). Regarding dysphagia, 92.70% in the first-round and 88.46% in the second-round considered the presence of moderate or severe dysphagia suggestive (sufficiently and absolutely determinant) of APD (Table 1). Moderate and/or severe dysarthria were considered as indicative (sufficiently and absolutely determinant) of APD for 77.40% of neurologists in the first-round and 76.92% in the second-round. The term moderate or severe dysphagia and dysarthria was defined in accordance with the UPDRS scale, part II.

In the second-round, nonmotor symptoms related to the disease such as symptomatic orthostatic hypotension (76.90%), dysautonomia (77.80%), and excessive daytime somnolence (69.20%) were some or sufficiently decisive in APD diagnosis. Although these nonmotor symptoms can be present in any stage of the disease, neurologists considered that their severity was a feature of advanced stages.

3.2.5. Neuropsychiatric and Cognitive Disorders. Neuropsychiatric and cognitive manifestations of the disease such as moderate/severe depression, mild cognitive impairment, chronic presence of hallucinations with preserved insight, moderate/severe apathy, and impulse control disorders were considered as possible features for APD diagnosis (Table 1).

In the second-round 57.70% of neurologists considered moderate/severe depression as no or little determinant, 69.2% established mild cognitive impairment as some, sufficiently, or absolutely determinant, 80.80% considered hallucinations with preserved insight as some, sufficiently (26.9%), or absolutely determinant (50.0%), 34.60% agreed on moderate/severe apathy as sufficiently or absolutely determinant, and 42.20% of participants established the presence of impulse control disorders as some, sufficiently, or absolutely determinant for APD diagnosis (Table 1).

In the first-round dementia was considered sufficiently or absolutely determinant for APD diagnosis by 91.30% (sufficiently: 33.90%; absolutely: 57.40%) and by 96.15% of responders of the second-round. Hallucinations without insight were also considered as sufficiently and absolutely decisive by 83.50% of first-round respondents and by 92.31% in second-round. The psychotic symptoms were also considered decisive to some degree (some, sufficiently, and absolutely) by 91.8% and 92.31% of the first- and second-round respondents, respectively (Table 1).

3.2.6. Symptoms as Indicative of APD. According to the answers obtained in the second-round and in the experience of the Scientific Committee, the following PD symptoms were

TABLE 1: Percentages of respondents in both rounds.

Symptoms	First-round		Second-round			Indicative symptoms of APD
	Sufficiently and absolutely	Some, sufficiently, and absolutely	Absolutely	Sufficiently and absolutely	Some, sufficiently, and absolutely	
(A) Motor symptoms related to treatment						
Motor fluctuations	68.30			88.46		
Duration of *off* periods > 25%	89.50		100.00			
Off disability	92.10		100.00			84.62
Limitation to perform instrumental activities			47.83			
Limitation to perform basic activities (but without help)			78.26			
Requiring help for daily living activities			100.00			
Durations of *on* dyskinesias > 25%	53.50					
Functional disability due to dyskinesias	88.70			76.92		76.92
Limitation to perform instrumental activities			50.00			
Limitation to perform basic activities (but without help)			90.00			
Requiring help for daily living activities			100.00			
(B) Motor symptoms related to the disease						
Recurrent falls	87.80			100.00		
Freezing of gait	82.60			96.15		
Alteration of postural reflexes and equilibrium	88.70			92.31		
Moderate or severe dysphagia	92.70			88.46		76.92
Moderate or severe dysarthria	77.40			76.92		
(C) Neuropsychiatric and cognitive disorders						
Moderate/severe depression	20.50	57.50		15.40	42.30	
Mild cognitive impairment	29.50	76.50		26.90	69.20	
Dementia	91.30	97.00		96.15		92.31
Chronic presence of hallucinations with preserved insight	39.50	83.80		50.00	80.80	
Hallucinations without insight	83.50	95.70		92.31		
Psychotic symptoms	73.50	91.80			92.31	
Moderate/severe apathy	45.60	76.50		34.60	69.20	
Impulse control disorders	29.10	65.20		38.40	42.20	

considered for themselves as indicative of APD: dementia (92.31%), disability requiring help for the activities of daily living (88.46%), *off* disability (84.62%), moderate or severe dysphagia (76.92%), functional disability due to dyskinesia (76.92%), and autonomic dysfunction (53.85%) (Table 1).

3.2.7. Response of APD Symptoms to Available Therapies. Regarding the degree of clinical benefit induced by different therapies on PD symptoms, 53.50% of neurologists in the

first-round and 96.15% in the second-round considered that moderate/severe axial symptoms (such as balance, speech, and gait disturbances) had poor or no benefit from the available therapies. Similarly, 94.3% and 92.31% of first- and second-round respondents, respectively, also considered that dementia does not improve or poorly responds to the existing therapies. Nonmotor symptoms were considered to have moderate or no response to the available therapies by most respondents (89.10% and 92.31% in the first- and second-round, resp.). Most participants agreed that motor fluctuations and dyskinesia significantly improve with current therapies. In the first-round 91.80% of neurologists established that motor fluctuations are markedly reduced by available treatments while in the second-round the percentage reached 96.15%. Dyskinesia had moderate to excellent response to available treatments for 99.20% first-round respondents and 84.00% for second-round participants. In summary, participants considered that motor fluctuations and dyskinesia could improve with current therapies while motor symptoms related to the disease and the majority of nonmotor symptoms have a poor or absent response to the existing therapies. Then, the lack of clinical benefit with the available therapies might be considered as a factor in defining APD.

3.2.8. Symptoms Classification and Final Definition. The results of the three rounds allowed us to define 3 different categories of PD symptoms that can help to define APD: definitive symptoms, probable symptoms, and possible symptoms. The symptoms were grouped in 6 different areas (general characteristics of the disease, disability, motor symptoms related to the treatment, motor symptoms related to the disease, nonmotor symptoms related to the disease, and neuropsychiatric and cognitive manifestations).

Definitive symptoms were considered those whose presence, even isolated, was enough to classify PD as APD. These included disability requiring help for the activities of daily living, presence of motor fluctuations with limitations to perform basic activities of daily living without help, severe dysphagia, recurrent falls, and dementia (Table 2).

Probable symptoms indicative of APD included time of evolution of the disease (around 10 years), limitation to perform basic activities of daily living, even if not requiring help, functional disability due to dyskinesia that covered more than 25% of waking day, moderate dysphagia, freezing of gait, moderate or severe dysarthria, and hallucinations without preserved insight (Table 2). The association of two probable symptoms of different areas made them a definite symptom.

Finally, possible symptoms included postural and balance impairment, symptomatic dysautonomia (including symptomatic orthostatic hypotension), and excessive daytime somnolence, moderate or severe apathy, chronic presence of hallucinations with preserved insight, psychotic symptoms, and mild cognitive impairment (Table 2). The combination of one possible "motor or nonmotor symptom related with the disease" areas with one possible symptom of the "neuropsychiatric and cognitive" area made them a probable symptom.

This classification of symptoms was confirmed by the majority of the neurologists of the third-round (92.00% were in complete or quite agreement), while a minority of participants was in slight (7.38%) or poor agreement (0.67%). Therefore, based on these results, APD can be defined as an advanced stage of PD in which certain symptoms and complications are present, with a detrimental influence on the overall patient's health conditions and with a poor response to conventional treatments (Table 2).

4. Discussion

Current evidence suggests that both motor and nonmotor symptoms significantly contribute to health status and quality of life in PD [8].

A progressive limitation for carrying out the usual activities of daily living (disability) with disease progression is very common in PD. Such limitation results from a combination of motor impairment and complications, but also from nonmotor symptoms that can restrict the activity through a diversity of ways (fatigue, apathy, cognitive impairment, pain, etc.) and aging [16, 17]. As the disability increases, patients require to be helped for carrying out basic activities of daily living and, finally, are totally dependent of caring by others, leading to a great negative impact on patients and caregivers life [18]. Therefore, disability must be considered a fundamental feature for grading PD stage, although other characteristics as the disease duration, usually longer than 10 years, or the incapacity to obtain enough clinical benefit from conventional therapies are also important in defining APD.

Today, however, there is no agreement among neurologists concerning the clinical features that PD should exhibit to be considered as APD [4, 5].

Using the Delphi methodology in a large sample of neurologists we have obtained a consensus on the definition and clinical characteristics that PD patients exhibit in the advanced stage of PD. Most importantly, we have been able here to describe some definitive symptoms of PD that, when present, are sufficient to classify patients as having APD. In addition, this study has allowed us to identify certain symptoms that, when combined, could allow identifying possible and probable APD patients.

We found that both motor and nonmotor symptoms were definitive for the diagnosis of APD, either related to the evolution of the disease or related to the long-term levodopa therapy. In fact, the appearance of certain intrinsic motor symptoms of PD, as recurrent falls and severe dysphagia were definitive determinants for the diagnosis of APD, while moderate dysphagia and freezing of gait were probable symptoms for APD diagnosis. Classically, these manifestations have been associated with advanced disease and, frequently, parallel the appearance of cognitive decline [19, 20].

The development of severe motor fluctuations with disabling "off" periods was also considered a definitive factor for APD diagnosis. These motor complications can appear early in the course of the disease, particularly in young patients, and rethought to reflect the extent of nigrostriatal degeneration. These motor manifestations can dramatically improve with currently available therapies like DBS, continuous subcutaneous apomorphine infusion, or the infusion of levodopa/carbidopa intestinal gel.

Accordingly, we can suggest that APD would be reached when the underlying pathological substrate of PD is widespread but also when PD patients develop the characteristic complications associated with long-term levodopa treatment [20, 21]. In both instances the common feature is the impact they have on disability and quality of life. In fact, in our study the disability created either by the

TABLE 2: Results obtained in the third-round.

Level of relevance	General characteristics	Disability	Motor symptoms related with treatment	Motor symptoms related with the disease	Nonmotor symptoms related with the disease	Neuropsychiatric and cognitive symptoms
Definitive symptoms		Requiring help to perform daily living activities	Presence of motor fluctuations with an *off* time > 25%, with limitation to perform basic activities, without requiring help	Severe dysphagia Recurrent falls		Dementia
Probable* symptoms	Evolution time (around 10 years)	Limitation to perform basic activities, although not requiring help	Functional disability due to dyskinesias with an *on* time > 25%	Moderate dysphagia Freezing of gait Moderate-severe dysarthria		Hallucinations without preserved insight
Possible** symptoms				Postural and equilibrium disorders	Symptomatic dysautonomia, including orthostatic symptomatic hypotension, excessive daytime somnolence	Moderate-severe apathy Chronic presence of hallucinations with preserved insight Psychotic symptoms Mild cognitive impairment

*The association of two probable symptoms of different areas (general characteristics, disability, motor symptoms related to treatment, etc.) makes them a definite symptom.
**The association of one possible motor or nonmotor symptom related with the disease areas with one possible symptom of the neuropsychiatric and cognitive area makes them a probable symptom.

disease or by long-term levodopa therapy was considered for 100% of participants as a definitive factor for APD diagnosis.

Neuropsychiatric manifestations are common in both nondemented and demented PD patients [22]. Most participants established that dementia and hallucinations without insight are, respectively, definitive and probable symptoms for APD diagnosis. This is consistent with studies showing that more than 80% of PD patients develop dementia after 20 years of the disease evolution and also with reports describing that hallucinations are probably the clinical symptom most consistently associated with progressive cognitive deterioration and dementia in PD [23].

The number and severity of the nonmotor symptoms, as a whole, increase with PD progression, although in a variable manner [24–26]. Nonetheless, in late stages of the disease, the nonmotor symptoms may be the dominant problem in many patients [27] and have a huge impact on patient's health state, quality of life, and instrumental functionality [28–30].

Finally, in order to assess the real impact of this consensus in clinical practice we should now evaluate whether or not the 3 different categories of symptoms (definitive, probable, and possible) ascribed to APD clearly classify PD patients in different stages of the disease in the clinical practice.

Disclosure

AbbVie Spain S.L.U., Avenida de Burgos, 91, 28050 Madrid, has given support to the Scientific Committee to finance meetings and group activities/logistics, without taking part in the design, collection of information, data analysis, or preparation of this manuscript.

Acknowledgments

The authors acknowledge the statistical and technical secretary by Grupo Saned. C/Capitán Haya 60, 1ª Planta, 28020 Madrid. Thanks are due to all members of the Spanish Movement Disorders Group of the Spanish Society of Neurology for their participation in the study.

References

[1] L. M. de Lau and M. M. Breteler, "Epidemiology of Parkinson's disease," *Lancet Neurology*, vol. 5, no. 6, pp. 525–535, 2006.

[2] R. L. Nussbaum and C. E. Ellis, "Alzheimer's disease and Parkinson's disease," *The New England Journal of Medicine*, vol. 348, no. 14, pp. 1356–1364, 2003.

[3] S. M. Calne, "The psychosocial impact of late-stage Parkinson's disease," *The Journal of Neuroscience Nursing*, vol. 35, no. 6, pp. 306–313, 2003.

[4] M. Coelho and J. J. Ferreira, "Late-stage Parkinson disease," *Nature Reviews Neurology*, vol. 8, no. 8, pp. 435–442, 2012.

[5] D. Weintraub, C. L. Comella, and S. Horn, "Parkinson's disease—Part 3: neuropsychiatric symptoms," *The American Journal of Managed Care*, vol. 14, supplement 2, pp. S59–S69, 2008.

[6] P. J. García-Ruiz and M. R. Luquin, "Limits of conventional oral and transdermal medication in Parkinson's disease," *Revista de Neurología*, vol. 55, supplement 1, pp. S3–S6, 2012.

[7] C. G. Goetz, G. T. Stebbins, and L. M. Blasucci, "Differential progression of motor impairment in levodopa-treated Parkinson's disease," *Movement Disorders*, vol. 15, no. 3, pp. 479–484, 2000.

[8] C. Hinnell, C. S. Hurt, S. Landau et al., "Nonmotor versus motor symptoms: how much do they matter to health status in Parkinson's disease?" *Movement Disorders*, vol. 27, no. 2, pp. 236–241, 2012.

[9] S. W. Pedersen, J. Clausen, and M. M. Gregerslund, "Practical guidance on how to handle levodopa/carbidopa intestinal gel therapy of advanced PD in a movement disorder clinic," *The Open Neurology Journal*, vol. 6, no. 1, pp. 37–50, 2012.

[10] C. Okoli and S. D. Pawlowski, "The Delphi method as a research tool: an example, design considerations and applications," *Information & Management*, vol. 42, no. 1, pp. 15–29, 2004.

[11] G. J. Skulmoski, F. T. Hartman, and J. Krahn, "The Delphi method for graduate research," *Journal of Information Technology Education*, vol. 6, pp. 1–21, 2007.

[12] C. Cook, J.-M. Brismée, R. Fleming, and P. S. Sizer Jr., "Identifiers suggestive of clinical cervical spine instability: a Delphi study of physical therapists," *Physical Therapy*, vol. 85, no. 9, pp. 895–906, 2005.

[13] J. Kulisevsky, M. R. Luquin, J. M. Arbelo et al., "Advanced Parkinson's disease: clinical characteristics and treatment (part 1)," *Neurologia*, vol. 28, no. 8, pp. 503–521, 2013.

[14] M. P. Pérez-Campanero, *Cómo Detectar las Necesidades de Intervención Socioeducativa*, Editorial Narcea, Madrid, Spain, 1991.

[15] J. McDonnell, A. Meijler, J. P. Kahan, S. J. Bernstein, and H. Rigter, "Panellist consistency in the assessment of medical appropriateness," *Health Policy*, vol. 37, no. 3, pp. 139–152, 1996.

[16] S. Martínez-Horta, J. Pagonabarraga, R. Fernández De Bobadilla, C. García-Sanchez, and J. Kulisevsky, "Apathy in Parkinson's disease: more than just executive dysfunction," *Journal of the International Neuropsychological Society*, vol. 19, no. 5, pp. 571–582, 2013.

[17] P. A. Kempster, S. S. O'Sullivan, J. L. Holton, T. Revesz, and A. J. Lees, "Relationships between age and late progression of Parkinson's disease: a clinico-pathological study," *Brain*, vol. 133, no. 6, pp. 1755–1762, 2010.

[18] M. Coelho, M. J. Marti, C. Sampaio et al., "Dementia and severity of parkinsonism determines the handicap of patients in late-stage Parkinson's disease: the Barcelona-Lisbon cohort," *European Journal of Neurology*, vol. 22, no. 2, pp. 305–312, 2015.

[19] B. R. Bloem, J. M. Hausdorff, J. E. Visser, and N. Giladi, "Falls and freezing of Gait in Parkinson's disease: a review of two interconnected, episodic phenomena," *Movement Disorders*, vol. 19, no. 8, pp. 871–884, 2004.

[20] A. Diamond and J. Jankovic, "Treatment of advanced Parkinson's disease," *Expert Review of Neurotherapeutics*, vol. 6, no. 8, pp. 1181–1197, 2006.

[21] B. Pillon, B. Dubois, G. Cusimano, A.-M. Bonnet, F. Lhermitte, and Y. Agid, "Does cognitive impairment in Parkinson's disease result from non-dopaminergic lesions?" *Journal of Neurology Neurosurgery & Psychiatry*, vol. 52, no. 2, pp. 201–206, 1989.

[22] J. Kulisevsky, J. Pagonbarraga, B. Pascual-Sedano, C. García-Sánchez, and A. Gironell, "Prevalence and correlates of neuropsychiatric symptoms in Parkinson's disease without dementia," *Movement Disorders*, vol. 23, no. 13, pp. 1889–1896, 2008.

[23] J. Pagonabarraga and J. Kulisevsky, "Cognitive impairment and dementia in Parkinson's disease," *Neurobiology of Disease*, vol. 46, no. 3, pp. 590–596, 2012.

[24] P. Martinez-Martin, A. H. V. Schapira, F. Stocchi et al., "Prevalence of nonmotor symptoms in Parkinson's disease in an international setting; study using nonmotor symptoms questionnaire in 545 patients," *Movement Disorders*, vol. 22, no. 11, pp. 1623–1629, 2007.

[25] A. Antonini, P. Barone, R. Marconi et al., "The progression of non-motor symptoms in Parkinson's disease and their contribution to motor disability and quality of life," *Journal of Neurology*, vol. 259, no. 12, pp. 2621–2631, 2012.

[26] K. R. Chaudhuri, J. M. Rojo, A. H. V. Schapira et al., "A proposal for a comprehensive grading of Parkinson's disease severity combining motor and non-motor assessments: meeting an unmet need," *PLoS ONE*, vol. 8, Article ID e57221, 2013.

[27] M. A. Hely, J. G. L. Morris, W. G. J. Reid, and R. Trafficante, "Sydney Multicenter Study of Parkinson's disease: non L-dopa-responsive problems dominate at 15 years," *Movement Disorders*, vol. 20, no. 2, pp. 190–199, 2005.

[28] J. Kulisevsky, R. Fernández de Bobadilla, J. Pagonabarraga et al., "Measuring functional impact of cognitive impairment: validation of the Parkinson's disease cognitive functional rating scale," *Parkinsonism & Related Disorders*, vol. 19, no. 9, pp. 812–817, 2013.

[29] M. A. Lee, W. M. Prentice, A. J. Hildreth, and R. W. Walker, "Measuring symptom load in Idiopathic Parkinson's disease," *Parkinsonism & Related Disorders*, vol. 13, no. 5, pp. 284–289, 2007.

[30] P. Martinez-Martin, C. Rodriguez-Blazquez, M. M. Kurtis, and K. R. Chaudhuri, "The impact of non-motor symptoms on health-related quality of life of patients with Parkinson's disease," *Movement Disorders*, vol. 26, no. 3, pp. 399–406, 2011.

Permissions

List of Contributors

Yongpan Huang
Information Security and Big Data Research Institute, Central South University, Changsha, Hunan, China
Department of Pharmacology, Institute of Chinese Medicine, Hunan Academy of Chinese Medicine, Changsha, Hunan, China

Minhan Yi
Information Security and Big Data Research Institute, Central South University, Changsha, Hunan, China
Department of Ecology and Evolutionary Biology, University of Michigan, Ann Arbor, MI, USA

Langmei Deng
Department of Emergency, The Third Xiangya Hospital and School of Life Sciences, Central South University, Changsha, Hunan, China

Yanjun Zhong
ICU Centre, Second Xiangya Hospital, Central South University, Changsha, Hunan, China

Yiğit Çanga, Ayşe Emre, Mehmet Baran Karataş Nizamettin Selçuk Yelgeç, UfukGürkan, Ali Nazmi Çalık and Sait Terzi
Department of Cardiology, Dr. Siyami Ersek Cardiovascular and oracic Surgery Center, Istanbul, Turkey

Gülbün Asuman Yüksel and Hülya Tireli
Department of Neurology, Haydarpasa Numune Training and Research Hospital, Istanbul, Turkey

Kam-Wa Chan, Ka-Ho Chan and Kim-Pong Tse
School of Chinese Medicine, Hong Kong Baptist University, Kowloon, Hong Kong

Ka-Kit Chua, Zhao-Xiang Bian, Liang-Feng Liu, Lei-Lei Chen, Ju-Xian Song and Min Li
School of Chinese Medicine, Hong Kong Baptist University, Kowloon, Hong Kong
Mr. and Mrs. Ko Chi Ming Centre for Parkinson's Disease Research, Hong Kong Baptist University, Kowloon, Hong Kong

Adrian Wong, Yin-Kei Lau, Anne Chan, Justin Wu and Vincent Mok
Institutes of Integrative Medicine, Department of Medicine and Therapeutics, The Chinese University of Hong Kong, Sha Tin, Hong Kong

Jia-Hong Lu
State Key Laboratory of Quality Research in Chinese Medicine, Institute of Chinese Medical Sciences, University of Macau, Macau

Li-Xing Zhu
Department of Mathematics, Statistics Research and Consultancy Centre, Faculty of Science, Hong Kong Baptist University, Kowloon, Hong Kong

Peter S. Hanson
Medical Toxicology Centre and NIHR Health Protection Research Unit in Chemical and Radiation Threats and Hazards, Newcastle University, Wolfson Building, Claremont Place, Newcastle NE2 4AA, UK

Preeti Singh
Medical Toxicology Centre and NIHR Health Protection Research Unit in Chemical and Radiation Threats and Hazards, Newcastle University, Wolfson Building, Claremont Place, Newcastle NE2 4AA, UK
NIHR Biomedical Research Unit in Lewy Body Disorders, Newcastle University, Edwardson Building, Institute of Neuroscience, Newcastle upon Tyne NE4 5PJ, UK

Christopher M. Morris
Medical Toxicology Centre and NIHR Health Protection Research Unit in Chemical and Radiation Threats and Hazards, Newcastle University, Wolfson Building, Claremont Place, Newcastle NE2 4AA, UK
NIHR Biomedical Research Unit in Lewy Body Disorders, Newcastle University, Edwardson Building, Institute of Neuroscience, Newcastle upon Tyne NE4 5PJ, UK
NIHR Biomedical Research Centre in Ageing and Chronic Disease, Newcastle University, Biomedical Research Building, Campus for Ageing and Vitality, Newcastle upon Tyne NE4 5PJ, UK

S. Zabberoni and A. Costa
1Department of Psychology, Niccol`o Cusano University, Rome, Italy

A. Peppe
IRCCS Fondazione Santa Lucia, Rome, Italy

G. A. Carlesimo and C. Caltagirone
IRCCS Fondazione Santa Lucia, Rome, Italy
Department of Systems Medicine, Tor Vergata University, Rome, Italy

Bilge Kocer, Hayat Guven, Selim Selcuk Comoglu and Sennur Delibas
Department of Neurology, Diskapi Yildirim Beyazit Training and Research Hospital, 06110 Ankara, Turkey

Isik Conkbayir
Department of Radiology, Diskapi Yildirim Beyazit Training and Research Hospital, 06110 Ankara, Turkey

Mehmet Sorar, Sahin Hanalioglu, Muhammed Taha Eser and Hayri Kertmen
Department of Neurosurgery, Diskapi Yildirim Beyazit Training and Research Hospital, Health Sciences University, Ankara, Turkey

Bilge Kocer and Selim Selcuk Comoglu
Department of Neurology, Diskapi Yildirim Beyazit Training and Research Hospital, Health Sciences University, Ankara, Turkey

Teresa Paolucci, Federico Zangrando, Giulia Piccinini, Rossella Basile, Enrico Bruno, Emigen Buzi and Vincenzo M. Saraceni
Complex Unit of Physical Medicine and Rehabilitation, Policlinico Umberto I Hospital, "Sapienza" University of Rome, Piazzale Aldo Moro 5, 00185 Rome, Italy

Laura Deidda
Department of Physical Medicine and Rehabilitation, San Camillo-Forlanini Hospital, Circonvallazione Gianicolense 87,00151 Rome, Italy

Alice Mannocci
Department of Public Health and Infectious Diseases, "Sapienza" University of Rome, Piazzale Aldo Moro 5, 00185 Rome, Italy

Franca Tirinelli
Department of Physical Medicine and Rehabilitation, A.C.I.S.M.O.M., San Giovanni Battista Hospital, Via Luigi Ercole Morselli 13,00148 Rome, Italy

Shalom Haggiag and Ludovico Lispi
Department of Neurology, San Camillo-Forlanini Hospital, Circonvallazione Gianicolense 87, 00151 Rome, Italy

Ciro Villani
University Department of Anatomic, Histologic, Forensic and Locomotor Apparatus Sciences, Section of Locomotor Apparatus Sciences, Policlinico Umberto I Hospital, "Sapienza" University of Rome, Piazzale Aldo Moro 5, 00185 Rome, Italy

Raja Mehanna
University of Texas Health Science Center, Houston, TX, USA

Jawad A. Bajwa
Parkinson's, Movement Disorders and Neurorestoration Program, National Neuroscience Institute, King Fahad Medical City, Riyadh, Saudi Arabia

Hubert Fernandez
Center for Neurological Restoration, Cleveland Clinic, Cleveland, OH, USA

Aparna Ashutosh Wagle Shukla
University of Florida, Gainesville, FL, USA

Maria Sperens
Department of Community Medicine and Rehabilitation, Occupational Therapy, Umeå University, 901 87 Umeå, Sweden

Gun-Marie Hariz
Department of Community Medicine and Rehabilitation, Occupational Therapy, Umeå University, 901 87 Umeå, Sweden
Department of Pharmacology and Clinical Neuroscience, Umeå University, 90 187 Umeå, Sweden

Katarina Hamberg
Department of Public Health and Clinical Medicine, Family Medicine, Umeå University, 901 87 Umeå, Sweden

S. Coe, J. Collett, D. Boyle, A. Meaney, R. Chantry, P. Esser and H. Dawes
Department of Sport, Health Sciences and Social Work, Oxford Brookes University, Headington Rd., Oxford OX3 0BP, UK

M. Franssen
Nuffield Department of Primary Care Health Sciences, University of Oxford, Radcliffe Primary Care Building, Oxford OX2 6GG, UK

H. Izadi
School of Engineering, Computing and Mathematics, Oxford Brookes University, Wheatley, Oxford OX33 1HX, UK

Song-bin He, Lin-di Chen, Wei-guo Tang and Bin-da Wang
Department of Neurology, Zhoushan Hospital, Wenzhou Medical University, Zhoushan 316021, China

Chun-yan Liu
Department of Critical Care Medicine, Huzhou Central Hospital, Huzhou 313000, China

Zhi-nan Ye and Ya-ping Zhang
Department of Neurology, Taizhou Municipal Hospital, Taizhou 318000, China

Xiang Gao
Department of Nutritional Sciences, *e Pennsylvania State University, USA

Rafiqua Ben El Haj and Asmae Skalli
Research Team in Neurology and Neurogenetics, Medical School and Pharmacy, Mohammed V University, Rabat, Morocco

Ahmed Bouhouche, Ali Benomar, Mohammed Yahyaoui and Wafa Regragui
Research Team in Neurology and Neurogenetics, Medical School and Pharmacy, Mohammed V University, Rabat, Morocco
Department of Neurology and Neurogenetics, Specialties Hospital, Rabat, Morocco

Houyam Tibar, Khalil El Bayad, Sanaa Tazrout, Naima Bouslam and Loubna Elouardi
Department of Neurology and Neurogenetics, Specialties Hospital, Rabat, Morocco

Rachid Razine
Laboratory of Public Health, Medical School and Pharmacy, Mohammed V University, Rabat, Morocco

Pavel Šponer, Tomáš KuIera and Michal Grinac
Department of Orthopaedic Surgery, Charles University in Prague, Faculty of Medicine in Hradec Králové, Šimkova 870, 500 38 Hradec Králové, Czech Republic
Department of Orthopaedic Surgery, University Hospital Hradec Králové, Sokolská 581, 500 05Hradec Králové, Czech Republic

Aleš Bezrouk
Department of Medical Biophysics, Charles University in Prague, Faculty of Medicine in Hradec Králové, Šimkova 870, 500 38 Hradec Králové, Czech Republic

Daniel Waciakowski
Department of Orthopaedics and Traumatology, Kreiskrankenhaus Greiz GmbH, Wichmannstraße 12, 07973 Greiz, Germany

Yihui Xu
Second People's Hospital, Fujian University of Traditional Chinese Medicine, Fuzhou, Fujian Province 350003, China

Wei Lin
Academy of Integrative Medicine, Fujian University of Traditional Chinese Medicine, Fuzhou, Fujian Province 350122, China

Shuifen Ye
Longyan First Hospital Affiliated to Fujian Medical University, Longyan, Fujian Province 364000, China

Huajin Wang
Tibet Autonomous Region People's Hospital, Lhasa, Tibet Autonomous Region 850000, China

Tingting Wang Youyan Su Qian Xu and Jing Cai
College of Integrative Medicine, Fujian University of Traditional Chinese Medicine, Fuzhou, Fujian Province 350122, China

Liangning Wu
Graduate School, Fujian University of Traditional Chinese Medicine, Fuzhou, Fujian Province 350122, China

Yuanwang Wang
Quanzhou Orthopedic-Traumatological Hospital, Fujian University of Traditional Chinese Medicine, Quanzhou, Fujian Province 362000, China

Chuanshan Xu
School of Chinese Medicine, Faculty of Medicine, The Chinese University of Hong Kong, Shatin, Hong Kong

Donatas Lukšys, Gintaras Jonaitis and Julius Griškevičius
Faculty of Mechanics, Department of Biomechanical Engineering, Vilnius Gediminas Technical University, Basanavičiaus str. 28, LT-03224 Vilnius, Lithuania

Ya-Chao He, Pei Huang, Qiong-Qiong Li, Qian Sun, Dun-Hui Li, TianWang, Jun-Yi Shen, Juan-Juan Du, Shi-Shuang Cui, Chao Gao, Rao Fu and Sheng-Di Chen
Department of Neurology and Collaborative Innovation Center for Brain Science, Ruijin Hospital, Shanghai Jiao Tong University School of Medicine, Shanghai 200025, China

Daniel Glizer
MacDonald Lab, Brain and Mind Institute, University of Western Ontario, London, ON, Canada

Penny A. MacDonald
MacDonald Lab, Brain and Mind Institute, University of Western Ontario, London, ON, Canada
Clinical Neurological Sciences, Schulich School of Medicine and Dentistry, University of Western Ontario, London, ON, Canada

Michaela Karlstedt and Johan Lökk
Karolinska Institutet, Department of Neurobiology, Care Sciences and Society, Division of Clinical Geriatrics, Novum Pl 5, Blickagången 6/Hälsovägen 7, 14157 Huddinge, Sweden

Seyed-Mohammad Fereshtehnejad
Karolinska Institutet, Department of Neurobiology, Care Sciences and Society, Division of Clinical Geriatrics, Novum Pl 5, Blickagången 6/Hälsovägen 7, 14157 Huddinge, Sweden
Department of Neurology and Neurosurgery, McGill University, Montreal, QC, Canada

Dag Aarsland
Karolinska Institutet, Department of Neurobiology, Care Sciences and Society, Division of Neurogeriatrics, Novum Pl 5, Blickagången 6/Hälsovägen 7, 14157 Huddinge, Sweden

Anja Ophey, Richard Dano and Elke Kalbe
Department of Medical Psychology | Neuropsychology and Gender Studies and Center for Neuropsychological Diagnostics and Intervention (CeNDI), University Hospital Cologne, Kerpener Str. 68, 50937 Cologne, Germany

Carsten Eggers and Lars Timmermann
Department of Neurology, University Hospital Cologne, Kerpener Str. 62, 50937 Cologne, Germany
Department of Neurology, University Hospital Gießen Marburg, Baldingerstraße, 35043 Marburg, Germany

Oriol De Fabregues, Manuel Quintana and José Álvarez-Sabin
Movement Disorders Unit, Department of Neurology, Hospital Universitari Vall D'Hebron, Neurodegenerative Diseases Research Group-Vall D'Hebron Research Institute, Universitat Aut`onoma de Barcelona, Barcelona, Spain

Alex Ferré and Odile Romero
Sleep Unit, Department of Neurophysiology, Hospital Universitari Vall D'Hebron, Barcelona, Spain

Chuan Xu, Jiajun Chen, Yingyu Zhang and Jia Li
Department of Neurology (III), China-Japan Union Hospital of Jilin University, Changchun 130033, Jilin, China

Xia Xu
Yiwu Maternal and Child Health Hospital, Yiwu 322000, Zhejiang, China

Sándor Márki and Nikoletta Nagy
Department of Medical Genetics, University of Szeged, Somogyi u. 4, 6720 Szeged, Hungary

Márta Széll
Department of Medical Genetics, University of Szeged, Somogyi u. 4, 6720 Szeged, Hungary
MTA-SZTE Dermatological Research Group, University of Szeged, Korányi fasor 6, 6720 Szeged, Hungary

Eszter Szlávicz
Department of Dermatology and Allergology, University of Szeged, Korányi fasor 6, 6720 Szeged, Hungary

Anikó Göblös
Department of Dermatology and Allergology, University of Szeged, Korányi fasor 6, 6720 Szeged, Hungary
MTA-SZTE Dermatological Research Group, University of Szeged, Korányi fasor 6, 6720 Szeged, Hungary

Nóra Török József Engelhardt and Péter Klivényi
Department of Neurology, University of Szeged, Semmelweis u. 6, 6725 Szeged, Hungary

László Vécsei
Department of Neurology, University of Szeged, Semmelweis u. 6, 6725 Szeged, Hungary
MTA-SZTE Neuroscience Research Group, University of Szeged, Semmelweis u. 6, 6725 Szeged, Hungary

Péter Balicza, Benjamin Bereznai and Mária Judit Molnár
Institute of Genomic Medicine and Rare Disorders, Semmelweis University, Tömö u. 25-29, 1083 Budapest, Hungary

Annamária Takáts
Department of Neurology, Semmelweis University, VIII. Balassa J. u. 6, 1083 Budapest, Hungary

Yang Yang
Department of Neurology, Xiangya Hospital, Central South University, Changsha, Hunan 410008, China
Key Laboratory of Hunan Province in Neurodegenerative Disorders, Central South University, Changsha, Hunan 410008, China

Bei-sha Tang and Ji-feng Guo
Department of Neurology, Xiangya Hospital, Central South University, Changsha, Hunan 410008, China
Key Laboratory of Hunan Province in Neurodegenerative Disorders, Central South University, Changsha, Hunan 410008, China
State Key Laboratory of Medical Genetics, Changsha, Hunan 410008, China
Neurodegenerative Disorders Research Center, Central South University, Changsha, Hunan 410008, China

Suisui Pang, Jia Li, Yingyu Zhang and Jiajun Chen
Department of Neurology, China–Japan Union Hospital of Jilin University, No. 126, Xian Tai Road, Changchun, Jilin 130033, China

Jing Cai
Department of Integrative Medicine, Fujian University of Traditional Chinese Medicine, Fuzhou 350122, China

Shuifen Ye
Department of Integrative Medicine, Fujian University of Traditional Chinese Medicine, Fuzhou 350122, China
Longyan First Hospital Affiliated to Fujian Medical University, Longyan 364000, China

Wen Fan
Department of Integrative Medicine, Fujian University of Traditional Chinese Medicine, Fuzhou 350122, China
Xiamen Haicang Hospital, Xiamen 361026, China

Yihui Xu
Department of Integrative Medicine, Fujian University of Traditional Chinese Medicine, Fuzhou 350122, China
Second People's Hospital, Fujian University of Traditional Chinese Medicine, Fuzhou 350003, China

Wei Wei
Department of Integrative Medicine, Fujian University of Traditional Chinese Medicine, Fuzhou 350122, China
No. 477 Hospital of Chinese People's Liberation Army, Xiangyang 441000, China

Ho Kee Koon
School of Chinese Medicine, Faculty of Medicine,The Chinese University of Hong Kong, Shatin, Hong Kong

Chuanshan Xu
School of Chinese Medicine, Faculty of Medicine,The Chinese University of Hong Kong, Shatin, Hong Kong
Shenzhen Research Institute,The Chinese University of Hong Kong, Shenzhen 518057, China

Tânia M. Bovolenta
Programa de Pós-Graduação, Hospital Israelita Albert Einstein, São Paulo, SP, Brazil

Sônia Maria Cesar de Azevedo Silva
Movement Disorders Department in Neurology, Universidade Federal de São Paulo (UNIFESP), São Paulo, SP, Brazil

Roberta Arb Saba, Vanderci Borges and Henrique Ballalai Ferraz
Universidade Federal de São Paulo (UNIFESP), São Paulo, SP, Brazil

Andre C. Felicio
Neurology Program, Hospital Israelita Albert Einstein, São Paulo, SP, Brazil

Kim Wieczorek Austin and Suzanne Weil Ameringer
Virginia Commonwealth University School of Nursing, 1100 East Leigh Street, Richmond, VA 23219, USA

Leslie Jameleh Cloud
Virginia Commonwealth University Parkinson's and Movement Disorders Center and VCU Health Neuroscience, Orthopaedic, and Wellness Center, 11958West Broad Street, Richmond, VA 23233, USA

Shalika Bohingamu Mudiyanselage, Jennifer J. Watts, Julie Abimanyi-Ochom and Lisa Lane
Centre for Population Health Research, School of Health and Social Development, Faculty ofHealth, Deakin University, Burwood, VIC 3125, Australia

Anna T. Murphy and Robert Iansek
Clinical Research Centre for Movement Disorders and Gait,The National Parkinson Foundation Centre of Excellence, Kingston Centre, Monash Health, Cheltenham, VIC 3192, Australia
School of Clinical Sciences Monash University, Clayton, VIC 3168, Australia

Meg E. Morris
Healthscope, Northpark Private Hospital, Plenty and Greenhills Roads, Bundoora, VIC 3083, Australia
School of Allied Health, La Trobe University, Bundoora, VIC 3083, Australia

Maria-Rosario Luquin
Department of Neurology, Clínica Universidad de Navarra, Universidad de Navarra, Pamplona, Spain

Jaime Kulisevsky
Department of Neurology, Movement Disorders Unit, Hospital de la Santa Creu i Sant Pau (IIB Sant Pau), Universitat Autònoma de Barcelona, UniversitatOberta de Catalunya (UOC), Barcelona, Spain
Centro de Investigaciòn Biomédica en Red sobre Enfermedades Neurodegenerativas (CIBERNED), Madrid, Spain

Pablo Martinez-Martin
Centro de Investigación Biomédica en Red sobre Enfermedades Neurodegenerativas (CIBERNED), Madrid, Spain
Area of Applied Research, National Center of Epidemiology, Carlos III Institute of Health, Madrid, Spain

Pablo Mir
Centro de Investigación Biomédica en Red sobre Enfermedades Neurodegenerativas (CIBERNED), Madrid, Spain
Unidad de Trastornos del Movimiento, Servicio de Neurologíay Neurofisiología Clínica, Instituto de Biomedicina de Sevilla, Hospital Universitario Virgen del Rocío/CSIC/Universidad de Sevilla, Seville, Spain

Eduardo S. Tolosa
Unidad de Trastornos del Movimiento, Servicio de Neurología y Neurofisiología Clínica, Instituto de Biomedicina de Sevilla, Hospital Universitario Virgen del Rocío/CSIC/Universidad de Sevilla, Seville, Spain
Neurology Service, Hospital Clínic, IDIBAPS, Universitat de Barcelona, Barcelona, Spain

Index

www.ingramcontent.com/pod-product-compliance
Lightning Source LLC
Chambersburg PA
CBHW061331190326
41458CB00011B/3962